AN ATLAS OF ANATOMY

AN ATLAS OF

By Regions: Upper Limb, Abdomen, Perineum,
Pelvis, Lower Limb, Vertebrae, Vertebral Column,
Thorax, Head and Neck,
Cranial Nerves and Dermatomes

Anatomy

J. C. BOILEAU GRANT

M.C., M.B., Ch.B., Hon. D. Sc. (Man.), F.R.C.S. (Edin.)

*Professor Emeritus of Anatomy in the University of Toronto
and Curator of the Anatomy Museum; Visiting Professor of Anatomy
in the University of California, Los Angeles; formerly Professor
of Anatomy in the University of Manitoba*

FIFTH EDITION

THE WILLIAMS & WILKINS CO.

Baltimore • 1962

COMPOSED AND PRINTED
AT THE WAVERLY PRESS, INC.
MT. ROYAL & GUILFORD AVES.
BALTIMORE 2, MD., U.S.A.

Title page illustration:
THE ANATOMY LESSON OF DR. NICOLAES TULP
by Rembrandt van Rijn
FROM A MEZZOTINT IN THE BETTMAN ARCHIVES

To Catriona

Preface to the Fifth Edition

This collection of illustrations depicts the structures of the human body, region by region, in much the same order as the student displays them by dissection.

In the execution of these illustrations the following preliminary steps were taken: each specimen was posed and photographed; from the negative film so obtained an enlarged positive film was made, usually one third larger than it would appear when reproduced; with the aid of a viewing box the outlines of the structures on the enlarged film were traced on tracing paper; and these outlines were scrutinized against the original specimen, in order to ensure that the shapes, positions and relative proportions of the various structures were correct. The outline tracing was then presented to the artist who transferred it to suitable paper and, having the original dissection beside her, proceeded to work up a plastic drawing in which the important features were brought out. Thus, little, if any, liberty has been taken with the anatomy; that is to say, the illustrations profess a considerable accuracy of detail.

In order that the student may be able to turn the pages and study figure after figure without requiring to re-orient himself, all illustrations of bilaterally symmetrical structures are from the right half of the body, unless it is stated otherwise.

Most of the specimens here depicted are in the Anatomy Museum of the University of Toronto.

The observations and comments that accompany the illustrations are designed to attract attention to salient points and to points of significance that might otherwise escape notice. Their purpose is to interpret the illustrations. They are not, nor are they intended to be, exhaustive descriptions.

The often recurring noun, musculus or muscle, is omitted from the names of the muscles, but by way of compensation the initial letters of the qualifying adjectives are printed in capitals, e.g., musculus trapezius and musculus rectus abdominis are printed thus: Trapezius and Rectus Abdominis.

As to terminology, the international nomenclature, Nomina Anatomica Parisiensia (N. A. P., 1955) is employed in place of the Birmingham Revision (B. R., 1933) of the Basle Nomina Anatomica (B. N. A., 1895) which was formerly in use. Where, however, the N. A. P. terms differ substantially from the revised B. N. A. terms—and this is in a small minority of instances—both terms are given, the discarded B. N. A. terms being set within parentheses ( ). Square brackets [ ] indicate a synonym approved by N. A. P. These are very few.

The Publishers, finding that better pictures could be produced than formerly if newer technical methods were applied to the original art-work, decided to use this opportunity to have every picture re-engraved. This has been done, and at the same time some have been enlarged, a few have been reduced in size, and seven have been replaced.

Further, a number of half-tone illustrations and photographs have been added to this edition. These include: breast on section (12.1), posterior wall of omental bursa & tributaries of portal vein (134 & 135), corrosion preparations of liver (137–141), exposure of bile duct, 11 (148), reflected spleen (151), segmental arteries of kidney (183.1 & 183.2), male perineum (194), urethral mucosa (199.1), vessels of female pelvis (238), acetabulum (278 & 283), lower end of spinal cord (484), Mylohyoid & Geniohyoid from below (544 & 545), sections through parotid region & temporo-mandibular joint (554 & 555), os Japonicum (557.1) and arteries of larynx (628.1 & 631.1).

Diagrams and line drawings of photographs, most of which have been borrowed from the author's *A Method of Anatomy*, appear, mostly in the lower corners, as secondary or supporting figures. It is hoped that these slight intrusions may help to define a term, make clear some point, or otherwise speed comprehension.

A guide to the plan of the book is to be found in the abbreviated list of illustrations on pages xi to xiii. As, however, most structures appear in two or more illustrations, this list is not a substitute for the index.

Source references immediately precede the index.

During the preparation of the various editions of this work I have received generous assistance from several colleagues, notably: Dr. C. G. Smith, who verified the bony attachments of the muscles of the limbs for the first edition, and who devised the schemes of the cranial nerves for the second; Dr. Allene I. Scott, who spent long hours making many of the most difficult dissections for the third edition; and Dr. J. E. Anderson, who has lavished care on some of the more intricate preparations and tracings for the fourth and fifth editions. To these I renew my thanks.

To Professor J. W. A. Duckworth, my successor in the Chair in the University of Toronto, I express my deep thanks for the facilities of the Department so kindly placed at my disposal.

I have been most fortunate in the expert assistance rendered me by a number of medical artists. I owe a particular debt to Mrs. Dorothy I. Chubb, a pupil of Max Brodel, who worked with me from the beginning, and also to Miss Nancy Joy, now Medical Artist to the Faculty of Medicine of the University of Manitoba, who soon joined Mrs. Chubb, for without their expert skill, patience in a laborious task, and the desire to achieve accuracy and effect, this book could hardly have been made. Mrs. Chubb was mainly responsible for the art-work of the first two editions; Miss Joy for the last three. To them I record again my grateful appreciation of their work so cheerfully and carefully done.

I gladly acknowledge the assistance of Miss Elizabeth Blackstock, of the Department of Art as applied to Medicine of this University, whose talent is apparent in the cross-sections of the upper limb, the paranasal sinuses, and the arteries of the stomach, pancreas, and bile passages. Mrs. E. Hopper Ross and Miss Marguerite Drummond, who also are associated with the Department of Art, have provided me with occasional and excellent illustrations, for which I am very grateful.

To Mr. James B. Francis and Mr. Douglas Baker, for their early and valued assistance with the bones and muscles of the lower limb, I express my thanks.

To Mr. Charles E. Storton, who has throughout given me general expert assistance, including the preliminary photographic work, which has been of very high order, and to Mr. H. Whittaker, who at times has undertaken the photographic work, my thanks are due for their willing and very skillful help.

Finally, to the Publishers, Messrs. Williams and Wilkins, who, through Mr. Francis E. Old, Jr., have with unfailing courtesy and consideration given me loose rein and have endeavoured to meet all my requests, I express my gratitude and thanks.

J. C. B. GRANT.

Illustrations

HEAD AND NECK

The Upper Limb

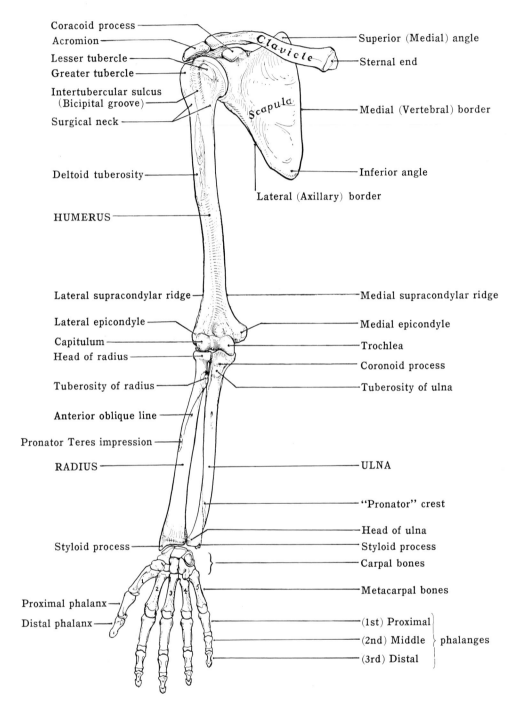

Coracoid process

Acromion

Lesser tubercle

Greater tubercle

Intertubercular sulcus
(Bicipital groove)

Surgical neck

Clavicle

Superior (Medial) angle

Sternal end

Scapula

Medial (Vertebral) border

Deltoid tuberosity

Inferior angle

Lateral (Axillary) border

HUMERUS

Lateral supracondylar ridge

Medial supracondylar ridge

Lateral epicondyle

Medial epicondyle

Capitulum

Trochlea

Head of radius

Coronoid process

Tuberosity of radius

Tuberosity of ulna

Anterior oblique line

Pronator Teres impression

RADIUS

ULNA

"Pronator" crest

Head of ulna

Styloid process

Styloid process

Carpal bones

Metacarpal bones

Proximal phalanx

Distal phalanx

(1st) Proximal

(2nd) Middle   phalanges

(3rd) Distal

1   Bones of the Upper Limb, from the front

(For bones of hand, see figs. 62 & 95; for attachments of muscles, see figs. 11, 29 & 58.)

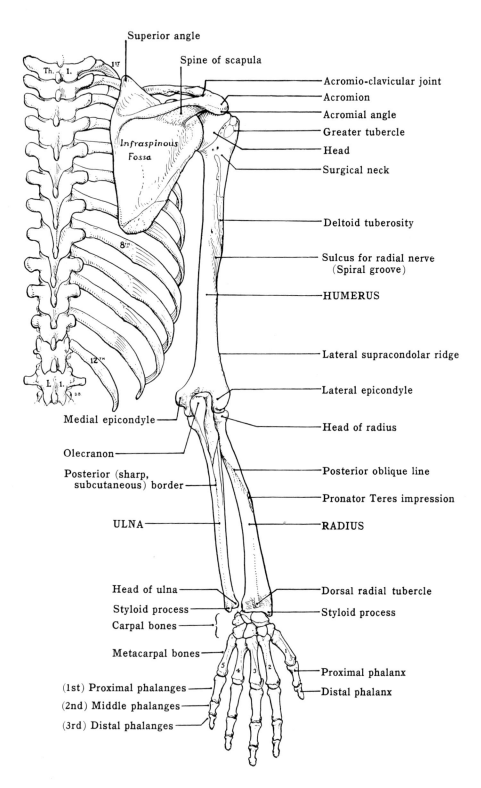

Superior angle

Spine of scapula

Acromio-clavicular joint

Acromion

Acromial angle

Greater tubercle

Head

Surgical neck

Infraspinous Fossa

Deltoid tuberosity

Sulcus for radial nerve (Spiral groove)

HUMERUS

Lateral supracondolar ridge

Lateral epicondyle

Head of radius

Medial epicondyle

Olecranon

Posterior (sharp, subcutaneous) border

Posterior oblique line

Pronator Teres impression

ULNA

RADIUS

Head of ulna

Dorsal radial tubercle

Styloid process

Styloid process

Carpal bones

Metacarpal bones

Proximal phalanx

Distal phalanx

(1st) Proximal phalanges

(2nd) Middle phalanges

(3rd) Distal phalanges

2   Bones of the Upper Limb, from behind

(For bones of hand, see fig. 86; for attachments of muscles, see figs. 30 & 77.)

Transverse cervical a.
[Transversa colli a.]

SUBCLAVIAN ARTERY

Suprascapular a.

Acromion

Thoraco-acromial a.

Lateral thoracic a.
Posterior humeral circumflex a.

Anterior humeral circumflex a.

ascending branch

Profunda brachii a.

Interosseous recurrent a.

Radial recurrent a.
Common interosseous a.

Posterior interosseous a.

RADIAL ARTERY

Scalenus Anterior

Thyro-cervical trunk

COMMON CAROTID ARTERY

Clavicle

1st rib

AXILLARY

Aortic arch

BRACHIO-CEPHALIC TRUNK (INNOMINATE ART.)

Pectoralis Minor

Teres Major

Subscapular a.

BRACHIAL ARTERY

Superior ulnar collateral a.

Inferior ulnar collateral a. (Supratrochlear a.)

Ant. & post. ulnar recurrent aa.

ULNAR ARTERY

Anterior interosseous a.

Dorsal carpal br.

Palmar carpal arch

Pisiform bone

Deep palmar arch

Palmar metacarpal aa.

Superf. palmar arch

Common palmar digital aa.

Palmar digital aa.

Transverse cervical a.

Suprascapular a.

Levator

Intercostal aa.

Teres Major

Circumflex scapular br. subscapular

SCAPULAR REGION

3 Diagram of the Named Arteries of the Upper Limb

Radius

Posterior interosseous a.

4

3

Anterior interosseous a.

Dorsal carpal br.

Dorsal carpal rete

Perforating brs.

Dorsal metacarpal aa.

Dorsal digital aa.

2

1

RADIAL ARTERY

Dorsales pollicis

Dorsalis indicis

ANTERIOR VIEW

SAGITTAL SECTION

POSTERIOR VIEW

3 Arteries of the Upper Limb

The stem artery of the upper limb is the subclavian artery. Now, the right subclavian artery springs from the brachio-cephalic trunk (innominate artery) behind the right sterno-clavicular joint, whereas the left subclavian artery springs directly from the aortic arch and ascends behind the left sterno-clavicular joint. From this point onward the arteries of the two sides are symmetrical.

The subclavian artery arches over the apex of the lung and pleura, rising about an inch above the clavicle, and it leaves the root of the neck at the lateral border of the 1st rib to enter the axilla, as the axillary artery. The axillary artery leaves the axilla at the lower border of the Teres Major to enter the arm or brachium as the brachial artery. About 1″ below the crease of the elbow the brachial artery bifurcates into the radial and ulnar arteries, which traverse the forearm or antebrachium and enter the palm where each ends as an arterial arch. The ulnar artery forms the superficial palmar arch, which descends to the level of the web of the thumb where it is completed by a slender branch of the radial artery—commonly its superficial palmar branch. The radial artery, after crossing the floor of the "snuff box" (i.e., the hollow at the root of the thumb), to reach the dorsum of the hand, passes through the 1st intermetacarpal space and so enters the palm. It there forms the deep palmar arch, which lies half an inch proximal to the superficial palmar arch. The deep palmar arch is completed by a slender artery, the deep palmar branch of the ulnar artery.

Subdivisions: The subclavian artery is divided into 3 unequal parts by the Scalenus Anterior, and the axillary artery is similarly divided by the Pectoralis Minor.

Relationship to bone: The axillary artery passes within a finger's breadth of the tip of the coracoid process. The brachial artery lies medial to the humerus proximally and anterior to it distally. At the wrist the ulnar artery (and nerve) is sheltered from injury by the pisiform bone; its deep palmar branch curves round the lower border of the hamate bone. The radial artery is identified at the wrist by its pulse, which beats against the lower end of the radius.

Branches: The limbs are organs of locomotion and prehension, and the muscles are the motors that move them. Hence, most of the blood delivered to the limbs is for the supply of the muscles and little for the skin, fasciae, bones, and joints. The branches of the arteries are numerous, and they are for the most part muscular and nameless. Most of the named branches in the limbs are muscular too, but their claim to recognition depends mainly on the anastomoses they effect, for these are important surgically, and on their size.

Anastomoses: (a) It should be safe to tie either the subclavian or the axillary artery between the thyro-cervical trunk and the subscapular artery because of the anastomoses around the scapula; (b) it should be safe to tie the brachial artery distal to the inferior ulnar collateral artery because of the anastomoses around the elbow; (c) and it should be safe to tie either the radial or the ulnar artery in the forearm because these arteries are united by 2 palmar arches and by 2 carpal arches.

Arches: The superficial palmar arch lies deep only to skin and palmar aponeurosis—it is well-named. The three other arches lie on the skeletal plane, that is to say, on bones, joints, ligaments or interosseous membranes. Their order of magnitude (1, 2, 3, 4) is indicated. The deep palmar arch not only unites the radial and ulnar arteries, but it anastomoses with the interosseous arteries of the forearm, of the dorsum of the hand, and of the digits.

Calibers: The caliber of the axillary artery diminishes considerably just beyond the origin of the subscapular and posterior circumflex arteries, which are large arteries. The caliber of the ulnar artery is reduced to that of the radial artery beyond the origin of the common interosseous artery.

The anterior interior interosseous artery does duty for the posterior interosseous artery in the distal half of the back of the forearm.

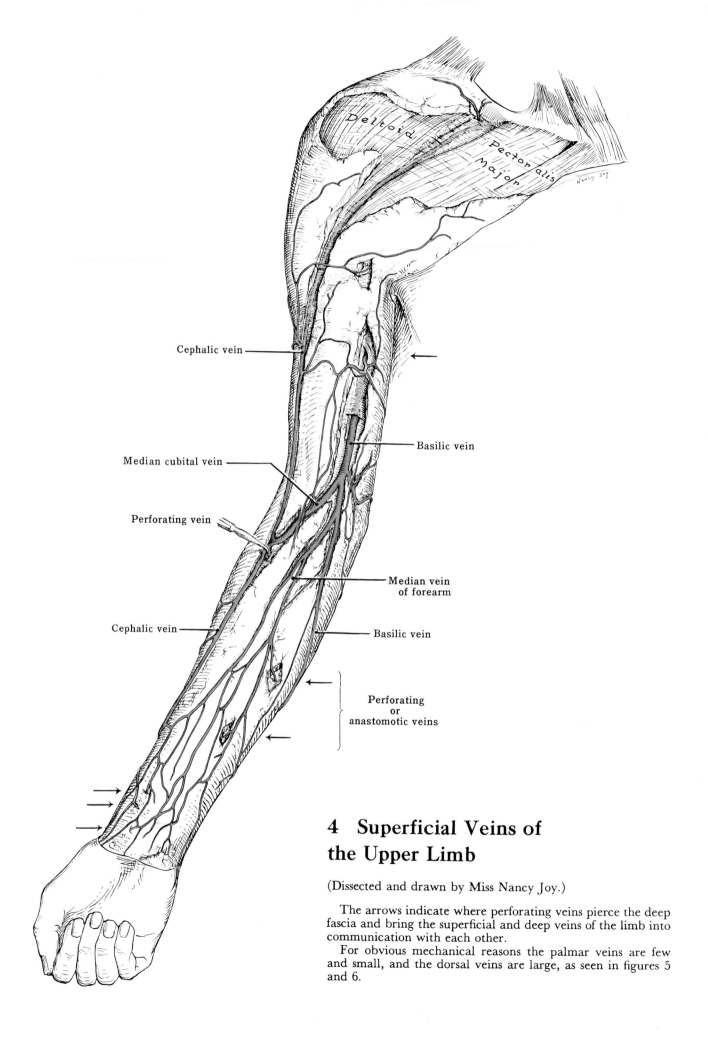

Cephalic vein

Median cubital vein

Perforating vein

Cephalic vein

Basilic vein

Median vein
of forearm

Basilic vein

Perforating
or
anastomotic veins

Deltoid

Pectoralis Major

Nancy Joy

4 Superficial Veins of the Upper Limb

(Dissected and drawn by Miss Nancy Joy.)

The arrows indicate where perforating veins pierce the deep fascia and bring the superficial and deep veins of the limb into communication with each other.

For obvious mechanical reasons the palmar veins are few and small, and the dorsal veins are large, as seen in figures 5 and 6.

Palmar digital veins

Intercapitular veins

Transverse anastomoses

Perforating
veins

Cephalic
vein

Basilic vein

5 Palmar Aspect

Dorsal digital
veins

Dorsal digital
venous arches

Intercapitular
veins

Perforating
veins

Superficial dorsal
veins

Dorsal venous
arch

Basilic vein

Perforating vein

Cephalic vein

6 Dorsal Aspect

Superficial Veins
of the Hand

(Dissected and drawn by Miss Nancy Joy.)
See legend attached to figure 4.

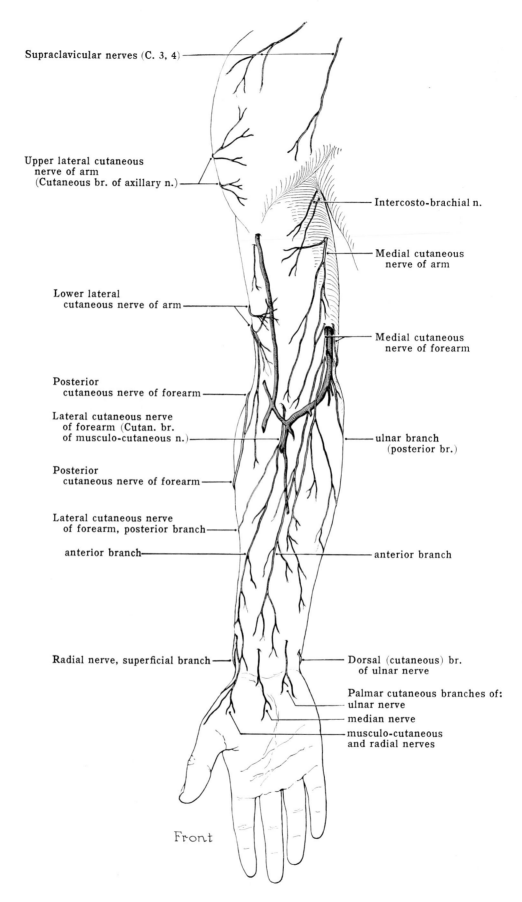

Supraclavicular nerves (C. 3, 4)

Upper lateral cutaneous
nerve of arm
(Cutaneous br. of axillary n.)

Intercosto-brachial n.

Medial cutaneous
nerve of arm

Lower lateral
cutaneous nerve of arm

Medial cutaneous
nerve of forearm

Posterior
cutaneous nerve of forearm

Lateral cutaneous nerve
of forearm (Cutan. br.
of musculo-cutaneous n.)

ulnar branch
(posterior br.)

Posterior
cutaneous nerve of forearm

Lateral cutaneous nerve
of forearm, posterior branch

anterior branch

anterior branch

Radial nerve, superficial branch

Dorsal (cutaneous) br.
of ulnar nerve

Palmar cutaneous branches of:
ulnar nerve
median nerve
musculo-cutaneous
and radial nerves

Front

7 Cutaneous Nerves of the Upper Limb

Of the 5 terminal branches of the brachial plexus, viz. musculo-cutaneous, median, ulnar, radial, and axillary (circumflex) nerves, the first 4 reach the hand.

The posterior cord of the plexus is represented by 5 cutaneous nerves. Of these (a) one, the upper lateral cutaneous n. of the arm, is a branch of the axillary n.;

Supraclavicular nerves (C. 3, 4)

Intercosto-brachial n.

Upper lateral cutaneous
nerve of arm
(Cutaneous br. of axillary n.)

Posterior
cutaneous nerve of arm

Lower lateral cutaneous
nerve of arm

Medial cutaneous
nerve of forearm,
ulnar (posterior) brs.

Posterior cutaneous nerve
of forearm

Posterior cutaneous nerve
of forearm

Lateral cutaneous nerve
of forearm, posterior
branch

Dorsal (cutaneous)
br. of ulnar nerve

Radial nerve,
superficial branch

Back

8   Cutaneous Nerves of the Upper Limb

(b) whereas 4 are branches of the radial n. They are: the posterior cutaneous n. of the arm, the lower lateral cutaneous n. of the arm, the posterior cutaneous n. of the forearm, and the superficial branch of the radial nerve.

See figures 13 (pectoral region), 24 (back), 44 (elbow), 83 (hand).

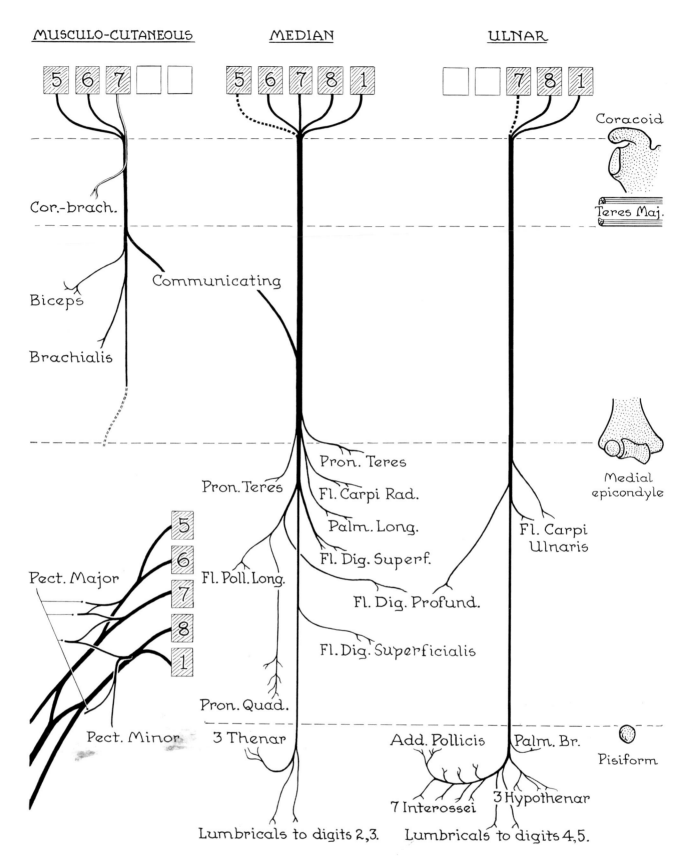

9 Scheme of the Motor Distribution of the Ventral Nerves of the Limb

The average levels at which the motor branches leave the stems of the main nerves are shown with reference to the lower border of the axilla (Teres Major), elbow joint (medial epicondyle), and wrist (pisiform bone).

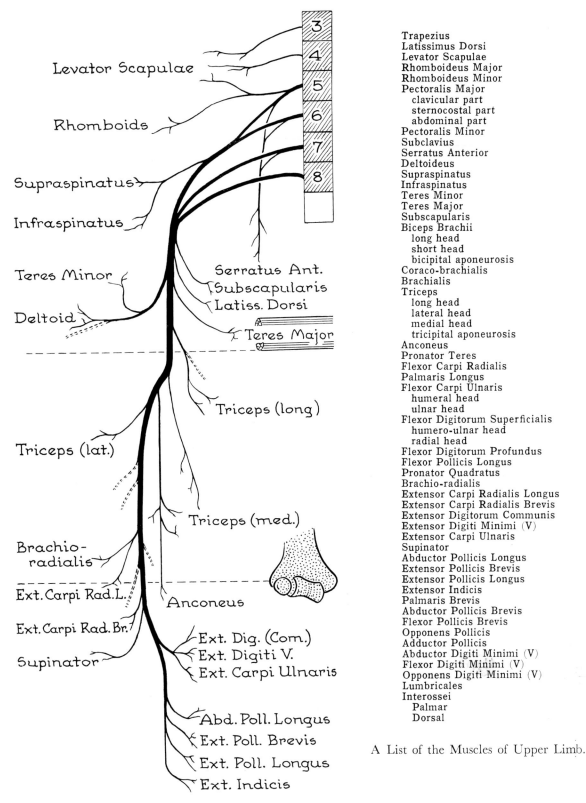

Levator Scapulae

Rhomboids

Supraspinatus

Infraspinatus

Teres Minor

Deltoid

Triceps (lat.)

Brachio-
radialis

Ext. Carpi Rad. L.

Ext. Carpi Rad. Br.

Supinator

Serratus Ant.
Subscapularis
Latiss. Dorsi
Teres Major

Triceps (long)

Triceps (med.)

Anconeus

Ext. Dig. (Com.)
Ext. Digiti V.
Ext. Carpi Ulnaris

Abd. Poll. Longus
Ext. Poll. Brevis
Ext. Poll. Longus
Ext. Indicis

Trapezius
Latissimus Dorsi
Levator Scapulae
Rhomboideus Major
Rhomboideus Minor
Pectoralis Major
  clavicular part
  sternocostal part
  abdominal part
Pectoralis Minor
Subclavius
Serratus Anterior
Deltoideus
Supraspinatus
Infraspinatus
Teres Minor
Teres Major
Subscapularis
Biceps Brachii
  long head
  short head
  bicipital aponeurosis
Coraco-brachialis
Brachialis
Triceps
  long head
  lateral head
  medial head
  tricipital aponeurosis
Anconeus
Pronator Teres
Flexor Carpi Radialis
Palmaris Longus
Flexor Carpi Ulnaris
  humeral head
  ulnar head
Flexor Digitorum Superficialis
  humero-ulnar head
  radial head
Flexor Digitorum Profundus
Flexor Pollicis Longus
Pronator Quadratus
Brachio-radialis
Extensor Carpi Radialis Longus
Extensor Carpi Radialis Brevis
Extensor Digitorum Communis
Extensor Digiti Minimi (V)
Extensor Carpi Ulnaris
Supinator
Abductor Pollicis Longus
Extensor Pollicis Brevis
Extensor Pollicis Longus
Extensor Indicis
Palmaris Brevis
Abductor Pollicis Brevis
Flexor Pollicis Brevis
Opponens Pollicis
Adductor Pollicis
Abductor Digiti Minimi (V)
Flexor Digiti Minimi (V)
Opponens Digiti Minimi (V)
Lumbricales
Interossei
  Palmar
  Dorsal

A List of the Muscles of Upper Limb.

10 Scheme of the Motor Distribution of the Dorsal Nerves of the Limb

The average levels of origin of the motor branches are shown as in figure 9.

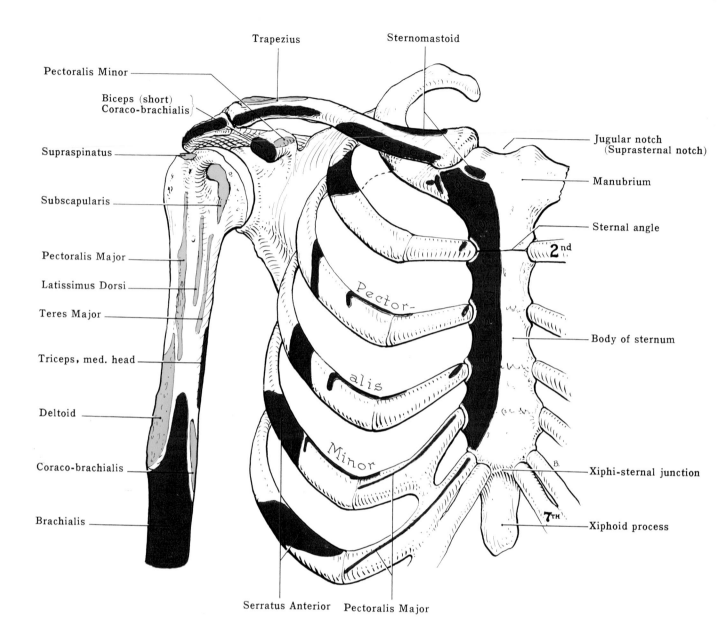

Pectoralis Minor

Biceps (short)
Coraco-brachialis

Supraspinatus

Subscapularis

Pectoralis Major

Latissimus Dorsi

Teres Major

Triceps, med. head

Deltoid

Coraco-brachialis

Brachialis

Trapezius

Sternomastoid

Jugular notch
(Suprasternal notch)

Manubrium

Sternal angle

2nd

Body of sternum

Xiphi-sternal junction

7TH

Xiphoid process

Serratus Anterior   Pectoralis Major

11   Bones of the Pectoral Region and Axilla

Observe:

1. The following muscles attached in line with each other: (a) Trapezius and Sternomastoid;
   (b) Deltoid and clavicular head of Pectoralis Major; (c) Supraspinatus, Pectoralis Major
   and anterior part of Deltoid; and (d) Subscapularis and Latissimus Dorsi and Teres Major.
2. Pectoralis Major having a crescentic origin from the clavicle, sternum and 5th and (or)
   6th costal cartilages.
3. Pectoralis Minor here arising from the 3rd, 4th and 5th ribs. It commonly arises also from
   either the 2nd or the 6th rib.

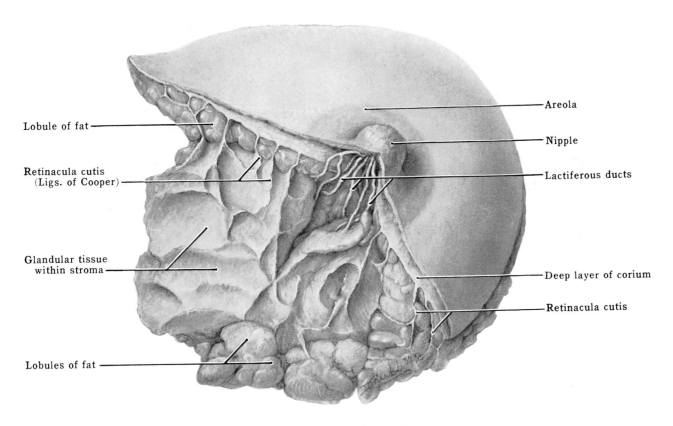

Areola

Nipple

Lobule of fat

Retinacula cutis
(Ligs. of Cooper)

Lactiferous ducts

Glandular tissue
within stroma

Deep layer of corium

Retinacula cutis

Lobules of fat

12   Mammary Gland of the Female

(Dissection by Dr. Ross G. MacKenzie)

With the rounded handle of the scalpel collections of superficial fat were scooped out of their compartments on the surface of the glandular tissue. The glandular tissue was incised in order to allow the ducts to be traced. A fringe of the deeper layer of the skin projects.

Observe:

1. The nipple rising from the centre of the pigmented areola.
2. The 7 of the 15 to 20 lactiferous ducts that are displayed. Traced in retrograde direction, they run at first dorsally in the long axis of the nipple, enveloped in an areolar cuff, and then spread radially and branch to the glandular tissue.
3. The glandular tissue within a dense (fibro-) areolar stroma from which septa, retinacula cutis, which imprison lobules of superficial fat, extend to the deeper layers of the skin.

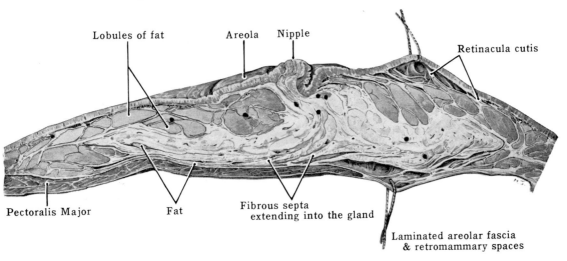

Lobules of fat   Areola   Nipple

Retinacula cutis

Pectoralis Major   Fat   Fibrous septa
extending into the gland

Laminated areolar fascia
& retromammary spaces

12.1   Mammary Gland of the Female, on antero-posterior section

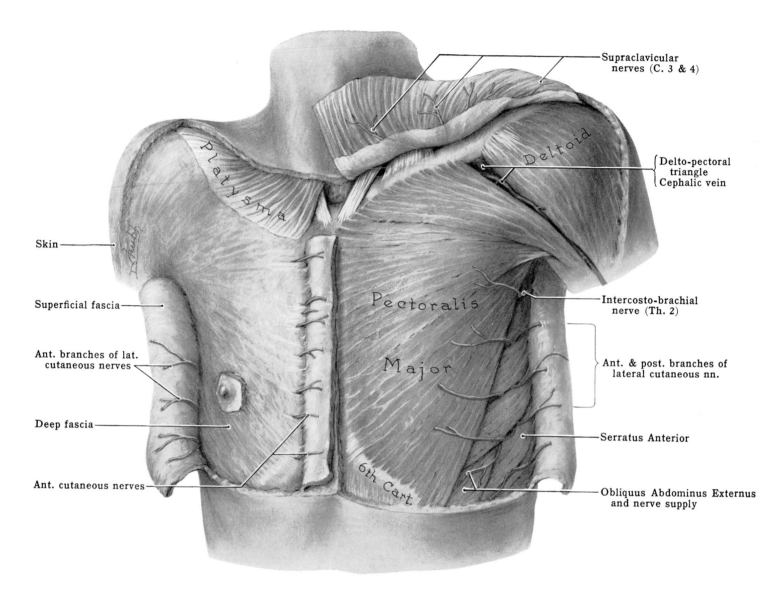

Labels on figure:
- Supraclavicular nerves (C. 3 & 4)
- Delto-pectoral triangle Cephalic vein
- Deltoid
- Platysma
- Skin
- Superficial fascia
- Pectoralis Major
- Intercosto-brachial nerve (Th. 2)
- Ant. branches of lat. cutaneous nerves
- Ant. & post. branches of lateral cutaneous nn.
- Deep fascia
- Serratus Anterior
- Ant. cutaneous nerves
- 6th Cart.
- Obliquus Abdominus Externus and nerve supply

13   Superficial Dissection of the Pectoral Region

Platysma, which descends to the 2nd or 3rd rib, is cut short on the left side of the picture; it, together with the supraclavicular nerves, is thrown up on the right side.

Observe:

1. The deep fascia covering Pectoralis Major is filmy.
2. The intermuscular bony strip running along the clavicle is both subcutaneous and subplatysmal.
3. The two heads of Pectoralis Major meeting at the sterno-clavicular joint.
4. The cephalic vein traversing the delto-pectoral triangle.

Note:—The brachial plexus (C.5, 6, 7, 8 and Th. 1) does not supply cutaneous branches here, hence the break in the numerical sequence, i.e., branches of nerves C.3 & 4 meet those of Th.2.

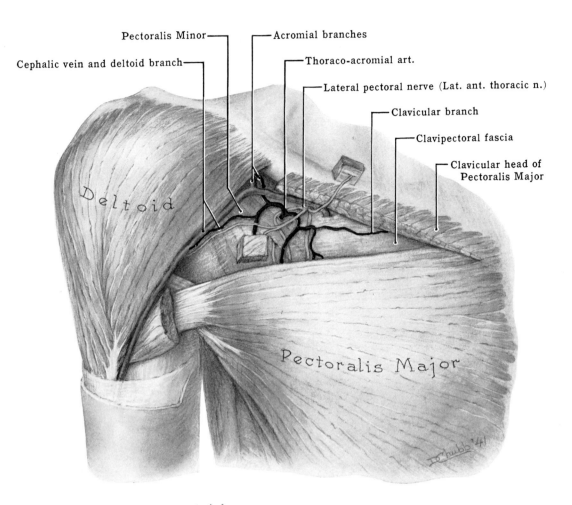

Pectoralis Minor — ─ Acromial branches

Cephalic vein and deltoid branch — ─ Thoraco-acromial art.

─ Lateral pectoral nerve (Lat. ant. thoracic n.)

─ Clavicular branch

─ Clavipectoral fascia

─ Clavicular head of Pectoralis Major

Deltoid

Pectoralis Major

14   Clavipectoral Fascia (Coraco-clavicular Fascia)

Clavicular head of Pectoralis Major is excised, but cubes of muscle identify its nerves. The thoraco-acromial veins are removed.

Observe:

1. The part of the clavipectoral fascia above Pectoralis Minor—the costocoracoid membrane (fig. 14.1)—pierced by the lateral pectoral nerve and its companion vessels.

2. The part of the fascia embracing Pectoralis Minor. Here muscle and fascia are pierced by the medial pectoral nerve (not labelled).

3. The trilaminar insertion of Pectoralis Major.

4. The course of the cephalic vein.

5. The two cubes of muscle attached to the lateral pectoral nerve are cut from the clavicular head of Pectoralis Major.

14.1

Diagram of anterior wall of axilla, on sagittal section.

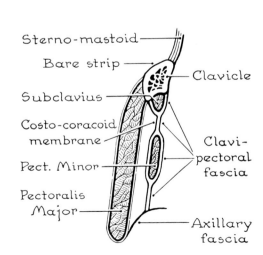

Sterno-mastoid

Bare strip

Clavicle

Subclavius

Costo-coracoid membrane

Clavi-pectoral fascia

Pect. Minor

Pectoralis Major

Axillary fascia

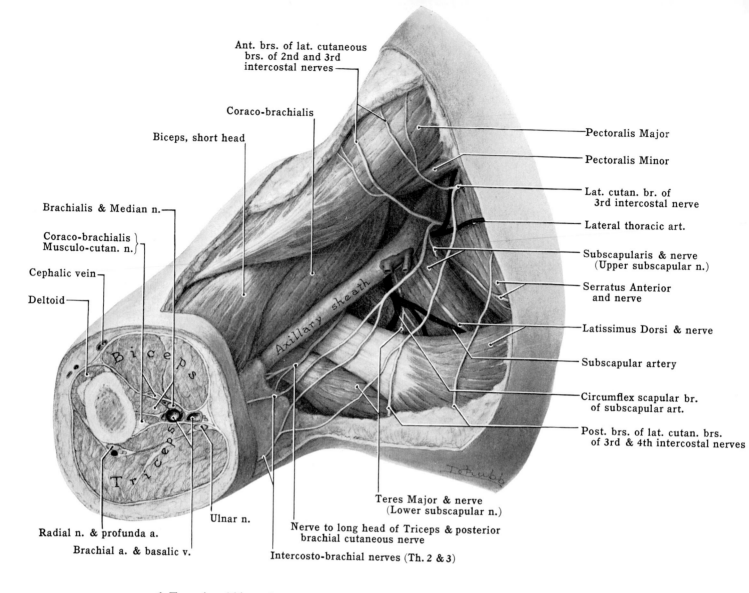

Ant. brs. of lat. cutaneous
brs. of 2nd and 3rd
intercostal nerves

Coraco-brachialis

Biceps, short head

Brachialis & Median n.

Coraco-brachialis }
Musculo-cutan. n. }

Cephalic vein

Deltoid

Biceps

Triceps

Axillary sheath

Pectoralis Major

Pectoralis Minor

Lat. cutan. br. of
3rd intercostal nerve

Lateral thoracic art.

Subscapularis & nerve
(Upper subscapular n.)

Serratus Anterior
and nerve

Latissimus Dorsi & nerve

Subscapular artery

Circumflex scapular br.
of subscapular art.

Post. brs. of lat. cutan. brs.
of 3rd & 4th intercostal nerves

Radial n. & profunda a.

Brachial a. & basalic v.

Ulnar n.

Teres Major & nerve
(Lower subscapular n.)

Nerve to long head of Triceps & posterior
brachial cutaneous nerve

Intercosto-brachial nerves (Th. 2 & 3)

15 Axilla, from below: Cross Section of the Arm

Observe:

1. The three muscular walls of the axilla:
   (a) Anterior wall—Pectoralis Major, Pectoralis Minor and Subclavius, but only the lower borders of Pectorales are in view.
   (b) Posterior wall—Subscapularis, Latissimus Dorsi and Teres Major.
   (c) Medial wall—Serratus Anterior.
   (d) The lateral or bony wall—intertubercular sulcus (bicipital groove of the humerus)— is concealed by Biceps and Coraco-brachialis.

2. The axillary sheath and the cutaneous nerves crossing Latissimus Dorsi. The most lateral of these nerves also, and alone, supplies long head of Triceps.

3. The axillary sheath of great vessels and nerves is a neuro-vascular bundle.

15.1

Diagram of the walls of the axilla, on cross section.

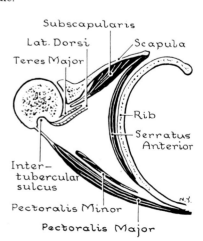

Subscapularis

Lat. Dorsi

Scapula

Teres Major

Rib

Serratus
Anterior

Inter-
tubercular
sulcus

Pectoralis Minor

Pectoralis Major

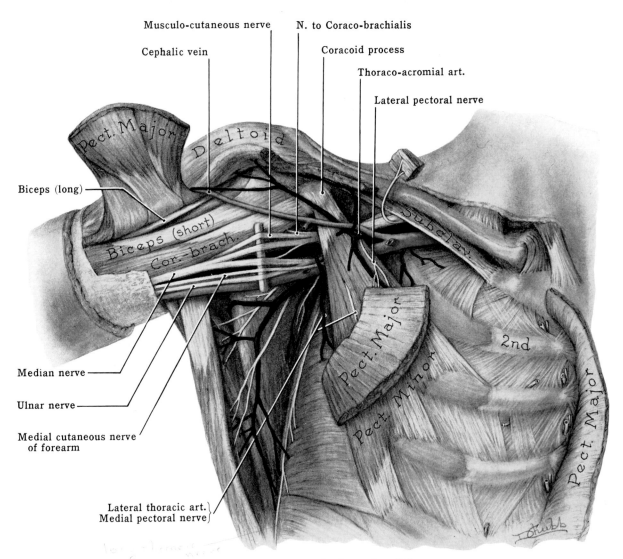

Musculo-cutaneous nerve

N. to Coraco-brachialis

Cephalic vein

Coracoid process

Thoraco-acromial art.

Lateral pectoral nerve

Biceps (long)

Median nerve

Ulnar nerve

Medial cutaneous nerve
of forearm

Lateral thoracic art.
Medial pectoral nerve

16 Anterior Structures of the Axilla

Pectoralis Major is reflected and the clavi-pectoral fascia removed.

Observe:

1. Subclavius and Pectoralis Minor, the two deep muscles of the anterior wall.

2. The axillary artery lying behind Pectoralis Minor a finger's breadth from the tip of the coracoid process and having the lateral cord lateral to it and the medial cord medial.

3. The axillary vein lying medial to the axillary artery.

4. The median nerve, followed proximally, leading by its lateral root to the lateral cord and the musculo-cutaneous nerve, and by its medial root to the medial cord and the ulnar nerve. [These and the medial cutaneous nerve of the forearm are raised on a stick.]

5. The nerve to Coraco-brachialis arising within the axilla.

6. The supreme thoracic artery (not labelled) passing to the 1st and 2nd intercostal spaces.

7. The cube of muscle above the clavicle is cut from the clavicular head of Pectoralis Major.

Note:—The lateral root of the median nerve may be in several strands.
Here there is one small extra strand.

16.1

Diagram of the contents of the axilla, on cross section.

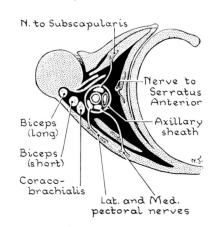

N. to Subscapularis

Nerve to
Serratus
Anterior

Axillary
sheath

Biceps
(long)

Biceps
(short)

Coraco-
brachialis

Lat. and Med.
pectoral nerves

Axillary (Circumflex) n. & Subscapular art.

Anterior & posterior circumflex humeral aa.

Pect. Major

Lateral thoracic art.
Medial pectoral nerve
(Med. ant. thoracic n.)

Suprascapular nerve
Thoraco-acromial art.

Lateral pectoral nerve
(Lat. ant. thoracic n.)

Subclavius

Posterior cord

Supreme thoracic art.

Intercosto-brachial nerve

Subscapularis & nerve
(Upper subscap. n.)

Serratus Anterior & nerve
[Long thoracic n.]

Basilic vein

Triceps, long head, & nerve

Posterior cutaneous n. of arm

Radial nerve

Circumflex scapular art.

Teres Major & nerve
(Lower subscap. n.)

Latissimus & nerve
[Thoraco-dorsal n.]

17 Posterior and Medial Walls of the Axilla

Pectoralis Minor is excised; the lateral and medial cords are retracted; the axillary vein is removed.

Observe:

1. The posterior cord and its terminal branches viz. radial and axillary nerves, lying behind the axillary artery.
2. The nerves to the 3 posterior muscles. Of these:
   (a) Nerve to Latissimus Dorsi enters the deep surface of its muscle $\frac{1}{2}''$ from its free border at a point mid-way between the chest and the abducted arm.
   (b) Nerve to Subscapularis lies parallel to (a) but above it.
   (c) Nerve to Teres Major lies parallel to (a) but below it.
3. Nerve to Serratus Anterior clinging to its muscle throughout.
4. Suprascapular nerve passing towards the root of the coracoid process.
5. Subscapular artery, the largest branch of the axillary artery. Here it is somewhat high; usually it arises at the lower border of Subscapularis.
6. Posterior circumflex humeral artery accompanying the axillary nerve through the quadrangular space.

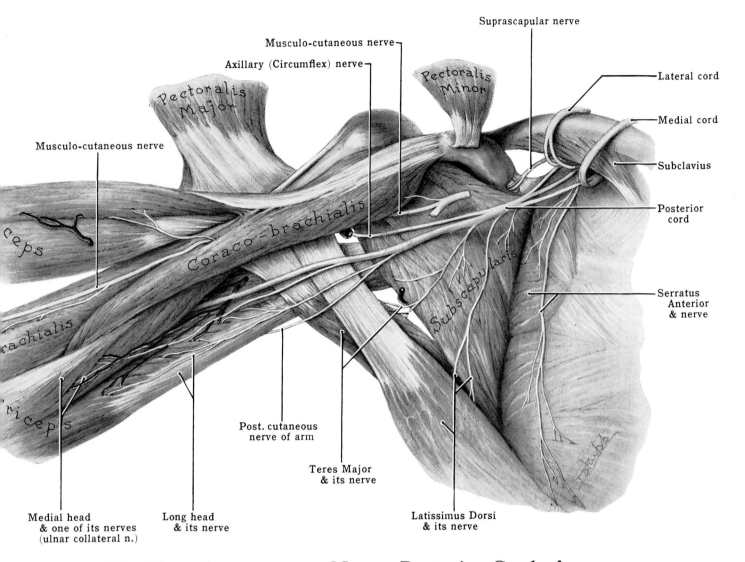

Suprascapular nerve

Musculo-cutaneous nerve

Axillary (Circumflex) nerve

Pectoralis Major

Pectoralis Minor

Lateral cord

Medial cord

Subclavius

Musculo-cutaneous nerve

Coraco-brachialis

Posterior cord

Subscapularis

Serratus Anterior & nerve

Post. cutaneous nerve of arm

Teres Major & its nerve

Latissimus Dorsi & its nerve

Medial head & one of its nerves (ulnar collateral n.)

Long head & its nerve

18 Musculo-cutaneous Nerve: Posterior Cord of the Brachial Plexus: Posterior Wall of the Axilla

Pectoralis Major and Pectoralis Minor are thrown laterally; the lateral and medial cords of the brachial plexus are thrown upwards; the arteries, veins, and median and ulnar nerves are removed.

Observe:

1. Coraco-brachialis arising with the short head of Biceps from the tip of the coracoid process and inserted half way down the humerus.

2. The musculo-cutaneous nerve piercing Coraco-brachialis, and supplying it, Biceps and Brachialis before becoming cutaneous.

3. The posterior cord of the plexus formed by the union of the 3 posterior divisions, supplying the 3 muscles of the posterior wall of the axilla, and soon ending as the radial and axillary nerves.

4. The radial nerve giving off, in the axilla, the nerve to the long head of Triceps and a cutaneous branch, and, in this specimen, the ulnar collateral branch to the medial head of Triceps. It then enters the spiral groove of the humerus with the profunda brachii artery.

5. The axillary nerve traversing the quadrangular space with the posterior circumflex humeral artery. The circumflex scapular artery traversing the triangular space.

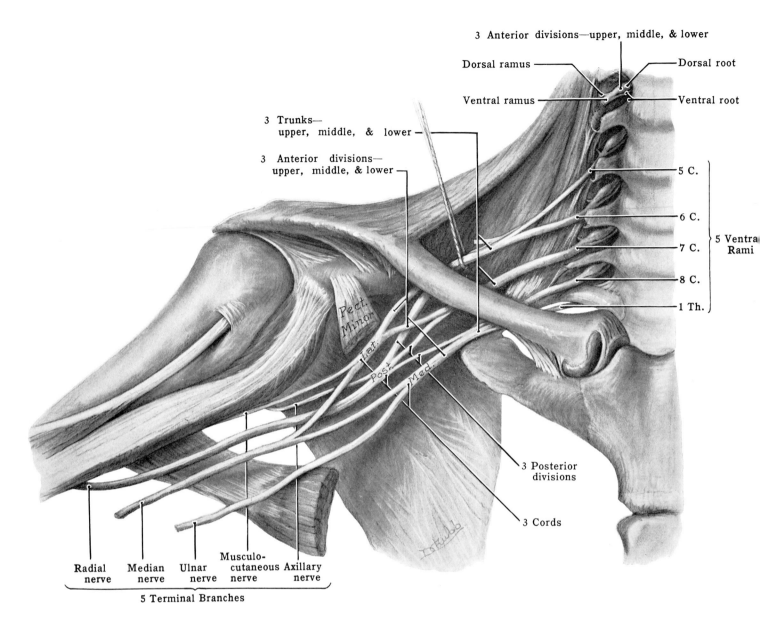

3 Anterior divisions—upper, middle, & lower

Dorsal ramus

Dorsal root

Ventral ramus

Ventral root

3 Trunks—
upper, middle, & lower

3 Anterior divisions—
upper, middle, & lower

5 C.

6 C.

7 C.

8 C.

1 Th.

5 Ventral
Rami

Pect. Minor

Lat.

Post.

Med.

3 Posterior divisions

3 Cords

Radial nerve | Median nerve | Ulnar nerve | Musculo-cutaneous nerve | Axillary nerve

5 Terminal Branches

19 Brachial Plexus: Ligaments of the Clavicle

Observe:

1. A dorsal (sensory) root of a spinal nerve larger than a ventral (motor) root.
2. The 2 roots uniting beyond the ganglion to form a very short mixed spinal nerve.
3. The mixed nerve at once dividing into a small dorsal ramus and a large ventral ramus.
4. The 5 ventral rami forming the brachial plexus. (Of these the middle ramus C.7, is the largest.)
5. These 5 rami uniting to form the 3 trunks of the plexus.
6. Each trunk dividing into 2 divisions, an anterior and a posterior.
7. These 6 divisions becoming 3 cords—a lateral, a medial, and a posterior.
8. The 3 cords lying behind Pectoralis Minor.
9. The posterior cord and the radial nerve derived from segments C.5, 6, 7 and 8, and slightly from Th.1.
10. The median nerve derived from segments C.6, 7, 8 and Th.1, and slightly from C.5.

Note: The ligaments of the clavicle and the structures of the sterno-clavicular joint are depicted but not labelled (fig. 36).

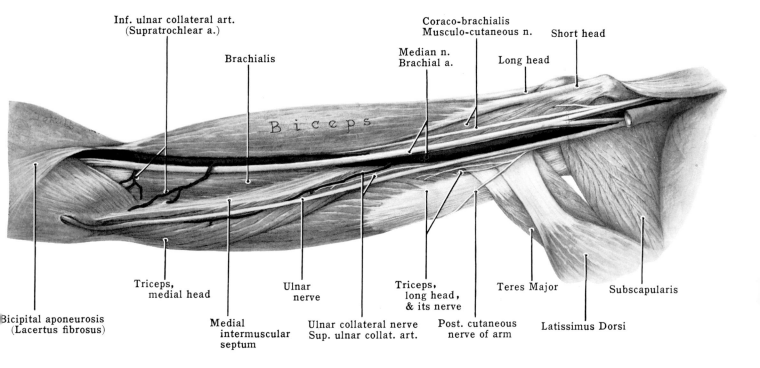

Inf. ulnar collateral art.
(Supratrochlear a.)

Brachialis

Coraco-brachialis
Musculo-cutaneous n.

Short head

Median n.
Brachial a.

Long head

Triceps,
medial head

Ulnar
nerve

Triceps,
long head,
& its nerve

Teres Major

Subscapularis

Bicipital aponeurosis
(Lacertus fibrosus)

Medial
intermuscular
septum

Ulnar collateral nerve
Sup. ulnar collat. art.

Post. cutaneous
nerve of arm

Latissimus Dorsi

20 Upper Arm or Brachium, medial view

Observe:

1. Biceps Brachii, Coraco-brachialis and Brachialis occupying the front of the arm; Triceps Brachii occupying the back.

2. The medial intermuscular septum separating these two muscle groups in the distal $\frac{2}{3}$ of the brachium.

3. The great artery of the limb lying a finger's breadth from the tip of the coracoid process, and applied to the medial side of Coraco-brachialis above, and to the front of Brachialis below.

4. In the axilla the lateral and medial cords of the brachial plexus and their end branches making an M-shaped display about the front of the artery.

5. The median nerve applied to the artery throughout and crossing it from lateral to medial side.

6. The ulnar nerve applied to the medial side of the artery as far as the middle of the arm, then passing behind the medial septum, and descending subfascially on the medial head of Triceps.

7. The superior ulnar collateral art. and the ulnar collateral branch of the radial nerve (to medial head of Triceps) accompanying the ulnar nerve.

8. The musculo-cutaneous nerve supplying Coraco-brachialis, following the lateral side of the artery, and disappearing between Biceps and Brachialis. More commonly it pierces Coraco-brachialis as in figure 18.

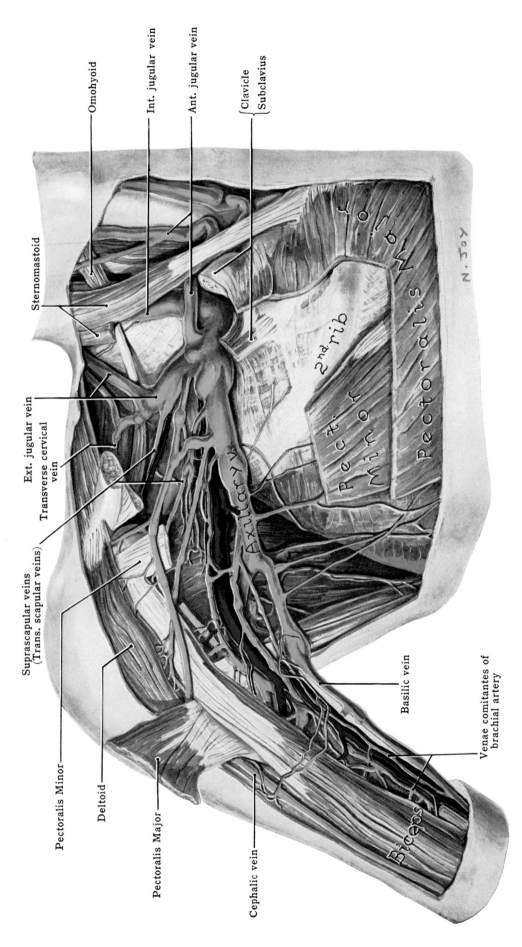

Omohyoid

Int. jugular vein

Ant. jugular vein

Clavicle
Subclavius

Sternomastoid

Ext. jugular vein

Transverse cervical
vein

Suprascapular veins
(Trans. scapular veins)

Pectoralis Minor

Deltoid

Pectoralis Major

Cephalic vein

Pectoralis Major

Pectoralis Minor

2nd rib

Axillary v.

Biceps

Basilic vein

Venae comitantes of
brachial artery

N. Joy

21 Veins of the Axilla

Observe:

1. The basilic vein becoming the axillary vein at the lower border of Teres Major; the axillary vein becoming the subclavian vein at the 1st rib; and the subclavian joining the internal jugular to become the brachiocephalic vein (innominate v.) behind the sternal end of the clavicle. Over 40 venous valves are shown. Note 1 in the basilic vein, 3 in the axillary, and 1 in the subclavian where it rests upon the 1st rib—the last valve on the road to the heart.

2. Venae comitantes of the brachial artery uniting and joining the axillary vein near the middle of the axilla.

3. The cephalic vein here bifurcating to end both in the axil-

4. The profunda brachii, posterior humeral circumflex, and circumflex scapular venae comitantes united and, as one large vein, joining the axillary vein.

5. Several subscapular veins, tenuous because the latex injection failed to force their valves.

6. Three suprascapular veins—1 from below the suprascapular ligament to the axillary vein, and 2 from above the ligament to the external jugular vein.

Note:—anastomotic veins are in view; obviously those on the dorsum of the scapula joining circumflex scapular and suprascapular veins cannot be seen.

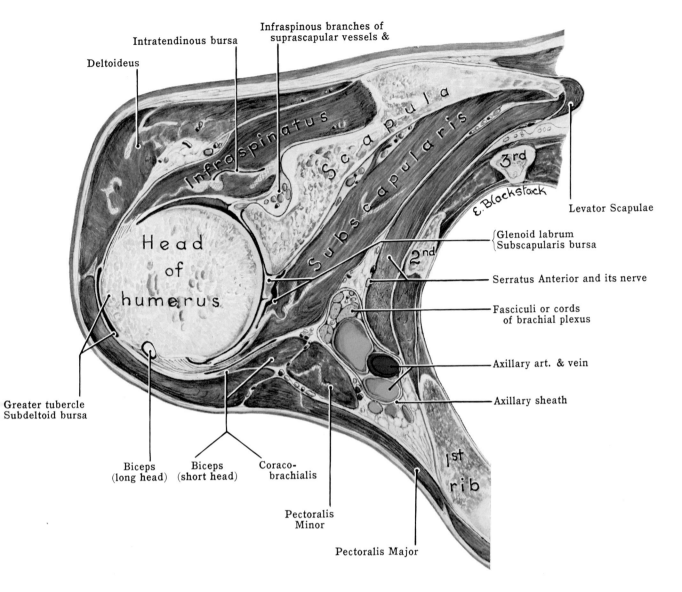

Deltoideus

Intratendinous bursa

Infraspinous branches of
suprascapular vessels &

Infraspinatus

Scapula

Subscapularis

3rd

E. Blackstock

Head
of
humerus

Greater tubercle
Subdeltoid bursa

Levator Scapulae

Glenoid labrum
Subscapularis bursa

Serratus Anterior and its nerve

Fasciculi or cords
of brachial plexus

2nd

Axillary art. & vein

Axillary sheath

1st
rib

Biceps
(long head)

Biceps
(short head)

Coraco-
brachialis

Pectoralis
Minor

Pectoralis Major

22 Cross-section through the Shoulder Joint
and the Axilla, near its apex

Observe:

1. The long head (tendon) of Biceps, in its synovial sheath, facing anteriorly. The short head of Biceps and the Coracobrachialis and Pectoralis Minor evidently sectioned close below their attachment to the coracoid process.

2. The cartilage of the head of the humerus, extensive and very thin peripherally.

3. The glenoid cavity of the scapula, small and with glenoid labrum attached loosely in front but firmly behind where it is part-origin of the long head of Biceps.

4. Delicate synovial folds projecting from the labra between head and glenoid cavity.

5. The fibrous capsule, thin posteriorly and partly fused with the tendon of Infraspinatus; thicker anteriorly (glenohumeral ligaments).

6. Bursae: (a) Subdeltoid bursa, between Deltoid and greater tubercle (continuous above with subacromial bursa, fig. 35); (b) Subscapular bursa, between Subscapularis tendon and the scapula (fig. 36) (communicating with the joint cavity); (c) Coraco-brachialis bursa, between Coraco-brachialis and Subscapularis; (d) an Intra-Infraspinatus bursa (present).

7. Walls of axilla near apex, formed by Subscapularis and scapula posteriorly; Serratus Anterior, thick at this high level, ribs and Intercostales medially; and Pectorales Major et Minor anteriorly. There is no bone in the anterior wall.

8. The axillary sheath of areolar tissue, delicate and enclosing the axillary artery and vein and the 3 cords or fasciculi of the brachial plexus (and here an extra vein) to form a neurovascular bundle, surrounded with axillary fat.

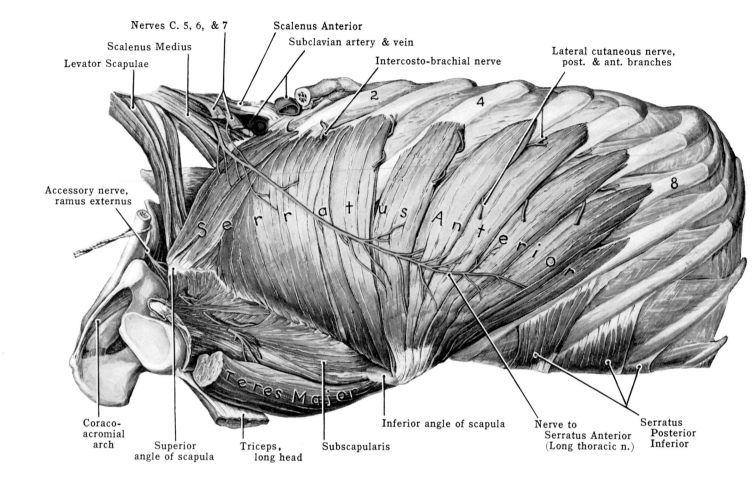

Nerves C. 5, 6, & 7
Scalenus Medius
Levator Scapulae
Scalenus Anterior
Subclavian artery & vein
Intercosto-brachial nerve
Lateral cutaneous nerve,
post. & ant. branches
Accessory nerve,
ramus externus
Coraco-
acromial
arch
Superior
angle of scapula
Triceps,
long head
Subscapularis
Inferior angle of scapula
Nerve to
Serratus Anterior
(Long thoracic n.)
Serratus
Posterior
Inferior

23   Serratus Anterior

Observe:

1. Serratus Anterior, which forms the medial wall of the axilla, having an extensive fleshy origin from the upper 8 (here 9) ribs far forward, and an insertion into the whole length of the medial border of the scapula. The fibres from the 1st rib and from the arch between the 1st and 2nd ribs converging on the superior angle, those from the 2nd and 3rd ribs diverging to spread thinly along the medial border, and the remainder (from 4th to 9th ribs), which forms the bulk of the muscle, converging on the inferior angle and therefore having a tendinous insertion. (For bony attachments see figs. 11 & 29.)

2. The nerve to Serratus Anterior, called the long thoracic nerve, arising from C.5, 6, and 7 and applied to the whole length of the muscle. The fibres from C.5 and 6 piercing Scalenus Medius and appearing lateral to the brachial plexus; those from C.7 descending between Scalenus Medius and the plexus.

3. Teres Major applied to the lateral border of Subscapularis; the nerve to Teres Major helping to supply Subscapularis.

4. The brachial plexus and the subclavian artery appearing between Scalenus Anterior and Scalenus Medius; the subclavian vein separated from the artery by Scalenus Anterior.

5. The term "Serratus Anterior" implies the existence of a "Serratus Posterior"; and the inferior part of this is seen attached to the lower 4 ribs.

Occipitalis

Occipital artery
Occipital lymph
nodes

Levator Scapulae

Rhomboideus Minor

Rhomboideus Major

Deltoideus

Accessory nerve

Trapezius

Latissimus Dorsi

Obliquus Abdominis
Externus

Lumbar triangle

Fascia covering
Gluteus Medius

Gluteus Maximus

Greater occipital nerve
(dorsal ramus C. 2)

3rd occipital nerve
(dorsal ramus C. 3)

Lesser occipital nerve
(ventral ramus C. 2)

Cutaneous branches of
dorsal rami

Triangle of
auscultation

Cutaneous branches of
dorsal (posterior) rami

Posterior branches of
lateral cutaneous nn.

Lateral cutaneous br. of ilio-
hypogastric n. (ventral
ramus L. 1)

Cutaneous branches of
dorsal rami of L. 1, 2, & 3
[Superior clunial nerves]

24   Cutaneous Nerves of the Back: The First Two Layers of Muscles

Trapezius is severed and reflected on the left side.

Observe:

1. The cutaneous branches of the dorsal (posterior) nerve rami.

2. Trapezius and Latissimus Dorsi of the 1st layer; Levator Scapulae and Rhomboidei of the 2nd layer.

3. The triangle of auscultation and the lumbar triangle.

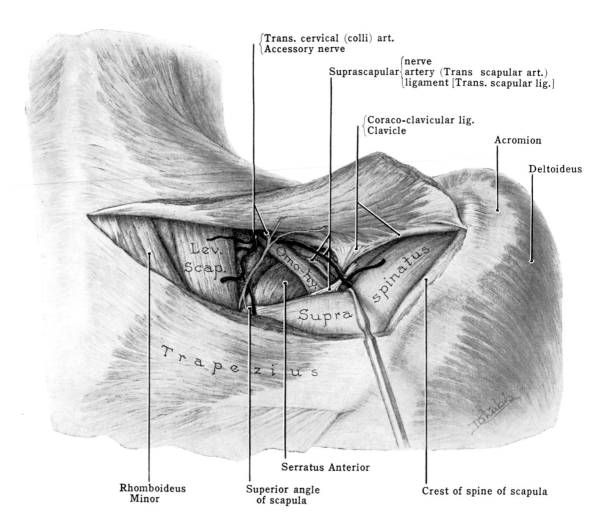

Trans. cervical (colli) art.
Accessory nerve

Suprascapular { nerve
artery (Trans scapular art.)
ligament [Trans. scapular lig.]

Coraco-clavicular lig.
Clavicle

Acromion

Deltoideus

Lev. Scap.

Omo-hy.

Supra spinatus

Trapezius

Rhomboideus Minor

Superior angle of scapula

Serratus Anterior

Crest of spine of scapula

25 Suprascapular Region

The horizontal fibres of Trapezius, at the level of the superior (medial) angle of the scapula, are separated and the incision is carried forwards along the crest of the spine of the scapula.

Observe:

1. The accessory nerve crossing the superior angle of the scapula.

2. The transverse cervical artery split by Levator Scapulae into a superficial and a deep branch, one following the accessory nerve, the other the nerve to Rhomboids (not shown).

3. The finger tip, placed on the superior angle, may trace a U-shaped course—laterally along the sharp superior border of the scapula and along the sharp suprascapular ligament to the coracoid process, thence cranially along the conoid ligament to the clavicle, and thence medially behind the smooth posterior surface of the clavicle.

4. The suprascapular artery running behind the clavicle, and therefore having a retro-clavicular course, before crossing above the suprascapular ligament.

5. The suprascapular nerve crossing below the ligament.

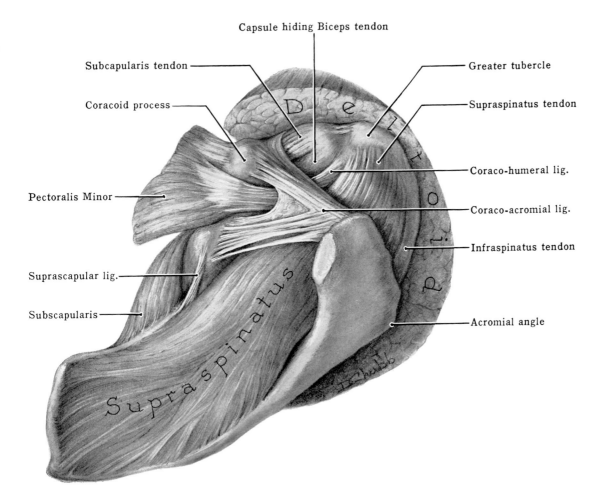

Capsule hiding Biceps tendon

Subcapularis tendon

Coracoid process

Pectoralis Minor

Suprascapular lig.

Subscapularis

Greater tubercle

Supraspinatus tendon

Coraco-humeral lig.

Coraco-acromial lig.

Infraspinatus tendon

Acromial angle

Supraspinatus

26 Supraspinous and Subdeltoid Regions

Observe:

1. The clavicular facet on the acromion. It is small, oval and obliquely set.

2. The triangular coraco-acromial ligament arching from the lateral border of the horizontal part of the coracoid process to the acromion between the facet and the tip.

3. Part of Pectoralis Minor tendon here (as commonly) dividing this ligament into 2 limbs and continuing, as the anterior part of the coraco-humeral ligament, to the greater tubercle (tuberosity) of the humerus.

4. Supraspinatus passing under the coraco-acromial arch, and then lying between Deltoid above and the capsule of the shoulder joint below. Supraspinatus and the middle fibres of Deltoid are the abductors of the joint. Though the middle part of the Deltoid is thin, it is multipennate and powerful.

(For subacromial and subdeltoid bursae see figures 35 & 38.1.)

A **Absence of Sternocostal Head of Right Pectoralis Major** associated with compensatory hypertrophy of Latissimus Dorsi is not rare. It is revealed on pressing downwards, e.g., on the arms of a chair.

(Courtesy of Squadron Leader David Christie.)

B **A Sternalis Muscle,** in line with Rectus Abdominis and Sternomastoid, was found in 6% of 535 cadavera (R. N. Barlow).

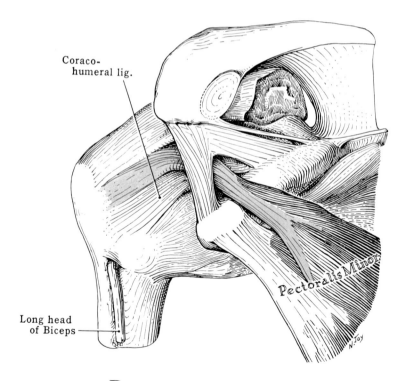

C **An Axillary Arch.** This occasional muscle crosses the base of the axilla superficially and joins Latissimus Dorsi to the tissues deep to Pectoralis Major.

D **Pectoralis Minor** inserted into Humerus; in about 15% of limbs (G. A. Seib) part of the tendon of the Minor passes over the coracoid process and between the two limbs of the coraco-acromial ligament to re-inforce the coraco-humeral ligament. See figure 26.

27 **Variations and Anomalies**

A Coracobrachialis Superior: Attrition of Biceps Tendon. Coracobrachialis is usually split by the musculocutaneous nerve into two parts, but occasionally, as here, it has a third part.

The margin of the head of the humerus is commonly hypertrophic, and the tendon of the long head of Biceps is worn through, pulled down, and loosely attached to the intertubercular sulcus, as here and in figure 28-B.

Margin of head

Musculo-cutaneous nerve

Short head of Biceps

Long head of Biceps

Coraco-brachialis

Margin of head

Long head of Biceps

B

The Biceps Brachii with a Third Head.
A third or humeral head occurs in about 5% of limbs.

Biceps

3rd head of Biceps

Brachialis

Lat. Dorsi

Brachial artery

Communicating branch from the musculo-cutaneous nerve

Ulnar artery

Biceps

Median nerve

Radial artery

C

5%   82%   13%

Developmental Explanation of the Variable Relationship of Median Nerve to Brachial Artery.

Of the two primitive brachial arteries, both persisted in 5% of 307 limbs; the posterior persisted in 82%, and the anterior in 13%. (*J.C.B.G.*)

High Division of the Brachial Artery into radial and ulnar arteries, with the median nerve passing between them. The musculocutaneous and median nerves very commonly, as here, communicate.

28   Variations and Anomalies

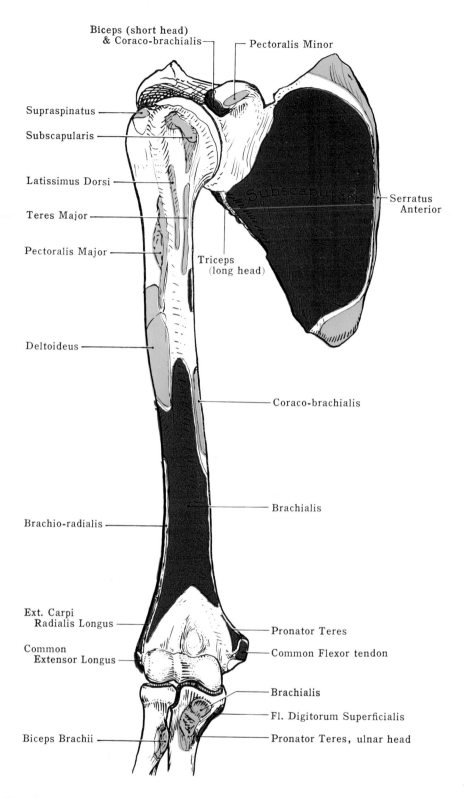

Biceps (short head) & Coraco-brachialis

Pectoralis Minor

Supraspinatus

Subscapularis

Latissimus Dorsi

Teres Major

Pectoralis Major

Triceps (long head)

Subscapularis

Serratus Anterior

Deltoideus

Coraco-brachialis

Brachialis

Brachio-radialis

Ext. Carpi Radialis Longus

Common Extensor Longus

Pronator Teres

Common Flexor tendon

Brachialis

Fl. Digitorum Superficialis

Biceps Brachii

Pronator Teres, ulnar head

29 Bones of the Upper Limb showing Attachments of Muscles, anterior view.

Origins (red), insertions (blue)

(For Bones of Forearm, anterior view, see fig. 58.)

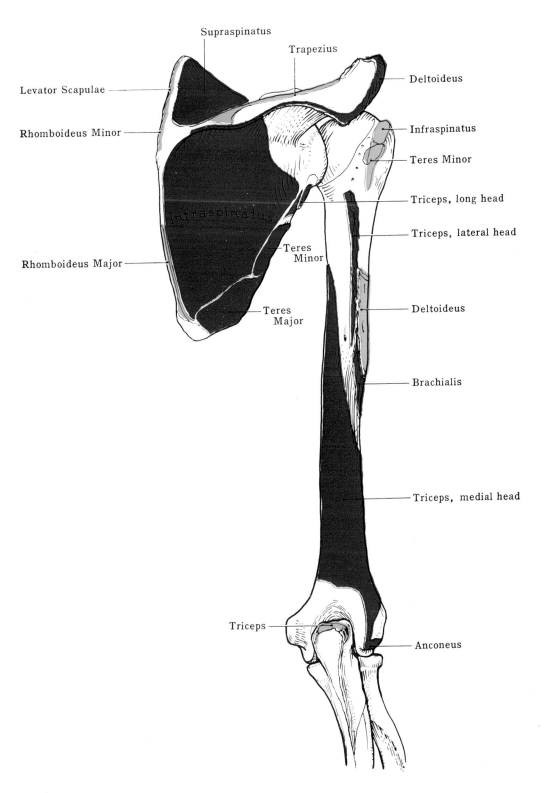

Supraspinatus

Trapezius

Deltoideus

Levator Scapulae

Infraspinatus

Rhomboideus Minor

Teres Minor

Triceps, long head

Triceps, lateral head

Infraspinatus

Teres
Minor

Rhomboideus Major

Deltoideus

Teres
Major

Brachialis

Triceps, medial head

Triceps

Anconeus

**30   Bones of the Upper Limb showing Attach-
ments of Muscles, posterior view**

(*For Bones of Forearm, posterior view, see fig. 77.*)

Deltoideus

long head

lateral head

Triceps Brachii

Biceps Brachii

Brachialis

Brachio-radialis

Lateral epicondyle

Olecranon

Extensor Carpi Radialis Longus

Fascia covering Anconeus and Common Extensor tendon

Extensor Carpi Radialis Brevis

31 Muscles of the Arm, lateral view

Note: The multipennate structure of the middle part of Deltoid, and the more parallel arrangement of the fibres of the anterior and posterior parts.

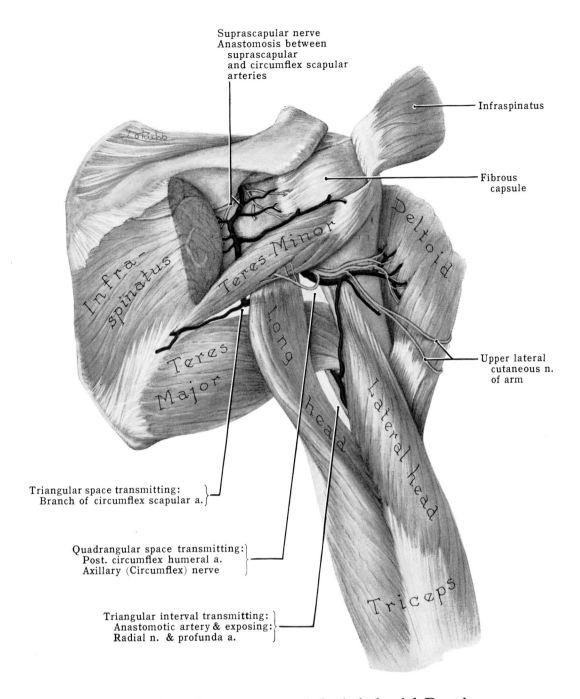

Suprascapular nerve
Anastomosis between
suprascapular
and circumflex scapular
arteries

Infraspinatus

Fibrous
capsule

Upper lateral
cutaneous n.
of arm

Triangular space transmitting:
Branch of circumflex scapular a.

Quadrangular space transmitting:
Post. circumflex humeral a.
Axillary (Circumflex) nerve

Triangular interval transmitting:
Anastomotic artery & exposing:
Radial n. & profunda a.

32 Posterior Scapular and Subdeltoid Regions

Observe:

1. The thickness of Infraspinatus, which, aided by Teres Minor and posterior fibres of Deltoid rotates the humerus laterally.

2. Long head of Triceps passing between Teres Minor (a lateral rotator) and Teres Major (a medial rotator).

3. Long head of Triceps separating the quadrangular space from the triangular space.

4. Teres Major separating the quadrangular space from another triangular space.

5. The arterial anastomoses behind the scapula and behind the Teres Major.

6. The distribution of the suprascapular and axillary nerves. Each comes from C. 5 & 6 (fig. 18); each supplies two muscles (Supraspinatus and Infraspinatus—Teres Minor and Deltoid); each supplies the shoulder joint (figs. 32 & 39); but only one has cutaneous branches.

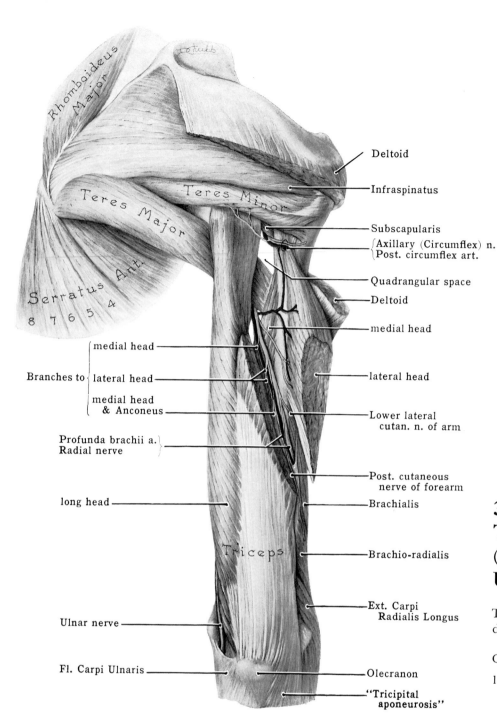

Deltoid

Infraspinatus

Subscapularis

{ Axillary (Circumflex) n.
{ Post. circumflex art.

Quadrangular space

Deltoid

medial head

lateral head

Lower lateral
cutan. n. of arm

Post. cutaneous
nerve of forearm

Brachialis

Brachio-radialis

Ext. Carpi
Radialis Longus

Olecranon

"Tricipital
aponeurosis"

Rhomboideus
Major

Teres Major

Teres Minor

Serratus Ant.

8 7 6 5 4

{ medial head

Branches to { lateral head

{ medial head
{ & Anconeus

Profunda brachii a.
Radial nerve

long head

Triceps

Ulnar nerve

Fl. Carpi Ulnaris

33 Triceps and its Three Related Nerves (Axillary, Radial, Ulnar), posterior view

The lateral head of Triceps is divided and displaced.

Observe:

1. The long and lateral heads of Triceps lying side by side behind the medial head. The radial nerve, passing in the plane between, has long and lateral heads behind it, medial head and bone in front of it.

2. The lateral head of Triceps rising to the level of Teres Minor.

3. An upward prolongation of Brachialis into the spiral groove separating the radial nerve from the insertion of Deltoid.

4. The radial nerve here supplying lateral and medial heads and Anconeus.

5. Triceps inserted into the upper aspect of the olecranon and also into deep fascia of the forearm (fig. 56).

6. Teres Major, Rhomboideus Major and Serratus Anterior mainly inserted into the inferior angle of the scapula, which is the end of a lever. The fibres of the two latter muscles are in alignment.

34 Cross-section through the Arm, below its mid-point

(The insertion of Coraco-brachialis is seen, but no Deltoid is visible nor is Brachio-radialis; consult fig. 29.)

Observe:

1. The body of the humerus, nearly circular; its cortex being thickest here.

2. The 3 heads of Triceps, in the posterior compartment of the arm, i.e., behind the medial and lateral intermuscular septa.

3. The radial nerve and its companion vessels in contact with the bone.

4. The 2 heads of Biceps, the Brachialis, and the insertion of Coraco-brachialis in the anterior compartment of the arm, i.e., in front of the medial and lateral intermuscular septa.

5. The musculocutaneous nerve and its companion vessels in the septum between Biceps and Brachialis.

6. The median nerve crossing to the medial side of the brachial artery and its venae comitantes; the ulnar nerve moving posteriorly on to the side of Triceps. The basilic vein (here as 2 vessels) has pierced the deep fascia.

7. The skin and subcutaneous tissues, thicker postero-laterally where exposed to injury than antero-medially where protected.

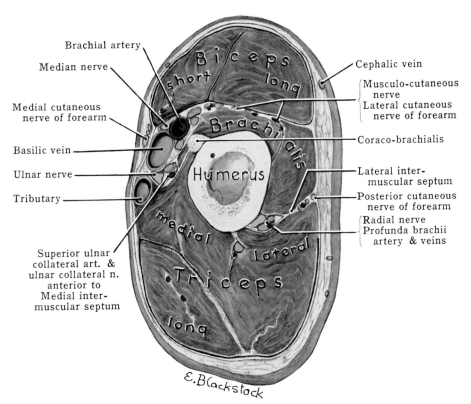

Brachial artery
Median nerve
Medial cutaneous nerve of forearm
Basilic vein
Ulnar nerve
Tributary
Superior ulnar collateral art. & ulnar collateral n. anterior to Medial intermuscular septum
Cephalic vein
Musculo-cutaneous nerve
Lateral cutaneous nerve of forearm
Coraco-brachialis
Lateral intermuscular septum
Posterior cutaneous nerve of forearm
Radial nerve
Profunda brachii artery & veins

Biceps short long
Brachialis
Humerus
medial
lateral
Triceps
long

E. Blackstock

35 Subacromial Bursa, superolateral view

(Injected with latex.)

Note:

1. The term "subacromial bursa" is usually understood to include the subdeltoid bursa, for the two bursae are usually combined.

2. Superficial to the bursa are parts of the Deltoid, acromion, and coraco-acromial ligament and the acromio-clavicular joint.

3. Deep to the bursa are the greater tubercle of the humerus and the Supraspinatus tendon (not in view).

4. The bursa may extend more widely under the acromion, and it may through attrition (fig. 42) communicate with the shoulder joint and also with the acromioclavicular joint.

5. The acromial branches of the thoraco-acromial and suprascapular arteries are seen contributing to the acromial rete (network); the branches of the circumflex artery are destroyed.

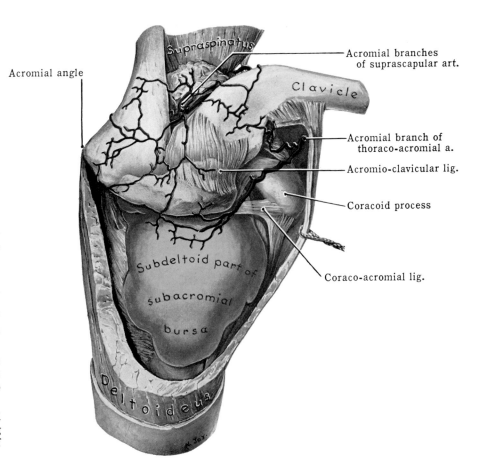

Acromial angle
Supraspinatus
Acromial branches of suprascapular art.
Clavicle
Acromial branch of thoraco-acromial a.
Acromio-clavicular lig.
Coracoid process
Subdeltoid part of subacromial bursa
Coraco-acromial lig.
Deltoideus

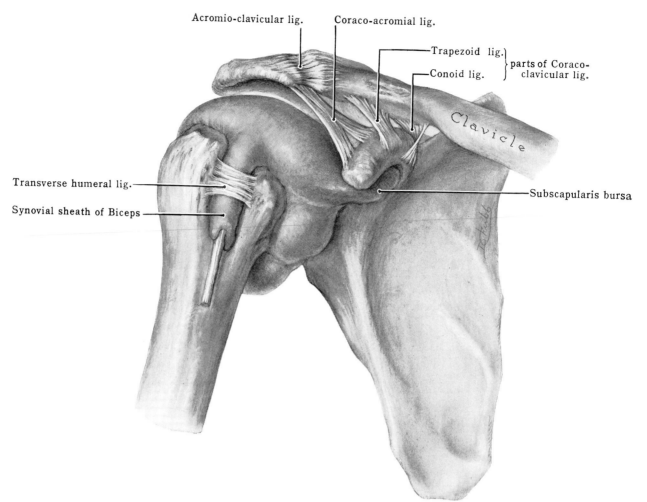

Acromio-clavicular lig. Coraco-acromial lig.

Trapezoid lig. } parts of Coraco-
Conoid lig.   } clavicular lig.

Clavicle

Transverse humeral lig.—

Synovial sheath of Biceps—

Subscapularis bursa

36   Synovial Capsule of the Shoulder Joint: Ligaments at the Lateral End of the Clavicle

Observe:

1. The capsule cannot extend on to the lesser and greater tubercles of the humerus, because the 4 short muscles (Subscapularis, Supraspinatus, Infraspinatus, and Teres Minor) are inserted there, but it can and does extend inferiorly on to the surgical neck.

2. The capsule has two prolongations: (a) where it forms a synovial sheath for the tendon of the long head of Biceps in its osseo-fibrous tunnel, and (b) below the coracoid process where it forms a bursa between Subscapularis tendon and the margin of the glenoid cavity.

3. The conoid and trapezoid ligaments are so directed that the clavicle shall hold the scapula laterally.

36.1

Demonstrating that so long as the coraco-clavicular ligament is intact, the acromion cannot be driven under the clavicle. This ligament, however, does not prevent protraction and retraction of the acromion.

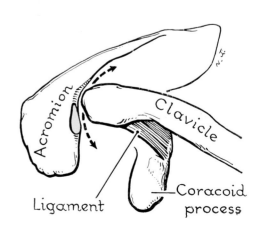

Acromion

Clavicle

Ligament

Coracoid process

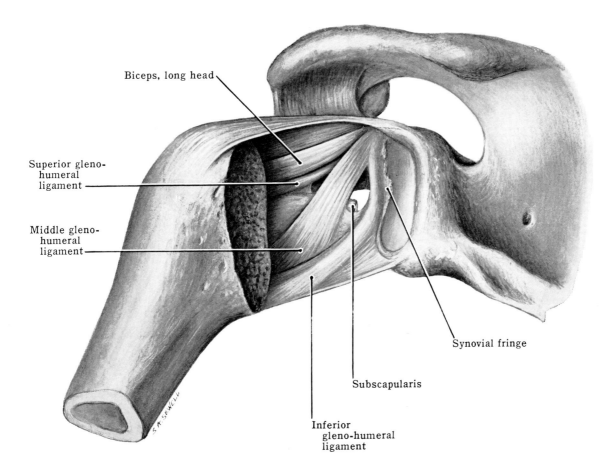

Biceps, long head

Superior gleno-
humeral
ligament

Middle gleno-
humeral
ligament

Synovial fringe

Subscapularis

Inferior
gleno-humeral
ligament

37   Interior of the Left Shoulder Joint

Exposed from behind by cutting away the posterior part of the capsule and sawing
off the head of the humerus.

Observe:

1. The 3 thickenings of the anterior part of the fibrous capsule,
   called the gleno-humeral ligaments, which are visible from
   within the joint, but not from without.

2. How these 3 ligaments and the long tendon of Biceps converge on the supraglenoid tubercle.

3. The slender superior ligament parallel to the Biceps tendon;
   the middle ligament free medially due to the fact that the
   Subscapularis bursa communicates with the joint cavity
   both above this ligament and below it; the inferior ligament
   contributing largely to the anterior lip of the glenoid
   labrum, much as the Biceps contributes to the posterior lip
   (see fig. 38).

4. The synovial fringe, constantly present, that overlies the
   anterior part of the glenoid cavity.

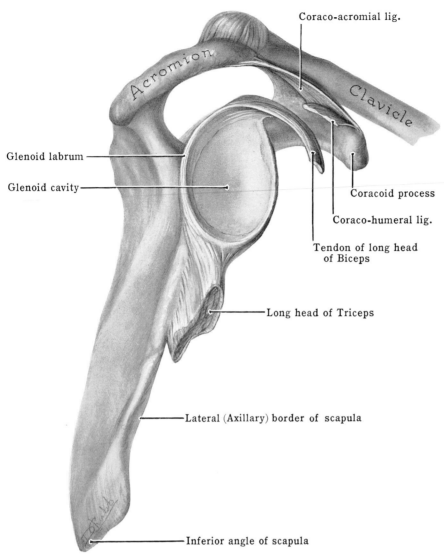

Coraco-acromial lig.

Acromion

Clavicle

Glenoid labrum

Glenoid cavity

Coracoid process

Coraco-humeral lig.

Tendon of long head
of Biceps

Long head of Triceps

Lateral (Axillary) border of scapula

Inferior angle of scapula

38 Glenoid Cavity, lateral view: Orientation of the Scapula

Observe:

1. The cavity overhung by the resilient coraco-acromial arch (i.e., coracoid process, coraco-acromial lig., and acromion), which prevents upward displacement of the head of the humerus.

2. The long head of Triceps arising just below the glenoid cavity.

3. The long head of Biceps arising just above the glenoid cavity. Proximally it is continued as the posterior lip of the glenoid labrum; distally it curves across the front of the head of the humerus—not above it.

4. The orientation of the scapula insures that should the head of the humerus be dislocated downwards it would pass on to the costal surface of the scapula.

Supra-spinatus

Acromion   Deltoid

Bursa

2"

N.T.

Teres Major

Triceps (long)

Quadrangular space

38.1 Diagram of the shoulder region, on coronal section, showing the relations of the subacromial bursa.

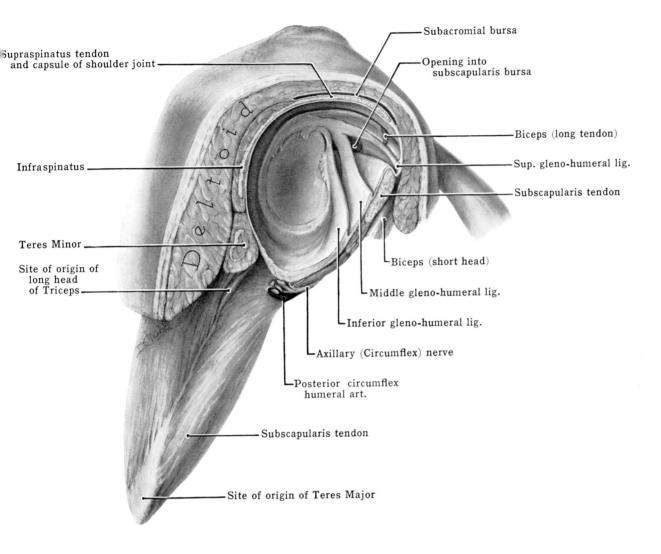

Supraspinatus tendon
and capsule of shoulder joint

Subacromial bursa

Opening into
subscapularis bursa

Biceps (long tendon)

Sup. gleno-humeral lig.

Subscapularis tendon

Infraspinatus

Teres Minor

Site of origin of
long head
of Triceps

Deltoid

Biceps (short head)

Middle gleno-humeral lig.

Inferior gleno-humeral lig.

Axillary (Circumflex) nerve

Posterior circumflex
humeral art.

Subscapularis tendon

Site of origin of Teres Major

39 Glenoid Cavity and the Relations of the Shoulder Joint, side view

Observe:

1. The fibrous capsule of the joint thickened in front by the three gleno-humeral ligaments which converge from the humerus to be attached with the long tendon of Biceps to the supraglenoid tubercle.

2. Four short muscles (Teres Minor, Infraspinatus, Supraspinatus, and Subscapularis) crossing the joint, blending with the capsule, and retaining the head of the humerus in its socket.

3. The subacromial bursa between the acromion and Deltoid above and the tendon of Supraspinatus below.

4. In contact with the capsule inferiorly, the axillary nerve and the posterior circumflex humeral artery. The nerve giving a twig to the capsule.

5. The Subscapularis bursa (of fig. 36) opening above and below the middle gleno-humeral ligament. Several synovial folds overlapping the glenoid cavity.

40   Unfused Acromial Epiphysis

In 16 of 194 dissecting room subjects ag[ed] over thirty years, the acromial epiphysis h[ad] failed to fuse. The epiphyseal line was transve[rse] and passed either through or just behind t[he] clavicular facet. The condition was bilateral in [5] subjects (10 limbs) and unilateral in 11 subje[cts] (7 being on the right side only and 4 on the l[eft] only). (*J.C.B.G.*)

41   Circumflex and Profunda Arteries

Four types of variations in origin of t[he] posterior humeral circumflex and profund[a] brachii arteries; in 2.9% the arteries we[re] otherwise irregular. Percentages are based o[n] 235 specimens. (*J.C.B.G.*)

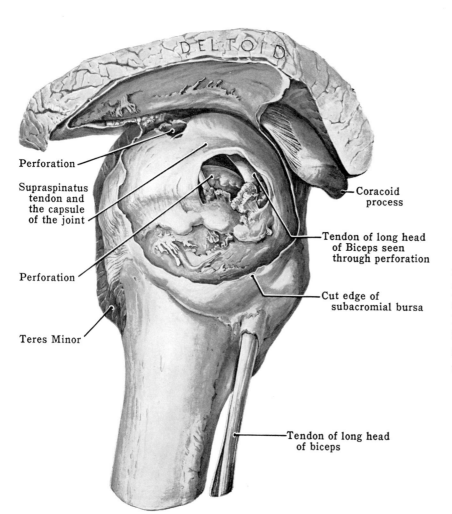

Perforation

Supraspinatus tendon and the capsule of the joint

Perforation

Teres Minor

Coracoid process

Tendon of long head of Biceps seen through perforation

Cut edge of subacromial bursa

Tendon of long head of biceps

42   Attrition of the Supraspinatus Tendon

As a result of wearing away of the Supr[a]spinatus tendon and underlying capsule, t[he] subacromial bursa and the shoulder joint co[me] into wide-open communication. The intraca[p]sular part of the long tendon of the Biceps b[e]comes frayed—even worn away—leaving [it] adherent to the intertubercular sulcus, as [in] figures 28, A and D.

Of 95 dissecting room subjects of proved ag[e] none of the 18 under fifty years of age had [a] perforation, but 4 of the 19 between fifty an[d] sixty years, and 23 of the 57 over sixty yea[rs] had perforations. The perforation was bilater[al] in 11 subjects (22 limbs) and unilateral in 1[4] subjects (8 being on the right side only and 6 o[n] the left only). (*J.C.B.G.* and *C.G.S.*)

VARIATIONS

43 Variations in the Anterior Part of the Shoulder Joint, in older subjects

(PREPARATIONS BY DR. ROSS G. MACKENZIE.)

Observe:

I. The tendon of Subscapularis almost alone guarding the front of the shoulder joint. The middle gleno-humeral ligament in miniature and blending with the inferior glenohumeral ligament to form the anterior part of the glenoid labrum. These two ligaments making individual contributions to the thickness of the fibrous capsule. A large pouch-like subscapularis bursa, above Subscapularis and covering the root of the coracoid process.

II. The middle glenohumeral ligament broad, with free borders, and with its apex converging on the supraglenoid tubercle, largely concealing the tendon of Subscapularis. These two guarding the front of the joint. The inferior ligament forming only the lower half of the anterior part of the labrum; there is here no upper half.

III. The tendon of Subscapularis very thick. The middle and inferior glenohumeral ligaments poorly developed and contributing little to the thickness of the fibrous capsule. The joint cavity extending between the upper part of the margin of the glenoid cavity and the glenoid labrum with the result that the labrum is loosely suspended by a "synovial mesentery".

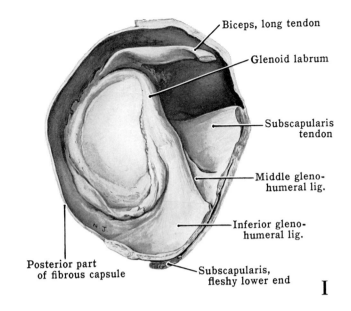

Biceps, long tendon

Glenoid labrum

Subscapularis tendon

Middle gleno-humeral lig.

Inferior gleno-humeral lig.

Posterior part of fibrous capsule

Subscapularis, fleshy lower end

I

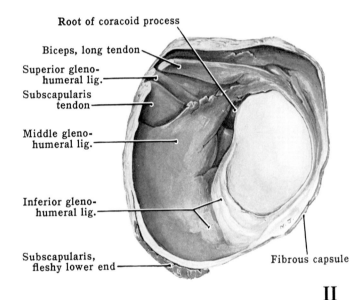

Root of coracoid process

Biceps, long tendon

Superior gleno-humeral lig.

Subscapularis tendon

Middle gleno-humeral lig.

Inferior gleno-humeral lig.

Subscapularis, fleshy lower end

Fibrous capsule

II

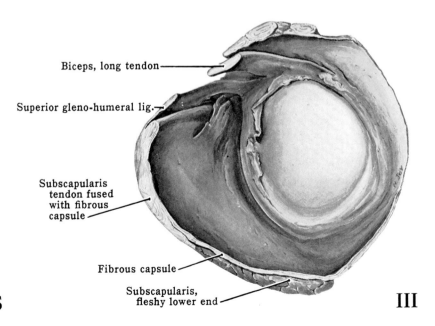

Biceps, long tendon

Superior gleno-humeral lig.

Subscapularis tendon fused with fibrous capsule

Fibrous capsule

Subscapularis, fleshy lower end

III

VARIATIONS

Cephalic vein

Lateral
cutaneous nerve
of forearm

Median vein
of forearm

Cephalic vein

Medial
cutaneous nerve
of forearm

Basilic vein

Cubital lymph node

Medial cubital vein

Basilic vein

Perforating vein

Bicipital aponeurosis
(Lacertus fibrosus)

44 Superficial Structures at the Front of the Elbow

Observe:

1. In the forearm, the superficial veins—cephalic, median, basilic and their connecting channels—making a (variable) M-shaped pattern.

2. The median cubital vein separated from the brachial artery only by the bicipital aponeurosis.

3. A perforating vein, lateral to the bicipital aponeurosis, connecting the deep veins to the median cubital vein.

4. In the arm, the cephalic and basilic veins occupying the bicipital furrows.

5. In the lateral bicipital furrow, the lateral cutaneous nerve of the forearm becoming cutaneous 1″ to 2″ above the elbow-crease.

6. In the medial bicipital furrow, the medial cutaneous nerve of the forearm becoming cutaneous at the mid point of the arm.

7. Cutaneous nerves mainly on a deeper plane than superficial veins.

8. The most distal superficial lymph node of the upper limb lying about 1″ above the medial epicondyle.

Superficial fascia

Deep fascia

Muscle fascia

Biceps

Brachialis

Lat. cutan. nerve
of forearm

Brachio-radialis

Branch of superior
ulnar collateral a.

Inf. ulnar collateral a.
(Supratrochlear a.)

Brachial artery and
venae comitantes

Median nerve

Flexors

Large perforating
or communicating vein

Bicipital aponeurosis

45 Cubital Fossa

The cubital fossa is the triangular space below the elbow crease. It is bounded laterally by the extensor muscles (represented by Brachio-radialis) and medially by the flexor muscles (represented by Pronator Teres). The apex is where these two muscles meet below.

Observe:

1. The large perforating vein piercing the deep fascia at the apex of the fossa.
2. The 3 chief contents—Biceps tendon, brachial artery, and median nerve.
3. Biceps tendon rotating through a right angle, and the bicipital aponeurosis springing from the tendon.

Musculo-cutaneous n.

Radial nerve

Brachio-radialis

Extensor Carpi
Radialis Longus

Post. interosseous n.
(Deep br. of radial n.)
Radial recurrent art.

Extensor Carpi
Radialis Brevis

Superficial branch
of radial nerve

Radial artery

Biceps

Brachialis

Supinator

Medial
intermuscular septum

Inferior
ulnar collateral art.

Ulnar nerve

Biceps tendon
Brachial artery
Median nerve

Pronator Teres

Ulnar artery

Deep head of
Pronator Teres

Fl. Carpi Radialis

46 Deeper Structures at the Front of the Elbow

Part of Biceps is excised and the cubital fossa is opened widely.

Observe:

1. The floor of the cubital fossa—Brachialis and Supinator.
2. The brachial artery lying between Biceps tendon and median nerve, and dividing into 2 nearly equal branches—the ulnar and radial arteries.
3. The median nerve supplying flexor muscles; hence its motor branches arising from its medial side,—the twig to the deep head of Pronator Teres excepted.

4. The radial nerve supplying extensor muscles; hence its motor branches arising from its lateral side,—the twig to Brachialis excepted. [The radial nerve has been displaced laterally, so its lateral branches appear in the drawing to run medially.]
5. The posterior interosseous nerve piercing Supinator.

Biceps

Ulnar nerve
Sup. ulnar
collateral a.

Supracondylar
process

Median nerve
Inf. ulnar
collateral a.

A

Pronator
Teres

N.J.

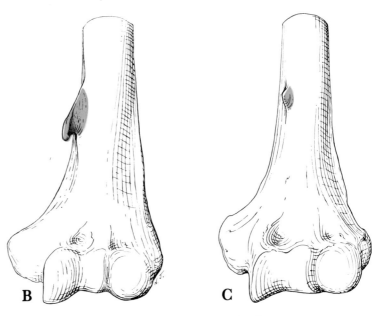

B   C

47   Supracondylar Process of the Humerus

A and B are from opposite sides of the same subject. C is a left-sided specimen. A fibrous band joins this process or spine to the medial epicondyle. Through the foramen so-formed the median nerve passes, as here, and the brachial artery may go with it. A process was found in 7 of 1000 living subjects (R. J. Terry).

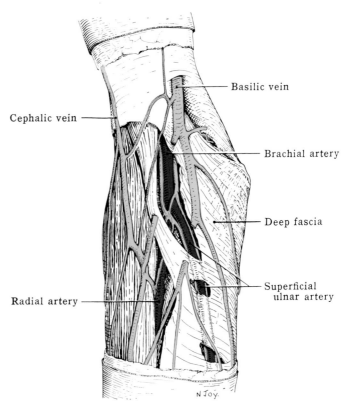

Cephalic vein

Basilic vein

Brachial artery

Deep fascia

Superficial
ulnar artery

Radial artery

N Joy.

N.J.

48   Supratrochlear Foramen

This hole, closed in life by membrane, was found in 4.2% of white people and 12.8% of American Negroes. It was more common on the left side than on the right, and in females than in males. (M. Trotter.)

48.1   Superficial Ulnar Artery

The ulnar artery descended superficial to the flexor muscles in 3.1% of 188 dissected limbs (paired) and in 2.7% of 542 students' limbs (paired). Of these 21 superficial arteries found in 730 limbs, 3 were present bilaterally, 8 in the right limb only, and 7 in the left only. (J. W. Hazlett.)

VARIATIONS AND ANOMALIES

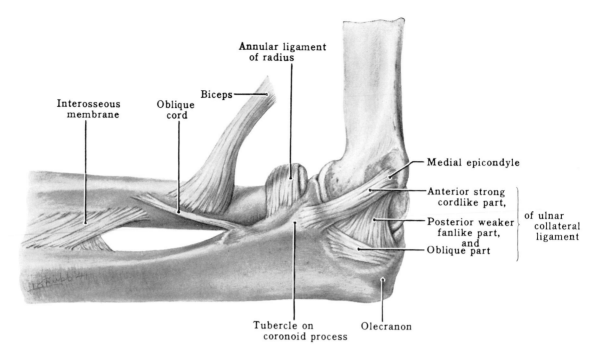

Interosseous membrane — Oblique cord — Biceps — Annular ligament of radius — Medial epicondyle — Anterior strong cordlike part, — Posterior weaker fanlike part, and Oblique part — of ulnar collateral ligament — Tubercle on coronoid process — Olecranon

49 Ulnar Collateral Ligament of the Elbow Joint (Medial Lig.)

The anterior part is a strong, round cord, taut in extension of the joint; the posterior part is a weak fan, taut in flexion of the joint; the oblique fibres merely deepen the socket for the trochlea of the humerus. Fl. Digitorum Superficialis arises from the cord and from an area of bone at each end of the cord; it also arises from the anterior oblique line of the radius.

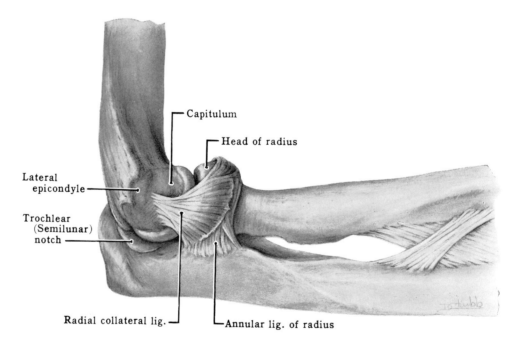

Capitulum — Head of radius — Lateral epicondyle — Trochlear (Semilunar) notch — Radial collateral lig. — Annular lig. of radius

50 Radial Collateral Ligament of the Elbow Joint (Lateral Lig.)

The fan-shaped lateral ligament is attached to the annular ligament, but its superficial fibres are continued onwards to the radius as Supinator—hence the ragged edge. Supinator also arises from the annular ligament and the supinator crest of the ulna, which limits the supinator fossa posteriorly.

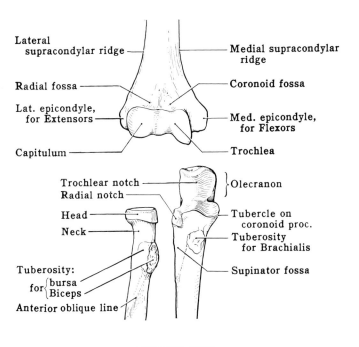

Lateral supracondylar ridge

Medial supracondylar ridge

Radial fossa

Coronoid fossa

Lat. epicondyle, for Extensors

Med. epicondyle, for Flexors

Capitulum

Trochlea

Trochlear notch

Radial notch

Olecranon

Head

Neck

Tubercle on coronoid proc.

Tuberosity for Brachialis

Supinator fossa

Tuberosity: for { bursa Biceps

Anterior oblique line

ANTERIOR VIEW

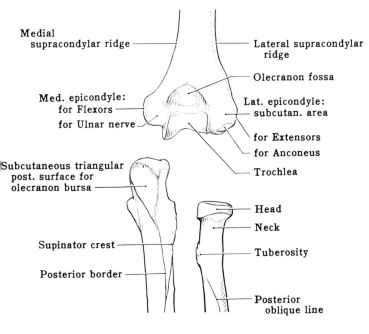

Medial supracondylar ridge

Lateral supracondylar ridge

Olecranon fossa

Med. epicondyle: for Flexors for Ulnar nerve

Lat. epicondyle: subcutan. area

for Extensors

for Anconeus

Trochlea

Subcutaneous triangular post. surface for olecranon bursa

Head

Neck

Supinator crest

Tuberosity

Posterior border

Posterior oblique line

POSTERIOR VIEW

51 Bones of the Elbow Region

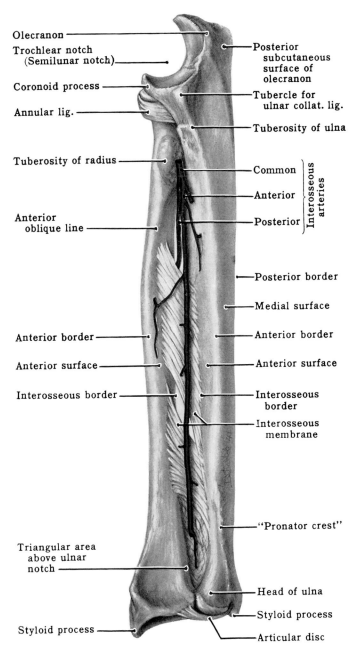

Olecranon

Trochlear notch (Semilunar notch)

Coronoid process

Annular lig.

Tuberosity of radius

Anterior oblique line

Anterior border

Anterior surface

Interosseous border

Triangular area above ulnar notch

Styloid process

Posterior subcutaneous surface of olecranon

Tubercle for ulnar collat. lig.

Tuberosity of ulna

Common

Anterior

Posterior

} Interosseous arteries

Posterior border

Medial surface

Anterior border

Anterior surface

Interosseous border

Interosseous membrane

"Pronator crest"

Head of ulna

Styloid process

Articular disc

52 Flexor Aspect of Radius and Ulna: Ligaments of the Radio-ulnar Joints: Interosseous Arteries

The ligament of the proximal radio-ulnar joint is the annular ligament; that of the distal joint is the articular disc; that of the middle joint is the interosseous membrane. The general direction of the fibres of the membrane is such that an upward thrust of the hand, and therefore received by the radius, is transmitted to the ulna. The membrane is attached to the interosseous borders of the radius and ulna, but it also spreads on to their surfaces.

Non-articular area overlaid with synovial pad of fat

Radial notch of ulna

Radial collateral lig.

Synovial fold

Annular ligament of radius

Olecranon

Synovial pad of fat

Oblique part of ulnar collateral lig.

Coronoid process

53 Socket for Head of Radius and Trochlea of Humerus, from above

The annular ligament keeps the head of the radius applied to the radial notch of the ulna, and with it forms a cup-shaped socket (i.e. wide above, narrow below); hence the head of the radius cannot be pulled distally through its socket. The annular ligament is bound to the humerus by the radial collateral ligament of the elbow, and a crescentic synovial fold occupies the angular space between the head of the radius and the capitulum of the humerus. Similarly, synovial folds containing fat occupy the 2 angular non-articular areas between the coronoid process and the olecranon.

Humerus

Annular lig.

Sacciform recess

Radius

Ulna

54 Articular Cavity of the Elbow and Proximal Radio-ulnar Joints, Injected with Wax, anterior view

The cavity was distended with wax. The fibrous capsule has been removed; the synovial capsule remains.

The sacciform recess that encircles the neck of the radius serves a similar function to a similar recess at the distal radio-ulnar joint (fig. 90).

(For posterior view see fig. 57.)

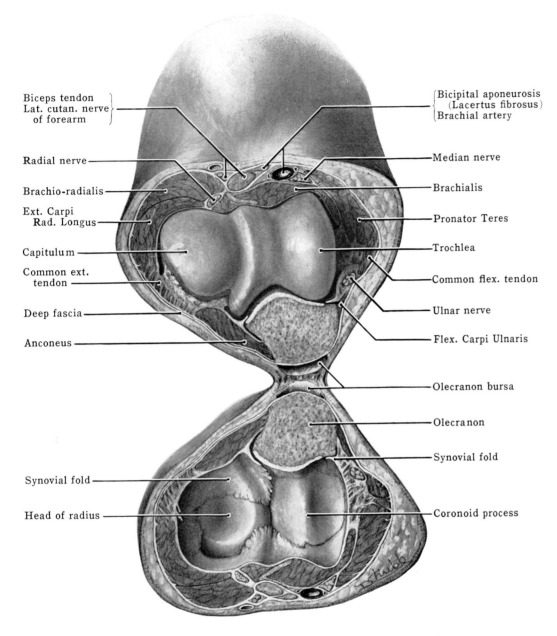

Biceps tendon
Lat. cutan. nerve
of forearm

Bicipital aponeurosis
(Lacertus fibrosus)
Brachial artery

Radial nerve

Brachio-radialis

Ext. Carpi
Rad. Longus

Capitulum

Common ext.
tendon

Deep fascia

Anconeus

Median nerve

Brachialis

Pronator Teres

Trochlea

Common flex. tendon

Ulnar nerve

Flex. Carpi Ulnaris

Olecranon bursa

Olecranon

Synovial fold

Coronoid process

Synovial fold

Head of radius

55   Cross Section through the Elbow Joint

Nerves:—The radial nerve is in direct contact with the capsule of the joint; the ulnar nerve is in contact with the ulnar collateral ligament; the median nerve is separated from the capsule by a film of fleshy fibres of Brachialis.

Synovial folds, containing fat, overlie the periphery of the head of the radius and also the non-articular indentations on the trochlear notch of the ulna.

A fracture across the olecranon brings the subcutaneous olecranon bursa into communication with the articular cavity.

Triceps

Medial epicondyle

Ulnar nerve

Posterior ulnar
recurrent a.

Olecranon

Fl. Carpi Ulnaris

Brachio-radialis

Extensor Carpi
Radialis Longus

Lateral epicondyle

Common
extensor tendon

Anconeus

Tricipital
aponeurosis
(Fascia covering
Anconeus)

56 Elbow, from behind—I

The "tricipital aponeurosis" is cut and lifted up to expose Anconeus.

Observe:

1. Triceps inserted not only into the upper surface of the olecranon but also, via the deep fascia covering Anconeus—"tricipital aponeurosis"—into the lateral border of the olecranon.

2. The subcutaneous and palpable posterior surfaces of—the medial epicondyle, lateral epicondyle, and olecranon.

3. The ulnar nerve, also palpable, running subfascially behind the medial epicondyle. Distal to this point it disappears deep to the two heads of Fl. Carpi Ulnaris.

4. The two heads of Fl. Carpi Ulnaris: one arising from the common flexor tendon, the other from the medial border of the olecranon and posterior border of the shaft of the ulna.

5. The continuous linear origin from the humerus of the superficial extensor muscles. These are Brachio-radialis, Ext. Carpi Radialis Longus, common extensor tendon and, Anconeus.

Medial intermuscular septum

Lateral intermuscular septum

Ulnar nerve

Anconeus

Ext. Carpi Ulnaris

Ulnar collateral lig. (Medial lig.)

Fl. Digitorum Superficialis

Annular ligament

Post. ulnar recurrent art.

Interosseous recurrent art.

Fl. Digitorum Profundus

Anconeus

Fl. Carpi Ulnaris

Supinator

Post. interosseous nerve

Ext. Carpi Ulnaris

57 Elbow, from behind—II

The lower portion of Triceps is removed. The upper portion, seen on cross section, is somewhat flattened because the subject had been lying on its back.

Observe:

1. The ulnar nerve descending first, within the posterior compartment of the arm, applied to the medial head of Triceps, and behind the medial intermuscular septum and medial epicondyle; secondly, applied to the medial ligament of the joint; lastly, between Fl. Carpi Ulnaris and Fl. Digitorum Profundus.

2. The first branches of the ulnar nerve distributed to Fl. Carpi Ulnaris, half of Profundus, and the joint.

3. Laterally, the synovial membrane protruding below the annular ligament as a sacciform recess. The joint is here covered with Anconeus and the common extensor tendon, including Ext. Carpi Ulnaris.

4. The posterior interosseous nerve appearing through Supinator 2½″ below the head of the radius.

Brachio-radialis

Ext. Carpi Radialis Longus

Common Extensor tendon

Pronator Teres

Common Flexor tendon

Fl. Digitorum Superficialis

Brachialis

Pronator Teres, ulnar head

Biceps Brachii

Supinator

Fl. Digitorum Superficialis

Pronator Teres

Fl. Pollicis Longus

Fl. Digitorum Profundus

Pronator Quadratus

Pronator Quadratus

Brachio-radialis

Add. Poll. Obliquus

Fl. Carpi Ulnaris
Abd. Digiti V

Fl. Carpi Radialis

Piso-hamate lig.
Piso-metacarpal lig.

Abd. Poll. Longus

Opponens Pollicis

Ext. Carpi Ulnaris

Fl.
Abd. }Poll. Brevis

Opponens

Adductor Pollicis

Digiti V

Fl. Poll. Longus

Abductor
Fl. Brevis

Add. Poll. Trans.

Interossei

Fl. Digit. Superfic.

Fl. Digitorum Profundus

58 Bones of the Forearm and Hand showing Attachment of Muscles, anterior view

Note that the origins of the Palmar Interossei are indicated by the letters P,P,P, the origins of the 4 Dorsal Interossei by colour only the origins of the 3 Thenar and 2 the Hypothenar muscles are omitt (*For posterior view, see fig. 77. F humerus, see figs. 29 & 30.*)

Superficial Mus-
...s on the Front of
...e Forearm: Palmar
...oneurosis

...rve:

...t the elbow, the brachial artery ly-
...g between Biceps tendon and median
...rve, and there bifurcating into the
...dial and ulnar arteries.

...t the wrist, the radial artery lateral
... Fl. Carpi Radialis tendon and the
...lnar artery lateral to Fl. Carpi Ul-
...aris tendon.

...n the forearm, the radial artery lying
...etween two muscle groups or two
...otor territories. The muscles lateral
... the artery are supplied by the radial
...erve; those medial to it, by the me-
...ian and ulnar nerves: so, no motor
...erve crosses the radial artery.

...he lateral group of muscles, repre-
...nted by Brachio-radialis, slightly
...verlapping the radial artery which
...therwise is superficial.

...he medial or flexor group of muscles
...in three layers: superficial (shown
...ere), middle, and deep.

...he four superficial muscles, viz.,
...ronator Teres, Fl. Carpi Radialis,
...almaris Longus and Fl. Carpi Ul-
...aris, radiating from the medial epi-
...ondyle. The muscle of the middle
...yer Fl. Digitorum Superficialis, is
...artially in view.

...almaris Longus continued into the
...alm as the palmar aponeurosis, which
...ceives an accession of fibres from the
...exor retinaculum and divides into 4
...ngitudinal bands, one for each fin-
...er. These bands are crossed on their
...eep surface by transverse fibres.

...almaris Brevis arising from this apo-
...eurosis.

Biceps — Brachialis
Brachialis — Brachial artery / Median nerve
Musculo-cutaneous n. — Pronator Teres
Bicipital aponeurosis
Radial artery — Fl. Carpi Radialis
Brachio-radialis — Palmaris Longus
Radial artery — Flexor Carpi Ulnaris
Superficial br. of radial nerve — Fl. Digitorum Sublimis or Superficialis
Flexor Pollicis Longus — Median nerve
Pronator Quadratus — Ulnar art. & nerve
Abd. Pollicis Longus — Palmaris Brevis
Superficial palmar branch — Palmar aponeurosis
Palmar digital arteries & nerves
Superficial transverse ligament of palm

Biceps
Brachial artery
Median nerve

Ulnar nerve
Triceps
Medial intermuscular septum

Pronator Teres

Fl. Carpi Radialis

Brachio-radialis

Brachialis

Radial nerve:
superficial br.

post. interosseous
(deep br.)

Radial recurrent a.

Nerves to:
Fl. Carpi Ulnaris &
Fl. Digit. Profundus

Supinator

Pronator Teres

Fl. Carpi Ulnaris

Radial artery

Ulnar n. & art.

Fl. Digit. (Sublimis)
Superficialis,
radial head

Fl. Digit. Profundus

Fl. Pollicis Longus

Pronator Quadratus

Pronator Quadratus

Dorsal (cutaneous) br.

Dorsal carpal. br.

Palmar carpal br.

Fl. Digit. Profundus

Superf. palmar br.
Palmar radio-
carpal lig.

Persisting median a.
Median nerve

Fl. Carpi
Radialis

Palmaris Longus

Sublimis

60 Flexor Digitorum Superficialis (Sublimis) and Related Structures

Observe:

1. The oblique origin of Superficialis from—(a) the medial epicondyle of the humerus, (b) the ulnar collateral ligament of the elbow, (c) the tubercle of the coronoid process, (d) the anterior oblique line of the radius and perhaps the anterior border below it.

2. Superficialis, which like the 3 muscles in front of it and the $2\frac{1}{2}$ muscles behind it, is supplied by the median nerve.

3. The muscles lateral to Superficialis supplied by the radial nerve.

4. The $1\frac{1}{2}$ muscles medial to Superficialis, supplied by the ulnar nerve.

5. The sequence of muscles crossed by the radial artery. At the wrist the artery crosses the radius and the palmar radio-carpal lig.

6. The radial artery having muscular and 3 anastomotic branches (recurrent, palmar carpal, and superficial palmar). Neither muscle nor motor nerve crosses the artery, but Brachio-radialis overlaps it.

7. The ulnar artery descending obliquely behind Superficialis to join the ulnar nerve.

8. The ulnar nerve descending vertically near the medial border of Superficialis and exposed by splitting the septum between Superficialis and Fl. Carpi Ulnaris.

9. The median nerve descending vertically behind Superficialis, clinging to it, and appearing at its lateral border.

10. The digital tendons at the wrist—3 and 4 large and side by side, 5 slender and 2 behind (fig. 64).

11. The median artery, here persisting.

61 Deep Flexors of the Digits and the Related Structures

Observe:

1. The two deep, digital flexor muscles, viz., Fl. Pollicis Longus and Fl. Digitorum Profundus, forming a sheet of muscle that arises from the flexor aspects of the radius, interosseous membrane, and ulna between the origin of Superficialis proximally and Pronator Quadratus distally.

2. The portion of Profundus for the index, here free above the wrist; the portions for digits III, IV, and V, fused.

3. The median nerve crossing in front of the ulnar artery at the elbow and behind the flexor retinaculum at the wrist.

4. The ulnar nerve entering the forearm behind the medial epicondyle, descending on Profundus, joined by the ulnar artery, continuing on Profundus to the wrist, and there passing in front of the flexor retinaculum. At the elbow it supplies Fl. Carpi Ulnaris and ½ Profundus; above the wrist it gives off its dorsal branch.

5. The recurrent, common interosseous, and dorsal carpal branches as well as muscular branches of the ulnar artery.

6. The 4 Lumbricals arising from Profundus tendons, seen better in figure 68.

Brachio-radialis
Radial recurrent a.

Radial nerve { Post. inteross. br.
Superficial br.

Ext. Carpi Rad. Longus
Ext. Carpi Rad. Brevis

Supinator

Pronator Teres

Fl. Digitorum Superficialis, (radial head, cut)

Fl. Pollicis Longus

Radial artery

Pronator Quadratus

Radius

Palmar radio-carpal lig.

Flexor retinaculum

Opponens Pollicis

Fl. Pollicis Brevis

Abd. Pollicis Brevis

Brachialis

Biceps tendon
Brachial artery
Median nerve

Fl. Digitorum Superficialis

Anterior interosseous n.

Post. ulnar recurrent a.
Ant. interosseous a.

Fl. Carpi Ulnaris

Ulnar art. & nerve

III, IV, V
Indicis } Flexor Digitorum Profundus

Dorsal (cutan.) branch of ulnar nerve

Dorsal carpal branch of ulnar artery

Median nerve

Deep branch of ulnar nerve & artery

Opponens Digiti V

Abductor Digiti V

L1 L2 L3 L4

- Rough for finger-pad
- for Fl. Digit. Profundus
- for { Fibrous sheath
      { Fl. Digit. Superfic.
- for Fibrous sheath

Distal end
Head (Trochlea)
Head (Trochlea)
Head
Tubercle

Trapezoid

Hook of hamate
Pisiform
Triquetrum
Lunate
Tubercle (Crest) of trapezium (gtr. multangular)
Tubercle of scaphoid (navicular)

62 Bones of the Hand, palmar aspect

(See also fig. 95.)

(For dorsal aspect, see fig. 86.)

62.1 Muscles attached to the Anterior Aspect of the Radius and Ulna

Observe:

1. The anterior aspect of the ulna clothed with (a) Brachialis, which is inserted into the coronoid process, and distal to this with (b) Fl. Digitorum Profundus, which arises as far distally as Pronator Quadratus. Profundus also arising from the upper $\frac{2}{3}$ of the medial aspect and with Fl. Carpi Ulnaris arising from the deep fascia.

2. The anterior aspect of the radius clothed with (a) Supinator above the anterior oblique line and, distal to this, with (b) Fl. Pollicis Longus as far as Pronator Quadratus. Fl. Digitorum Superficialis, here removed, arises from the oblique line.

3. The 5 tendons of the deep digital flexors, side by side, converging on the carpal tunnel, and, having traversed it, diverging to the 5 terminal phalanges.

4. Biceps inserted into the medial aspect of radius, hence it can rotate laterally, i.e., supinate; whereas Pronator Teres by invading the lateral surface can rotate medially, i.e., pronate.

Radial nerve
Layer of fat
Brachialis
Post. inteross. n.
Superficial br.
Supinator
Ant. oblique line of radius
Pronator Teres
Flexor Pollicis Longus
Brachioradialis
Pronator Quadratus
Radial art.
Abd. Pollicis Longus
Flexor retinaculum
Opponens Pollicis

Biceps Brachii & burs
Ulnar ne
Anterior interos
Common interos
Anterior interos nerve
Flexor Carp Ulnaris
Flexor Digitorum Profundus
Median nerve
Pisiform bone
Ulnar nerve & a.
Abductor Digiti V
Opponens Digiti V

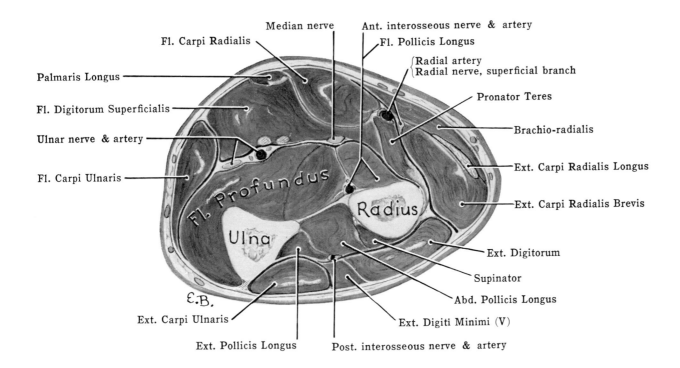

Median nerve

Fl. Carpi Radialis

Ant. interosseous nerve & artery

Fl. Pollicis Longus

Palmaris Longus

Radial artery
Radial nerve, superficial branch

Fl. Digitorum Superficialis

Pronator Teres

Ulnar nerve & artery

Brachio-radialis

Fl. Carpi Ulnaris

Ext. Carpi Radialis Longus

Ext. Carpi Radialis Brevis

Fl. Profundus

Radius

Ulna

Ext. Digitorum

Supinator

E.B.

Abd. Pollicis Longus

Ext. Carpi Ulnaris

Ext. Digiti Minimi (V)

Ext. Pollicis Longus

Post. interosseous nerve & artery

63 Cross-section through the middle of the Forearm (at level of insertion of the Pronator Teres)

Observe:

1. The interosseous membrane stretching from the interosseous (lateral) border of the ulna to a fibro-cartilaginous labrum along the interosseous (medial) border of the radius and spreading far on to the surface anterior (fig. 52) and less far on to the posterior surface of the radius.

2. The ulnar nerve and artery and the median nerve lying in the areolar septum between the superficial and deep digital flexors, i.e., between Fl. Digitorum Superficialis and and Flexores Digitorum Profundus et Pollicis Longus. The ulnar nerve, as usual, clinging to Profundus and supplying its medial part; the median nerve clinging to Superficialis and supplying it. The anterior interosseous branch of the median nerve, placed on the skeletal plane.

3. The radial artery overlapped by Brachio-radialis.

4. The superficial branch of the radial nerve following the anterior border of Extensor Carpi Radialis Brevis; the posterior interosseous nerve lying between the superficial and deep layers of digital extensors.

5. Flexores Digitorum Profundus et Pollicis Longus wrapped around the medial and anterior surfaces of the ulna and the anterior surface of the radius—this being Flexor Territory. Pronator Teres inserted into the lateral surface of the radius—and therefore invading Extensor Territory; hence its ability to pronate.

6. Artificial Spaces, readily created: (a) The space deep to Flexor Carpi Ulnaris extending dorsally to where Fl. Carpi Ulnaris and Fl. Profundus both arise from the deep fascia and through it from the posterior border of the ulna. (b) The space deep to Ext. Carpi Ulnaris. This mucle arises slightly from the deep fascia and through it from the posterior border of the ulna. (c) The space between the superficial and deep digital flexors, noted in item 2, above. (d) The space between the long extensors of the fingers and the deep muscles of the back of the forearm. (e) The space deep to the three lateral muscles of the forearm (Brachio-radialis, Ext. Carpi Radialis Longus et Brevis).

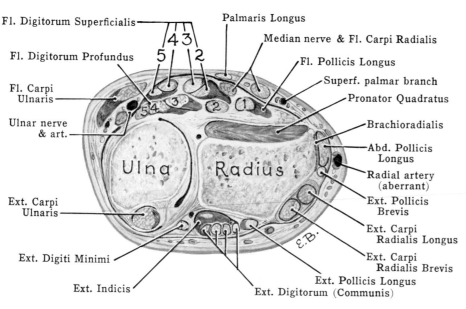

Labels on figure 64 (clockwise):
Fl. Digitorum Superficialis — 4 3
5
Fl. Digitorum Profundus
Fl. Carpi Ulnaris
Ulnar nerve & art.
Ext. Carpi Ulnaris
Ext. Digiti Minimi
Ext. Indicis
Palmaris Longus
Median nerve & Fl. Carpi Radialis
Fl. Pollicis Longus
Superf. palmar branch
Pronator Quadratus
Brachioradialis
Abd. Pollicis Longus
Radial artery (aberrant)
Ext. Pollicis Brevis
Ext. Carpi Radialis Longus
Ext. Carpi Radialis Brevis
Ext. Pollicis Longus
Ext. Digitorum (Communis)
Ulna   Radius
E.B.

64 Cross-section through the Forearm, above the wrist

Observe:

1. The synovial cavity of the distal ra ulnar joint.

2. Fl. Carpi Radialis, Palmaris Lon and Fl. Carpi Ulnaris constituting a face layer of flexors of the wrist.

3. Deep to these, the long flexors of digits: (a) The 4 tendons of Fl. Digito Superficialis lying two deep, those to middle and ring fingers being ant to those to the index and little fin (b) The 5 tendons of the deep di flexors, lying side by side, those to thumb (Fl. Pollicis Longus) and in being free.

4. The ulnar nerve and artery under c of Fl. Carpi Ulnaris where the puls the artery could not be felt. The me nerve at the mid-point on the fron the wrist, deep to Palmaris Longus, at the lateral border of Fl. Digito Superficialis. The radial artery is aberrant (see fig. 74), so its pulse m be missed.

5. Four tendons on the dorsum of wrist, large, because, being inserted metacarpal bones, they work as sy gists with the powerful flexors of digits, whereas the remaining tend being extensors of the digits, are slen

Labels on figure 65:
Mid-palmar spaces (medial and lateral)
Lumbricalis and digital art. & nerve
Long digital tendons of digit V
Palmar aponeurosis
Fl. Pollicis Longus
Abd. Pollicis Brevis
Fl. Pollicis Brevis
Abd. Digiti Minimi (V)
Opponens Digiti Minimi (V)
Princeps pollicis aa.
Sesamoid bone
Ext. Pollicis Longus
Dorsalis pollicis art.
Dorsalis indicis art.
Extensor tendons
Subaponeurotic areolar space
V, P3, D4, P2, IV, D3, III, D2, PI, II, D1, Add. Pollicis, I
E. Blackstock

65 Cross-section through the middle of the Palm

(The section passes through the head of the first metacarpal bone and, therefore, distal to Opponens Pollicis.)

Observe:

1. The 4 Dorsal Interossei (Abductors) filling the spaces between the 5 metacarpal bones.

2. The 3 Palmar Interossei (Adductors) arising from the palmar aspects of the 2nd, 4th and 5th metacarpal bones, and the Adductor Pollicis arising from the 3rd.

Note: All Interossei and the Adductor are supplied by the ulnar nerve.

3. Between the foregoing muscles and the palmar aponeurosis lie the long flexor tendons (superficial and deep) of the 4 fingers, the 4 Lumbricales, and the palmar digital nerves and arteries.

4. Fl. Pollicis Longus tendon, in its synovial

sheath, accompanied by its palmar digital arteries and nerves, and passing anterior to the palmar ligament (palmar plate) of the metacarpo-phalangeal joint

5. The tendons of Ext. Digitorum, flat tened, and within a membrane that ex tends from the 2nd to the 5th metacarpa bone, and the loose areolar subapo neurotic space deep to it.

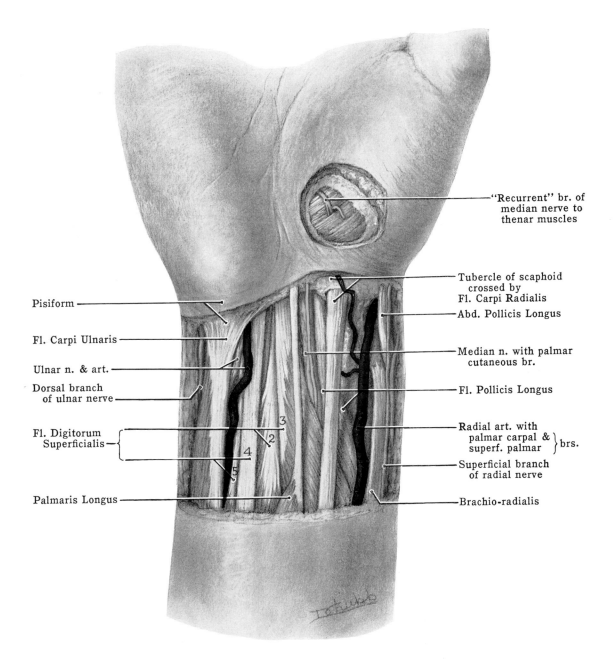

Pisiform

Fl. Carpi Ulnaris

Ulnar n. & art.

Dorsal branch
of ulnar nerve

Fl. Digitorum
Superficialis

Palmaris Longus

3
2
4
5

"Recurrent" br. of
median nerve to
thenar muscles

Tubercle of scaphoid
crossed by
Fl. Carpi Radialis

Abd. Pollicis Longus

Median n. with palmar
cutaneous br.

Fl. Pollicis Longus

Radial art. with
palmar carpal &
superf. palmar } brs.

Superficial branch
of radial nerve

Brachio-radialis

66 Structures at the Front of the Wrist

The distal transverse skin incision was made along the lowest skin-crease at the wrist. Medially this crease crosses the pisiform; and to this Fl. Carpi Ulnaris can be followed. At the junction of its lateral one-third with its medial two-thirds this crease crosses the tubercle of the scaphoid (navicular), and to this the conspicuous Fl. Carpi Radialis tendon is the guide.

Observe:

1. Palmaris Longus tendon bisecting the distal crease, exactly at the middle of the wrist. Deep to its lateral margin is the median nerve.

2. Abd. Pollicis Longus and Ext. Pollicis Brevis tendons forming the lateral margin of the wrist. They also form the anterior margin of the "snuff-box".

3. The radial artery disappearing deep to the Abductor.

4. The ulnar nerve and artery sheltered by Fl. Carpi Ulnaris

tendon and by the expansion this gives to the flexor retinaculum.

5. Fl. Digitorum Superficialis tendons to digits 3 and 4 somewhat anterior to those to digits 2 and 5.

6. The "recurrent" branch of the median nerve to the thenar muscles lying within a circle whose centre is from 1″ to 1½″ below the tubercle of the scaphoid. Seek it in the proper plane—between deep fascia and muscle fibres.

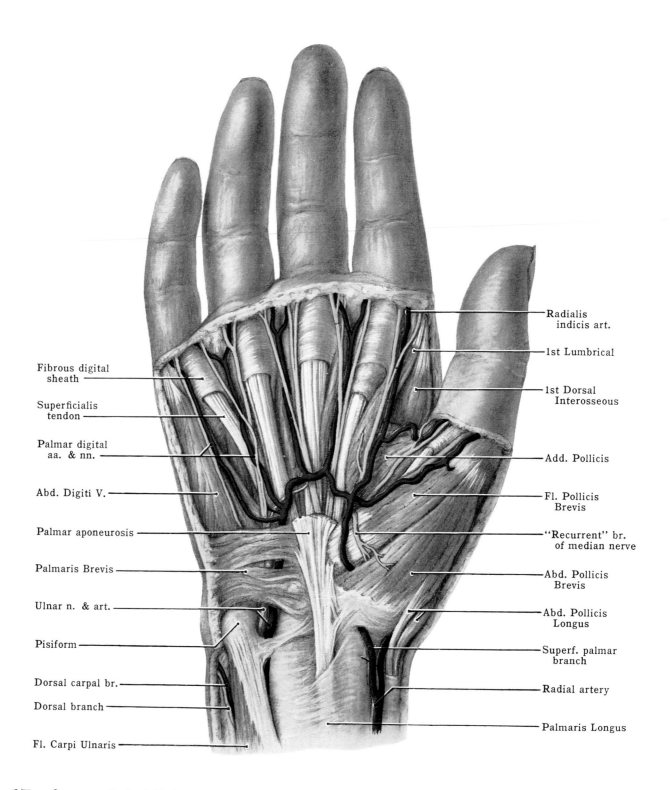

Radialis
indicis art.

1st Lumbrical

1st Dorsal
Interosseous

Add. Pollicis

Fl. Pollicis
Brevis

"Recurrent" br.
of median nerve

Abd. Pollicis
Brevis

Abd. Pollicis
Longus

Superf. palmar
branch

Radial artery

Palmaris Longus

Fibrous digital
sheath

Superficialis
tendon

Palmar digital
aa. & nn.

Abd. Digiti V.

Palmar aponeurosis

Palmaris Brevis

Ulnar n. & art.

Pisiform

Dorsal carpal br.

Dorsal branch

Fl. Carpi Ulnaris

67 Superficial Dissection of the Palm

The skin and the superficial fascia are removed; so are the palmar aponeurosis and the thenar and hypothenar fasciae (fig. 70).

The superficial palmar arch is formed by the ulnar artery and is completed by the superficial palmar branch of the radial artery. Only the foregoing structures and Palmaris Brevis cover the arch. It is truly superficial; so likewise are the digital vessels and nerves and the "recurrent" branch of the median nerve exposed in figure 66. The four Lumbricals lie behind digital vessels and nerves.

The prominent pisiform shelters the ulnar nerve and artery as they pass into the palm.

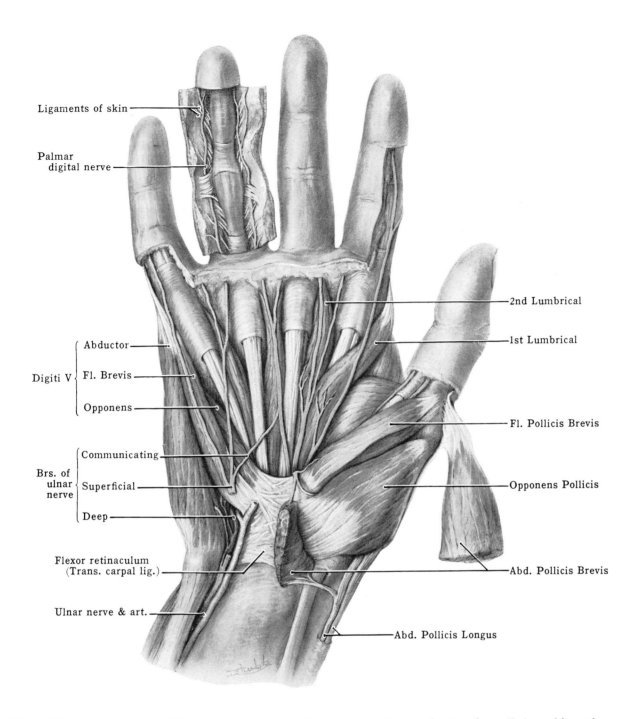

Ligaments of skin

Palmar digital nerve

Digiti V { Abductor / Fl. Brevis / Opponens

Brs. of ulnar nerve { Communicating / Superficial / Deep

Flexor retinaculum (Trans. carpal lig.)

Ulnar nerve & art.

2nd Lumbrical

1st Lumbrical

Fl. Pollicis Brevis

Opponens Pollicis

Abd. Pollicis Brevis

Abd. Pollicis Longus

68   Thenar and Hypothenar Muscles: Lumbricals: Distribution of the Median Nerve: Cutaneous Ligaments of the Fingers

The 3 thenar and 3 hypothenar muscles arise from the flexor retinaculum and from the 4 marginal carpal bones united by this retinaculum. Abd. Pollicis Brevis arises from Abd. Pollicis Longus tendon also; Abd. Digiti V arises from the pisiform only.

The 4 Lumbricals arise from the radial sides of the 4 Profundus tendons, and are inserted into the radial sides of the dorsal expansions (fig. 88) of the corresponding digits. The medial 2 Lumbricals, however, also arise from the medial sides of adjacent Profundus

tendons; and the 3rd Lumbrical is commonly inserted into two extensor expansions, as here.

The median nerve is distributed in the hand to 5 muscles (3 thenar and 2 lumbrical) and to 3½ digits, including parts of their dorsal aspects (fig. 83). All other short muscles in the hand are supplied by the deep branch of the ulnar nerve, Palmaris Brevis excepted (supplied by the superficial br.).

The skin of the fingers cannot be pulled off like a glove, on account of the oblique fibrous strands, cutaneous ligaments, that moor it.

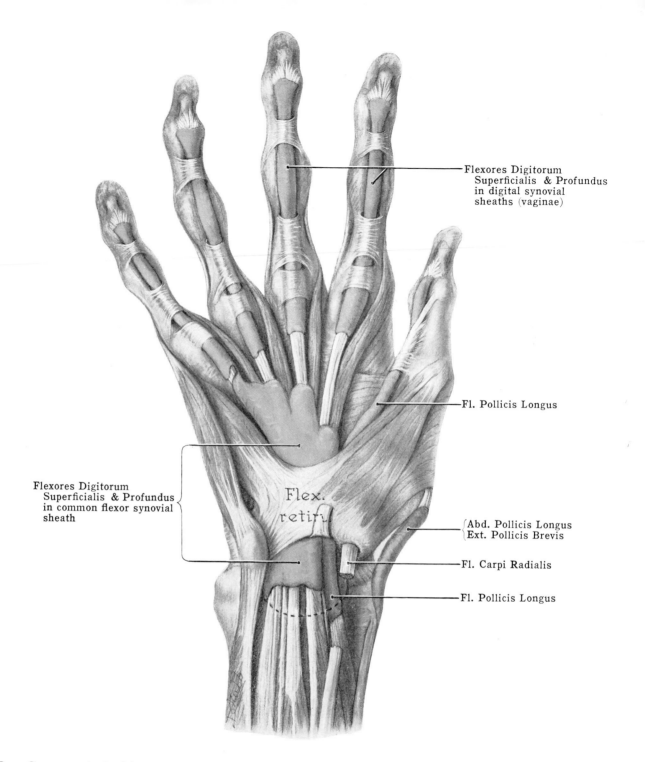

Flexores Digitorum
Superficialis & Profundus
in digital synovial
sheaths (vaginae)

Fl. Pollicis Longus

Flexores Digitorum
Superficialis & Profundus
in common flexor synovial
sheath

Flex.
retin.

{ Abd. Pollicis Longus
{ Ext. Pollicis Brevis

Fl. Carpi Radialis

Fl. Pollicis Longus

69 Synovial Sheaths of the Long Flexor Tendons of the Digits

These sheaths or tubular bursae are lubricating devices that envelope the long digital tendons where they pass through osseofibrous tunnels. There are 2 sets: (a) proximal or carpal, behind the flexor retinaculum; (b) distal or digital, behind the fibrous sheaths of the digital flexors.

The carpal synovial sheaths of the flexors of the fingers, though developmentally separate, unite with one another to form a common flexor sheath, and the carpal sheath of the thumb tendon usually communicates with it. This common flexor sheath extends ½″ to 1″ proximal to and distal to the flexor retinaculum, varying distally with the extent of the site of friction and with the degree of mobility of the corresponding metacarpal bone. These are greatest in the marginal digits (thumb and little finger). Further, the marginal metacarpals being the shortest, the common flexor sheath extends to, and is continuous with, the digital sheaths of thumb and little finger.

In the case of the thumb, union always occurs; the little finger usually.

Each digital sheath extends from the proximal end of the palmar lig. or plate (figs. 72 & 96) that covers a metacarpal head to the base of a distal phalanx.

Fluid injected into the digital sheath of the little finger will, therefore, usually flow through the common flexor sheath and on into the digital sheath of the thumb.

The flexor tendons play across the very prominent anterior border of the inferior articular surface of the radius; hence the common flexor sheath extends further proximally behind the tendons (broken line) than in front of them.

The median nerve (thrown down in the figure), not requiring lubrication, has no sheath. Fl. Carpi Radialis tendon has a sheath, not injected in this specimen.

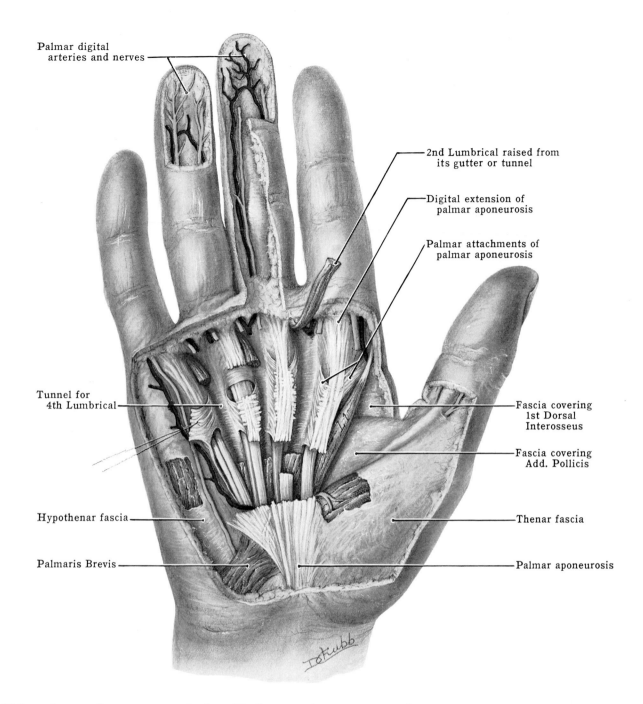

Palmar digital
arteries and nerves

2nd Lumbrical raised from
its gutter or tunnel

Digital extension of
palmar aponeurosis

Palmar attachments of
palmar aponeurosis

Tunnel for
4th Lumbrical

Fascia covering
1st Dorsal
Interosseus

Fascia covering
Add. Pollicis

Hypothenar fascia

Thenar fascia

Palmaris Brevis

Palmar aponeurosis

70 Attachments of the Palmar Aponeurosis:
Palmar Digital Vessels and Nerves

Skin and superficial fascia are removed and, in the palm, parts of the
palmar aponeurosis, digital vessels, and nerves, and Lumbricals are excised.

Observe:

1. From the palmar aponeurosis some longitudinal fibres descending to the fingers where they are lost; other fibres,
forming extensive fibro-areolar septa pass dorsally, not only
to the palmar ligaments, but also more proximally, to the
fascia covering the Interossei. Thus, two sets of tunnels exist
in the distal half of the palm: (1) tunnels for long flexor tendons, and (2) tunnels for Lumbricals, digital vessels and
digital nerves. The former are continued into the fingers; the
latter open on the dorsum of the hand behing the web.

2. In a finger, the digital artery and nerve lying on the side of
the fibrous digital sheath.

3. The absence of fat deep to the skin-creases of the fingers.

4. The 4 palmar spaces: (1) a "thenar", behind the thenar fascia; (2) a "hypothenar," behind the hypothenar fascia; between these (3) a "middle," behind the palmar aponeurosis;
and (4) a fourth, between Adductor Pollicis and 1st Dorsal
Interosseous. The middle space contains Superficialis and
Profundus tendons, Lumbricals, and digital vessels and
nerves. It is bounded behind by (a) the fascia covering Interossei and Add. Pollicis, (b) the palmar ligs. and (c) the
deep transverse metacarpal ligs. of the palm (fig. 72).

Proper palmar digital arteries

Radialis indicis artery

3 Common palmar digital arteries

3 Palmar metacarpal arteries

Digiti V { Abductor — Fl. Brevis — Opponens }

Add. Pollicis

Abd. Brevis
Fl. Brevis } Pollicis
Opponens

Ext. Carpi Ulnaris
Deep br. of ulnar
artery & nerve
Piso-hamate lig.

Recurrent branch of deep palmar arch
Trapezium (Gtr. multangular)

Ulnar artery

Superficial palmar br.

Palmar carpal arch

Palmar carpal br.

Fl. Digitorum Profundus

Fl. Pollicis Longus

Fl. Digit. Superficialis

Median nerve

Fl. Carpi Ulnaris

Fl. Carpi Radialis

Palmaris Longus

Radial artery

71 Deep Dissection of the Palm

Observe:

1. Superficialis bellies for digits 3 and 4 lying in front of those for digits 2 and 5. Pollicis and Profundus tendons lying side by side.

2. Fl. Pollicis Longus tendon making a spiral turn around Fl. Carpi Radialis tendon.

3. The anterior or palmar carpal arch and its connections lying on the skeletal plane.

4. The Opponens Pollicis and Opponens Digiti V inserted into the lengths of their respective metacarpals.

5. Adductor Pollicis arising from metacarpal 3 and the capitate, and inserted, via 2 sesamoids (fig. 72), into both sides of the proximal phalanx of the thumb. The radial artery divides it into a transverse and an oblique head.

6. The deep branch of the ulnar artery joining the radial artery to form the deep palmar arch.

Fibrous digital sheath

Superficialis

Profundus

nerve
artery } Palmar
vein } digital

Cutaneous lig.

Dorsal (ext.) expansion

Bone

71.1 Cross-section of a Finger, through the proximal phalanx

Observe:

1. The skin, thickest on the palmar surface.

2. The palmar digital nerve and vessels, applied to the fibrous sheath — not to the bone.

3. Ligaments, mooring skin to bone.

Palmar lig. or plate
(Accessory volar lig.)

Fibrous digital sheath

Palmar lig. or plate

Fl. Digitorum Profundus

Fl. Digitorum Superficialis

Fibrous digital sheath

Deep Transverse metacarpal lig.

Palmar lig. (Accessory volar lig.)

Attachment of palmar aponeurosis to palmar ligament

Twig to joint

Twig to 4th Lumbrical

Deep br. of ulnar nerve

Collateral lig.

Radial artery
3 Perforating aa.

Hook of hamate

Articular capsule

Piso-metacarpal } ligs.
Piso-hamate

Tubercle (Crest) of trapezium

Pisiform

Tubercle of scaphoid

Palmar radio-carpal lig.

Flex. retin.

Pronator Quadratus

Abd. Pollicis Longus

Brachio-radialis

Fl. Carpi Ulnaris

Fl. Carpi Radialis

D2   D1
D3   P1
P4
P3   P2

72   Deep Dissection of the Palm and Digits: Ulnar Nerve

Observe:

1. The flexor retinaculum (transverse carpal lig.) uniting the 4 marginal carpal bones, and having the ulnar nerve in front and the median nerve (not labelled) behind.

2. Fl. Carpi Radialis descending vertically in front of the navicular tubercle and along the groove on the trapezium to the 2nd metacarpal.

3. Fl. Carpi Ulnaris continuing beyond the pisiform as the piso-hamate and the piso-metacarpal ligament.

4. The loose capsule of the carpo-metacarpal joint of the thumb and the strong collateral ligament of its metacarpo-phalangeal joint.

5. 4 Dorsal and 3 Palmar Interossei.

6. The ulnar nerve crossing the hook of the hamate to be dis-

tributed by its deep branch to the 3 hypothenar muscles, all 7 Interossei, 2 Lumbricals, Adductor Pollicis and several joints. The superficial branch supplies Palmaris Brevis and 1½ digits.

7. The radial artery appearing in series with the 3 perforating arteries.

8. The palmar ligs., with the deep transverse metacarpal ligaments uniting them, and the septa from the palmar aponeurosis attached to them.

9. A Lumbrical passing in front of the deep transverse ligament, and Interossei passing behind.

10. On the index, a proximal and distal osseo-fibrous tunnel; on the middle finger, a Superficialis tendon spreading like a V and decussating like an X; on the ring finger, a Profundus tendon; and on the little finger, both tendons.

73 Radial Aspect of the Wrist—I

(The Anatomical Snuffbox, and the Dorsum of the Thumb and First Intermetacarpal Space.)

Observe:

1. The superficial veins and nerves crossing the snuffbox.
2. Perforating veins and articular nerves piercing the deep fascia.

74 Radial Aspect of the Wrist—II

Observe:

1. Three long tendons of the thumb forming the sides of the snuffbox.
2. The radial artery and its venae comitantes crossing the floor of the snuffbox and disappearing between the two heads of the 1st Dorsal Interosseous.
3. The 1st Dorsal Interosseus and the Adductor Pollicis.

Labels for left figure (top to bottom):
...uctor ...oll. Brevis — Adductor Pollicis
Metacarpal I — 1st Dorsal Inteross.
...xtensor Pollicis Brevis
...bductor Pollicus Longus — Extensor Poll. Longus
...caphoid bone — Ext. Carpi Rad. Brevis
...tyloid process — Ext. Carpi Rad. Longus
...adial artery
...l. Carpi Radialis
...rachio-radialis

Labels for right figure:
Extensor Pollicis Longus — 1st Dorsal Inteross.
Extensor Pollicis Brevis — Adductor Pollicis
Metacarpal I — 1st Dorsal Inteross.
Abductor Pollicis Longus — Ext. Carpi Radialis Longus
Trapezium — Trapezoid
Scaphoid
Styloid process — Dorsal radial tubercle
3 grooves for: Abd. Poll. Longus / Ext. Poll. Brevis
Ext. C. Rad. Longus / Ext. C. Rad. Brevis
Ext. Poll. Longus

75 Radial Aspect of the Wrist—III

Observe:

1. The scaphoid bone; the wrist joint (and radius) proximal to the scaphoid; and the midcarpal joint (and trapezium and trapezoid) distal to it.
2. The capsule of the 1st carpo-metacarpal joint.
3. The Abductor Pollicis Brevis and Adductor Pollicis partly inserted into the dorsal (extensor) expansion.

76 Bones of the Radial Aspect of the Hand Showing Muscle Attachments

Observe:

1. The anatomical snuffbox, limited proximally by the styloid process of the radius; distally by the base of the metacarpal of the thumb.
2. The 2 lateral marginal bones of the carpus (viz., scaphoid and trapezium) forming the floor of the snuff-box.

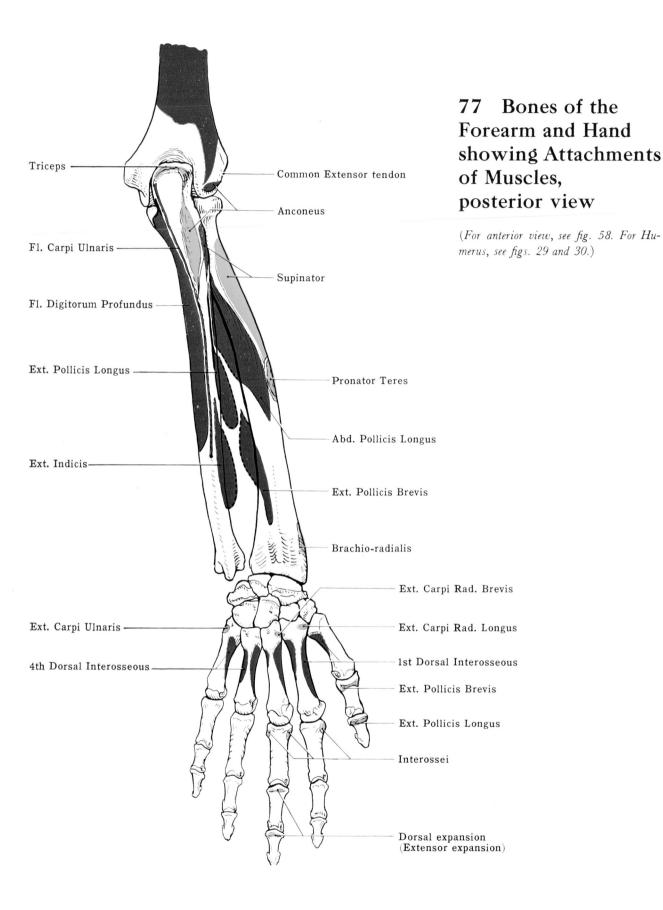

Triceps

Fl. Carpi Ulnaris

Fl. Digitorum Profundus

Ext. Pollicis Longus

Ext. Indicis

Ext. Carpi Ulnaris

4th Dorsal Interosseous

Common Extensor tendon

Anconeus

Supinator

Pronator Teres

Abd. Pollicis Longus

Ext. Pollicis Brevis

Brachio-radialis

Ext. Carpi Rad. Brevis

Ext. Carpi Rad. Longus

1st Dorsal Interosseous

Ext. Pollicis Brevis

Ext. Pollicis Longus

Interossei

Dorsal expansion
(Extensor expansion)

77 Bones of the Forearm and Hand showing Attachments of Muscles, posterior view

(*For anterior view, see fig. 58. For Humerus, see figs. 29 and 30.*)

nconeus
& its nerve

The 3 lateral muscles:
Brachio-radialis

Extensor Carpi
Radialis Longus

Extensor Carpi
Radialis Brevis

xt. Digitorum
(Communis)

xt. Digiti V
(Proprius)

xt. Carpi
Ulnaris

The 3 outcropping
muscles of the thumb;
Abd. Pollicis Longus

Ext. Pollicis Brevis

xt. Indicis
(Proprius)

Ext. Pollicis Longus

xt. retinaculum
(Dorsal carpal lig.)

orsal carpal br.
of ulnar artery

Radial artery in snuff-box

orsal carpal
arch or rete

Dorsal carpal br. of radial a.

Perforating aa.

Dorsales Pollicis aa.

orsal metacarpal aa.

Dorsalis Indicis a.

Dorsal digital aa.

78 Muscles of the Extensor Region (i.e., Dorsal and Lateral Aspects) of the Forearm: Arteries on the Dorsum of the Hand

The extensors of the fingers are reflected.

Observe:

1. Three muscles of the thumb outcropping between Ext. Carpi Radialis Brevis and Ext. Digitorum

2. The arteries seen are the radial, the dorsal carpal branch of the ulnar, and their branches. All these are undisturbed by the removal of muscles, since they lie on the skeletal plane (i.e., on bone, ligament, or fascia covering Interossei).

3. The radial artery disappearing between the two heads of the 1st Dorsal Interosseous where it is in series with the perforating arteries.

4. No muscle is attached to the back of a carpal bone. The 3 extensors of the wrist span the carpal bones to reach the bases of metacarpals 2, 3 and 5.

Anconeus

Intermuscular
septum

Post interosseous
recurrent artery

Post interosseous
nerve & artery

Ext. Digitorum
(Communis)

Ext. Digiti V
(Proprius)

Ext. Carpi
Ulnaris

Ext. Indicis
(Proprius)

Dorsal carpal
arch or rete

Dorsalis indicis art.

Radialis indicis art.

Insertion of {First Dorsal
Interosseous

Supinator

Post. interosseous
nerve

Brachio-radialis

Ext. Carpi Radialis
Longus

Ext. Carpi Radialis
Brevis

Pronator Teres

The 3 outcropping
thumb-muscles:
Abd. Pollicis Longus

Ext. Pollicis Brevis

Ext. Pollicis Longus

Radial artery
(in the "snuff-box")

Dorsales pollicis aa.

Adductor Pollicis

79 Exposure of the Dee
Structures at the Back o
the Forearm: The Three
Outcropping Muscles of
the Thumb, postero-later
view

The furrow from which the 3 musc
outcrop has been opened widely, up to t
lateral epicondyle. It crosses Supinator a
is a "line of safety" since the 3 latera
retracted muscles are supplied before t
posterior interosseous nerve enters the fles
tunnel in Supinator, whilst the others are su
plied after it emerges $2\frac{1}{2}''$ below the head
the radius.

The 3 outcropping muscles of the thur
pass to the epiphyses at the bases of t
metacarpal, proximal phalanx, and dis
phalanx of the thumb (fig. 104). Of the
thumb muscles, Ext. Longus is separated fr
Ext. Brevis and Abd. Longus by its pull
the dorsal radial tubercle (figs. 92 & 9
hence the "anatomical snuffbox" proxin
to the base of the 1st metacarpal, where t
radial artery lies on the scaphoid (navicula
and trapezium (greater multangular).

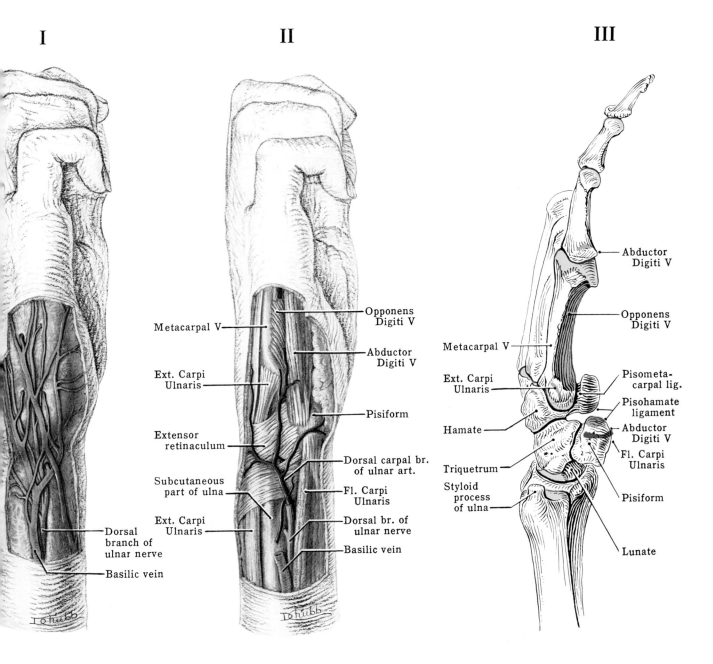

I   II   III

Figure I labels:

Metacarpal V

Ext. Carpi Ulnaris

Extensor retinaculum

Subcutaneous part of ulna

Ext. Carpi Ulnaris

Dorsal branch of ulnar nerve

Basilic vein

Figure II labels:

Opponens Digiti V

Abductor Digiti V

Pisiform

Dorsal carpal br. of ulnar art.

Fl. Carpi Ulnaris

Dorsal br. of ulnar nerve

Basilic vein

Figure III labels:

Abductor Digiti V

Opponens Digiti V

Metacarpal V

Pisometa-carpal lig.

Ext. Carpi Ulnaris

Pisohamate ligament

Hamate

Abductor Digiti V

Triquetrum

Fl. Carpi Ulnaris

Styloid process of ulna

Pisiform

Lunate

80   Ulnar Border of the Wrist

Observe:

. The superficial veins and their perforating branches.

. The superficial nerve appearing from under cover of Fl. Carpi Ulnaris.

81   Ulnar Border of the Wrist

Note: A vertical incision made along the medial subcutaneous surface of the ulna and along the medial border of the hand passes between two motor territories (Fl. Carpi Ulnaris, Abd. Digiti V, and Opponens Digiti V, supplied by the ulnar nerve; and Ext. Carpi Ulnaris by the post. interosseous nerve). Superficial veins, nerves, and arteries will be divided, but no motor nerves.

82   Bones of the Ulnar Border of the Hand, Showing Muscle Attachments

Observe:

Ext. Carpi Ulnaris inserted directly into the base of metacarpal V; Fl. Carpi Ulnaris inserted indirectly through the medium of the pisiform bone and piso-metacarpal lig.

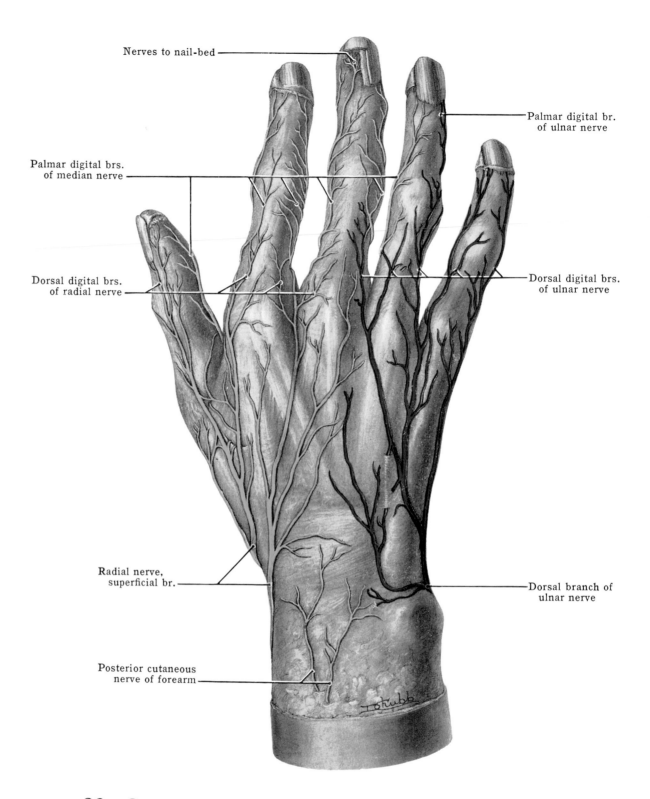

Nerves to nail-bed

Palmar digital brs. of median nerve

Dorsal digital brs. of radial nerve

Radial nerve, superficial br.

Posterior cutaneous nerve of forearm

Palmar digital br. of ulnar nerve

Dorsal digital brs. of ulnar nerve

Dorsal branch of ulnar nerve

83 Cutaneous Nerves of the Dorsum of the Hand

Observe:

1. The radial nerve and the dorsal branch of the ulnar nerve distributed nearly equally and symmetrically on the dorsum of the hand and digits. The radial nerve supplies the radial half of the dorsum and extends on the 2½ digits—in fact, all the way along the first digit; the dorsal branch of the ulnar nerve behaves similarly on the ulnar half. Each distribution is almost a looking-glass distribution of the other.

2. The palmar digital branches of the median and ulnar nerves (fig. 68) alone supply the distal halves of the three middle digits, including the nail beds.

3. Anastomoses between adjacent nerves are numerous.

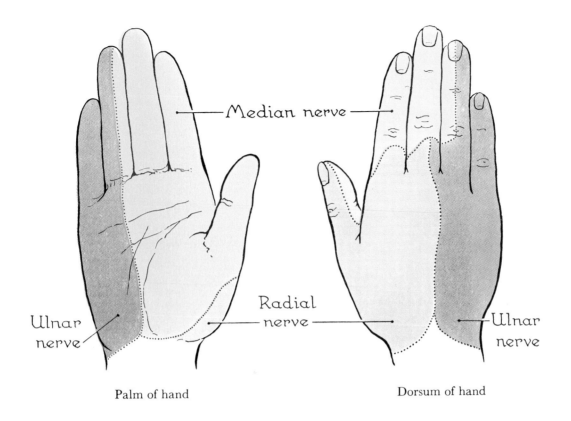

Palm of hand   Dorsum of hand

84   Distribution of the Cutaneous Nerves to the Palm and to the Dorsum of the Hand

85   Variations in the Pattern of the Cutaneous Nerves to the Dorsum of the Hand

(After Learmonth, Hutton, Hutton, and Appleton respectively.)

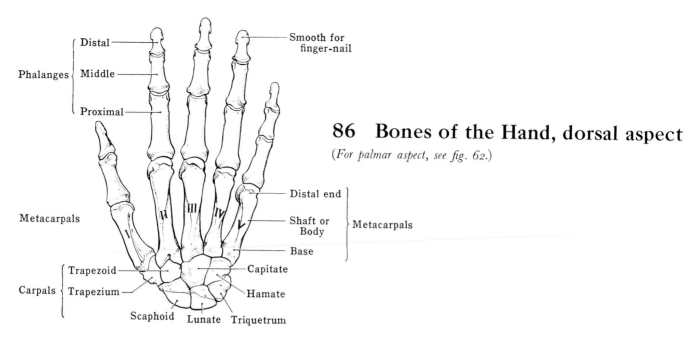

Distal ⎫
Middle ⎬ Phalanges
Proximal ⎭

Smooth for finger-nail

86   Bones of the Hand, dorsal aspect

(For palmar aspect, see fig. 62.)

Metacarpals

II III IV V

I

Distal end ⎫
Shaft or Body ⎬ Metacarpals
Base ⎭

Trapezoid
Trapezium ⎬ Carpals

Capitate
Hamate

Scaphoid   Lunate   Triquetrum

86.1   Synovial Sheaths of the Tendons on the Dorsum of the Wrist

Note:

These six sheaths occupy the six osseo-fibrous tunnels deep the extensor retinaculum.

They contain 9 tendons—3 for the thumb in two sheaths & 2); 3 for the extensors of the wrist in two sheaths (3 & 4); an 3 for the extensors of the fingers in two sheaths (5 & 6).

They may be studied in the foregoing order after the dors radial tubercle (figs. 2 & 94), which is the pulley for the Exter sor Pollicis Longus, has been located.

The tendons of the three extensors of the wrist are the strong est (fig. 64) because they work synergically with the flexors the digits.

Ext. Digiti V (6)

Ext. Carpi Ulnaris (4)

(3) Ext. Carpi Radiales:
Longus ⎫
Brevis ⎬

{ Ext. Digitorum (5)
{ Ext. Indicis

(1) Ext. Pollicis Longus

(2) Abd. Pollicis Longus ⎫
Ext. Pollicis Brevis ⎬

Tubercle

1 5 6 4
3
2   Radius   Ulna

86.2

Diagram of a cross section of the tendons on the dorsum of the wrist.

(Extensor expansion)
Dorsal expansion

Ext. Indicis
(Proprius)

1st Dorsal
Interosseous

Radial artery

Ext. Carpi Radialis
Longus

Ext. Carpi Radialis
Brevis

Radial nerve,
superficial br.

Ext. Pollicis Longus

Ext. Pollicis Brevis

Abd. Pollicis Longus

Dorsal digital vein

Ext. Digiti Quinti
(Proprius)

Ulnar nerve,
dorsal branch

Ext. retinaculum
(Dorsal carpal lig.)

Ext. Carpi Ulnaris

Ext. Indicis (Proprius)

Ext. Digiti Quinti
(Proprius)

Ext. Digitorum
(Communis)

87 Tendons on the Dorsum of the Hand and the Extensor Retinaculum (Dorsal Carpal Lig.)

Observe:

1. The disposition of the tendons of the 9 muscles at the back of the wrist and hand.
2. The deep fascia, here thickened and called the extensor retinaculum, stretching obliquely from one ridge on the radius to another. Medially it passes distal to the ulna to be attached to the pisiform and triquetrum, as depicted in figure 81.
3. The bands connecting the tendons of the digital extensor tendons and thereby denying the fingers independent action
4. The digital veins passing to the dorsum of the hand where they are not subjected to pressure.
5. The body of the 2nd metacarpal is not covered with an extensor tendon.

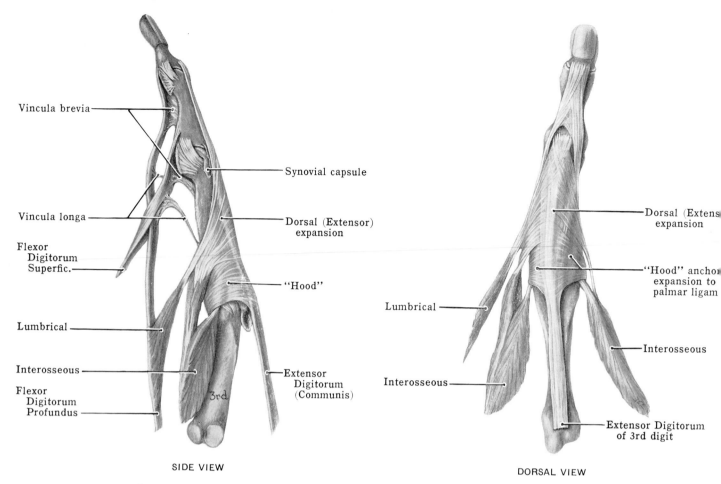

Vincula brevia

Vincula longa

Flexor
Digitorum
Superfic.

Lumbrical

Interosseous

Flexor
Digitorum
Profundus

Synovial capsule

Dorsal (Extensor)
expansion

"Hood"

3rd

Extensor
Digitorum
(Communis)

SIDE VIEW

Dorsal (Extens
expansion

"Hood" anchor
expansion to
palmar ligam

Lumbrical

Interosseous

Interosseous

Extensor Digitorum
of 3rd digit

DORSAL VIEW

88 Extensor (Dorsal) Expansion of the Middle Digit

Observe:

1. Interossei in part inserted into the bases of the proximal phalanx (figs. 76–79) and in part into the expansion.

2. Lumbrical inserted wholly into the radial side of the expansion.

3. The hood covering the head of the metacarpal. It is moored to the palmar ligament (figs. 72 and 96).

4. The expansion extending to the bases of the middle and distal phalanges, and giving a strong areolar band to the base of the proximal phalanx, here not in view, (Kaplan).

5. (On side view) the vincula longa et brevia, which are all that remain of the primitive mesotendons.

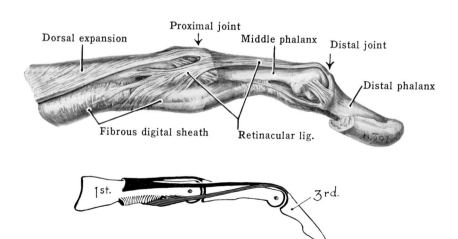

Dorsal expansion

Proximal joint

Middle phalanx

Distal joint

Distal phalanx

Fibrous digital sheath

Retinacular lig.

1st.

3rd.

89 Retinacular Ligament

Observe:

1. This delicate fibrous band runs from the 1st o proximal phalanx and the fibrous digital sheat obliquely across the 2nd phalanx and the two inter phalangeal joints to join the dorsal expansion and so to the 3rd or distal phalanx.

2. On flexing the distal joint either passively (as in th cadaver) or voluntarily, the retinacular ligamen becomes taut and pulls the proximal joint int flexion.

3. Similarly, on extending the proximal joint, th distal joint is pulled by the retinacular ligamen into nearly complete extension. (J. M. F Landsmeer.)

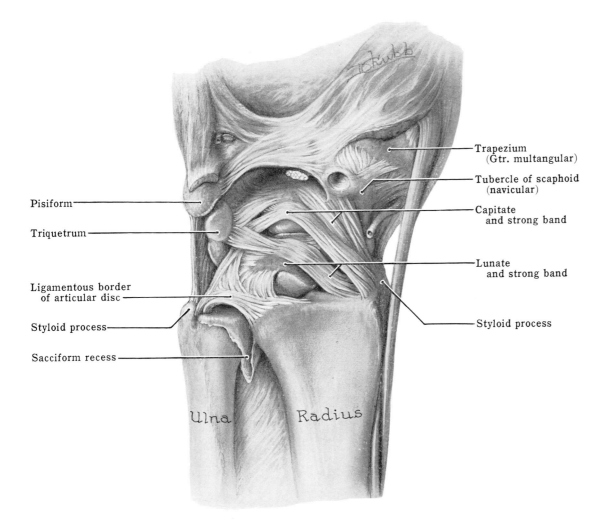

Pisiform

Triquetrum

Ligamentous border
of articular disc

Styloid process

Sacciform recess

Trapezium
(Gtr. multangular)

Tubercle of scaphoid
(navicular)

Capitate
and strong band

Lunate
and strong band

Styloid process

Ulna   Radius

90 Ligaments of the Distal Radio-ulnar, Radio-carpal and Intercarpal Joints, front view

The hand is forcibly extended.

Observe:

1. The sacciform recess of the distal radio-ulnar joint (similar to the recess of the proximal joint, fig. 54) and the ligamentous anterior border of the disc.

2. The anterior or palmar ligaments, passing from the radius to the two rows of carpal bones, strong and so directed that the hand shall follow the radius during supination. The dorsal ligaments take the same direction, hence the hand is obedient during pronation also.

3. The proximal articular surface of the triquetrum applied to the medial ligament of the wrist.

4. The unlabelled deep branch of the ulnar artery and nerve; median nerve; tunnel for Fl. Carpi Radialis; and the radial artery.

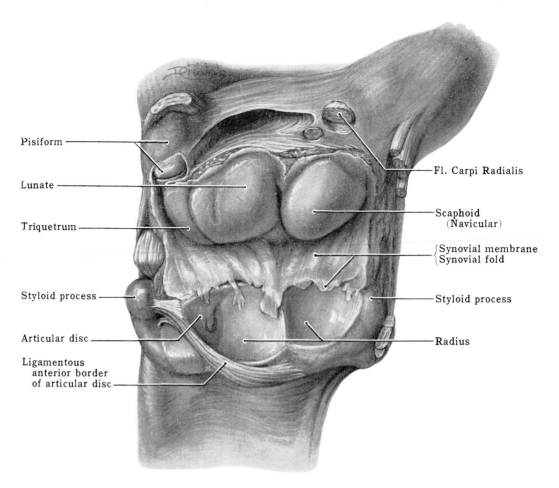

Pisiform

Lunate

Triquetrum

Styloid process

Articular disc

Ligamentous
anterior border
of articular disc

Fl. Carpi Radialis

Scaphoid
(Navicular)

Synovial membrane
Synovial fold

Styloid process

Radius

91 Surfaces of the Radio-carpal or Wrist Joint, opened from front

Observe:

1. The nearly equal proximal articular surfaces of the scaphoid and lunate.
2. The lunate articulating with the radius and the articular disc. Only during adduction of the wrist does the triquetrum come into articulation with the disc.
3. Transparent synovial folds, like cellophane, projecting between the bony surfaces.

4. The perforation in the disc and the associated roughened surface of the lunate. This is a common occurrence.
5. The pisiform joint communicating with the radio-carpal joint.
6. The interosseous ligament between the scaphoid and the lunate, partly absorbed. In such a specimen—and they are common—infection could spread widely.

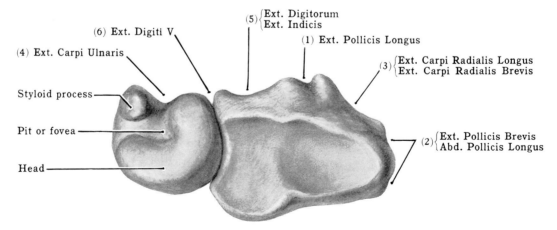

(6) Ext. Digiti V

(4) Ext. Carpi Ulnaris

(5) {Ext. Digitorum
Ext. Indicis

(1) Ext. Pollicis Longus

(3) {Ext. Carpi Radialis Longus
Ext. Carpi Radialis Brevis

Styloid process

Pit or fovea

Head

(2) {Ext. Pollicis Brevis
Abd. Pollicis Longus

92 Distal Ends of Radius and Ulna, from below

Observe:

1. The 4 features of the distal end of the ulna—head, fovea, process, and groove for the tendon of Ext. Carpi Ulnaris.
2. The 6 grooves for the 9 tendons at the back of the wrist. Figure 86.1 shows these tendons in their synovial sheaths.

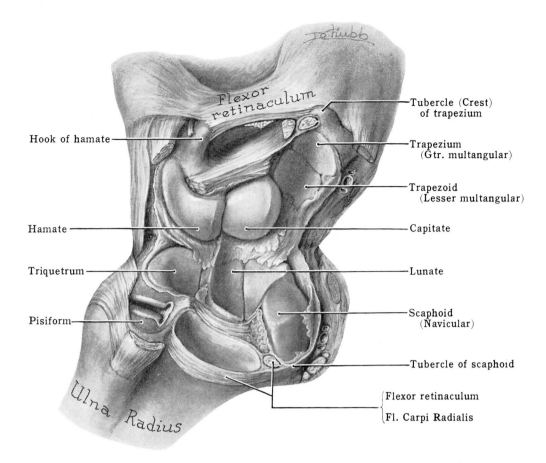

Flexor retinaculum

Hook of hamate

Tubercle (Crest) of trapezium

Trapezium (Gtr. multangular)

Trapezoid (Lesser multangular)

Hamate

Capitate

Triquetrum

Lunate

Pisiform

Scaphoid (Navicular)

Tubercle of scaphoid

Flexor retinaculum
Fl. Carpi Radialis

Ulna Radius

93 Surfaces of the Midcarpal Joint (Transverse Carpal Joint)

The flexor retinaculum (transverse carpal lig.) is divided.

Observe:

1. The sinuous surfaces of the opposed bones: the trapezium and trapezoid together presenting a concave, oval surface to the scaphoid; the capitate and hamate together presenting a convex surface to the scaphoid, lunate and triquetrum, which is slightly broken by the linear facet on the apex of the hamate for its counterpart on the lunate.

2. Synovial folds projecting into the joint.

3. The relative weakness of the proximal part of the flexor retinaculum, which stretches from the movable pisiform to the scaphoid, and the strength of the distal part, which stretches from the hook of the hamate to the tubercle (crest) of the trapezium.

4. Locations of the unlabelled deep branch of the ulnar nerve, median nerve, Fl. Pollicis Longus, and Fl. Carpi Radialis.

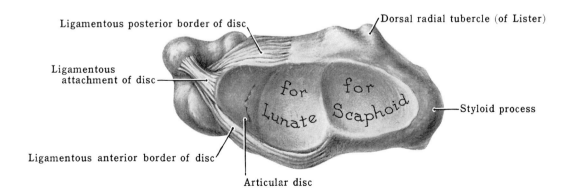

Ligamentous posterior border of disc

Dorsal radial tubercle (of Lister)

Ligamentous attachment of disc

for Lunate

for Scaphoid

Styloid process

Ligamentous anterior border of disc

Articular disc

94 Articular Disc of the Distal Radio-ulnar Joint, from below

This disc is the bond of union between the lower ends of the radius and ulna. It is fibro-cartilaginous, smooth, and stiff at the triangular area compressed between the head of the ulna and the lunate bone (figs. 52 & 91), but it is ligamentous and pliable elsewhere. The cartilaginous part is commonly fissured, as here, but the ligamentous parts are not.

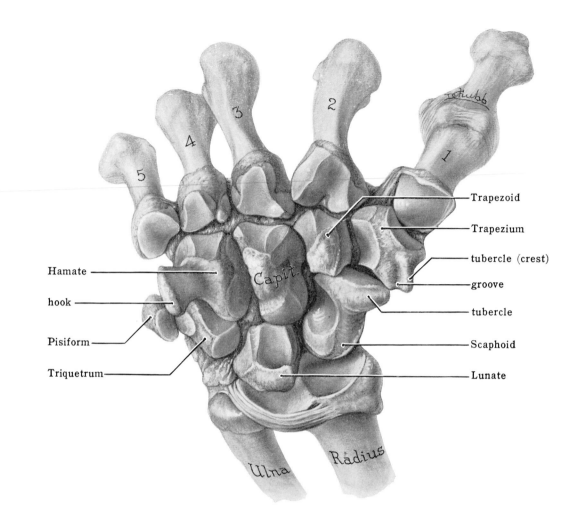

Labels on figure: 5, 4, 3, 2, Chubb, 1, Trapezoid, Trapezium, tubercle (crest), groove, tubercle, Scaphoid, Lunate, Hamate, hook, Pisiform, Triquetrum, Capit., Ulna, Radius

95 Carpal Bones and the Bases of the Metacarpal Bones, front view

The dorsal ligaments remain as a binding that allows the bones to be "opened and closed".

Observe:

1. One bone (radius) supporting two proximal carpals (scaphoid and lunate); these in turn supporting three distal carpals (trapezium, trapezoid, and capitate) and articulating with the apex of the hamate; the four distal carpals supporting the five metacarpals. The triquetrum is unsupported.

2. The marginal projections (pisiform, hook of hamate, tubercle of scaphoid, and tubercle of trapezium) which afford attachment to the flexor retinaculum.

3. The triquetrum having an isolated facet for the pisiform.

4. Of the eight carpals only the lunate is wider in front than behind.

5. The capitate articulating with three metacarpals (2nd, 3rd, and 4th).

6. The second metacarpal articulating with three carpals (trapezium, trapezoid, and capitate).

7. The basal surfaces of the 2nd and 3rd metacarpals individually about as large as those of the 4th and 5th collectively.

8. The 2nd and 3rd carpo-metacarpal joints practically immobile; the 1st, saddle-shaped; the 4th and 5th, hinge-shaped.

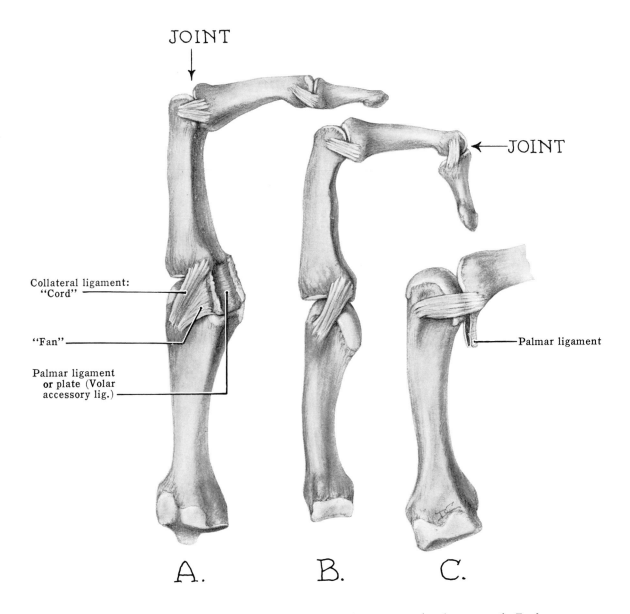

JOINT

JOINT

Collateral ligament:
"Cord"

"Fan"

Palmar ligament
or plate (Volar
accessory lig.)

Palmar ligament

A.   B.   C.

96 Metacarpo-phalangeal and Interphalangeal Joints

Observe:

1. A fibro-cartilaginous plate, the palmar ligament, hanging from the base of the proximal phalanx; fixed to the head of the metacarpal by the weaker, fanlike part, of the collateral ligament; and moving like a visor across the metacarpal head.

   Figure 72 shows the transverse ligaments that unite the plates, and the insertions of the palmar aponeurosis into them.

2. The extremely strong, cordlike parts of the collateral ligaments of this joint, being eccentrically attached to the metacarpal heads. They are slack during extension and taut during flexion; hence the fingers cannot be spread (abducted) unless the hand is open.

   The interphalangeal joints have corresponding ligaments but, the distal ends of the 1st and 2nd phalanges, being flattened anteroposteriorly and having two small condyles (cf., distal end of femur), permit neither adduction nor abduction.

A. Long Communicating Branch from Ulnar to Median Nerve

B. Persisting Median Artery

C. Extensor Digitorum Brevis

This muscle, constant on the dor[sum] of the foot, is found occasionally on [the] dorsum of the hand, usually as a si[ngle] bundle.

D. Palmaris Longus: misplaced or absent

The fleshy belly occasionally migrates distally and comes to lie close above the wrist, as here.

Palmaris Longus was absent in 98 of 716 dissected limbs (i.e., in 13.7% of 358 paired limbs, 26 times in both limbs, 26 in the right only, and 20 in the left only. (*R. K. George*).

E. Separate Styloid Process of 3rd Metacarpal

LEFT SIDE   RIGHT SIDE

F. Fused Lunate and Triquetr[um]

97 VARIATIONS AND ANOMALIES
of occasional occurrence

98 Bones of Upper Limb at Birth

The diaphyses of the long bones and the scapula are well ossified; but the epiphyses have not started to ossify nor have the carpal bones—except occasionally the head of the humerus and the capitate (and hamate) in the female. The coracoid process, the medial border of the scapula and the acromion are cartilaginous.

(All ages given in figures 98—104 are for males.)

99 Epiphysis of the Clavicle

The Clavicle has a thin epiphysis covering its sternal end. This may start to fuse at any time between the 18th and 25th years. Between the 23rd and 31st years (mostly between 26th and 29th) all undergo terminal fusion. It is the last of the long bone epiphyses to fuse. (*McKern and Stewart.*)

Coracoid process

AGED ABOUT 3 YEARS.

THE CORACOID PROCESS, FUSING,
AGED ABOUT 15 YEARS.

AGED ABOUT 17 YEARS.

100 Ossification of the Scapula

The Coracoid Process. A single ossific center appears in the coracoid during the 1st year; another center for the upper end of the glenoid cavity and adjacent part of the coracoid appears about the 10th year. These fuse with the scapula about the 15th year.

The Acromion has two ossific centers; the medial border and the inferior angle have separate centers.

These appear about puberty and usually start to fuse before the 17th year. Fusion of all three is usually complete between the 18th and 20th years and always by the 23rd year (McK. & S.).

(For ununited acromial epiphysis, see fig. 40.)

OSSIFICATION—EPIPHYSES

ANTERIOR VIEW   POSTERIOR VIEW

101   Humerus, proximal epiphysis

The proximal epiphysis fits on to the billowy conical end of the diaphysis. It develops from three centres, (a) one for the head during the 1st year (occasionally before birth), (b) one for the greater tubercle before the end of the 3rd year, (c) and one for the lesser tubercle before the 5th year. These have fused to form a single mass before the 7th year. This mass, or proximal epiphysis, is in some cases completely fused to the diaphysis by the 17th to 18th year and in all cases by the 24th year. (McKern and Stewart.) The centres for the head and lesser tubercle lie on the medial side of the cone; the greater tubercle lies on the lateral side. The epiphyseal plate lies well above the level of the surgical neck, and it cuts through the head medially, i.e., the articular cartilage of the head extends for 2 or 3 mm. on to the diaphysis; hence, the epiphyseal plate cuts into the shoulder joint.

102   Epiphyses at the Elbow Region

The Humerus, distal end:—The lower border of the diaphysis is oblique. It lies well below the levels of the radial, coronoid, and olecranon fossae. Its roller-like surface is ridged and pitted and the distal epiphysis fits it like a trough. There are 4 centres of ossification: for (a) lateral epicondyle, (b) capitulum and lateral part of trochlea, (c) medial part of trochlea, and (d) medial epicondyle. a, b, & c appear about the 12th, 1st, and 10th years respectively and they fuse into a single mass which is probably in all cases completely fused to the diaphysis before the end of the 17th year. It is the first of all long bone epiphyses to fuse. The epiphysis for the medial epicondyle appears about the 6th year and is completely fused to the side of the diaphysis by the end of the 19th year. (McK. & S.) It is quite independent of the main epiphysis.

The Ulna and Radius, proximal ends:—These have one centre each: for (a) olecranon, and (b) head of radius. The olecranon epiphysis is the traction epiphysis of the Triceps. It appears about the 11th year. It may be quite large, in which case it cuts into the trochlear notch (see dotted line). The centre for the head of the radius appears about the 7th year and, like the olecranon epiphysis, is usually completely fused by the 17th or 18th year and always by the 19th year. (McK. & S.) The diameters of the head and neck of a young radius are about equal; but after the 6th or 7th year the head enlarges.

Medial epicondyle

POSTERIOR VIEWS
WITHOUT AND WITH EPIPHYSES

ANTERIOR VIEWS
WITHOUT AND WITH EPIPHYSES

Medial epicondyle

Medial epicondyle

ANTERIOR VIEW

MEDIAL VIEW

ANTERIOR VIEW

MEDIAL VIEW

OSSIFICATION—EPIPHYSES

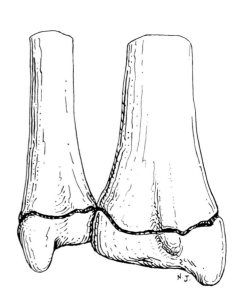

FRONT VIEW   DORSAL VIEW

103   Ulna and Radius, distal ends

The epiphyseal plates of the ulna and radius lie at the same level and cut into the distal radio-ulnar joint. The centre for the radius appears at the end of the 1st year; that for the ulna appears about the 7th year (C. C. Francis). Early stages of fusion occur from the 17th to 20th year; thereafter all cases are either fused or in late stages of fusion, fusion being always complete by the 23rd year (McK. & S.).

OSSIFICATION—EPIPHYSES

104 Bones of the Hand

The capitate starts to ossify soon after birth, or in the female at birth or even before. It is at once followed by the hamate. The triquetrum usually starts at $2\frac{1}{2}$ years; the lunate at $3\frac{1}{2}$ years; the scaphoid, trapezium, and trapezoid (usually in that order) between 5 and 6 years; and the pisiform, which is the last to start, at 10 years.

The metacarpal bones and the phalanges have each one epiphysis. These epiphyses are situated at the distal ends of the metacarpals and at the proximal ends of the phalanges. The metacarpal of the thumb behaves as a phalanx. These epiphyses usually start to ossify before the age of 3 years, and they have fused with their diaphyses before the age of 18 years—the first to fuse being the epiphyses of the distal phalanges, at $15\frac{1}{2}$ years.

(*For details consult W. W. Greulich and S. I. Pyle.*)

OSSIFICATION—EPIPHYSES

Humerus

Radius and Ulna

104.1   Cross Sections of Humerus, Radius, and Ulna

These sections demonstrate the variations in thickness of compact and spongy bone at different levels and at different parts of the same level. They demonstrate also the extent of the medullary cavity.

The Abdomen

Serratus Anterior

5th costal cartilage

Anterior layer
of rectus sheath

Anterior layer
of rectus sheath

Rectus Abdominis

Obliquus Externus

Obliquus Externus

Lateral
cutaneous nerves

Tendinous
intersection

Anterior
cutaneous nerves

Anterior
superior spine

Aponeurosis of
Obliquus Externus

Superf. circumflex
iliac art. & vein

Superficial fascia,
membranous layer

Superf. epigastric
art. & vein

Intercrural fibres

(Superf.) External
pudendal a. & v.

Ilio-inguinal nerve
Spermatic cord

Great (Long)
saphenous vein

105   Anterior Abdominal Wall—I

The anterior layer of the left Rectus sheath is reflected.

Observe:

1. Obliquus Externus, aponeurotic medial to a line that curves upwards from a point 1″ lateral
to the ant. sup. iliac spine to the 5th rib. The aponeurosis gives origin to a slip of Pectoralis
Major.

2. The lateral border of Rectus Abdominis curving from the pubic tubercle, through the mid-
point between the navel and the ant. sup. spine, and across the chest margin to the 5th rib.

3. The anterior cutaneous nerves (Th. 7–12) piercing Rectus and the anterior layer of its
sheath. T. 10 supplies the region of the umbilicus or navel.

4. In the superficial fascia (of Camper), the three superficial inguinal branches of the femoral
artery and the three superficial inguinal tributaries of the great saphenous vein. Of these, the
external pudendal artery and vein cross the spermatic cord.

5. The membranous layer of the superficial fascia (of Scarpa) blending with the fascia lata a
finger's breadth below the inguinal ligament and thereby forming a gutter that empties into
the superficial perineal pouch (of Colles).

6. The spermatic cord and the ilio-inguinal nerve issuing through the superficial. (subcutaneous) inguinal ring.

Serratus Anterior

Anterior layer
of rectus sheath

Obliquus Externus
(cut edges)

Obliquus Internus

Anterior
superior spine

Ilio-hypogastric n.

Ilio-inguinal n.

Saphenous opening
(Fossa ovalis)

Great saphenous v.

Pectoralis Major

Rectus Abdominis

Obliquus Externus
(cut edge)

Superior epigastric
artery

Posterior layer
of rectus sheath

Transversus
Abdominis

Ant. cutaneous nn.

Obliquus Internus
(cut edges)

Arcuate line
(Semicircular line)

Inferior epigastric
artery

Rectus Abdominis

Coverings of
spermatic cord

7th cartilage

Linea Alba

106 Anterior Abdominal Wall—II

On the right side of the body, part of Obliquus Externus is excised. On the left,
Rectus Abdominis is excised and Obliquus Internus divided.

Observe:

1. Obliquus Internus fibers running horizontally at the level of the ant. sup. spine; running obliquely upwards above this level, and obliquely downwards below it.

2. The two anterior branches of nerve L. 1 piercing Obliquus Internus infero-medial to the
   ant. sup. spine and running forwards and medially; the upper branch then piercing Obliquus
   Externus aponeurosis; the lower lying within $\frac{1}{2}''$ of the inguinal lig. and passing through the
   superficial (subcutaneous) inguinal ring with the spermatic cord.

3. The arcuate line at the level of the ant. sup. iliac spine.

4. The anastomosis between the superior and inferior epigastric arteries which indirectly unites
   the arteries of the upper limb with those of the lower.

5. Nerves Th. 7–12, but not L. 1, entering the Rectus sheath. Of these nerves, the upper ones
   ascend, the lower ones descend.

6. Obliquus Externus attached a hand's breadth above the costal margin; Obliquus Internus
   to the margin; and Transversus within the margin.

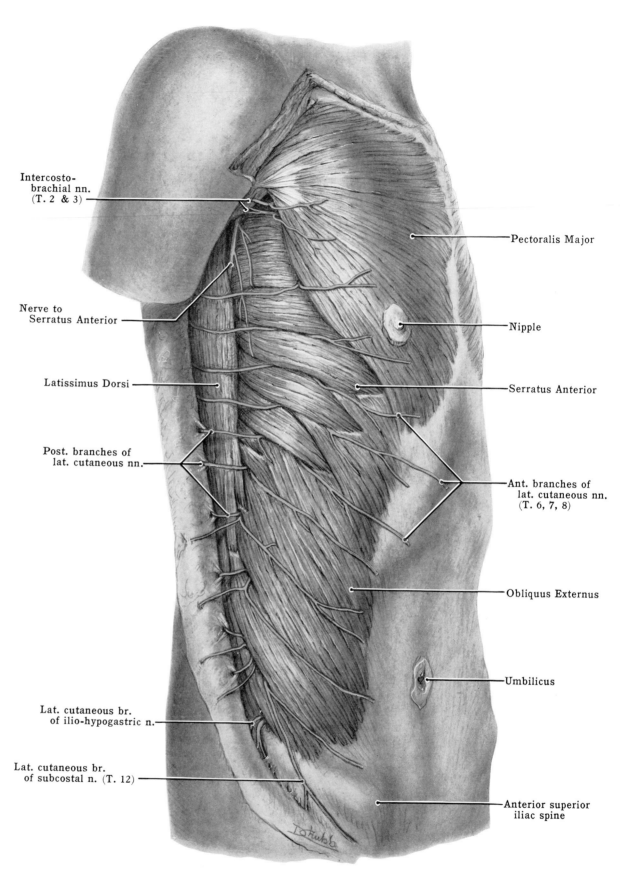

Intercosto-
brachial nn.
(T. 2 & 3)

Nerve to
Serratus Anterior

Latissimus Dorsi

Post. branches of
lat. cutaneous nn.

Lat. cutaneous br.
of ilio-hypogastric n.

Lat. cutaneous br.
of subcostal n. (T. 12)

Pectoralis Major

Nipple

Serratus Anterior

Ant. branches of
lat. cutaneous nn.
(T. 6, 7, 8)

Obliquus Externus

Umbilicus

Anterior superior
iliac spine

107   Lateral Cutaneous Nerves

Note twigs supplying Obliquus Externus. The shoulder is pushed forwards, hence
the nerve to Serratus is partly concealed by Latissimus.

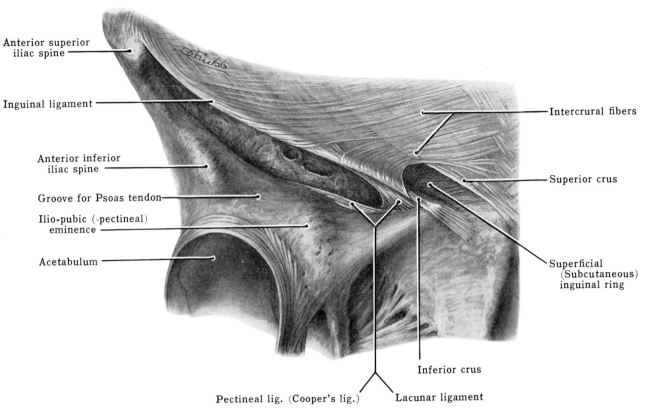

Anterior superior iliac spine

Inguinal ligament

Anterior inferior iliac spine

Groove for Psoas tendon

Ilio-pubic (-pectineal) eminence

Acetabulum

Intercrural fibers

Superior crus

Superficial (Subcutaneous) inguinal ring

Inferior crus

Pectineal lig. (Cooper's lig.)

Lacunar ligament

108 Inguinal Ligament, antero-inferior view

Observe:

1. The inguinal ligament extending from the medial part of the tip of the anterior superior iliac spine to the pubic tubercle, and receiving accessions of fibres from the lower part of the External Oblique.

2. The fibres of the ligament that, falling short of the pubic tubercle, find attachment to the pecten pubis as the lacunar ligament. This ligament forms the medial border of the lacuna, or space, called the femoral ring.

3. The unnamed fibres that, extending beyond the pubic tubercle, find attachment to the front of the body of the pubis.

4. The pectineal ligament whose fibres run along the pecten pubis (pectineal line).

5. The groove for Psoas tendon situated between the anterior inferior spine and the iliopubic eminence. Note that this groove descends to the acetabulum.

6. The inferior crus of the superficial inguinal ring formed by the inguinal ligament, which is rounded; the superior crus formed by the aponeurosis of External Oblique, which is sharp.

7. The space between the inguinal ligament and the hip bone. The lateral part transmits Iliacus, Psoas, femoral nerve, and lateral cutaneous nerve of the thigh. The medial part transmits the femoral artery, vein, and lymph vessels and the genital branch of the genitofemoral nerve (ext. spermatic nerve).

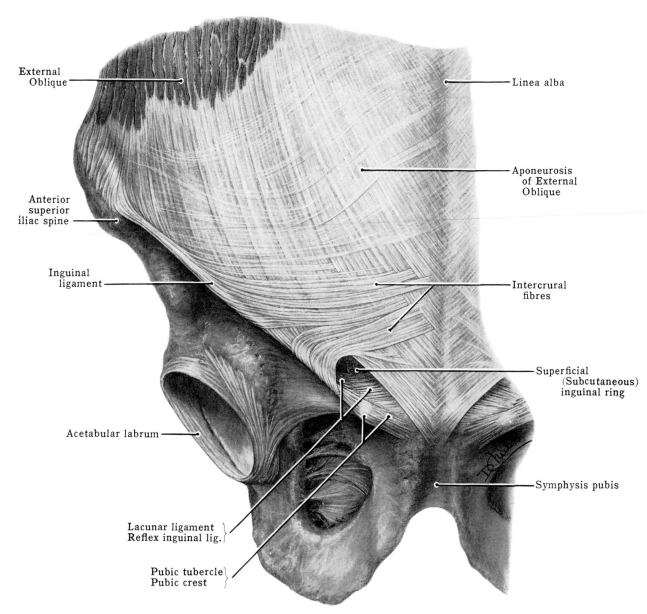

External Oblique

Linea alba

Anterior superior iliac spine

Aponeurosis of External Oblique

Inguinal ligament

Intercrural fibres

Superficial (Subcutaneous) inguinal ring

Acetabular labrum

Symphysis pubis

Lacunar ligament } Reflex inguinal lig. }

Pubic tubercle } Pubic crest }

109   Inguinal Region—I

Aponeurosis of External Oblique: Superficial Inguinal Ring.

Observe:

1. The linea alba to be not an unyielding ligament uniting the sternum to the symphysis pubis, but a line across which fibres decussate in bias and therefore extensible.

2. The intercrural fibres, well developed in this specimen, preventing the crura of the inguinal ring from spreading. (See also fig. 105.)

3. The superficial inguinal ring to be triangular in shape, its central point being above the pubic tubercle, its base being the lateral half of the pubic crest, its inferior side or crus being the inguinal ligament, and its superior side or crus being fibres of External Oblique aponeurosis which cross the pubic crest at its mid point.

4. Behind the ring, some fibres of External Oblique aponeurosis from the opposite side passing to the pubic crest and pecten pubis (pectineal line). These constitute the reflected inguinal ligament.

5. Most of the fleshy fibres, here shown, of External Oblique sending their tendinous fibres to join the inguinal ligament.

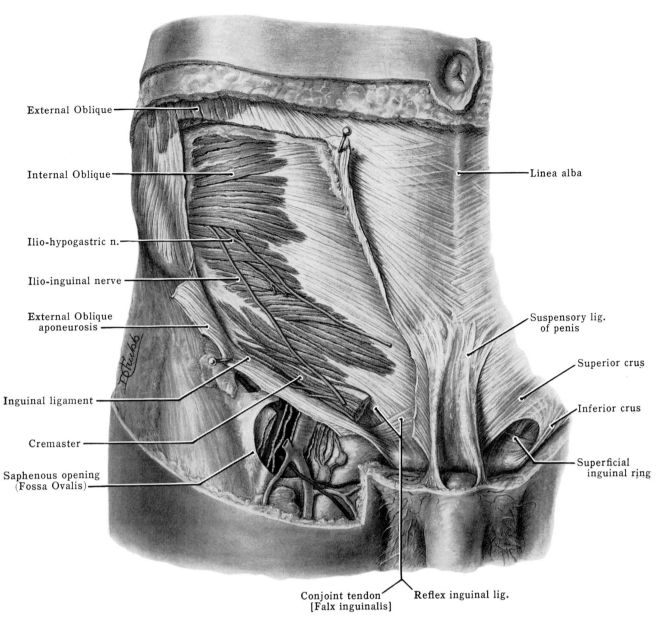

External Oblique

Internal Oblique

Ilio-hypogastric n.

Ilio-inguinal nerve

External Oblique
aponeurosis

Inguinal ligament

Cremaster

Saphenous opening
(Fossa Ovalis)

Linea alba

Suspensory lig.
of penis

Superior crus

Inferior crus

Superficial
inguinal ring

Conjoint tendon
[Falx inguinalis]

Reflex inguinal lig.

110 Inguinal Region—II

Internal Oblique and Cremaster Muscles.
(External Obliquue aponeurosis is partly cut away and the spermatic cord is cut short.)

Observe:

1. The laminated, suspensory lig. of the penis descending to the junction of the fixed and mobile parts of the organ.

2. The reflex inguinal lig., which represents External Oblique, lying anterior to the conjoint tendon [falx inguinalis] which represents Internal Oblique and Transversus.

3. The only two structures that course between External and Internal Obliques, namely, the ilio-hypogastric and ilio-inguinal branches of the 1st lumbar nerve segment. They are sensory from this point to their terminations.

4. The fleshy fibres of Internal Oblique at the level of the anterior superior spine running horizontally; those from the iliac crest passing medio-cranially; and those from the inguinal ligament arching medio-caudally.

5. The Cremaster muscle covering the cord and filling the arched space between conjoint tendon and inguinal ligament.

6. At the level of the navel, the aponeurosis of External Oblique blending with the aponeurosis of Internal Oblique near the lateral border of the Rectus, but in the suprapubic region free as far as the median plane.

7. The numerous lymph vessels (not labelled) streaming cranially around the femoral artery and vein.

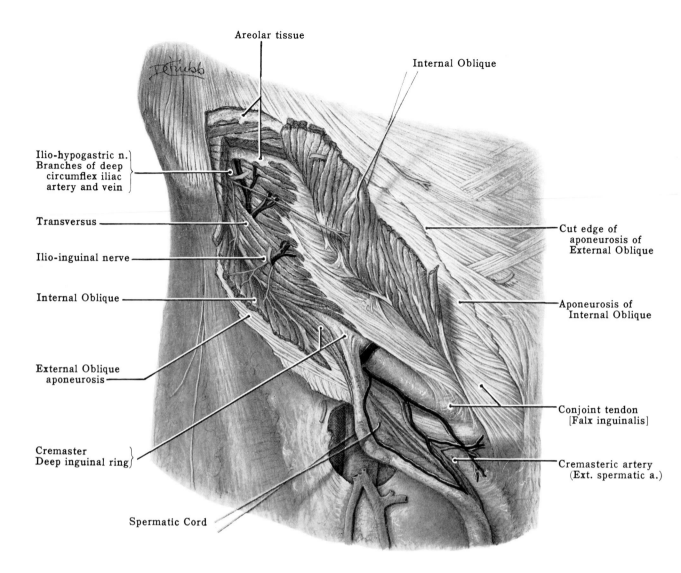

Areolar tissue

Internal Oblique

Ilio-hypogastric n.
Branches of deep
circumflex iliac
artery and vein

Transversus

Ilio-inguinal nerve

Internal Oblique

External Oblique
aponeurosis

Cremaster
Deep inguinal ring

Spermatic Cord

Cut edge of
aponeurosis of
External Oblique

Aponeurosis of
Internal Oblique

Conjoint tendon
[Falx inguinalis]

Cremasteric artery
(Ext. spermatic a.)

111 Inguinal Region—III

(Internal Oblique is reflected and the spermatic cord is retracted.)

Observe:

1. Transversus fibres taking, in this region, the same common medio-caudal direction as the fibres of External Oblique aponeurosis and Internal Oblique.
2. Transversus having a less extensive origin from the inguinal ligament than Internal Oblique.
3. The Internal Oblique portion of the conjoint tendon attached to the pubic crest; Transversus portion extending laterally along the pecten pubis (pectineal line).
4. Conjoint tendon not sharply defined from fascia transversalis, but blending with it.
5. Segment lumbar I, via the ilio-hypogastric and ilio-inguinal nerves, supplying the fibres of Internal Oblique and Transversus that control the conjoint tendon.
6. Fascia transversalis evaginated to form the tubular internal spermatic fascia. The mouth of the tube, called the deep (abdominal) inguinal ring, situated lateral to the inferior epigastric vessels.
7. The cremasteric artery (a branch of the inf. epigastric art.) which in figure 119 is seen to anastomose with the testicular artery and the artery to the deferent duct (vas deferens).
8. The Cremaster muscle arising from the inguinal ligament.

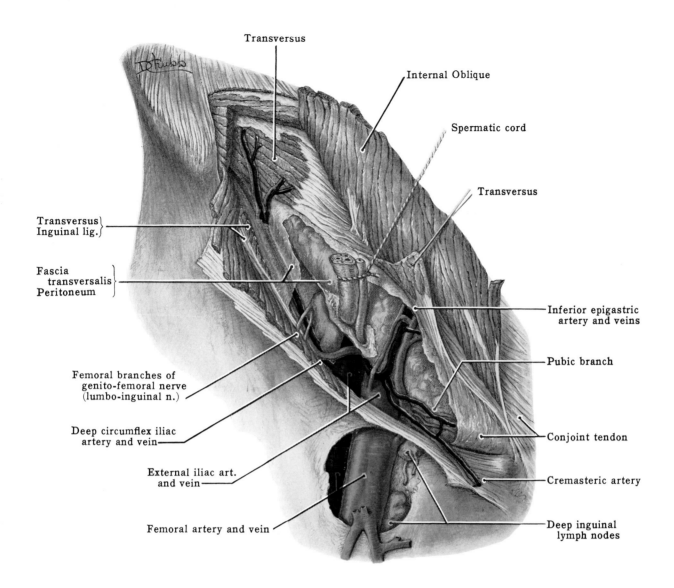

Transversus

Internal Oblique

Spermatic cord

Transversus

Transversus
Inguinal lig.

Fascia
transversalis
Peritoneum

Inferior epigastric
artery and veins

Pubic branch

Femoral branches of
genito-femoral nerve
(lumbo-inguinal n.)

Deep circumflex iliac
artery and vein

Conjoint tendon

External iliac art.
and vein

Cremasteric artery

Femoral artery and vein

Deep inguinal
lymph nodes

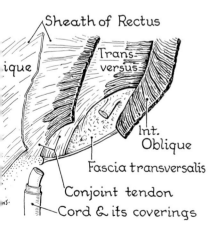

Sheath of Rectus

Trans-
versus

ique

Int.
Oblique

Fascia transversalis

Conjoint tendon

Cord & its coverings

11.1

emonstrating the continuity of Rectus
eath with conjoint tendon.

112   Inguinal Region—IV

(The inguinal part of Transversus and fascia transversalis are partly cut away and the spermatic cord is retracted.)

Observe:

1. The lower limit of the peritoneal sac. It lies some distance above the inguinal ligament laterally but close to it medially.

2. The location of the deep (abdominal) inguinal ring—a finger's breadth above the inguinal ligament at the midpoint between the anterior superior spine and the pubic tubercle.

3. The testicular vessels and the deferent duct (retracted) starting to part company at the deep inguinal ring.

4. The proximity of the external iliac artery and vein to the inguinal canal.

5. The only two branches of the external iliac artery, namely, the deep circumflex iliac artery and the inferior epigastric artery; also the cremasteric and pubic branches of the latter.

Peritoneum ——————8.
Subperitoneal fat ————7.
Fascia transversalis ——6.
Transversus ——————5.
Internal Oblique ————4.
External Oblique ————3.
  aponeurosis
Subcutaneous fat ————2.
Skin ———————————I.

Inferior epigastric art.   Obliterated umbilical art.   Urac. or Blad.

Constituents of the cord { 8 7
Coverings of the cord { 6 5. 4 3

Scrotum:
  Colles' fascia }
  Dartos muscle} — 2
Skin — I

113 Scheme of the Inguinal Canal

The Eight Layers of the Abdominal Wall and their Evaginations.

(In this schematic horizontal section, the scrotum and testis are assumed to have been raised to the level of the superficial inguinal ring.)

The evaginations become the scrotum, the coverings of the spermatic cord, and two of the contents of that cord.

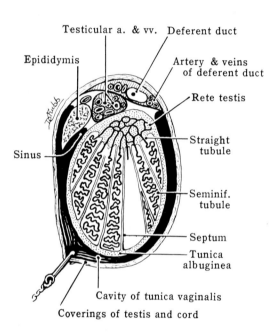

Testicular a. & vv.   Deferent duct
Epididymis
Artery & veins of deferent duct
Rete testis
Straight tubule
Sinus
Seminif. tubule
Septum
Tunica albuginea
Cavity of tunica vaginalis
Coverings of testis and cord

114 Testis on Cross Section

(RIGHT TESTIS, VIEWED FROM ABOVE.)

Observe:

1. The cavity of the tunica vaginalis testis surrounding the testis in front and at the sides and extending between testis and epididymis as the sinus of the epididymis.

2. The epididymis lying postero-lateral to the testis. It indicates to which side a testis belongs, for it is on the right side of a right testis and on the left side of a left testis.

3. The deferent duct with its fine lumen and thick wall lying postero-medial to the testis.

4. The 3 groups of longitudinal veins (a) around the testicular artery, (b) medial to the duct with the artery of the duct, and (c) lateral to it.

5. The pyramidal compartments for the seminiferous tubules, shown semi-diagrammatically. Each of the 250 compartments contains two or three hair-like seminiferous tubules which join in the mediastinum testis to form a rete.

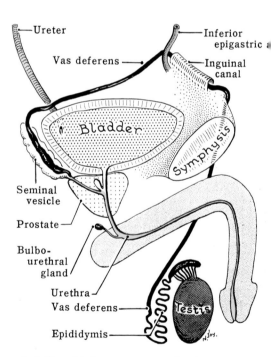

Ureter
Vas deferens
Inferior epigastric a.
Inguinal canal
Bladder
Symphysis
Seminal vesicle
Prostate
Bulbo-urethral gland
Urethra
Vas deferens
Testis
Epididymis

115 Diagram of the Male Genital System

indicating the course of the deferent duct. (The ejaculatory duct and the utriculus, both within the prostate, are not labelled.)

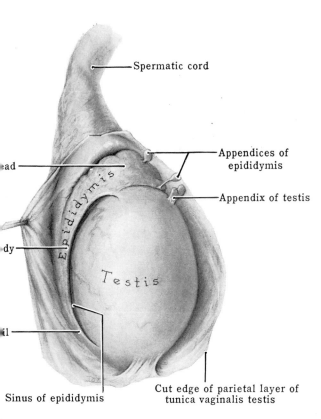

Spermatic cord

Appendices of
epididymis

Appendix of testis

ad

Epididymis

dy

Testis

l

Sinus of epididymis

Cut edge of parietal layer of
tunica vaginalis testis

16 Testis, lateral view

e tunica vaginalis testis has been incised longitudinally.

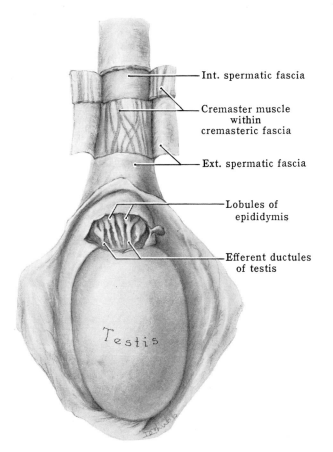

Int. spermatic fascia

Cremaster muscle
within
cremasteric fascia

Ext. spermatic fascia

Lobules of
epididymis

Efferent ductules
of testis

Testis

117 Coverings of Spermatic Cord: Efferent Ductules

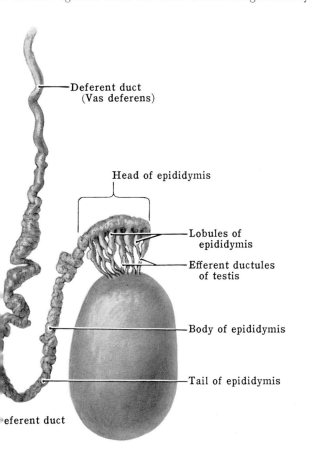

Deferent duct
(Vas deferens)

Head of epididymis

Lobules of
epididymis

Efferent ductules
of testis

Body of epididymis

Tail of epididymis

eferent duct

18 Epididymis

te the eight efferent ductules uniting the epididymis to
upper pole of the testis.

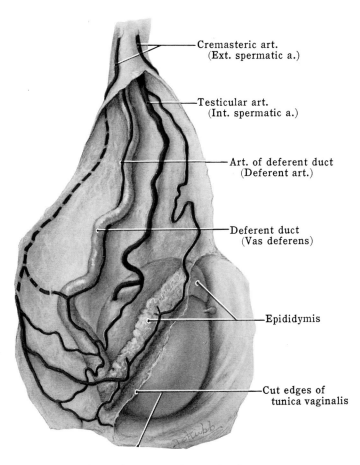

Cremasteric art.
(Ext. spermatic a.)

Testicular art.
(Int. spermatic a.)

Art. of deferent duct
(Deferent art.)

Deferent duct
(Vas deferens)

Epididymis

Cut edges of
tunica vaginalis

119 Blood Supply of the Testis

The epididymis is displaced slightly to the lateral side. Note
the free anastomosis between the three arteries.

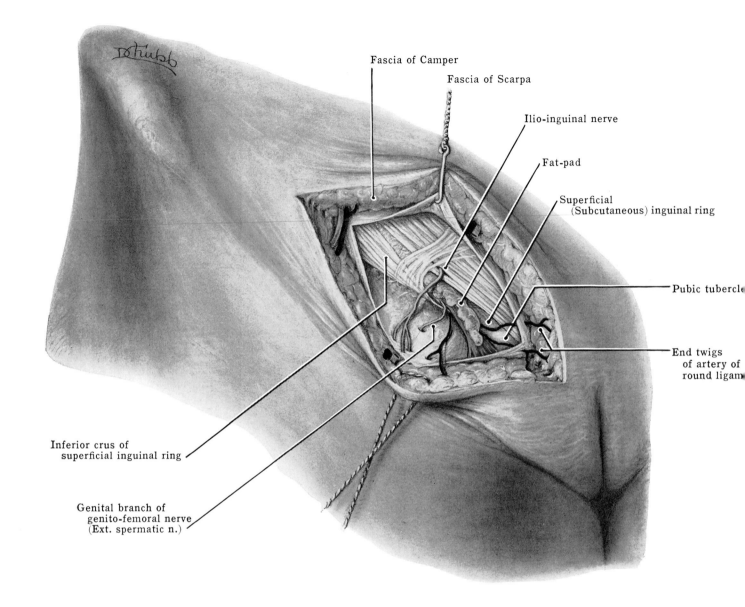

Fascia of Camper

Fascia of Scarpa

Ilio-inguinal nerve

Fat-pad

Superficial
(Subcutaneous) inguinal ring

Pubic tubercle

End twigs
of artery of
round ligam

Inferior crus of
superficial inguinal ring

Genital branch of
genito-femoral nerve
(Ext. spermatic n.)

120, 121, 122, and 123 Stages in the Dissection of the Female Inguinal Canal

Observe:

1. In 120, the superficial inguinal ring, small and its crura prevented by the intercrural fibres from spreading.

2. Issuing from the superficial inguinal ring: (a) the round ligament of the uterus (lig. teres uteri), (b) a closely applied pad of fat, (c) the genital branch of the genito-femoral nerve, and (d) the artery of the round ligament of the uterus. This artery is homologous with the cremasteric artery in the male shown in figure 112.

3. The ilio-inguinal nerve, here as commonly, perforating the superior crus of the superficial inguinal ring.

4. In 121, the Cremaster muscle, not extending beyond the ring.

5. In 122, the round ligament breaking up into strands as it leaves the inguinal canal and approaches the labium majus.

6. In 123, the close relationship of the external iliac artery and vein to the inguinal canal.

Fig. 121

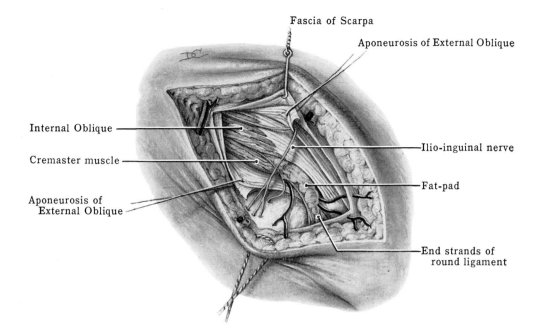

Fascia of Scarpa

Aponeurosis of External Oblique

Internal Oblique

Cremaster muscle

Aponeurosis of
External Oblique

Ilio-inguinal nerve

Fat-pad

End strands of
round ligament

Fig. 122

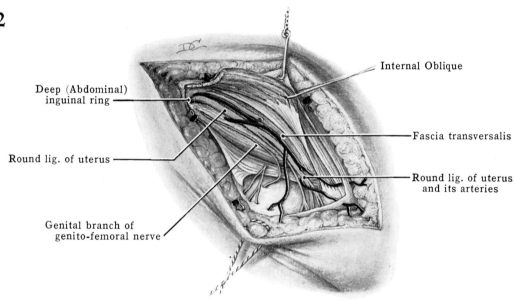

Deep (Abdominal)
inguinal ring

Internal Oblique

Round lig. of uterus

Fascia transversalis

Genital branch of
genito-femoral nerve

Round lig. of uterus
and its arteries

Fig. 123

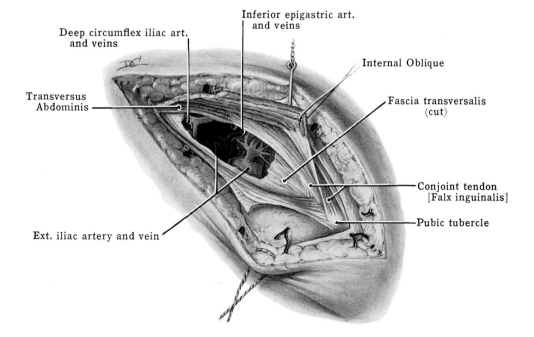

Deep circumflex iliac art.
and veins

Inferior epigastric art.
and veins

Internal Oblique

Transversus
Abdominis

Fascia transversalis
(cut)

Conjoint tendon
[Falx inguinalis]

Pubic tubercle

Ext. iliac artery and vein

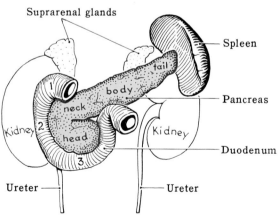

Digestive System Apparatus

This system extends from the li
to the anus.

Here is a list of its chief parts:

CAVITY OF THE MOUTH OR CAVUM ORIS
Vestibule of mouth
  Lips or labia
  Cheeks or buccae
  Gums or gingivae
  Teeth or dentes
Cavity proper of mouth
Palate
  hard
  soft
Tongue or lingua
Salivary glands
  Parotid
  Sublingual
  Submandibular
Palato-glossal arch

CAVITY OF THE PHARYNX
Oral part
  Palatine tonsil
Laryngeal part
  Entrance, or aditus, to larynx

ALIMENTARY CANAL
Esophagus
  Cervical part
  Thoracic part
  Abdominal part
Stomach or Ventriculus or Gaste
  Cardiac orifice
  Incisura cardiaca
  Greater curvature
  Lesser curvature
    Incisura angularis
  Fundus
  Body
  Pyloric part
    Pyloric antrum
    Pyloric canal
    Pylorus
      Pyloric orifice
Small intestine
  Duodenum
    1st or superior part
    2nd or descending part
    3rd or inferior part
      horizontal part
      ascending part (4th)
  Duodeno-jejunal flexure
  Jejunum
  Ileum
  Ileo-cecal orifice and valve
Large intestine
  Vermiform appendix
  Cecum
  Ascending colon
  Right colic flexure
    (Hepatic flexure)
  Transverse colon
  Left colic flexure
    (Splenic flexure)
  Descending colon
  Sigmoid colon
  Rectum
  Anal canal
  Anus

ASSOCIATED ORGANS
Liver or Hepar
  Gall bladder
    fundus, body, and neck
  Biliary passages
Pancreas
  head, neck, body, tail, and du
Spleen or Lien

124 Diagram of the Main Parts of the Digestive System

In the lower figure, 3 organs—spleen, pancreas, and duodenum—are uncovered by removal of the stomach and the transverse colon.

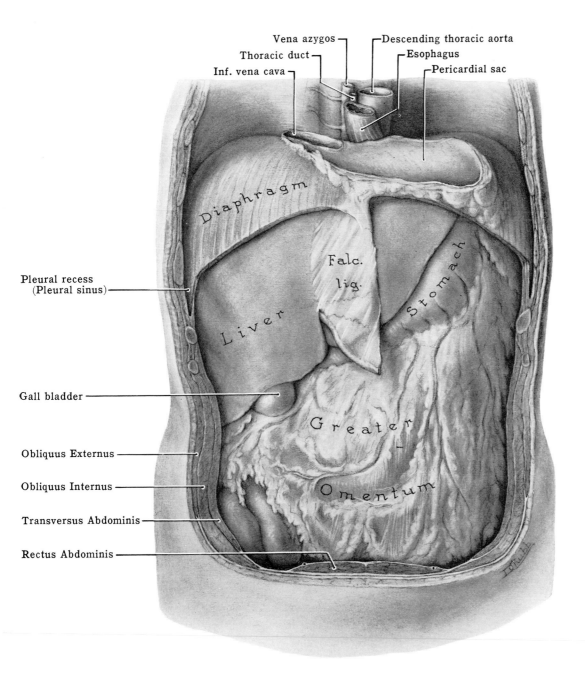

Vena azygos —
Thoracic duct —
Inf. vena cava —
Descending thoracic aorta
Esophagus
Pericardial sac

Diaphragm

Falc. lig.

Stomach

Pleural recess (Pleural sinus) —

Liver

Gall bladder —

Greater

Obliquus Externus —

Obliquus Internus —

Omentum

Transversus Abdominis —

Rectus Abdominis —

125 Abdominal Contents, undisturbed

The anterior abdominal and thoracic walls are cut away.

Observe

1. The falciform lig., with the lig. teres in its free edge, severed at its attachment to the abdominal wall and Diaphragm in the median plane. Its attachment to the liver is its own width to the right of the median plane.

2. The gall bladder projecting below the sharp, inferior border of the liver.

3. The two Recti meeting in the median plane above the pubis.

4. Obliquus Internus, the thickest of the three flat abdominal muscles.

5. The pleural cavities separating the upper abdominal viscera from the body wall.

6. Two thirds of the pericardial sac lying to the left of the median plane; its apex, i.e. the lowest and leftmost point, overlying the stomach. Behind are the two lungs (removed), esophagus and aorta.

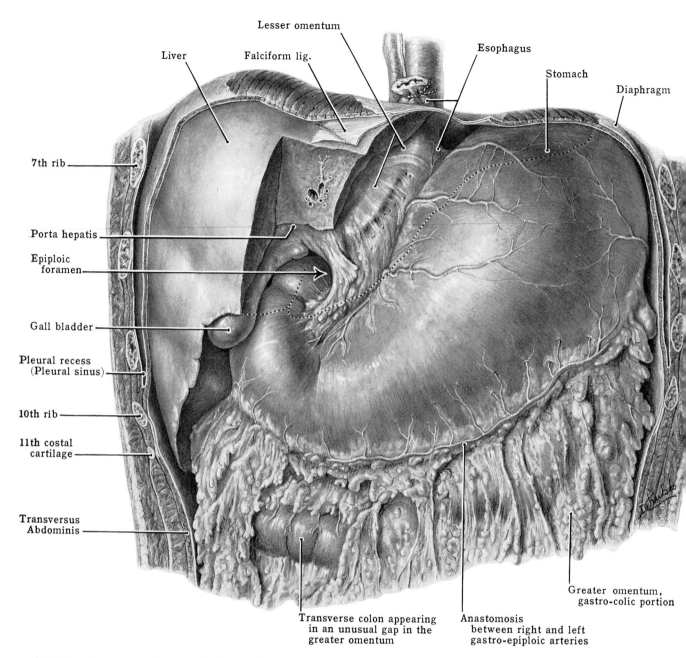

Lesser omentum

Liver   Falciform lig.   Esophagus

Stomach

Diaphragm

7th rib

Porta hepatis

Epiploic foramen

Gall bladder

Pleural recess (Pleural sinus)

10th rib

11th costal cartilage

Transversus Abdominis

Transverse colon appearing in an unusual gap in the greater omentum

Anastomosis between right and left gastro-epiploic arteries

Greater omentum, gastro-colic portion

126   Stomach and the Omenta, front view

The stomach is inflated with air; the left part of the liver is cut away.

Observe:

1. The pyloric end of the stomach which has moved to the right and has come to lie below, or rather infero-posterior to, the gall bladder; the 1st or superior part of the duodenum—placed behind the arrow head—almost occluding the epiploic foramen (mouth of the lesser sac).

2. The medial or left border of the gall bladder, followed cranially, leading to the free margin of the lesser omentum, and hence acting as a guide to the epiploic foramen, which lies behind the free margin.

3. The lesser omentum passing from the lesser curvature of the stomach and first inch of the duodenum to the fissure for the lig. venosum and porta hepatis. This omentum thickened at its free margin but elsewhere like gossamer, much perforated, and with the caudate lobe of the liver visible through it.

4. The greater omentum hanging from the greater curvature of the stomach.

5. The right cupola of the diaphragm rising higher than the left cupola, which is usual.

6. The relative thinness of the Transversus Abdominis. The pleural recess, about two fingers breadth above the costal margin in the mid-lateral line.

127 Stomach, front view

The cardiac notch and the angular notch [incisura angularis] are here well marked. The pyloric antrum is here not demarcated from the tubular pyloric canal.

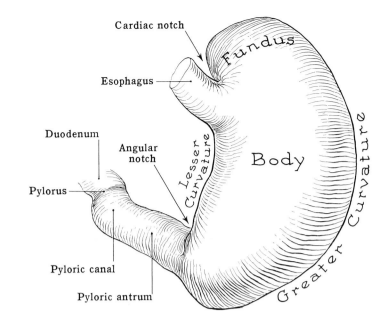

128 Mucous Membrane of the Stomach

Along the lesser curvature several longitudinal ridges extend from esophagus to pylorus, elsewhere the mucous membrane is rugose when the stomach is empty.

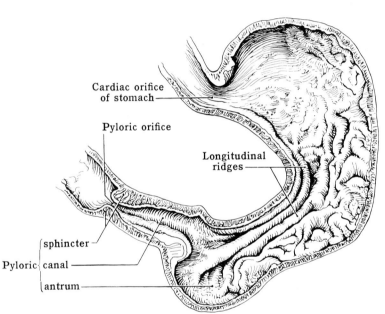

129 Muscular Coat of the Stomach, from within

The stomach is cut along the greater curvature and the loosely adherent mucous and submucous coats are dissected off.

The fibres of the innermost or oblique muscle layer form ⋂-shaped loops that extend over the fundus and down both surfaces of the stomach as far as the antrum. Their medial limit is at the cardiac notch, hence the fibres of the middle or circular layer become the innermost layer along the lesser curvature and in the pyloric region; at the pylorus they are thickened to form the pyloric sphincter. They are present everywhere except at the fundus. The fibres of the outermost or longitudinal layer (not seen) are best marked along the curvatures.

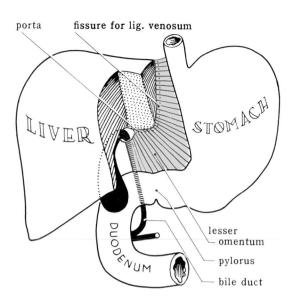

porta   fissure for lig. venosum

LIVER   STOMACH

DUODENUM

lesser omentum

pylorus

bile duct

130   Diagram of the Attachments of the Lesser Omentum

Two sagittal cuts have been made through the liver—one at the fissure for the lig. venosum; the other at the right limit of the porta hepatis. These two cuts have been joined by a coronal cut.

Note:

1. The lesser omentum may be regarded as the "mesentery" of the bile passages, seeing they occupy its free edge.
2. The lesser omentum extends from the lesser curvature of the stomach and first inch of the duodenum to the fissure for the lig. venosum and to the porta. The part attached to the body of the stomach passes to the fissure; the part attached to the pyloric part of the stomach and duodenum passes to the porta.

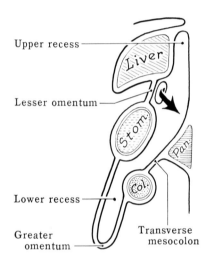

Upper recess

Liver

Lesser omentum

Stom.

Pan.

Col.

Lower recess

Greater omentum

Transverse mesocolon

130.1   Diagram Showing the Vertical Extent of the Omental Bursa (Lesser Sac) in the median plane

The arrow passes from the greater sac of peritoneum through the epiploic foramen (mouth of the lesser sac) into the lesser sac.

Note the 3 approaches to the lesser sac: it may be opened by tearing through (a) the lesser omentum, (b) the greater omentum, or (c) the transverse mesocolon.

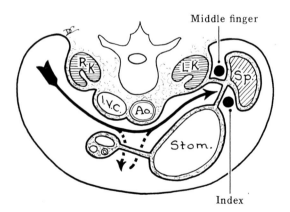

Middle finger

R.K.   L.K.   Sp.

I.V.C.   Ao.

Stom.

Index

130.2   Diagram Showing the Horizontal Extent of the Omental Bursa (Lesser Sac) at the Level of its Mouth, the Epiploic Foramen. The Pedicle of the Spleen

Instructions:

1. While standing on the right side of the body, run your right middle finger upwards between the left kidney and the spleen, and your right index upwards between the stomach and the spleen. The 'pedicle or stalk' of the spleen now lies in the cleft between these two fingers, as though in a clamp. The pedicle has a free lower border (and a free upper border), or you could not grasp it as you are doing. Its linear site of attachment to the spleen is around the hilus.
2. Clamped between your index and middle finger are four layers of peritoneum. Of this you can satisfy yourself by passing your left index through the epiploic foramen and across the abdomen, behind the stomach, till it touches the spleen between your two right fingers. If your left index will not reach all the way, pass it as far as it will go, tear through the lesser omentum over its tip, withdraw the finger, and reinsert it at the half-way opening just made. The hilus of the spleen, which you are palpating, is situated at the left extremity of the omental bursa.

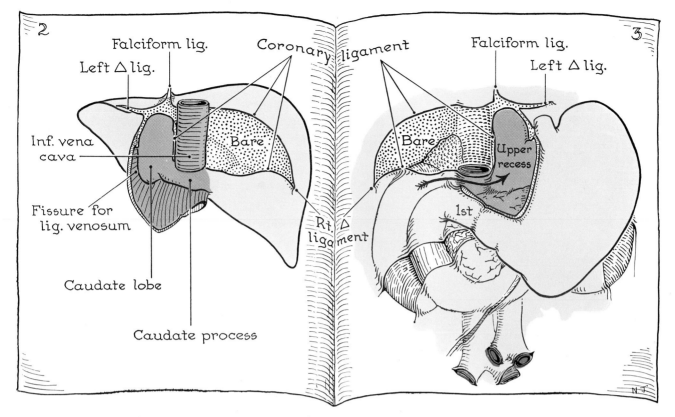

131 Diagram of the Peritoneal Ligaments of the Liver

(The attachments of the liver are cut through and the liver is turned to the right side of the cadaver, i.e. to the left of the picture, as you would turn the page of a book. Hence, the posterior aspect of the liver is shown on page 2 and its posterior relations on page 3.

Note:

1. The arrow passing from the greater sac of peritoneum (yellow) into the lesser sac (orange).

2. The upper recess of the lesser sac, or omental bursa, occupies the median plane of the body. Dorsally lies the descending thoracic aorta, diaphragm intervening (fig. 131.1). Ventrally is the lesser omentum. On the left is esophagus, and on the right is inf. vena cava, both of which lie bare on the diaphragm.

3. The inferior vena cava occupies the left or medial limit of the bare area of the liver.

4. The bare area is triangular; hence, the so-called coronary ligament is not a corona, but is three-sided. Its left side or

base is between the i.v. cava and the caudate lobe; it is palpated when the right index is inserted into the upper recess.

5. Its apex is at the right triangular ligament, where the cranial and caudal layers of the coronary ligament meet.

6. The lower or caudal layer of the ligament is reflected from the liver on to the diaphragm, right kidney, and right suprarenal gland. It is called the hepato-renal ligament by the surgeon. Followed medially this layer crosses the i.v. cava at the mouth of the lesser sac, and turning cranially becomes the left or basal layer of the ligament (fig. 177).

7. The lesser omentum is divided close to the stomach. It is not labelled, nor is the kidney, nor the suprarenal gland.

131.1

Diagram of the upper recess of the omental bursa (lesser sac) on cross-section to show its relations, viewed from below.

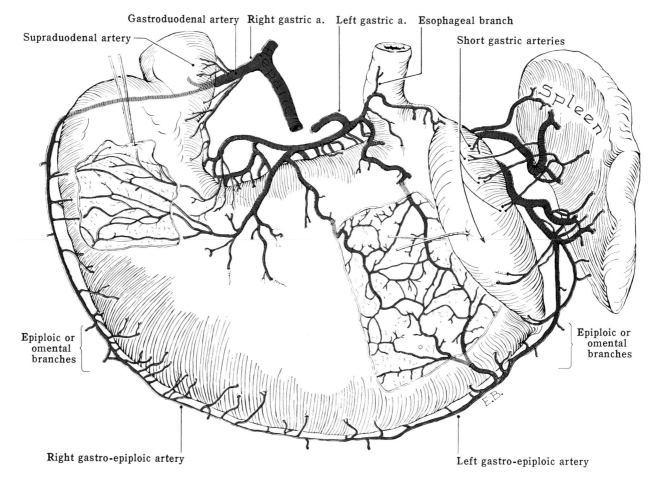

Supraduodenal artery — Gastroduodenal artery — Right gastric a. — Left gastric a. — Esophageal branch — Short gastric arteries — Spleen — Epiploic or omental branches — Epiploic or omental branches — Right gastro-epiploic artery — Left gastro-epiploic artery

132   Dissection of the Arteries of the Stomach and Spleen

The serous and muscular coats are removed from two areas of the stomach, thereby revealing the anastomotic networks in the submucous coat.

Observe:

1. The arterial arch on the lesser curvature formed by the larger left gastric artery and completed by the much smaller right gastric artery.
2. The arterial arch on the greater curvature formed equally by the right and the left gastro-epiploic artery. The anas-

tomosis between their two trunks is attenuated; commonly it is absent.

3. The anastomoses between the branches of the two foregoing arterial arches taking place in the submucous coat two-thirds of the distance from lesser to greater curvature.
4. Four or five tenuous short gastric arteries leaving the terminal branches of the splenic artery close to the spleen; and the left gastro-epiploic artery, belonging to the short gastric artery series, arising within 2.5 cm. of the hilus of the spleen.

(For details consult Michels, N. A.)

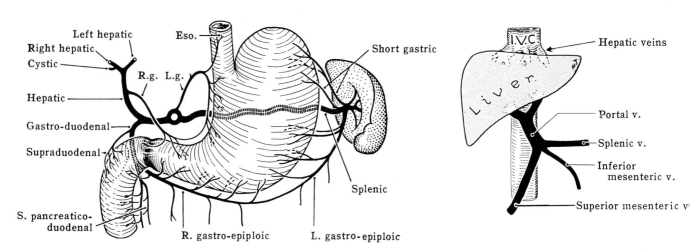

Left hepatic — Right hepatic — Cystic — Eso. — Short gastric — R.g. L.g. — Hepatic — Gastro-duodenal — Supraduodenal — S. pancreatico-duodenal — R. gastro-epiploic — L. gastro-epiploic — Splenic — I.V.C — Liver — Hepatic veins — Portal v. — Splenic v. — Inferior mesenteric v. — Superior mesenteric v.

132.1   Scheme of the distribution of the celiac trunk (artery).

132.2   Diagram of the blood from the gastro-intestinal apparatus entering the liver via the portal vein and leaving it via the hepatic veins to enter the inf. vena cava.

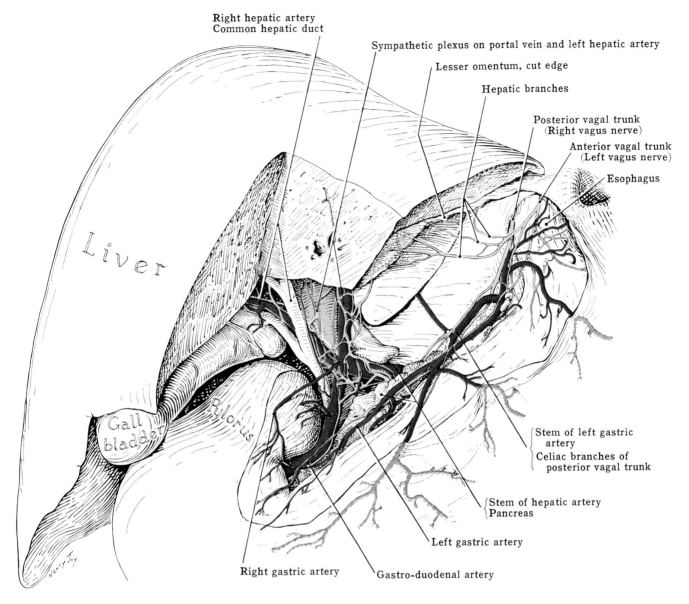

Right hepatic artery
Common hepatic duct

Sympathetic plexus on portal vein and left hepatic artery

Lesser omentum, cut edge

Hepatic branches

Posterior vagal trunk
(Right vagus nerve)

Anterior vagal trunk
(Left vagus nerve)

Esophagus

Liver

Gall bladder

Pylorus

Stem of left gastric
artery

Celiac branches of
posterior vagal trunk

Stem of hepatic artery
Pancreas

Left gastric artery

Right gastric artery

Gastro-duodenal artery

133 Vagus Nerves within the Abdomen

The liver is divided, as in figure 130-A. The lesser omentum is removed, except at its attachment to the fissure for the lig. venosum where a fringe remains; this fringe lies ventral to the caudate lobe (not labelled). The two ends of the stomach and the lesser curvature are in view.

Observe:

1. The posterior vagal trunk and the anterior vagal trunk applied to the esophagus and entering the abdomen through the esophageal hiatus in the diaphragm.

2. These two nerves then running near each other along the lesser curvature of the stomach, communicating with each other, supplying the respective surfaces of the stomach, and extending to the pyloric antrum.

3. The stout celiac branch of the posterior vagal trunk, dividing and descending along the stem of the left gastric artery

to the celiac ganglia (fig. 180). Thence it is distributed mostly with the sympathetic plexuses along the blood vessels to the abdominal viscera (spleen, pancreas, kidneys, and intestines as far as the left colic flexure fig. 660).

4. The hepatic branches of the anterior vagal trunk running between the two layers of the lesser omentum to the liver, and there joining sympathetic fibres from the celiac plexus that are ascending with the hepatic artery to the liver.

5. A lower branch (not shown), in series with the hepatic branches, turns downwards in the lesser omentum from near the porta and sends twigs (a) to the pylorus and 1st part of duodenum, (b) with the right gastric artery to the pyloric canal, (c) with the gastroduodenal artery to the 2nd part of the duodenum and the head of the pancreas, and (d) a branch turns upwards on the hepatic artery to communicate with the sympathetic fibres passing to the gall bladder (E. D. McCrea)

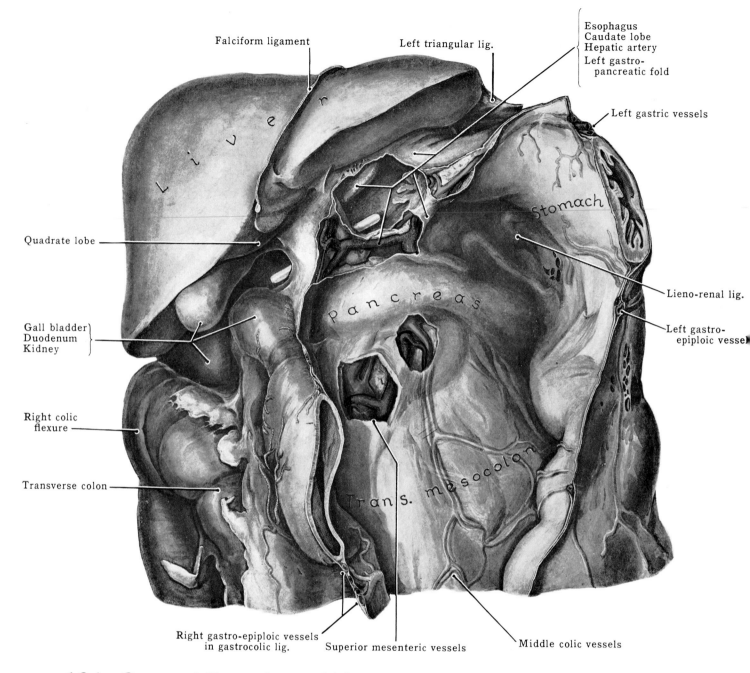

Falciform ligament

Left triangular lig.

Esophagus
Caudate lobe
Hepatic artery
Left gastro-
pancreatic fold

Left gastric vessels

Liver

Stomach

Quadrate lobe

Pancreas

Lieno-renal lig.

Gall bladder
Duodenum
Kidney

Left gastro-
epiploic vessel

Right colic
flexure

Transverse colon

Trans. mesocolon

Right gastro-epiploic vessels
in gastrocolic lig.

Superior mesenteric vessels

Middle colic vessels

134 Omental Bursa in an Older Subject, opened—I

The anterior wall of the bursa, consisting of the stomach with its two omenta and the vessels along its two curvatures, has been divided vertically and the two parts have been turned aside.

Observe:

1. The esophagus and body of the stomach on the left side of the cadaver, and the pyloric part and the superior (1st) part of the duodenum on the right side. This part of the duodenum running backwards, upwards and to the right, and having the gall bladder and quadrate lobe in contact with it above.

2. The kidney forming the posterior wall of the hepato-renal pouch, and the white rod passed from the pouch, through the epiploic foramen, into the omental bursa.

3. The pancreas on the posterior wall of the bursa, moulded on the vertebral column, and lying roughly horizontally. Below this, the transverse mesocolon, the root of which has slipped caudally from its attachment to the pancreas.

4. Above the pancreas, the left gastro-pancreatic fold, which is the "mesentery" of the left gastric vessels, separates the upper recess, into which the caudate lobe projects, from the splenic recess, which lies to the left.

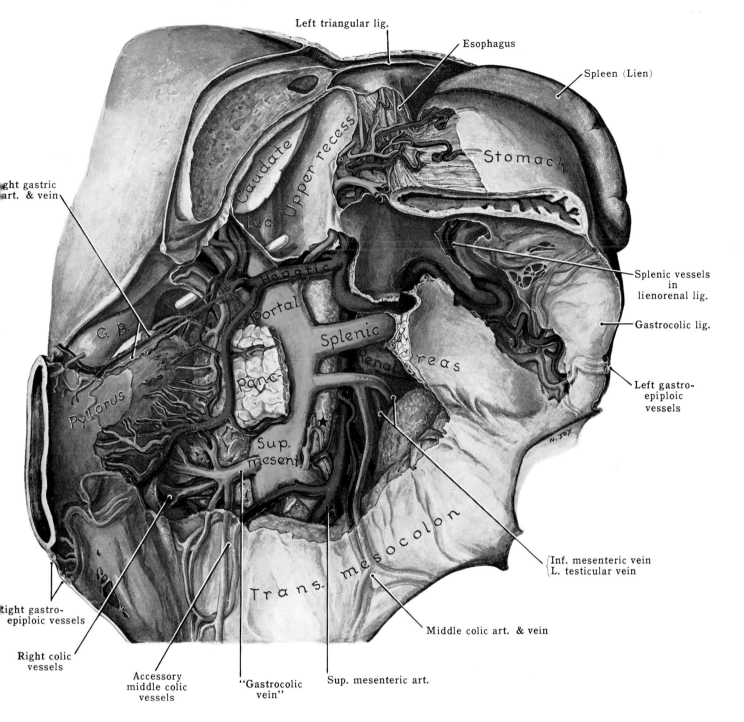

Left triangular lig.

Esophagus

Spleen (Lien)

Stomach

ght gastric
art. & vein

Caudate

Upper recess

l.v.c.

Hepatic

Portal

Splenic

enal

reas

Splenic vessels
in
lienorenal lig.

Gastrocolic lig.

Left gastro-
epiploic
vessels

G. B.

Pan-
creas

Pylorus

Sup.
mesent.

Inf. mesenteric vein
L. testicular vein

light gastro-
epiploic vessels

Trans. mesocolon

Middle colic art. & vein

Right colic
vessels

Accessory
middle colic
vessels

"Gastrocolic
vein"

Sup. mesenteric art.

135   Posterior Wall of the Omental Bursa in an Older Subject—II

The peritoneum of the posterior wall has largely been removed and a section of pancreas has been excised.

Observe:

1. The white rod passed through the epiploic foramen.

2. The esophagus and the left gastro-pancreatic fold bounding the left side of the upper recess.
   The esophageal branches of the left gastric vessels and the right and left vagal trunks applied to the esophagus.

3. The celiac trunk (not labelled) from which (a) the left gastric art. arches upwards, (b) the splenic art. runs tortuously to the left, and (c) the hepatic art. runs straight to the right to the front of the portal vein where it bifurcates like the letter Y or T set horizontally.

4. The right hepatic artery here arising early and passing dorsal to the portal vein (fig. 144 C). This was not obvious

in figure 134.

5. The portal vein formed behind the neck of the pancreas by the union of the superior mesenteric and splenic veins, with the inferior mesenteric vein joining at or near the angle of union. It here receives the left gastric vein, usually the right gastric vein (fig. 145) and the posterior superior pancreatico-duodenal vein (fig. 148) and one or two small duodenal or pancreatic veins.

6. The superior mesenteric vein receiving the gastro-colic trunk (Falconer and Griffiths) which is formed by (a) ant. sup. pancreatico-duodenal vein, (b) right gastro-epiploic vein, (c) a right colic vein, and (d) here two middle colic veins. The middle colic vein accompanying the middle colic artery here ends in the inferior mesenteric vein.

7. The left renal vein receiving the left testicular vein on a plane dorsal to the splenic vein.

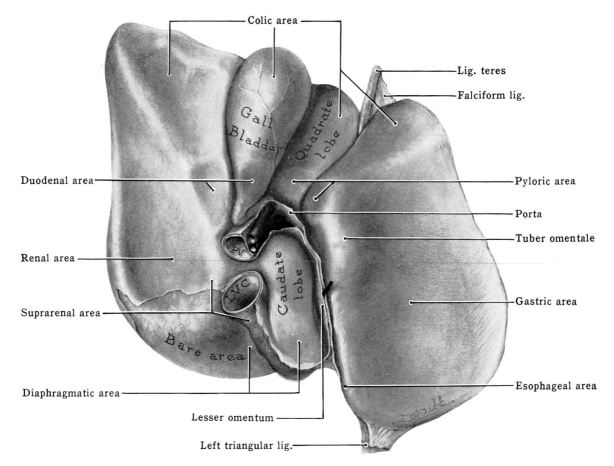

Colic area

Lig. teres

Falciform lig.

Gall Bladder

Quadrate lobe

Duodenal area

Pyloric area

Porta

Tuber omentale

Renal area

P.V.

Caudate lobe

I.V.C.

Suprarenal area

Gastric area

Bare area

Diaphragmatic area

Esophageal area

Lesser omentum

Left triangular lig.

136 The Inferior and Posterior Surfaces of the Liver

You are standing on the right side of the cadaver and facing the head. The attachments of the liver are divided and the sharp, inferior border is raised.

Observe:

1. The visceral areas: (a) for esophagus, stomach, pylorus, and duodenum; (b) for transverse colon; and (c) for right kidney and right suprarenal gland. The gall bladder rests on the transverse colon and on the duodenum (fig. 126).
2. The posterior surface comprising: (a) the bare area, occupied on its left by the inf. vena cava, (b) the caudate lobe, and (c) the groove for the esophagus.
3. The caudate lobe separated from the quadrate lobe by the porta, and joined to the right lobe by the caudate process (not labelled) which is squeezed between the inf. vena cava and the portal vein.

4. The cut edge of the peritoneum: At the right end of the bare area the right triangular lig. (not labelled) bifurcates into the upper and the lower layer of the coronary lig. The lower layer crosses the renal and suprarenal areas, and, after passing in front of the inf. vena cava, turns cranially as the left layer, or base, of the coronary lig. Followed to the left this layer of peritoneum forms the upper limit of the upper recess and then turns caudally as the posterior layer of the lesser omentum. This omentum is attached to the fissure for the lig. venosum and to the porta. In this specimen it contains an accessory hepatic artery, a branch of the left gastric artery.

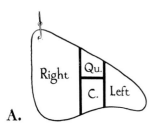

A.

The 4 lobes of the liver—right, quadrate, caudate, and left.

B.

The H-shaped deep fissures and wide sulci, defining the lobes.

C.

The occupants of the fissures and sulci.

136.1

In C, the arrow traverses the epiploic foramen. Behind it lies the inf. vena cava; in front, the portal vein; and above (at the roof) a narrow isthmus, the caudate process, joins the caudate lobe to the right lobe.

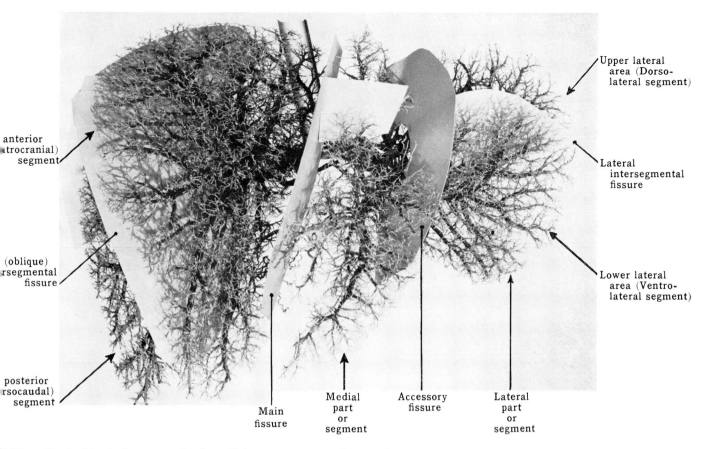

anterior
(trocranial)
segment

(oblique)
rsegmental
fissure

posterior
rsocaudal)
segment

Main
fissure

Medial
part
or
segment

Accessory
fissure

Lateral
part
or
segment

Upper lateral
area (Dorso-
lateral segment)

Lateral
intersegmental
fissure

Lower lateral
area (Ventro-
lateral segment)

37 Subdivisions of the Liver, anterior view (Courtesy of Douglas Bilbey.)

rrosion specimen of the portal structures.

The main fissure divides the liver into almost equal ves, "the right and left portal lobes", served by right l left portal veins, hepatic arteries, and bile passages. surface markings are the right sagittal sulci and an aginary line, 3 or 4 cmm from the falciform lig.

The right half is divided into an anterior and a posior segment; the left half is divided into a medial and a lateral segment by the accessory fissure, whose surface markings are the left sagittal fissures and the attachment of the falciform lig.

Each of these 4 segments is subdivisible into an upper and a lower area (segment), as revealed by the inserted slips of paper and the branches seen in figs. 138 & 140. Notable are the upper and lower lateral areas.

37.1 Large Hepatic eins, anterior view

These 3 veins are intersegmental, as pulmonary veins. They occupy the in, the right and the accessory and eral intersegmental fissures. (The rtal vein is injected white.)

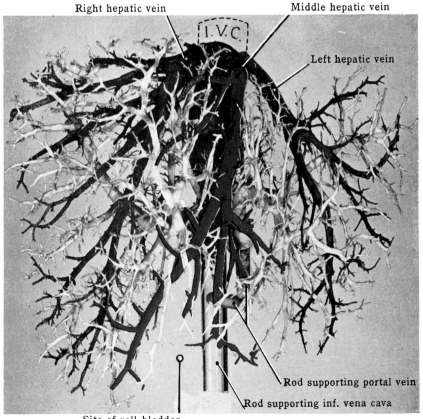

Right hepatic vein

I.V.C.

Middle hepatic vein

Left hepatic vein

Rod supporting portal vein

Rod supporting inf. vena cava

Site of gall bladder

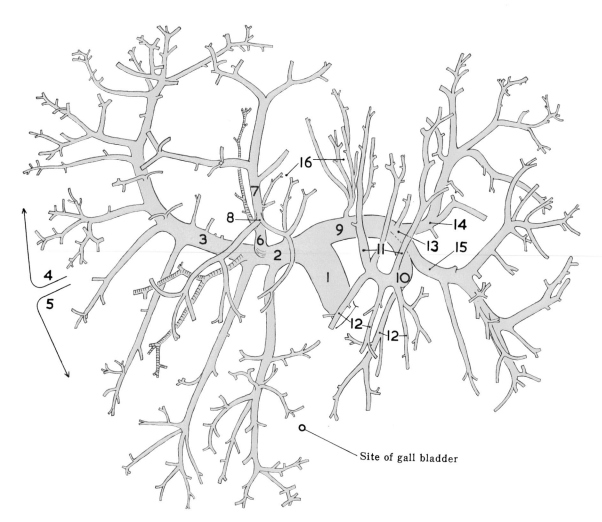

Site of gall bladder

138 Portal Vein and its Branches, left antero-inferior view

(Figures 138 & 140 were traced from a projected koda-chrome of a corrosion specimen. Photograph by Professor Duckworth. The specimen was tilted slightly in various directions to bring structures more fully into view.)

Perhaps it is simplest to regard the portal vein as branching and re-branching dichotomously. If branches 10 & 15 were split back to where 14 arises (broken line), branch 13 would be created. This figure of the portal vein would then serve equally as a plan of the hepatic artery and of the bile passages, as figure 140 shows.

1 = portal vein; 2 & 9—right & left portal veins; 16—caudate veins.
3 = Posterior (Dorso-caudal), 13 = Lateral ⎱ Segmental
6 = Anterior (Ventro-cranial), 10 = Medial ⎰ veins

Area veins ⎰ Upper 4 ⎱ 3
⎱ Lower 5 ⎰
⎰ Upper 7 ⎱ 6
⎱ Lower 8 ⎰
2 1 9
13 ⎰ 14 Upper (Dorso-lateral) ⎱ Area
⎱ 15 Lower (Ventro-lateral) ⎰ veins
10 ⎰ 11 Upper (Central) ⎱
⎱ 12 Lower (Quadrate) ⎰

(Numbering is after Healey, Schroy and Sorensen. Terminology is after J. E. Healey et al.; and C. H. Hjortsjo who should be consulted for details and variations.)

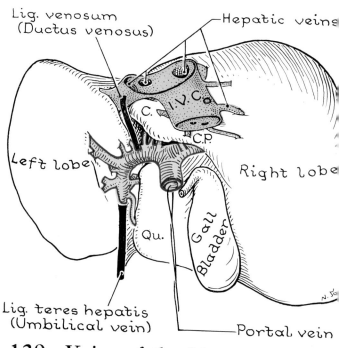

Lig. venosum (Ductus venosus)
Hepatic veins
I.V.C.
C.
C.P.
Left lobe
Right lobe
Qu.
Gall Bladder
Lig. teres hepatis (Umbilical vein)
Portal vein

139 Veins of the Liver, posterior view

Note the branches of the portal vein (yellow) entering the liver, and 3 large and several small hepatic veins (blue) leaving it to join the inf. vena cava. (C. = caudate lobe; C.P. = caudate process.)

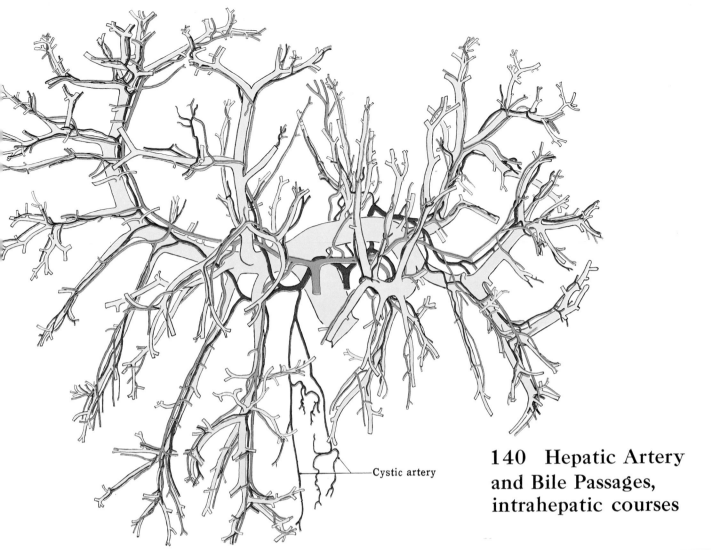

Cystic artery

140 Hepatic Artery and Bile Passages, intrahepatic courses

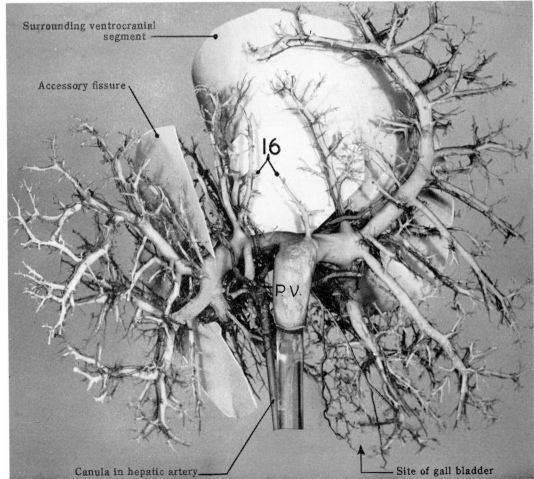

Surrounding ventrocranial segment

Accessory fissure

16

P.V.

141 Portal Structures, intrahepatic courses, posterior view

(From same specimen as used for figure 140. A lens may aid you.)

Canula in hepatic artery

Site of gall bladder

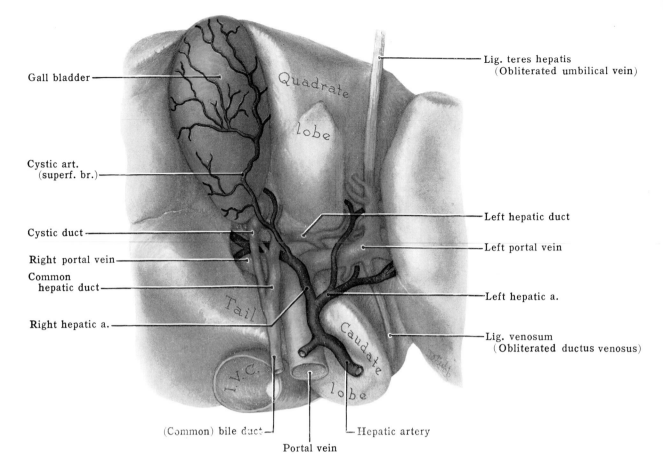

Gall bladder

Cystic art. (superf. br.)

Cystic duct

Right portal vein

Common hepatic duct

Right hepatic a.

Quadrate lobe

Tail

I.V.C.

Caudate lobe

(Common) bile duct

Portal vein

Hepatic artery

Lig. teres hepatis (Obliterated umbilical vein)

Left hepatic duct

Left portal vein

Left hepatic a.

Lig. venosum (Obliterated ductus venosus)

142   Porta Hepatis and the Cystic Artery

1. The tail of the caudate lobe forming the roof of the epiploic foramen, and lying between the upper end of the portal vein, and the inf. vena cava.

2. The relation of structures as they ascend to the porta—duct to the right, artery to the left, vein behind.

3. The order of structures at the porta—duct, artery, vein—from before backwards.

4. The left portal vein and left hepatic artery supplying the quadrate and caudate lobes en route to the left lobe, and

accompanied by tributaries of the left hepatic duct.

5. The lig. teres hepatis passing to the left portal vein, and the lig. venosum arising opposite it and ascending to the inf. vena cava.

6. The cystic artery springing from the right hepatic artery and dividing into a superficial and a deep branch which arborise on the respective surfaces of the bladder.

7. The cystic duct, sinuous at its origin.

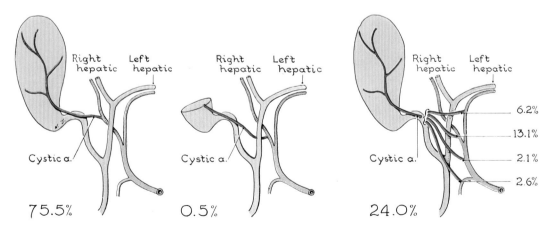

Right hepatic   Left hepatic

Cystic a.

75.5%

Right hepatic   Left hepatic

Cystic a.

0.5%

Right hepatic   Left hepatic

Cystic a.

6.2%

13.1%

2.1%

2.6%

24.0%

143   Variations in the Origin and Course of the Cystic Artery

The cystic art. usually arises from the right hepatic art. in the angle between the common hepatic duct and the cystic duct, and has no occasion to cross the common hepatic duct, as in figures 144 and 147. When, however, it arises on the

left of the bile passages, it almost always crosses anterior to the passages, as in figure 142, and only rarely (3 in 580 cases) does it cross behind. (Diagrams based on 580 cases by Daseler, Anson, Hambley and Reimann.)

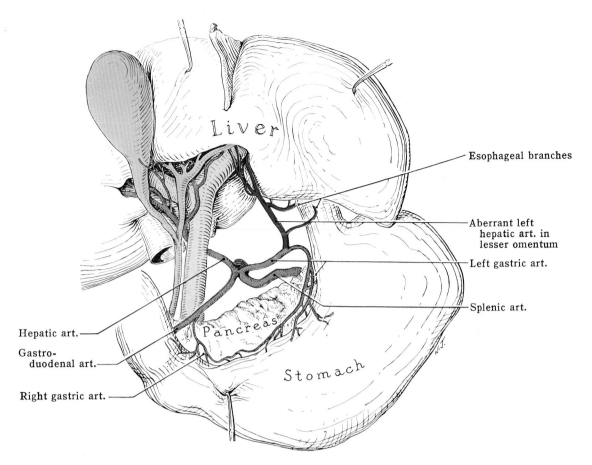

Esophageal branches

Aberrant left
hepatic art. in
lesser omentum

Left gastric art.

Splenic art.

Hepatic art.

Gastro-
duodenal art.

Right gastric art.

A. Aberrant Left Hepatic Artery.

The left hepatic artery was entirely replaced by a branch of the left gastric artery, as in this specimen, in 11.5 % of 200 cadavera, and in another 11.5 % it was partially replaced. (Michels, N. A.)

ight   Left
hepatic a. hepatic a.

R.H.   L.H.

R.H.   L.H.

Hepatic a.
24%

Hepatic a.
64%

R. Hepatic a.
12%

Right
hepatic a.

Portal
vein
91%

Right
hepatic a.

Portal
vein
9%

C. Right Hepatic Artery and Portal Vein.

The artery crossed ventral to the portal vein in 91 % of 165 specimens and dorsal in 9 %. (J.C.B.G.)

. Right Hepatic Artery and Bile Passages: Aber-
nt Right Hepatic Artery.

The right hepatic artery crossed ventral to the
le passages in 24 % of 165 specimens, and dorsal
64 %, whereas in 12 % it was aberrant, arising
om the superior mesenteric artery. (J.C.B.G.)

144   Variations in the Hepatic Arteries

VARIATIONS

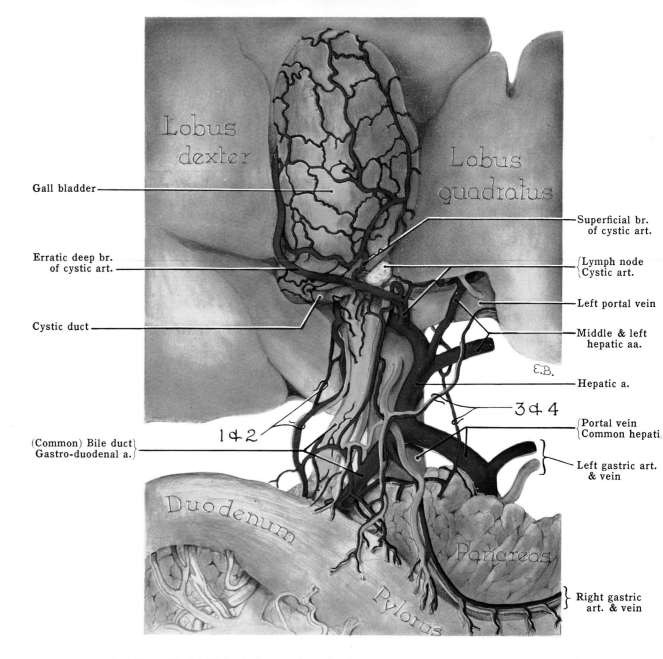

Gall bladder

Erratic deep br. of cystic art.

Cystic duct

(Common) Bile duct}
Gastro-duodenal a.}

Lobus dexter

Lobus quadratus

1 & 2

3 & 4

E.B.

Superficial br. of cystic art.

{Lymph node
{Cystic art.

Left portal vein

Middle & left hepatic aa.

Hepatic a.

{Portal vein
{Common hepati

Left gastric art. & vein

Duodenum

Pancreas

Pylorus

} Right gastric art. & vein

145 Gall Bladder, the Bile Passages, and the related Blood Vessels

The liver is turned up and the duodenum is pulled down. (*Preparation by Dr. A. J. A. Noronha.*)

Observe:

1. The network of arteries on the gall bladder. Most of the smaller arteries lying on a deeper plane than the larger arteries.

2. A large erratic, deep branch of the cystic artery, crossing superficial to the neck of the gall bladder.

3. The cystic lymph node.

4. Many fine sinuous arterial twigs supplying the bile passages and springing from nearby arteries.

5. The right gastric artery, here arising very low—indeed, from the gastro-duodenal artery.

6. The right gastric vein, here ending high in the portal vein.

7. Several, here 5, anastomotic arteries capable of bringing blood from various gastric and pancreatic arteries to the porta hepatis. 4 of these have been retracted, 1 of them passing to the left lobe.

8. Veins (not all shown), accompanying faithfully most arteries.

9. A middle hepatic artery, seen here, passing to the quadrate lobe is common (Michels).

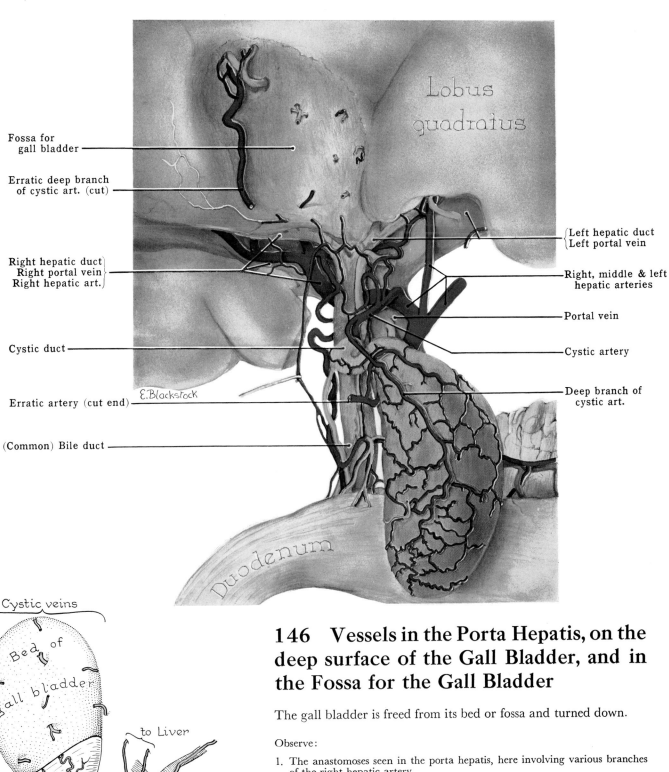

Fossa for gall bladder

Erratic deep branch of cystic art. (cut)

Right hepatic duct)
Right portal vein }
Right hepatic art.)

Cystic duct

E. Blackstock

Erratic artery (cut end)

(Common) Bile duct

Lobus quadratus

Left hepatic duct
Left portal vein

Right, middle & left hepatic arteries

Portal vein

Cystic artery

Deep branch of cystic art.

Duodenum

Cystic veins

Bed of gall bladder

to Liver

to Left portal v.

nt. cystic v.

ost. cystic v.

ystic duct

Common hepatic duct

R. gastric v.

ile duct

ost. sup.
ancreatico-
uodenal v.

146 Vessels in the Porta Hepatis, on the deep surface of the Gall Bladder, and in the Fossa for the Gall Bladder

The gall bladder is freed from its bed or fossa and turned down.

Observe:

1. The anastomoses seen in the porta hepatis, here involving various branches of the right hepatic artery.
2. A very large anastomotic artery passing behind the origin of the common hepatic duct; several smaller arteries forming a network (rete) in front of the ducts. From the network, twigs passing to the subcapsular arterial plexus.
3. The deep branch of the cystic artery, aided by a branch of the erratic deep cystic artery, ramifying on the deep or attached surface of the gall bladder, anastomosing with twigs of the superficial branch of the cystic artery, and sending twigs into the bed of the gall bladder. (The cut ends of the arterial and venous twigs can be seen.)
4. The erratic artery plunging into the bed.

146.1 Veins of the Extrahepatic Bile Passages and Gall bladder

Note: The venous twigs draining the passages and the neck of the bladder join veins which, clinging to the passages, connect gastric, duodenal and pancreatic veins partly to the liver directly and partly via a portal vein. The veins of the fundus and body, here 8, plunge directly into the liver.

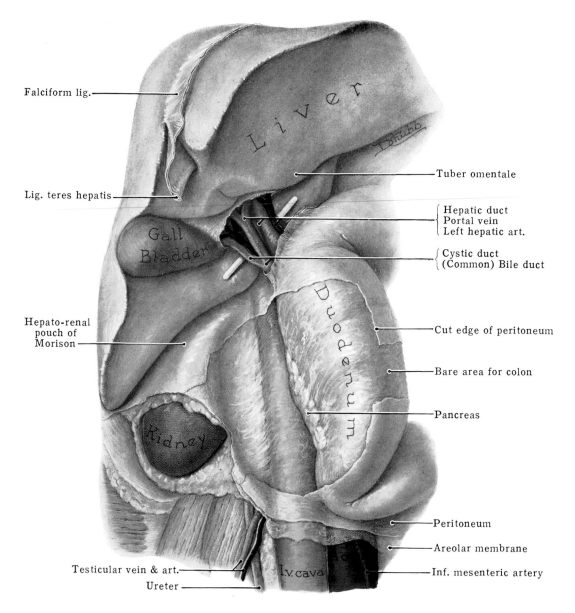

Falciform lig.

Liver

Tuber omentale

Lig. teres hepatis

{ Hepatic duct
Portal vein
Left hepatic art. }

Gall Bladder

{ Cystic duct
(Common) Bile duct }

Hepato-renal
pouch of
Morison

Duodenum

Cut edge of peritoneum

Bare area for colon

Pancreas

Kidney

Peritoneum

Areolar membrane

Testicular vein & art.

I.v. cava

Inf. mesenteric artery

Ureter

147 Exposure of the (Common) Bile Duct, posterior aspect—I

A rod is passed through the epiploic foramen. The lesser omentum is removed. The transverse colon is separated from the front of the descending, or 2nd, part of the duodenum and thrown down; the peritoneum is cut along the right or convex border of the 2nd part of the duodenum, and this part of the duodenum is swung forwards like a door on a hinge.

Note:

1. The space opened up is virtually a bursal space, comparable to the retropubic space where two smooth areolar membranes are applied to each other. Here one membrane covers the posterior aspect of the 2nd part of the duodenum and the head of the pancreas; the other covers the aorta, inf. vena cava, renal vessels and perinephric fat. The duodenum can expand and contract, but, being

suspended from the liver by the structures entering the porta, it cannot descend unless the liver either alters its shape or descends with it.

2. To find the epiploic foramen either: (a) follow the liver, at the upper limit of the hepato-renal pouch, medially to the caudate process (tail of the caudate lobe), which forms the roof of the foramen and which lies in front of the inf. vena cava, which forms the posterior wall; or (b) follow the gall bladder to the cystic duct, which occupies the free edge of the lesser omentum, which forms the anterior wall of the foramen.

3. Of the three main structures in the anterior wall—the portal vein is posterior, the hepatic artery ascends from the left, and the bile passages descend to the right (fig. 142).

4. In this specimen the right hepatic artery springs from the superior mesenteric artery. (For data on this common variant, see fig. 144 B.)

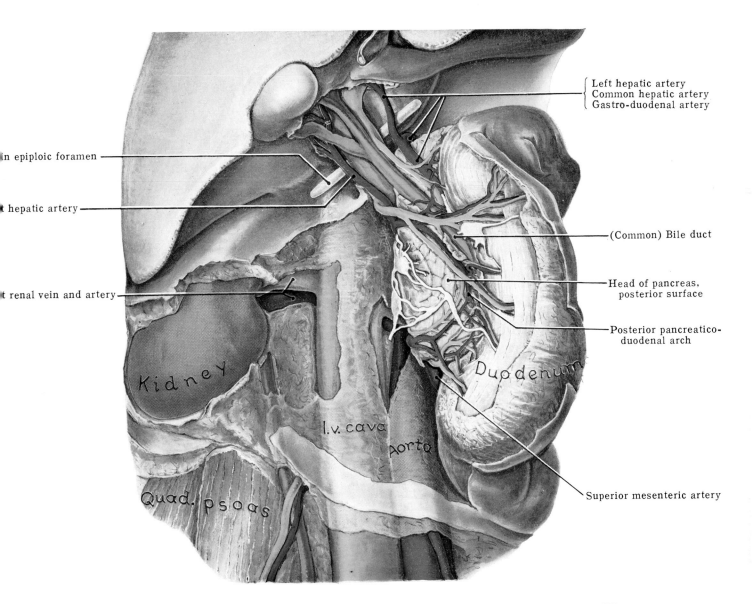

In epiploic foramen

t hepatic artery

t renal vein and artery

Kidney

I.v. cava

Aorta

Quad. psoas

Left hepatic artery
Common hepatic artery
Gastro-duodenal artery

(Common) Bile duct

Head of pancreas,
posterior surface

Posterior pancreatico-
duodenal arch

Duodenum

Superior mesenteric artery

148   Exposure of the (Common) Bile Duct, posterior aspect—II

The duodenum is swung still further forwards and to the left, taking the head of the pancreas with it. In effect, the epiploic foramen has been enlarged caudally. The areolar membrane covering these two organs is largely removed; that covering the great vessels is in part removed.

Observe:

1. The right renal vein to be short, and the right artery, which passes behind the inf. vena cava, to be long.
2. The bile duct descending in a groove on the head of the pancreas, and a tongue of that head (reflected) lying behind the end of the duct.
3. Vasa recta, accompanied by veins and lymph vessels, passing from the posterior pancreatico-duodenal arch to the duodenum.

4. Of the two posterior pancreatico-duodenal arteries that form the posterior arch, the inferior springing from the superior mesenteric artery, and the superior here springing from the right hepatic artery, but usually from the gastro-duodenal artery, as in figure 159.

5. The posterior superior pancreatico-duodenal vein ending in the portal vein.

6. The very close posterior relationship of the inf. vena cava to the portal vein and the bile duct.

7. The duct ending at the level of the hilus of the kidney, and the ureter beginning at the same level.

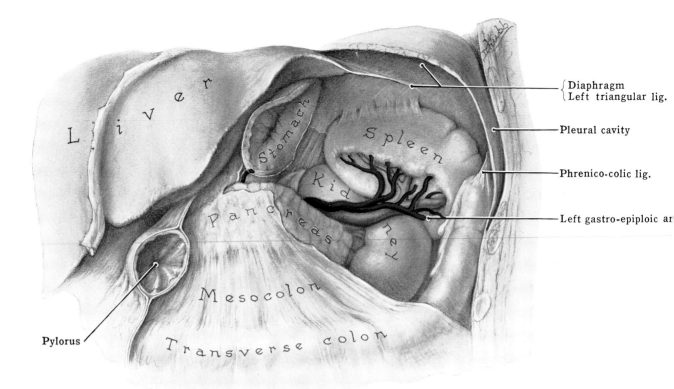

Diaphragm
Left triangular lig.

Pleural cavity

Phrenico-colic lig.

Left gastro-epiploic ar

149 Stomach Bed

The stomach is excised. The peritoneum of the omental bursa, or lesser sac, covering the stomach bed is largely removed; so is the peritoneum of the greater sac covering the lower part of the kidney and pancreas.

The pancreas is unusually short; the adhesions binding the spleen to Diaphragm are pathological but not unusual.

Unlabelled are:—1. The branch of the posterior vagal trunk that descends on the right side of the left gastric artery to the celiac plexus. 2. The left suprarenal gland. 3. The three short gastric branches of the splenic artery. 4. The tuber omentale of the liver and that of the pancreas, which fit into the lesser curvature of the stomach. 5. The lesser omentum attached to the upper border of the pylorus and the greater omentum to the lower border.

Note the pleural cavity separating the spleen and Diaphragm from the thoracic wall.

150 Spleen or Lien, visceral surfac

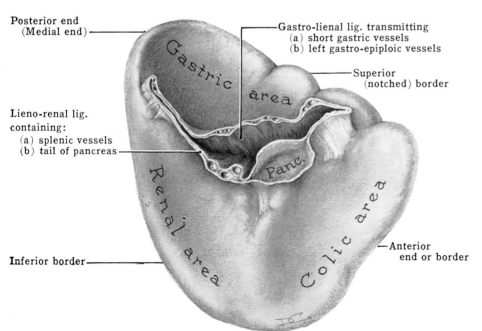

Posterior end
(Medial end)

Gastro-lienal lig. transmitting
(a) short gastric vessels
(b) left gastro-epiploic vessels

Superior
(notched) border

Lieno-renal lig.
containing:
(a) splenic vessels
(b) tail of pancreas

Inferior border

Anterior
end or border

For orientation see figure 149.

Observe:

1. A "circumferential border" comprising the inferior, superior, and anterior borders, a
   separating the visceral surface from the d
   phragmatic surface.

2. The notches characteristic of the super
   border.

3. The left limit of the omental bursa at the h
   of the spleen, between the lieno-renal and g
   trolienal ligs.

4. The spleen taking the impressions of the str
   tures in contact with it. The large colic area s
   here is reduced in figure 152—presumably
   the one case the colon was full (of gas), and
   the other it was empty.

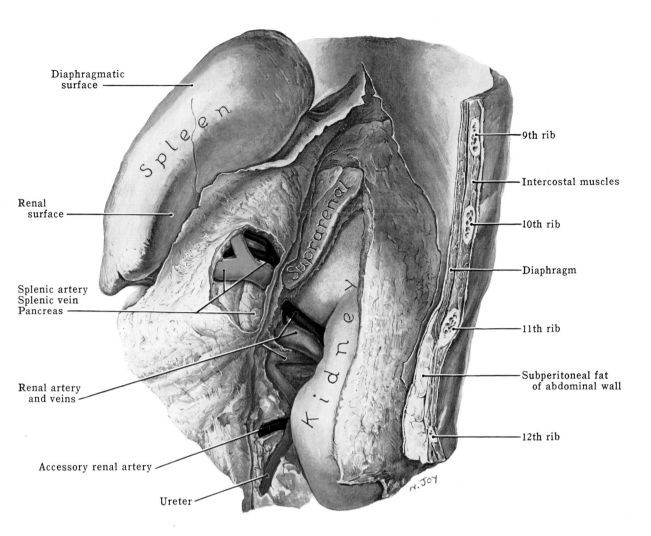

Diaphragmatic surface

Renal surface

Splenic artery
Splenic vein
Pancreas

Renal artery and veins

Accessory renal artery

Ureter

Spleen

Suprarenal

Kidney

9th rib

Intercostal muscles

10th rib

Diaphragm

11th rib

Subperitoneal fat of abdominal wall

12th rib

151 Reflexion of the Spleen: Exposure of the Left Kidney and Suprarenal Gland from the front

The spleen and the lieno-renal ligament are turned forwards and to the right, like the page of a book, taking the splenic vessels and the tail of the pancreas with them. Part of the fatty capsule of the kidney is cut away.

Observe:

The exposed left kidney, renal vessels, and ureter, also the left suprarenal gland, separated from the kidney by a thin layer of fat.

When in situ, the splenic vessels lie ventral to the renal vessels (fig. 149); but two areolar membranes, closely applied to each, and some fatty capsule are seen to intervene. There are two comparable membranes on the right side (figs. 147 & 148).

The subperitoneal fat of the abdominal wall stopping on reaching the diaphragm.

Note that this exposure is, in effect, a restoration to the embryological state.

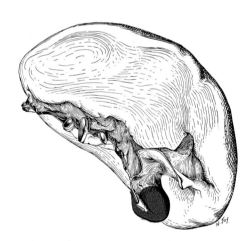

152 An Accessory Spleen

Accessory spleens resemble lymph nodes, about 1 cm. in diameter, but they are usually covered with peritoneum, as is the spleen itself. They lie along the course of the splenic artery or its gastro-epiploic branch, but they may be elsewhere. The commonest location is at or near the hilus of the spleen, but 1 in 6 are partially (or wholly) embedded in the tail of the pancreas. At 3000 necropsies on male veteran patients, 311, or 10%, had accessory spleens. Of these, 272 were solitary and 39 were multiple. (B. Halpert & F. Gyorkey; G. M. Curtis & D. Movitz.)

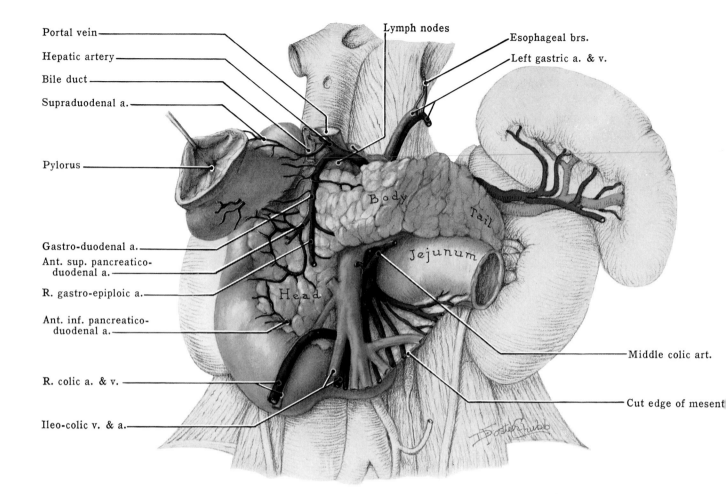

Portal vein
Hepatic artery
Bile duct
Supraduodenal a.
Pylorus
Gastro-duodenal a.
Ant. sup. pancreatico-duodenal a.
R. gastro-epiploic a.
Ant. inf. pancreatico-duodenal a.
R. colic a. & v.
Ileo-colic v. & a.

Lymph nodes
Esophageal brs.
Left gastric a. & v.

Body
Tail
Jejunum
Head

Middle colic art.
Cut edge of mesent

153 Duodenum and Pancreas in situ, front view

Observe:

1. *The duodenum* moulded around the head of the pancreas. Its 1st or superior part (retracted) overlapping the pancreas and passing backwards, upwards, and to the right. The remaining parts (2nd, 3rd & 4th) overlapped by the pancreas. Near the junction of its 3rd and 4th parts the duodenum is crossed by the superior mesenteric vessels. These appearing from under cover of the neck of the pancreas, descending in front of the uncinate process, and entering the root of the mesentery, which commonly, as here, constricts the duodenum and causes the 1st, 2nd & 3rd parts to be dilated.

2. *The pancreas*, here very short—its tail usually abuts on the spleen and is blunt (fig. 150). It is arched forwards because it crosses the vertebral column and aorta.

3. *The celiac trunk*, which lies behind the upper border of the pancreas, sending (a) the left gastric a. upwards on the diaphragm towards the cardiac orifice of the stomach to enter the lesser omentum; (b) the splenic a. to the left; and (c) the hepatic a. to the right. The hepatic a. passing on to the front of the portal vein and giving off the gastro-duodenal a., which descends between the duodenum and pancreas, less than an inch from the pylorus, and divides into the right gastroepiploic a. and the superior pancreatico-duodenal a. Note the single supraduodenal a. and the several retroduodenal aa. supplying the first inch of the duodenum.

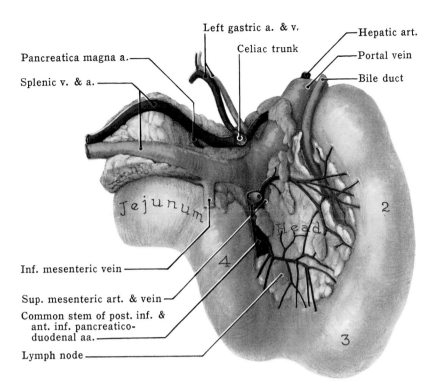

Pancreatica magna a.

Splenic v. & a.

Left gastric a. & v.

Celiac trunk

Hepatic art.

Portal vein

Bile duct

Jejunum

Head

2

Inf. mesenteric vein

Sup. mesenteric art. & vein

Common stem of post. inf. & ant. inf. pancreatico-duodenal aa.

Lymph node

4

3

154 Duodenum, Pancreas and Bile Duct, from behind

This is the reverse of the specimen depicted in figure 153.

Observe:

1. Only the end of the 1st or superior part of the duodenum is in view.
2. The bile duct here descending in a long fissure (opened up) in the posterior part of the head of the pancreas—contrast figure 148.
3. Arteries: In the absence of the usual posterior superior pancreatico-duodenal artery, the vasa recta that pass behind the duct springing from an accessory branch of the superior mesenteric artery—compare figure 159.

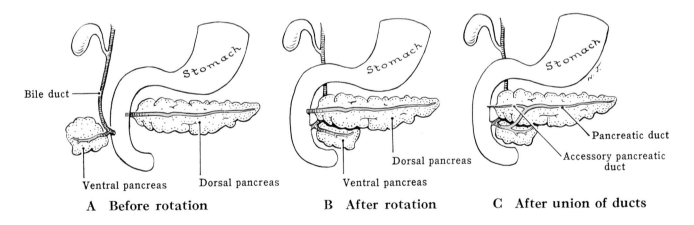

Bile duct

Stomach

Stomach

Stomach

Pancreatic duct

Accessory pancreatic duct

Ventral pancreas   Dorsal pancreas

A   Before rotation

Dorsal pancreas

Ventral pancreas

B   After rotation

C   After union of ducts

155 Developmental Explanation of Variability of Pancreatic Ducts

Note:

(a) A smaller primitive ventral bud arises in common with the bile duct, and a larger primitive dorsal bud arises independently from the duodenum, cranial to this.

(b) The 2nd or descending part of the duodenum rotates on its long axis, which brings the ventral bud and the bile duct behind the dorsal bud.

(c) A connecting segment unites the dorsal duct to the ventral duct, whereupon the duodenal end of the dorsal duct tends to atrophy and the direction of flow within it is reversed.

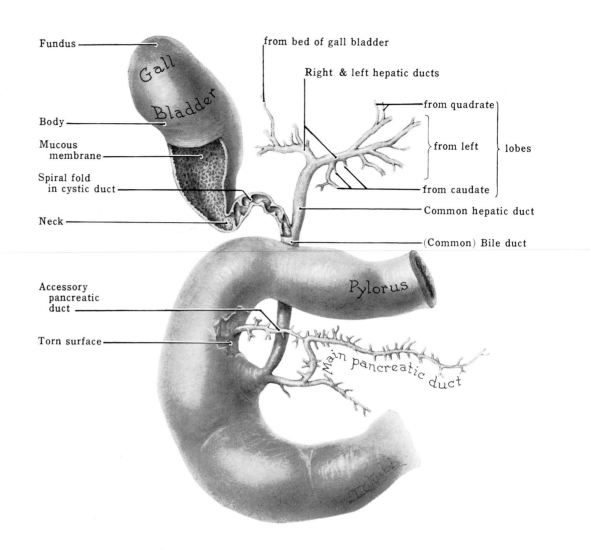

Fundus

Gall Bladder

Body

Mucous membrane

Spiral fold in cystic duct

Neck

Accessory pancreatic duct

Torn surface

from bed of gall bladder

Right & left hepatic ducts

from quadrate

from left } lobes

from caudate

Common hepatic duct

(Common) Bile duct

Pylorus

Main pancreatic duct

156   Extra-hepatic Bile Passages and the Pancreatic Ducts

Note: The right hepatic duct collects from the right lobe of the liver; the left hepatic duct collects from the left, quadrate and caudate lobes. The common hepatic duct unites with the cystic duct close above the duodenum. The mucous membrane of the gall bladder has a low honeycomb surface. The cystic duct is sinuous; its mucous membrane forms a spiral fold (spiral valve).

The bile duct, after descending behind the 1st part of the duodenum and the accessory pancreatic duct, is joined by the main pancreatic duct; these open on the duodenal papilla (fig. 168).

The main pancreatic duct with its tributaries bears semblance to a herring bone, and differs from the common hepatic duct with its tributaries which resembles a deciduous tree. The accessory pancreatic duct retains its anastomosis with the main duct. The pancreas invades the duodenal wall around the accessory duct, and cannot be removed without lacerating the duodenum.

157   Comments on the Pancreatic Ducts

Dimensions: The average length of 27 pancreases is 8.2″. The main duct begins 1″ from the tip of the tail and there the internal diameter is 0.5 mm.; at 2″ from the tip it ranges from 0.5 mm. to 1.5 mm.; at 4″ it ranges from 1.5 mm. to 3.0 mm.; and in the head the average diameter is 3.5 mm. The primary ductules narrow at their entrances to the main duct, and they approach it from all sides. Branches are fewest where the gland is narrowest, i.e., where it crosses the sup. mesenteric vessels, indeed, it may there be bald. (Horsey and Paul.)

Connections with Duodenum: In about 9% the primitive dorsal duct (fig. 155) persists, usually quite unconnected with the primitive ventral duct, as in fig. 157-D In about 44% the accessory duct loses its connection with the duodenum (fig. 157-A); or in 8% ends blindly at the duodenum; or in 9% retains only a negligibly small opening into the duodenum. In about 10%, however, the accessory duct is large enough to relieve an obstructed main duct (fig. 157-B), and in 20% it could probably substitute for it (fig. 157-C). Further in about 5% the bile and main pancreatic ducts open separately on the duodenal papilla (fig. 157-B). (Data based on radiograms of 200 specimens injected with radio-opaque material. E. Millbourn, 1950.)

157   Corrosion Preparations of the Pancreatic Ducts

(Prepared by W. J. Horsey and W. Paul, photographed by C. E. Storton.)

The pancreatic ducts were injected with plastic by retrograde flow, via the bile duct, and then corroded with acid. In specimens where the bile duct and the main pancreatic duct (of Wirsung) opened separately on to the duodenal papilla (of Vater) injection was made directly into the main duct.

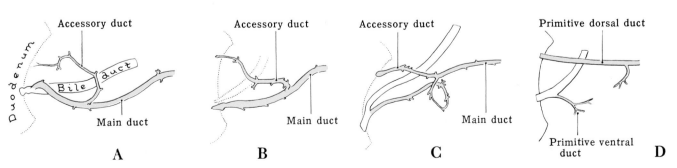

KEY TO FIGURE 157

For comments see opposite page.

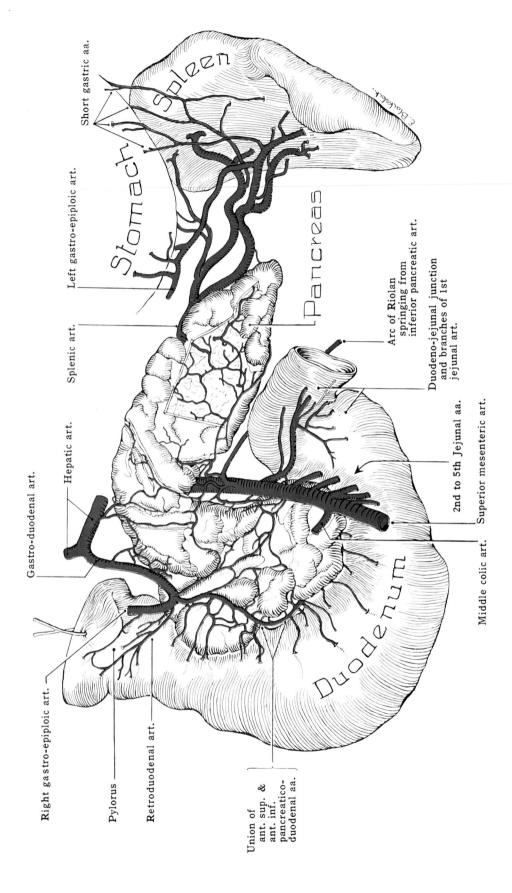

Short gastric aa.

Spleen

Stomach

Left gastro-epiploic art.

Pancreas

Splenic art.

Hepatic art.

Gastro-duodenal art.

Right gastro-epiploic art.

Pylorus

Retroduodenal art.

Union of
ant. sup. &
ant. inf.
pancreatico-
duodenal aa.

Duodenum

Arc of Riolan
springing from
inferior pancreatic art.

Duodeno-jejunal junction
and branches of 1st
jejunal art.

2nd to 5th Jejunal aa.

Superior mesenteric art.

Middle colic art.

E. Blacksto.

158 Blood Supply to the Pancreas, Duodenum, and Spleen, front view

Two or three short slices have been removed from the pancreas.

Observe:

1. This territory to be supplied by the hepatic, splenic, and superior mesenteric arteries.

2. Several retroduodenal branches springing from the right gastro-epiploic artery.

3. The anterior superior pancreatico-duodenal branch of the gastro-duodenal artery and the anterior inferior pancreatico-duodenal branch of the superior mesenteric artery forming an

continued on facing page

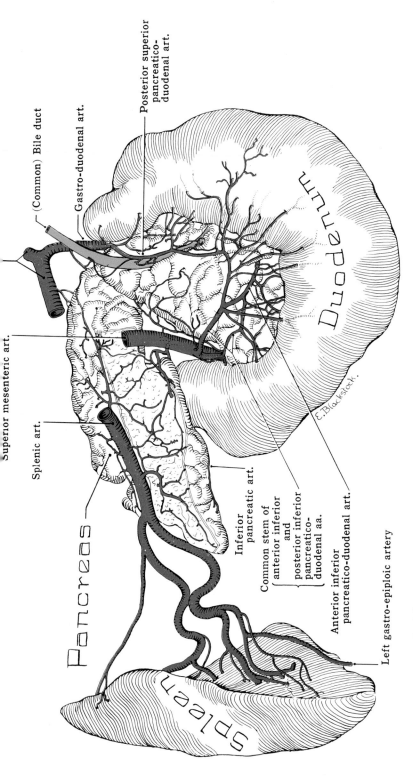

Superior mesenteric art.

Splenic art.

(Common) Bile duct

Gastro-duodenal art.

Posterior superior pancreatico-duodenal art.

Duodenum

Pancreas

Spleen

E.Blackstock.

Inferior pancreatic art.

Common stem of { anterior inferior and posterior inferior pancreatico-duodenal aa.

Anterior inferior pancreatico-duodenal art.

Left gastro-epiploic artery

159 Blood Supply to the Pancreas, Duodenum, and Spleen, back view

continued from facing page

arch in front of the head of the pancreas. The posterior superior and posterior inferior branches of the same two arteries forming another arch behind the pancreas. The 2 inferior arteries here, as usually, springing from a common stem. From each arch thus formed straight vessels, called vasa recta duodeni, passing to the anterior and posterior surfaces respectively of the 2nd, 3rd and 4th parts of the duodenum. The duodeno-jejunal junction supplied by the large branching vessel depicted.

4. The fine network of arteries that pervades the pancreas to be derived from: the stem of the hepatic artery, the gastro-duodenal artery, the pancreatico-duodenal arches, the splenic artery, and also from the superior mesenteric artery via its inferior pancreatic branch—this branch, in this specimen, springing from the arc of Riolan, below the neck of the pancreas, and effecting liaisons with the other branches.

5. The arc of Riolan, an occasional artery on the posterior abdominal wall, which connects the superior mesenteric artery to a branch of the inferior mesenteric artery.

(For more details see Michels; Woodburne.)

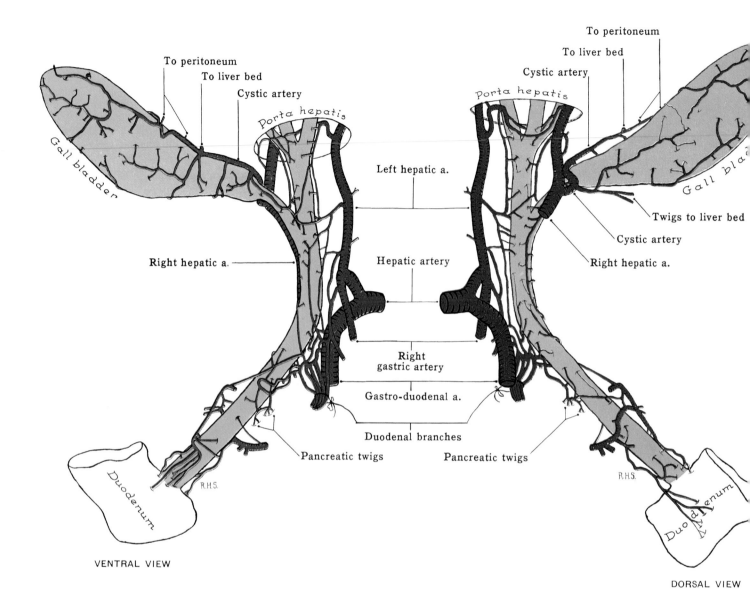

To peritoneum
To liver bed
Cystic artery
Porta hepatis
Gall bladder
Right hepatic a.

To peritoneum
To liver bed
Cystic artery
Porta hepatis
Gall bladder
Twigs to liver bed
Cystic artery
Right hepatic a.

Left hepatic a.

Hepatic artery

Right
gastric artery

Gastro-duodenal a.

Duodenal branches

Pancreatic twigs

Pancreatic twigs

R.H.S.

R.H.S.

Duodenum

Duodenum

VENTRAL VIEW

DORSAL VIEW

160   Blood Supply of the Bile Passages

(This illustration and the dissection were made by a skilful and diligent medical student, R. H. Sheppard.)

Observe:

1. The numerous fine arterial twigs seen to be derived from all vessels near by.

2. The right hepatic artery in this specimens springs from the superior mesenteric artery (for data see fig. 144 B.)

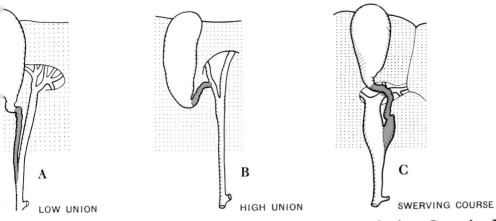

LOW UNION   HIGH UNION   SWERVING COURSE

—Variations in the Length and Course of the Cystic Duct

The cystic duct usually lies on the right of the common hepatic duct and joins it above the 1st part of the duodenum, but this varies as in a, b, c.

—Varieties of Accessory Hepatic Ducts

Accessory right hepatic ducts are common. Thus, of 95 gall bladders and bile passages injected in situ with melted paraffin wax and then dissected, 7 had accessory hepatic ducts in positions of surgical danger. Of these, 4 joined the common hepatic duct near the cystic duct (a); 2 joined the cystic duct (b); and 1 was an anastomosing duct (*J.C.B.G.*) "Accessory" ducts are now known to be not additional ducts but liver area or segmental ducts that arise early.

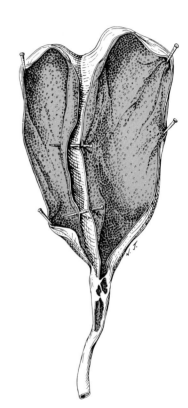

D—Double Gall Bladder

(By the courtesy of Professor William Boyd.)

The gall bladder was rarely double with two cystic ducts and very rarely was it bilobed. (Boyden, E. A.)

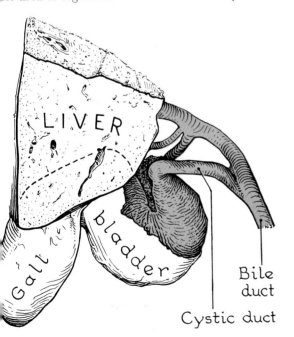

LIVER

Gall bladder

Bile duct

Cystic duct

C—Folded Gall Bladder

Radiologically, the body of the gall bladder was found to be folded, or kinked, upon itself in 14.5% of 165 persons. The fundus was folded upon the bladder in 3.5%, as in fig. A above. (Boyden, E. A.)

51   **Variations in the Bile Passages and Gall Bladder**

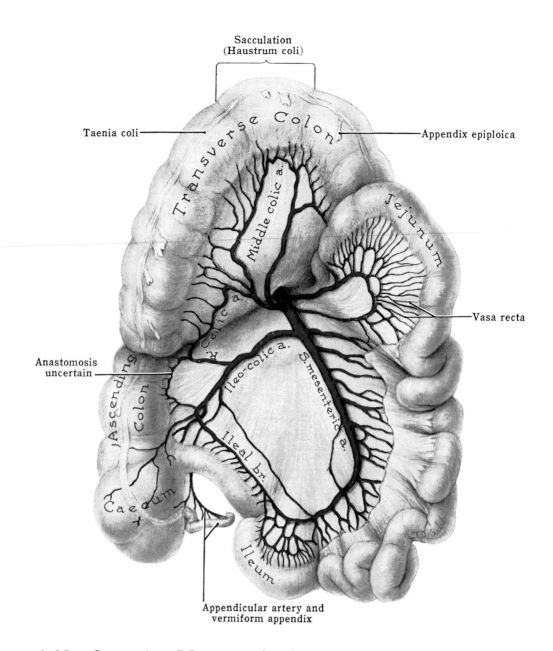

Sacculation
(Haustrum coli)

Taenia coli

Appendix epiploica

Transverse Colon

Middle colic a.

Jejunum

R. Colic a.

Vasa recta

Anastomosis
uncertain

Ileo-colic a.

S. mesenteric a.

Ascending Colon

Ileal br.

Caecum

Ileum

Appendicular artery and
vermiform appendix

162 Superior Mesenteric Artery

The peritoneum is in part stripped off.

Observe:

1. The sup. mesenteric artery ending by anastomosing with the ileal branch of the ileo-colic artery.

2. Its branches:

   (a) From its left side, twelve or more jejunal and ileal branches. These anastomose to form arcades from which vasa recta pass to the small gut.

   (b) From its right side, the middle colic, the ileo-colic, and commonly, but not here, an independent right colic artery. These anastomose to form a marginal artery (labelled in fig. 163) from which vasa recta pass to the large gut.

   (c) The two inferior pancreatico-duodenal arteries (not in view, but seen in fig. 154) arise from the main artery either directly or in conjunction with the 1st jejunal branch.

3. Taeniae coli, sacculations, and appendices epiploicae which distinguish the large gut from the smooth walled small gut.

(For variations in patterns of arteries see J. V. Basmajian.)

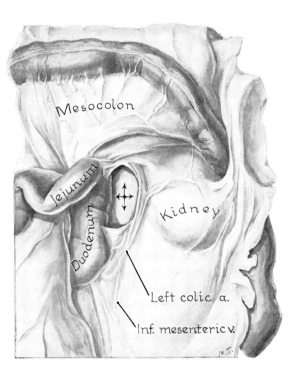

3 Inferior Mesenteric Artery

…mesentery has been cut at its root and discarded with the …um and ileum.

…ve:

…e inf. mesenteric artery arising behind the duodenum, $1\frac{1}{2}''$ …ove the bifurcation of the aorta. On crossing the left common …c artery, it becomes the superior rectal (haemorrhoidal) artery.

…branches:

(a) a single (superior) left colic artery and

(b) several sigmoid arteries (inf. left colic aa.) springing from its … side. In this specimen the two lowest sigmoid arteries spring …m the superior rectal artery. The point at which the last artery …the colon leaves the artery to the rectum is known as the critical …nt of Sudeck.

163.1 Duodenal Recesses

These occasional peritoneal fossae may pass either upwards or downwards or to the right or to left. The lower fold is bloodless. When present, the left fold does, and the upper fold may, contain the inferior mesenteric vein. The right recess is retro-duodenal.

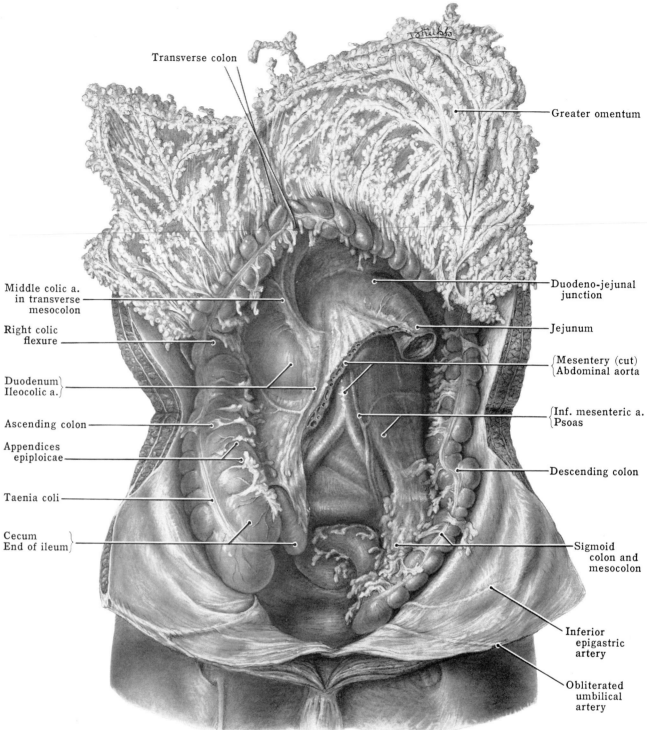

Transverse colon

Greater omentum

Middle colic a. in transverse mesocolon

Right colic flexure

Duodenum} Ileocolic a.}

Ascending colon

Appendices epiploicae

Taenia coli

Cecum } End of ileum }

Duodeno-jejunal junction

Jejunum

{Mesentery (cut) {Abdominal aorta

{Inf. mesenteric a. {Psoas

Descending colon

Sigmoid colon and mesocolon

Inferior epigastric artery

Obliterated umbilical artery

164 Intestines

The greater omentum is thrown upwards and with it go the transverse colon and transverse mesocolon. The jejunum and ileum are cut away, excepting their end pieces, and the mesentery is cut short. Examine in conjunction with figure 165 facing.

Observe:

1. The duodeno-jejunal junction, situated to the left of the median plane and immediately below the root of the transverse mesocolon.

2. The first few inches of the jejunum descending infero-sinistrally anterior to the left kidney. The last few inches of the ileum ascending supero-dextrally out of the pelvic cavity. Of these two parallel pieces of gut, the former being much the larger.

3. The root of the mesentery directed infero-dextrally and crossing in turn the junction of the 3rd and 4th parts of the duodenum, the inferior vena cava, the right ureter, and the right Psoas (fig. 165).

4. The large gut forming $3\frac{1}{2}$ sides of a square, or picture frame, around the jejunum and ileum (removed); the missing $\frac{1}{2}$ side being infero-dextral, between the cecum and the sigmoid colon.

5. The distinguishing features of the large gut: (a) its position around the small gut, (b) the taeniae coli or longitudinal muscle bands, (c) the sacculations or haustra, and (d) the appendices epiploicae.

6. The right colic flexure, which lies below the liver, placed at a lower level than the left colic flexure which lies below the spleen.

7. The vermiform appendix had been removed at operation.

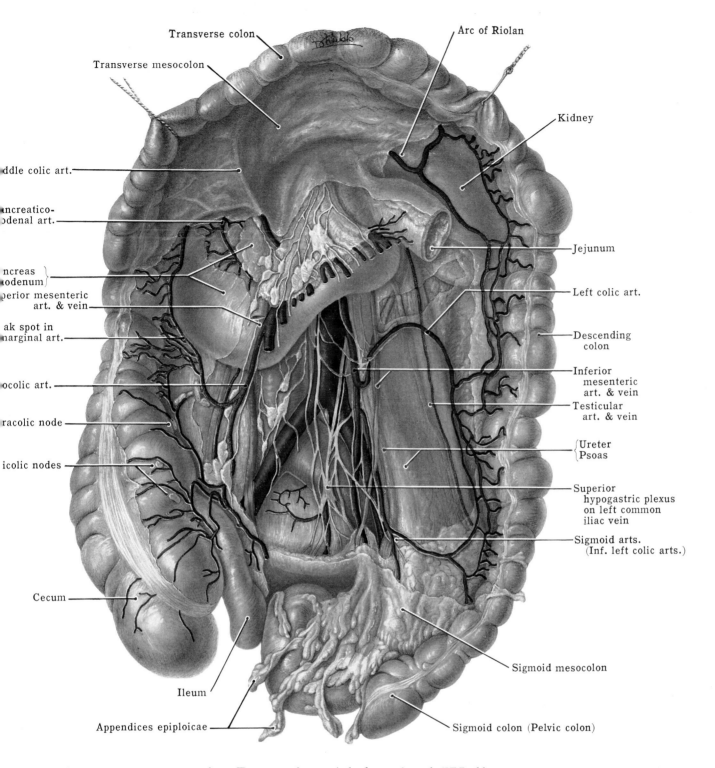

Transverse colon

Transverse mesocolon

Arc of Riolan

Kidney

ddle colic art.

ncreatico-
odenal art.

ncreas
odenum

perior mesenteric
art. & vein

ak spot in
marginal art.

ocolic art.

racolic node

icolic nodes

Jejunum

Left colic art.

Descending
colon

Inferior
mesenteric
art. & vein

Testicular
art. & vein

Ureter
Psoas

Superior
hypogastric plexus
on left common
iliac vein

Sigmoid arts.
(Inf. left colic arts.)

Cecum

Ileum

Appendices epiploicae

Sigmoid mesocolon

Sigmoid colon (Pelvic colon)

165 Structures on the Posterior Abdominal Wall

This is figure 164 enlarged and with much peritoneum removed.

Observe:

1. The duodenum, of large diameter before the site of crossing
of the superior mesenteric vessels, and narrow beyond. It is,
indeed, much wider than the descending colon.

2. The jejunal and ileal branches (cut) passing from the left
side of the superior mesenteric artery; the right colic artery,
here as commonly, being a branch of the ileocolic artery.

3. An accessory artery, called the arc of Riolan, which connects
the superior mesenteric artery to the left colic artery.

4. On the right side: small (epicolic) lymph nodes on the colon;

small (paracolic) nodes beside the colon; nodes along the
ileo-colic artery which drain into main nodes ventral to the
pancreas.

5. (a) The intestines and the intestinal vessels lying on a plane
anterior to (b) that of the testicular vessels, and these in turn
lying (c) anterior to the plane of the kidney, its vessels, and
the ureter.

6. The right and left ureters asymmetrically placed, in this
specimen.

7. The superior hypogastric plexus (presacral nerve) lying
within the fork of the aorta and ventral to the left common
iliac vein, the body of the 5th lumbar vertebra and the 5th
disc.

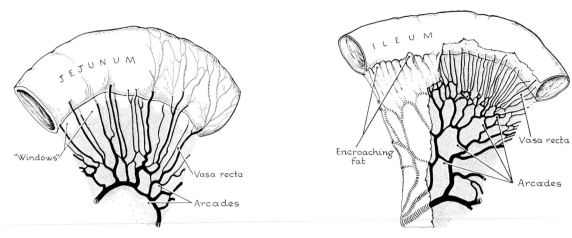

166   Jejunum contrasted with Ileum

Note whether: large diameter or small; thick wall or thin; one or two arterial arcades or several; long vasa recta or short; and translucent (fat-free) areas at the mesenteric border or fat encroaching on the wall of the gut.

Antimesenteric border of gut

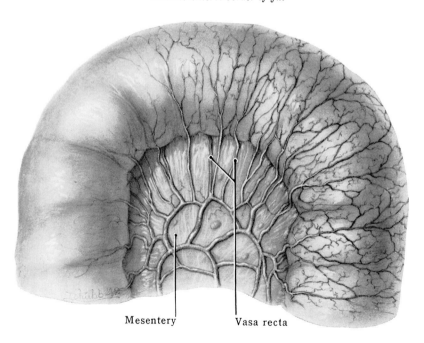

Segment of Intestinum Jejunum with Mesentery and Arteries.

167   Blood Supply of the Small Intestine

Observe.

1. The series of anastomotic arterial arches in the mesentery.
2. The vasa recta that proceed from the arches to the mesenteric border of the gut and then pass more or less alternately to opposite sides of the gut.

3. The arborisations of the vasa in the wall of the gut and the fine anastomoses effected between adjacent arborisations.

4. The efficient anastomoses across the anti-mesenteric border.

Stomach

Pyloric orifice

Duodenum

Pylorus

Upper part of Jejunum

Longitudinal fold

Hood

Papilla major

Papilla minor

Duodenum

Upper part of Ileum

Lower part of Ileum

168 Interior of the Small Intestine

Pylorus: The pylorus pouts into the 1st (superior) part of the duodenum and, having a fornix around it, resembles the cervix projecting into the vagina. The first $1\frac{1}{2}''$ of the duodenum has no plicae circulares, but the mucous membrane may be rugose.

Duodenum: The larger duodenal papilla (of Vater) projects into the 2nd (descending) part of the duodenum on the concave border $3\frac{1}{2}''$ from the pylorus (in fig. 156 it is at the apex of a conical evagination). On its tip is the orifice of the bile duct and, below this, the orifice of the pancreatic duct, but usually these 2 ducts open together (see fig. 157). A hood is thrown over the larger papilla, a longitudinal fold descends from it, and the smaller duo-

denal papilla, of the accessory pancreatic duct, lies $\frac{1}{4}''-\frac{3}{4}''$ antero-superior to it. Plicae circulares are pronounced.

Jejunum, upper part: The plicae circulares are tall, closely packed, and commonly branched.

Ileum, upper part: The plicae circulares are low and becoming sparse. The calibre of the gut is reduced and the wall is thinner.

Ileum, lower part: Plicae are now absent. Solitary lymph nodules stud the wall. [In youth, aggregated lymph nodules, up to $1\frac{1}{2}''$ long and $\frac{3}{4}''$ wide, are scattered along the antimesenteric border.]

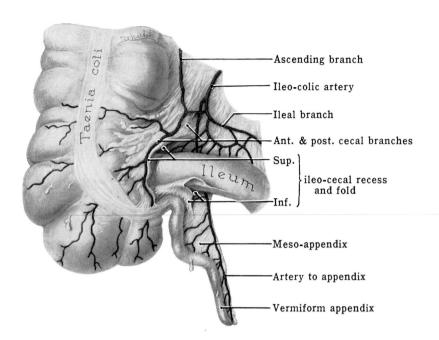

- Ascending branch
- Ileo-colic artery
- Ileal branch
- Ant. & post. cecal branches
- Sup.
- Inf. } ileo-cecal recess and fold
- Meso-appendix
- Artery to appendix
- Vermiform appendix

169 Ileo-cecal Region

Observe:

1. The appendix in one free border of the meso-pendix and the artery in the other.
2. The anterior taenia coli leading to the appen
3. The inferior ileocecal (bloodless) fold extend from ileum to meso-appendix.
4. The vascular cecal fold is the official name the superior ileocecal fold.

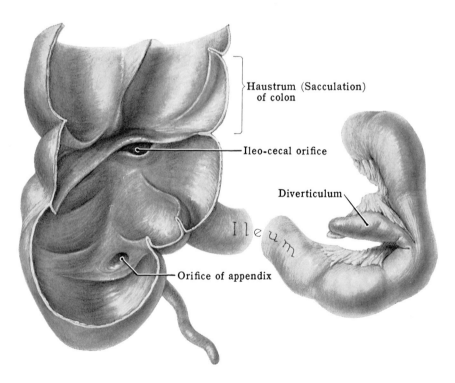

- Haustrum (Sacculation) of colon
- Ileo-cecal orifice
- Diverticulum
- Orifice of appendix

170 Interior of a Dried Cecum

This cecum was filled with air, dried, oper and varnished.

Observe:

1. The ileocecal valve guarding the ileoce orifice; its pouting upper lip overhanging lower lip; and the folds or frenula running ho zontally from the commissures of the lips.
2. The slight fold closing the upper part of the fice of the appendix.

170.1 A Meckel's Diverticulum

Meckel's diverticulum, found in 2% of pe sons, is the remains of the prenatal vitel intestinal duct. It projects from the si of the ileum (theoretically, from the an mesenteric border) and it is attached to it a short peritoneal fold. Usually less than inches in length, it may attain ten inch About 75% of diverticula are located with $3\frac{1}{2}$ feet of the ileocecal orifice, and 25% fro $3\frac{1}{2}$ to $5\frac{1}{2}$ feet. (G. D. Jay et al.).

171 Duodenal Diverticula

A.

Sites of 20 diverticula found in 15 of 133 duodena investigated. Melted wax, poured into the duodena, fills any diverticula that may be present; these are revealed when the wax hardens. (*J.C.B.G.*)

B.

Two diverticula, posterior to the bile and pancreatic ducts, posterior view.

C.

A single diverticulum, anterior to the bile and pancreatic ducts, posterior view.

Note that the mucous and submucous coats are herniated through the muscular coats.

172 Vermiform Appendix

A.

Locations and their Approximate Frequencies. (After Wakeley.) Like the hands of a clock, the appendix may be long or short, and it may occupy any position consistent with its length.

B.

A Retrocolic Appendix seven inches long.

B.

VARIATIONS AND ANOMALIES

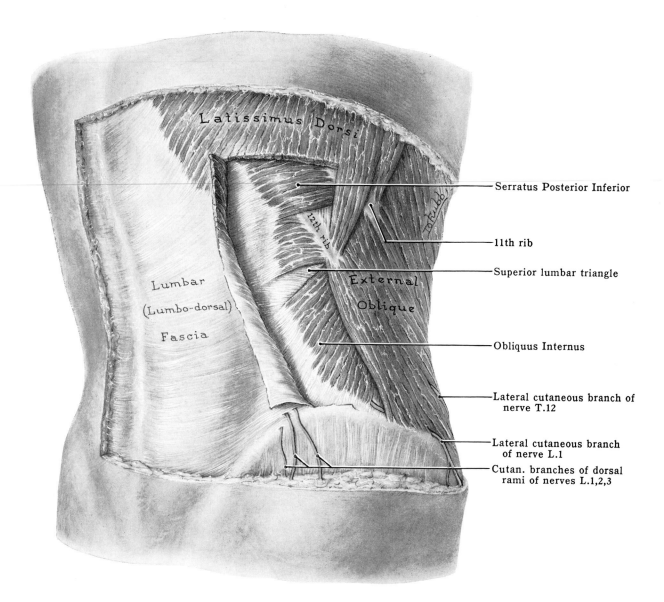

Latissimus Dorsi

Serratus Posterior Inferior

11th rib

Superior lumbar triangle

12th rib

External Oblique

Lumbar (Lumbo-dorsal) Fascia

Obliquus Internus

Lateral cutaneous branch of nerve T.12

Lateral cutaneous branch of nerve L.1

Cutan. branches of dorsal rami of nerves L.1,2,3

173   Posterior Abdominal Wall, postero-lateral view—I

Latissimus Dorsi is in part reflected.

Observe:

1. External Oblique having an oblique, free, posterior border at the mid-point of the iliac crest.

2. The small, triangular space between External Oblique, Latissimus Dorsi, and the iliac crest. This is the (inferior) lumbar triangle (fig. 24).

3. Internal Oblique extending behind External Oblique. It forms the floor of the lumbar triangle, creeps up on to the lumbar fascia, and has a triangle between it and Serratus Posterior Inferior. This is the "superior lumbar triangle".

   (In N. A. P. lumbo-dorsal fascia reads thoraco-lumbar fascia.)

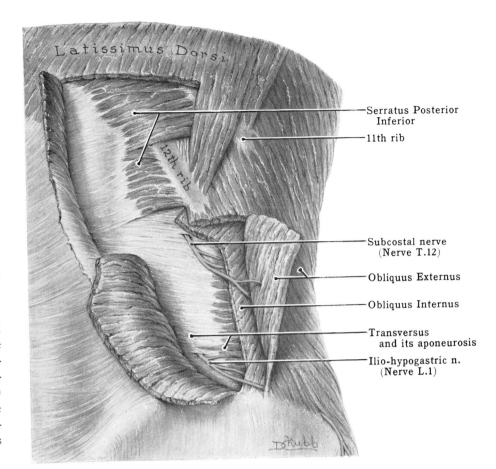

74 Posterior Abdominal Wall—II

When External Oblique has been incised and turned laterally, and Internal Oblique incised and turned medially, Transversus Abdominis and its posterior aponeurosis are exposed where pierced by the subcostal (T.12) and ilio-hypogastric (L.1) nerves. These nerves give off motor twigs and lateral cutaneous (iliac) branches, and continue forwards between Internal Oblique and Transversus.

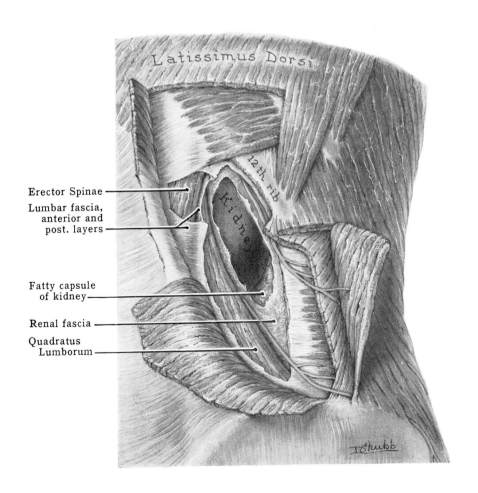

75 Posterior Abdominal Wall—III

On dividing the posterior aponeurosis of Transversus between the subcostal and ilio-hypogastric nerves, and lateral to the oblique lateral border of Quadratus Lumborum, the retroperitoneal fat surrounding the kidney is exposed. The renal fascia is within this fat. The portion of fat inside the renal fascia is termed fatty renal capsule (perinephric fat); the fat outside is paranephric fat.

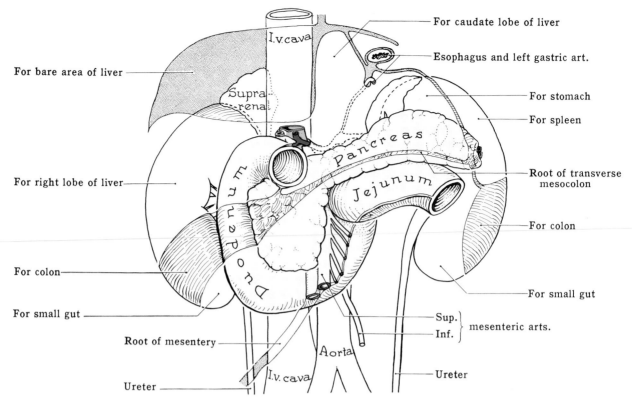

For bare area of liver

I.v.cava

Supra-renal

For caudate lobe of liver

Esophagus and left gastric art.

For stomach

For spleen

Pancreas

Duodenum

Jejunum

For right lobe of liver

Root of transverse mesocolon

For colon

For colon

For small gut

For small gut

Root of mesentery

Sup.
Inf. } mesenteric arts.

Aorta

I.v.cava

Ureter

Ureter

176 Duodenum and Pancreas, in situ

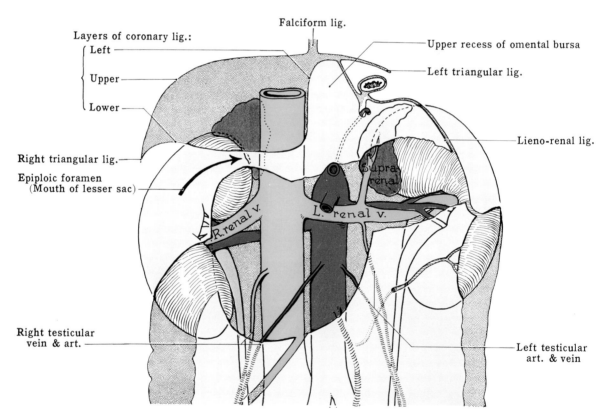

Falciform lig.

Layers of coronary lig.:
{ Left
Upper
Lower

Upper recess of omental bursa

Left triangular lig.

Right triangular lig.

Supra-renal

Lieno-renal lig.

Epiploic foramen
(Mouth of lesser sac)

R.renal v.

L. renal v.

Right testicular
vein & art.

Left testicular
art. & vein

177 Duodenum and Pancreas, removed

176 & 177 Posterior Abdominal Viscera and their Ventral Relations

Observe:

1. The peritoneal covering (yellow) of pancreas and duodenum.

2. The colic area of the right kidney, second part of duodenum, and head of pancreas; the line of attachment of the transverse mesocolon to the body and tail of the pancreas; and the colic area of the left kidney. (Figs. 153 and 154.)

4. The anterior relations of the kidneys and suprarenal glands.

5. The right suprarenal gland at the epiploic foramen.

6. The three layers of the coronary ligament, which enclose the bare area of the liver and are attached to the diaphragm except where the inferior vena cava, suprarenal gland, and kidney intervene.

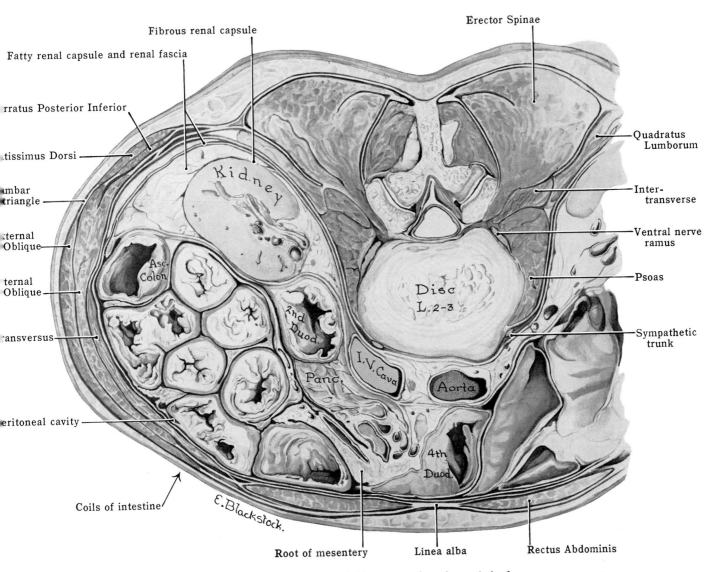

Fatty renal capsule and renal fascia — Fibrous renal capsule — Erector Spinae

rratus Posterior Inferior — tissimus Dorsi — mbar triangle — ternal Oblique — ternal Oblique — ansversus — eritoneal cavity — Coils of intestine

Quadratus Lumborum — Inter-transverse — Ventral nerve ramus — Psoas — Sympathetic trunk

Kidney — Asc. Colon — 2nd Duod. — Panc. — I.V.Cava — Aorta — Disc L.2-3 — 4th Duod. — E.Blackstock.

Root of mesentery — Linea alba — Rectus Abdominis

178 Transverse Section Through the Abdomen

at the level of the disc between the 2nd and 3rd lumbar vertebrae and between their transverse processes.

Observe:

1. The anterior aspect of the vertebral column, nearer to the ventral surface of the body than to the dorsal surface in this thin recumbent subject.

2. The coils of small intestine, not circular as seen at operation, but mutually compressed.

3. The mucous membrane of the small intestine—which in life is much more moist and succulent than in this hardened specimen—in loose folds which nearly completely occlude the lumen.

4. The ascending colon with an appendix epiploica, having no mesentery but being bare posteriorly.

5. The anterior and posterior surfaces of the kidney facing not ventrally and dorsally but ventro-laterally and dorso-medially.

6. The adipose renal capsule (perinephric fat) massed along the borders of the kidney and leaving the anterior surface close to the peritoneum.

7. The kidney projecting lateral to Quadratus Lumborum.

8. The 2nd or descending part of the duodenum overlapping this surface of the kidney.

9. The sympathetic trunk lying along the anterior border of Psoas; and on the right side behind the i. vena cava.

10. The lipping at the epiphyseal plate of the vertebral body which first begins to show itself before the age of 30 years.

11. The linea alba, band-like above the navel, though linear below it.

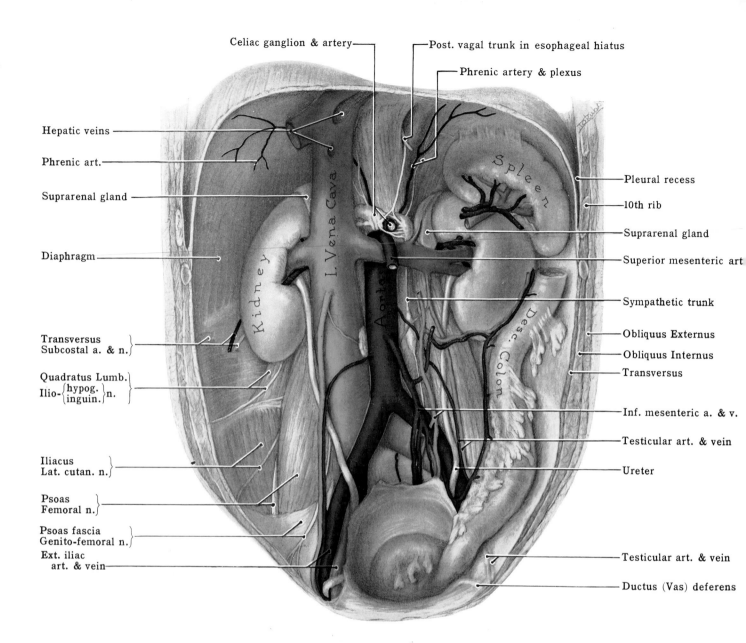

Celiac ganglion & artery

Post. vagal trunk in esophageal hiatus

Phrenic artery & plexus

Hepatic veins

Phrenic art.

Suprarenal gland

Diaphragm

Transversus
Subcostal a. & n.

Quadratus Lumb.
Ilio-{hypog.}n.
    {inguin.}

Iliacus
Lat. cutan. n.

Psoas
Femoral n.

Psoas fascia
Genito-femoral n.

Ext. iliac
    art. & vein

I. Vena Cava

Aorta

Spleen

Desc. Colon

Pleural recess

10th rib

Suprarenal gland

Superior mesenteric art

Sympathetic trunk

Obliquus Externus

Obliquus Internus

Transversus

Inf. mesenteric a. & v.

Testicular art. & vein

Ureter

Testicular art. & vein

Ductus (Vas) deferens

179   Great vessels: Kidneys: Suprarenal Glands

The abdominal aorta is shorter than the combined common and external iliac arteries, and it is much shorter and of smaller calibre than the inf. vena cava.

The celiac trunk is surrounded by the celiac plexus and has a celiac ganglion on each side. The ganglia receive a branch of the posterior vagal trunk. Wide of these are the suprarenal glands, the right gland being partly covered by the inf. vena cava.

The superior mesenteric artery arises just below the celiac artery, and in the angle it makes with the aorta runs the left renal vein. This indicates the level of the upper part of the hilus of the kidney. The left renal vein drains the left testis and left suprarenal as well as the left kidney. The renal arteries are behind their veins.

The inferior mesenteric artery arises 1½″ above the bifurcation of the aorta and crosses the left common iliac vessels to become the superior rectal (haemorrhoidal) artery.

The kidneys lie in front of Diaphragm, Transversus aponeurosis, Quadratus Lumborum and Psoas. *The ureter* crosses the external iliac artery just beyond the bifurcation of the common iliac artery and descends in the pelvis in front of the internal iliac artery.

The testicular vessels cross in front of the ureter and join the ductus deferens in front of the external iliac artery at the deep inguinal ring.

Note that the vessels to the intestine cross anterior to the testicular vessels, and these in turn cross anterior to the ureter.

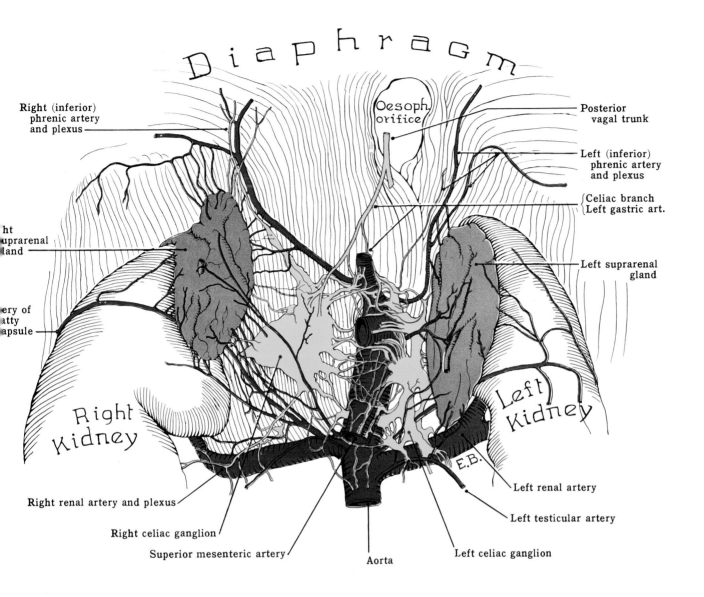

Labels on figure:

Diaphragm

Right (inferior) phrenic artery and plexus

Oesoph. orifice

Posterior vagal trunk

Left (inferior) phrenic artery and plexus

Celiac branch Left gastric art.

ht uprarenal land

Left suprarenal gland

ery of atty apsule

Right Kidney

Left Kidney

E.B.

Left renal artery

Left testicular artery

Right renal artery and plexus

Right celiac ganglion

Superior mesenteric artery

Aorta

Left celiac ganglion

180   Celiac Plexus, the Celiac Ganglia, and the Suprarenal Glands

(Arteries injected with latex. Dissection by Surgeon Lieutenant Ian B. MacDonald.)

Observe:

1. The celiac plexus of nerves surrounding the celiac trunk (not labelled) and connecting the right and the left celiac ganglion.

2. A stout branch from the posterior vagal trunk descending along the stem of the left gastric artery and conveying vagal (parasympathetic) fibres to the celiac ganglia.

3. Nerves extending along the arteries to the viscera, e.g., along left gastric, celiac, superior mesenteric, phrenic, suprarenal, and renal arteries, and down the aorta. The nerves to the suprarenal glands are few and very slender.

4. The suprarenal glands, abreast of the celiac trunk, two inches apart, but not equidistant from the medial plane.

5. The right suprarenal vein, about 5 mm long, ascending to join the i.v. cava; the left vein descending to join the left renal vein.

6. The very numerous thread-like branches of the phrenic artery, aorta, renal artery and artery of the fatty capsule of the kidney converging on the periphery of the suprarenal gland.

(*For variations on the blood vessels of the gland, see Kenneth Clark.*)

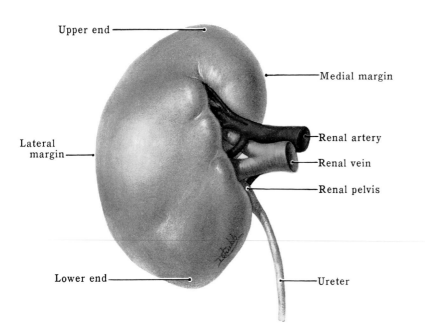

Upper end

Medial margin

Renal artery

Lateral margin

Renal vein

Renal pelvis

Lower end

Ureter

181   Right Kidney, front view

The order of structures at the hilus (entrance to the renal sinus) from before backwards is—vein, artery, duct (pelvis or ureter), and a branch of the artery crosses behind the pelvis.

The upper end of the kidney is usually wider than the lower, and closer to the median plane, as in figure 183.

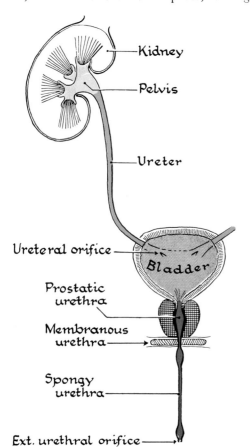

Kidney

Pelvis

Ureter

Ureteral orifice

Bladder

Prostatic urethra

Membranous urethra

Spongy urethra

Ext. urethral orifice

182   Diagram of the Male Urinary System

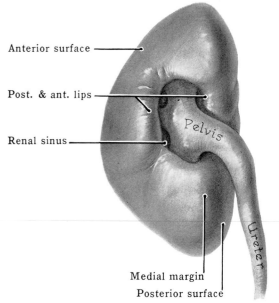

Anterior surface

Post. & ant. lips

Renal sinus

Pelvis

Medial margin

Posterior surface

Ureter

181.1   Sinus of the Kidney

The anterior surface has an upper and a lower inclin plane.

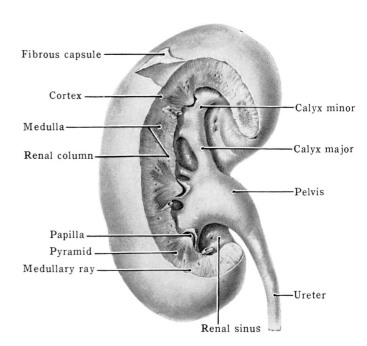

Fibrous capsule

Cortex

Medulla

Renal column

Calyx minor

Calyx major

Pelvis

Papilla

Pyramid

Medullary ray

Ureter

Renal sinus

183   Structure of the Kidney

The anterior lip of the sinus is cut away. The outer $\frac{1}{3}$ of the renal substance is cortex; the inner $\frac{2}{3}$ is medulla. Cortical tissue (glomeruli, convoluted tubules) is granular on section and extends, as renal columns (of Bertin), through the medulla to the sinus. The medulla contains 7 to 14 pyramids which are striated because they consist of converging tubules (collecting, loops of Henle). Each pyramid sends finger-like rays into the cortex and each ends as a papilla on which a dozen or more ducts open. One or two (or more) papillae project into each calyx minor; several calyces minores unite to form a calyx major. Of calyces majores there are usually two, an upper and a lower, but not uncommonly there are also one or two middle.

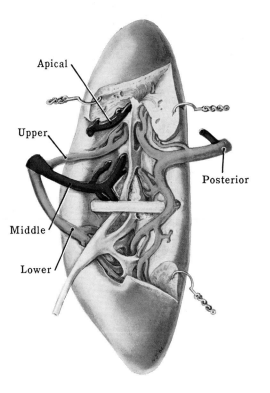

Apical

Upper

Middle

Lower

Posterior

3.1 Branches of the Renal
rtery within the Sinus

ypically, as shown, there are 5 such segmental ar-
es. The posterior lip of the sinus has been incised,
ve and below, near the limits of the territory of the
terior segmental artery. (Riches; Graves; and Rob-
.)

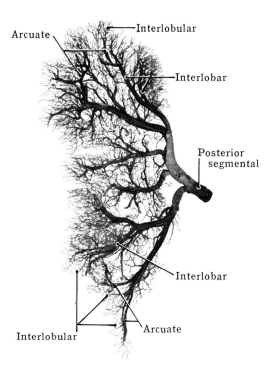

Arcuate

Interlobular

Interlobar

Posterior
segmental

Interlobar

Interlobular

Arcuate

3.2 A Segmental Artery

e that interlobar arteries are end arteries.

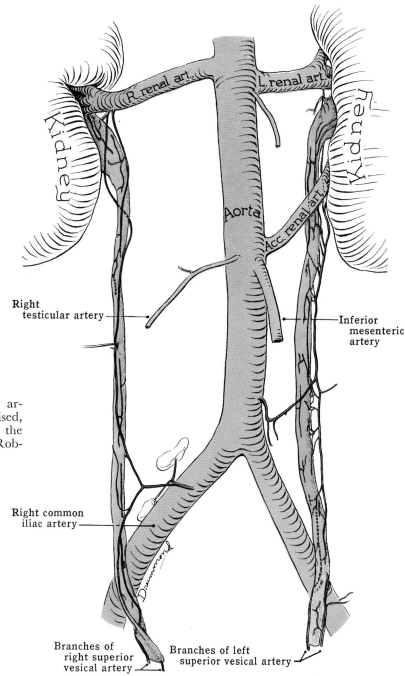

R. renal art.   L. renal art.

Kidney

Kidney

Aorta

Acc. renal art.

Right
testicular artery

Inferior
mesenteric
artery

Right common
iliac artery

Drummond

Branches of
right superior
vesical artery

Branches of left
superior vesical artery

184 Blood Supply to the Ureter

The arterial system was injected with latex by way of the
femoral artery. (*Dissection by W. R. Mitchell.*)

Observe:

1. The blood supply to the ureter coming from 3 main sources: (a) from the
   renal artery above, (b) from a vesical artery below, and (c) about the
   middle of its course either from the common iliac artery or from the aorta.

2. These branches approaching the ureter from the medial side. In this
   specimen an accessory renal artery also supplies branches. The testicular
   artery may also contribute a branch.

3. The excellent anastomotic chain made by these long, tenuous branches.

Right
suprarenal gland

Superior
mesenteric
artery

Left
suprarenal gland

Right common iliac vein

185   Left Postrenal Inferior Vena Cava

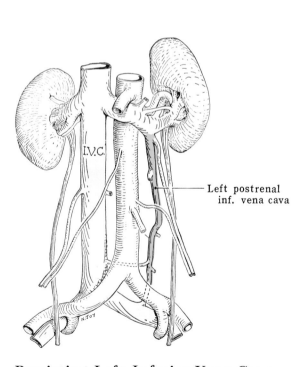

Left postrenal
inf. vena cava

185.1   Persisting Left Inferior Vena Cava

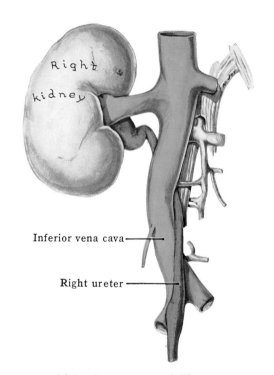

Inferior vena cava

Right ureter

186   Retrocaval Ureter

joins the left common iliac vein to the left renal vein. This
occasional vessel may be small, as in this specimen, or it may
be large.

There were only 34 isolated cases of retrocaval ureter
ported up to the year 1946 (Lowsley). The dissecting ro
specimen depicted here has not been recorded before.

Anomalies of the Inferior Vena Cava

Horseshoe Kidney

"In our 35,329 postmortems there were 4 cases, 1:376." (Bell, E. T.)

Multiple Renal Arteries and Fetal Lobulation

About 25% of kidneys receive directly from the aorta 2nd, 3rd, and even 4th branches. These enter either through the renal sinus or at the upper or lower pole. (Data from Adachi; Lloyd, L. W.)

Duplicated or Bifid Ureters

These may be either unilateral or bilateral, and either complete or incomplete.

In 32,360 postmortems 205 cases were found, 1:157. The incidence is probably higher. Of these, 167 were unilateral, 37 being complete; and 38 were bilateral, 11 being complete on both sides, and 3 on one side. (Bell, E. T.; also Campbell, M.)

ht ureter—— ——Left ureter

Ectopic Pelvic Kidney

Pelvic kidneys have no fatty capsule. During childbirth, they may both cause obstruction and suffer injury. Of 112 recorded cases, 97 were unilateral (mostly left), 10 were bilateral (either fused or separate), and 5 were solitary. (Anderson, Rice and Harris.)

Bifid Pelves

(*Dissections by Dr. C. A. Armstrong.*)

The pelves are almost replaced by two long calyces majores, which lie entirely within the sinus (left), and partly within and partly without (right).

187   Anomalies of the Kidney and Ureter

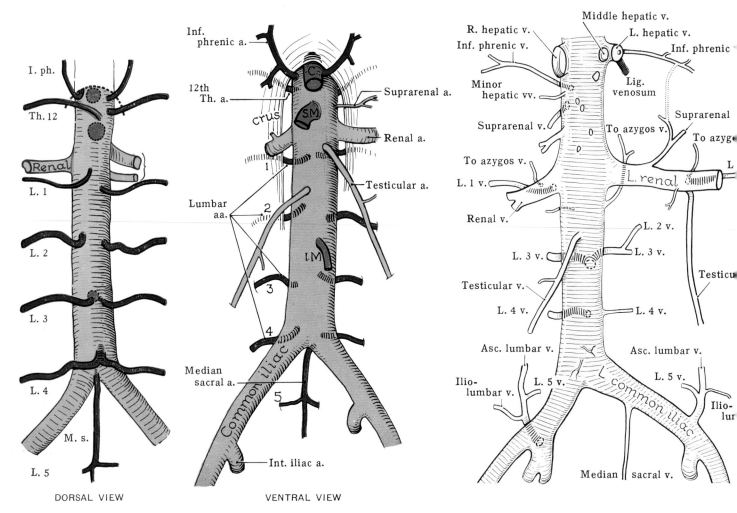

188 Abdominal Aorta and its Branches

(The dorsal and ventral views are of different specimens.)

DORSAL VIEW — VENTRAL VIEW

I. ph. — Th. 12 — Renal — L. 1 — L. 2 — L. 3 — L. 4 — M. s. — L. 5

Inf. phrenic a. — 12th Th. a. — crus — Lumbar aa. — Median sacral a. — Int. iliac a. — Common iliac

Suprarenal a. — Renal a. — Testicular a.

188.2 Inferior Vena Cava and its Tributaries

R. hepatic v. — Inf. phrenic v. — Minor hepatic vv. — Suprarenal v. — To azygos v. — L. 1 v. — Renal v. — L. 3 v. — Testicular v. — L. 4 v. — Asc. lumbar v. — Ilio-lumbar v. — L. 5 v.

Middle hepatic v. — L. hepatic v. — Inf. phrenic — Lig. venosum — Suprarenal — To azygos v. — L. renal — L. 2 v. — L. 3 v. — Testicu — L. 4 v. — Asc. lumbar v. — L. 5 v. — Ilio-lur — common iliac

Median sacral v.

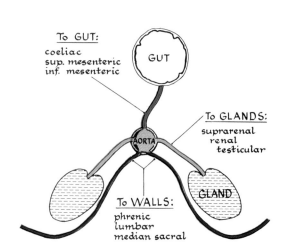

188.1 Its Branches Classified

To GUT:
coeliac
sup. mesenteric
inf. mesenteric

GUT

To GLANDS:
suprarenal
renal
testicular

AORTA

GLAND

To WALLS:
phrenic
lumbar
median sacral

188.3 Ascending Lumbar Vein

Azygos v. — Hemiazygos v. — Intercostal veins — I.V.C. — Lumbar vv. — Ascending lumbar v. — L. c. iliac — Ilio-lumbar vein

This intersegmental vein, which lies on the transverse processes, is interrupted in about 15% of cases (Seib, G. A.).

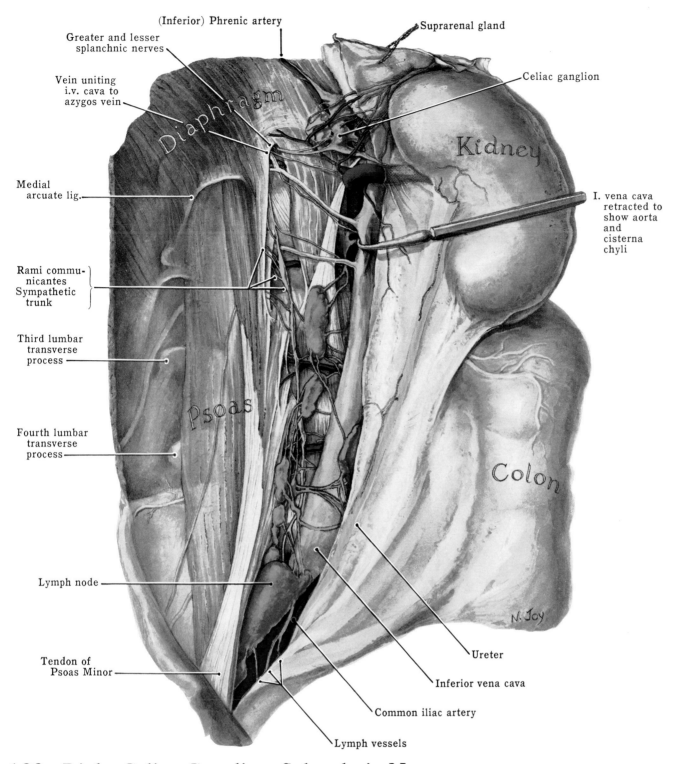

(Inferior) Phrenic artery

Greater and lesser splanchnic nerves

Vein uniting i.v. cava to azygos vein

Suprarenal gland

Celiac ganglion

Kidney

Medial arcuate lig.

Diaphragm

I. vena cava retracted to show aorta and cisterna chyli

Rami commu- nicantes Sympathetic trunk

Third lumbar transverse process

Psoas

Fourth lumbar transverse process

Colon

Lymph node

N. Joy

Tendon of Psoas Minor

Ureter

Inferior vena cava

Common iliac artery

Lymph vessels

189 Right Celiac Ganglion, Splanchnic Nerves, and Sympathetic Trunk

The right suprarenal gland, kidney, ureter, and colon are reflected; the inferior vena cava is pulled medially; and the third and fourth lumbar veins are removed.

Observe:

1. In this specimen a Psoas Minor.

2. A wide cleft in the right crus (not labelled) of the dia- phragm through which pass both splanchnic nerves, the sympathetic trunk, and a communicating vein. This un- usually wide cleft is present on the left side also.

3. The greater splanchnic nerve ending in the celiac ganglion; the lesser splanchnic nerve here ending in the renal plexus (aortico-renal ganglion). Usually, as in figure 190, the

greater splanchnic nerve pierces the crus at the level of the celiac trunk; the lesser nerve infero-lateral to this: and the sympathetic trunk enters with the Psoas.

4. The sympathetic trunk lying on the bodies of the vertebrae, the lumbar vessels alone intervening, and descending along the anterior border of the Psoas. The trunk is slender where it enters the abdomen; its ganglia are ill-defined: about eleven rami communicantes join it postero-laterally; and about six visceral branches, or lumbar splanchnic nerves, leave it antero-medially.

5. The 4 right lumbar arteries and cranial 2 veins (not la- belled); the tip of the 3rd lumbar transverse process project- ing further than the other transverse processes; and the right lumbar lymph nodes and vessels draining into the cisterna chyli.

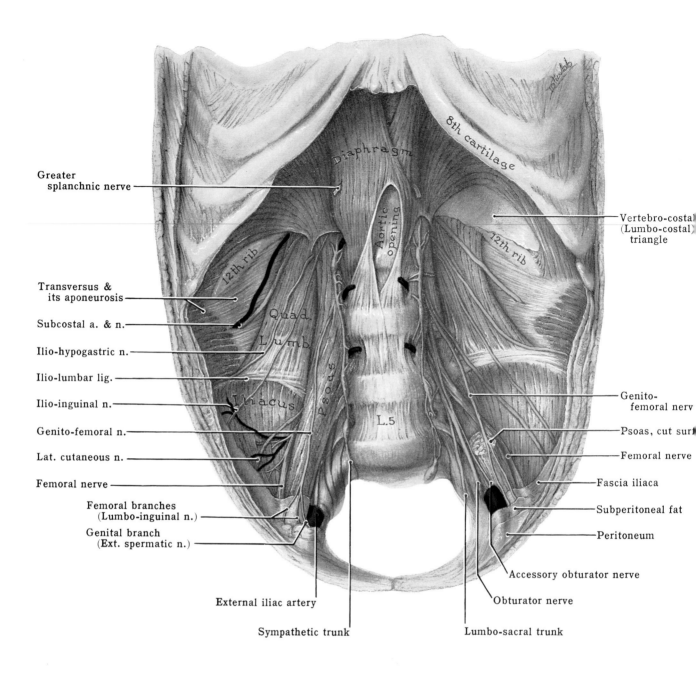

Greater splanchnic nerve

Transversus & its aponeurosis

Subcostal a. & n.

Ilio-hypogastric n.

Ilio-lumbar lig.

Ilio-inguinal n.

Genito-femoral n.

Lat. cutaneous n.

Femoral nerve

Femoral branches (Lumbo-inguinal n.)

Genital branch (Ext. spermatic n.)

External iliac artery

Sympathetic trunk

Diaphragm

8th cartilage

Aortic opening

12th rib

L.5

Quad. Lumb.

Iliacus

Psoas

Vertebro-costal (Lumbo-costal) triangle

Genito-femoral nerv

Psoas, cut surf

Femoral nerve

Fascia iliaca

Subperitoneal fat

Peritoneum

Accessory obturator nerve

Obturator nerve

Lumbo-sacral trunk

190 Posterior Abdominal Wall: Lumbar Plexus

Muscles: Transversus Abdominis becomes aponeurotic on a line dropped from the tip of the 12th rib. Quadratus Lumborum has an oblique lateral border; its fascia is thickened to form the lateral arcuate ligament (lumbo-costal arch) above, and the ilio-lumbar ligament below. Iliacus lies below the iliac crest. Psoas rises above the crest and extends above the medial arcuate ligament (lumbo-costal arch) which is thickened Psoas fascia.

Nerves: The subcostal nerve (T.12) passes behind the lateral arcuate lig. and runs at some distance below the 12th rib (with its artery). The next four nerves appear at the lateral border of Psoas. Of these, the ilio-hypogastric (T.12, L.1) takes the characteristic course here shown; the ilio-inguinal (L.1) and the lateral cutaneous of the thigh (L.2, 3) are variable; the femoral (L.2, 3, 4) descends in the angle between Iliacus and Psoas. The genito-femoral nerve (L.1, 2) pierces Psoas and its fascia anteriorly. The obturator nerve (L.2 3, 4) and a branch of L.4 that joins with L.5 to form the lumbo-sacral trunk appear at the medial border of Psoas, and, crossing the ala of the sacrum, enter the pelvis.

The Sympathetic Trunk enters the abdomen with Psoas from behind the medial arcuate lig., and descends along the line of the vertebral border of Psoas to enter the pelvis. Its rami communicantes run dorsally with, or near, the lumbar arteries to the lumbar plexus.

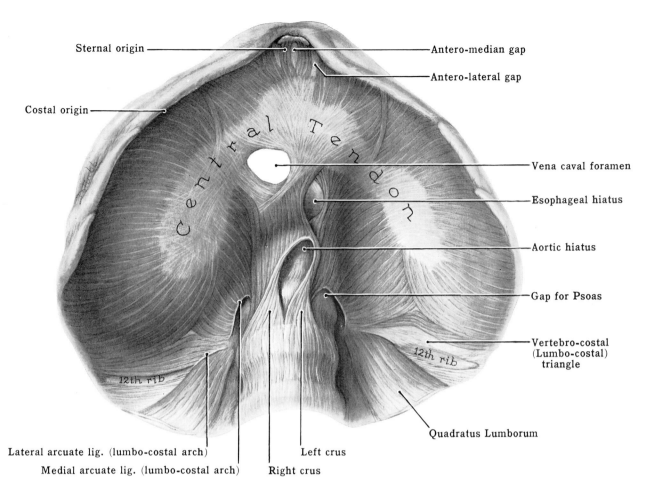

Sternal origin — — — — — — — — — — — — — Antero-median gap

— — — — — — — — — Antero-lateral gap

Costal origin — — — — — — —

Central Tendon

— — — — Vena caval foramen

— — — — Esophageal hiatus

— — — — Aortic hiatus

— — — — Gap for Psoas

12th rib — — — Vertebro-costal
(Lumbo-costal)
triangle

12th rib

Quadratus Lumborum

Lateral arcuate lig. (lumbo-costal arch)   Left crus

Medial arcuate lig. (lumbo-costal arch)   Right crus

191   Diaphragm, viewed from below

Observe:

1. The trefoil-shaped, aponeurotic insertion called the central tendon; and the fleshy fibres of the sternal, costal, and vertebral origins (crura) that converge on this tendon.

2. Three large openings: The foramen for the inferior vena cava in the central tendon. The elliptical esophageal hiatus, which is almost a canal, surrounded by fleshy fibres from one or both crura. The aortic hiatus lying postero-medianly behind the diaphragm.

3. The right and left crura, lying one on each side of the aortic

hiatus, and united in front of this opening by a fibrous arch called the median arcuate ligament. Also, thickenings of the Psoas fascia and of the Quadratus Lumborum fascia, called the medial and lateral arcuate ligaments. These ligaments afford origin to fibres of the Diaphragm.

4. The Diaphragm, in this specimen, failing to arise from the left lateral arcuate ligament; hence the area, called the vertebrocostal triangle, where only an areolar membrane separates the kidney and surrounding fat from the pleura. It marks the site occupied in the embryo by the pleuroperitoneal canal.

191.1   Diagram of the Nerve Supply to the Diaphragm

Each phrenic nerve (C.3, 4, and 5) is the sole motor nerve to its own half of the diaphragm. Each phrenic nerve is also sensory to the greater part of its own half of the diaphragm, including the pleura on the thoracic surface and the peritoneum on the abdominal surface; but the lower intercostal nerves are sensory to the peripheral fringe.

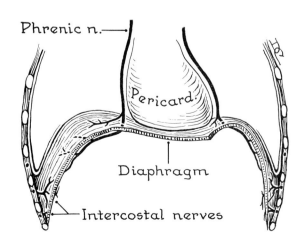

Phrenic n.—

Pericard.

Diaphragm

Intercostal nerves

The Perineum and Pelvis

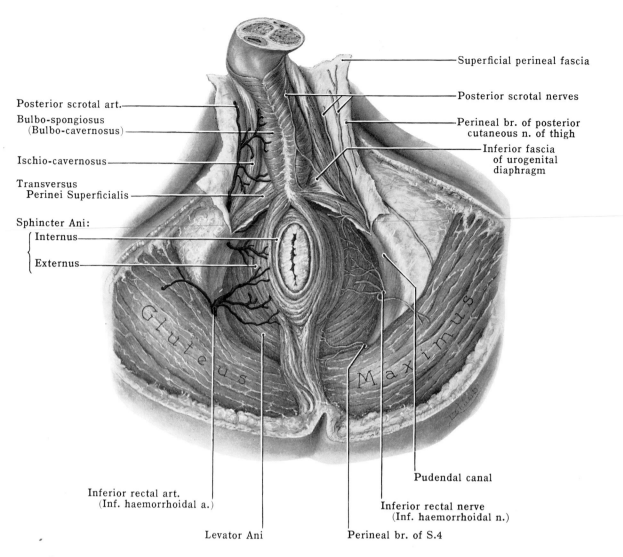

Superficial perineal fascia

Posterior scrotal nerves

Perineal br. of posterior cutaneous n. of thigh

Inferior fascia of urogenital diaphragm

Posterior scrotal art.

Bulbo-spongiosus (Bulbo-cavernosus)

Ischio-cavernosus

Transversus Perinei Superficialis

Sphincter Ani:
{ Internus
{ Externus

Gluteus

Maximus

Pudendal canal

Inferior rectal art. (Inf. haemorrhoidal a.)

Inferior rectal nerve (Inf. haemorrhoidal n.)

Levator Ani

Perineal br. of S.4

192 Male Perineum

Observe in the anal region or triangle:

1. The anal orifice at the center of the anal triangle, surrounded by Sphincter Ani Externus.
2. The superficial fibres of Sphincter Ani Externus anchoring the anus in front to the perineal body, or tendon of the perineum, and behind to the coccyx—here to the skin.
3. On each side, an ischio-rectal fossa, bounded medially by Levator Ani and Sphincter Ani Externus; laterally by Obturator Internus fascia; behind by Gluteus Maximus overlying the sacro-tuberous ligament; in front by the base of the perineal membrane. The apex or roof is where the medial and lateral walls meet. The base or floor, formed by tough skin and deep fascia, is removed.
4. The inferior rectal nerve leaving the pudendal canal and, with the perineal branch of S.4, supplying Sphincter Ani Externus. Its cutaneous twigs to the anus are removed. The branch turning round Gluteus Maximus is replacing the perforating cutaneous nerve.

Observe in the urogenital region or triangle:

5. The superficial perineal fascia (of Colles) incised in the midline, freed from its attachment to the base of the perineal membrane, and reflected.
6. The cutaneous nerves and artery in the superficial perineal pouch.
7. The three paired superficial perineal muscles—Bulbospongiosus, Ischiocavernosus, and Transversus Perinei Superficialis.
8. The exposed triangular portion of the perineal membrane or inf. fascia.

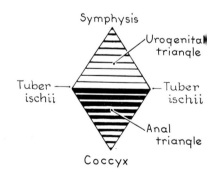

Symphysis

Urogenital triangle

Tuber ischii

Tuber ischii

Anal triangle

Coccyx

192.1

Diagram of the 2 parts of the diamond-shaped perineal region.

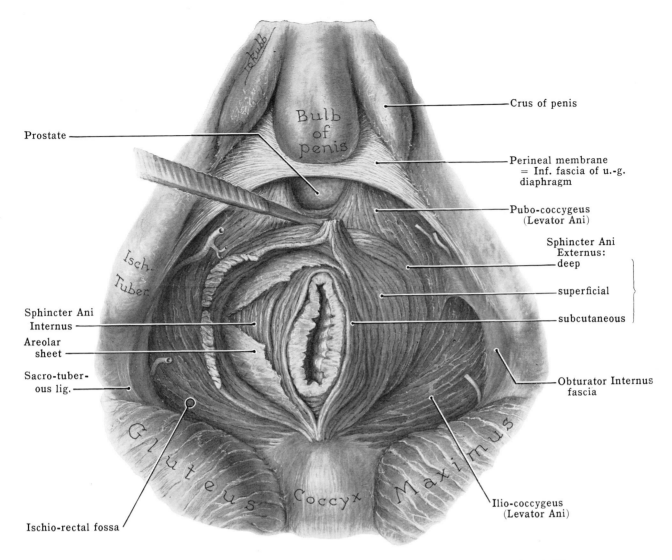

Prostate

Crus of penis

Perineal membrane
= Inf. fascia of u.-g.
diaphragm

Pubo-coccygeus
(Levator Ani)

Sphincter Ani
Externus:
deep

superficial

Sphincter Ani
Internus

subcutaneous

Areolar
sheet

Obturator Internus
fascia

Sacro-tuber-
ous lig.

Ilio-coccygeus
(Levator Ani)

Ischio-rectal fossa

193 Dissection of Sphincter Ani Externus

Observe the 3 parts of this voluntary sphincter: (a) subcutaneous—encircling the anal orifice and here uniting posteriorly with the next part; (b) superficial—anchoring the anus in the median plane by its attachments, here severed, to the perineal body in front and to the coccyx behind; and (c) deep—forming a wide encircling band.

On the right side the superficial and deep parts of the sphincter are reflected, and the underlying sheet, consisting of areolar tissue, Levator Ani fibres, and outer longitudinal muscle coat of the rectum, is cut, in order to reveal the inner circular muscle coat which is thickened to form an involuntary Sphincter Ani Internus.

Observe the anterior free borders of Levatores Ani meeting in front of the anal canal, and pressed backwards in order to give a view of the prostate.

Notice the remains of the "false roof" of the ischio-rectal fossa, i.e., a layer of fascia that stretches from Obturator Internus fascia to the thin fascia covering Levator Ani. It resembles the floor of an attic which, of course, lies below the true roof which latter is the site of origin of the Levator.

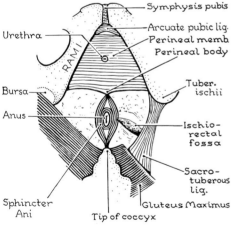

Urethra

Symphysis pubis

Arcuate pubic lig.

Perineal memb

Perineal body

Bursa

Anus

Tuber.
ischii

Ischio-
rectal
fossa

Sacro-
tuberous
lig.

Sphincter
Ani

Tip of coccyx

Gluteus Maximus

193.1

Diagram of the boundaries of the perineal region.

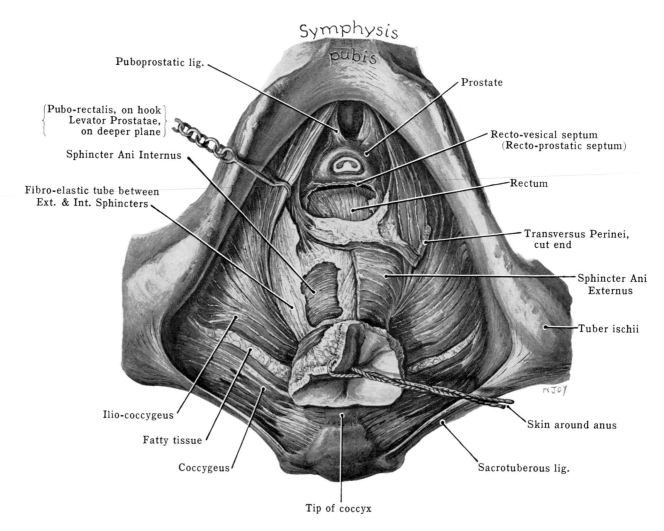

Puboprostatic lig.

{Pubo-rectalis, on hook
Levator Prostatae,
on deeper plane}

Sphincter Ani Internus

Fibro-elastic tube between
Ext. & Int. Sphincters

Symphysis pubis

Prostate

Recto-vesical septum
(Recto-prostatic septum)

Rectum

Transversus Perinei,
cut end

Sphincter Ani
Externus

Tuber ischii

Skin around anus

Sacrotuberous lig.

Ilio-coccygeus

Fatty tissue

Coccygeus

Tip of coccyx

194 Levatores Ani and Coccygei, perineal aspect, and Exposure of the Prostate

(For pelvic aspect of Levatores Ani, see fig. 209.)

Observe:

1. The anal canal guarded by two sphincters: Sphincter Ani Internus being a continuation of the circular muscle coat of the gut; it is smooth muscle. Sphincter Ani Externus extending below Sphincter Internus and having three parts; it is skeletal muscle.

2. Puborectalis, the sling-like muscle uniting with Sphincter Externus behind and at the sides. (It is better shown in figures 203 & 204).

3. The anal columns united half way down the Internal Sphincter by semilunar anal valves.

4. The pecten, or smooth zone of simple stratified epithelium, between the anal valves above and the lower border of the Internal Sphincter below. It is transitional between intestinal mucosa above and skin having dermal papillae and appendages below.

5. The longitudinal muscle coat of the rectum and its fascia blending with the Levator Ani and its fasciae to form a fibro-elastic tube which descends between the two Sphincters. From this tube septa pass through the Internal Sphincter to the submucous coat, through the External Sphincter to the skin, and, as the anal intermuscular septum, below the Internal Sphincter. (*Wilde, F. R.*)

(See also figures 196 and 196.1.)

195 Arteries of the Rectum and Anal Canal, front view

(The Levatores Ani are semidiagrammatic.)

Observe:

1. The branches of the right and left divisions of the superior rectal artery obliquely encircling the rectum, much as the branches of the dorsal arteries of the penis encircle the penis (fig. 199).
2. The middle rectal arteries (branches of the int. iliac arteries) are usually small. In this specimen the right artery is small, but the left one is large and partly replaces the left division of the superior rectal artery.
3. The inferior rectal arteries (branches of the int. pudendal arteries are largely expended on the anal canal.

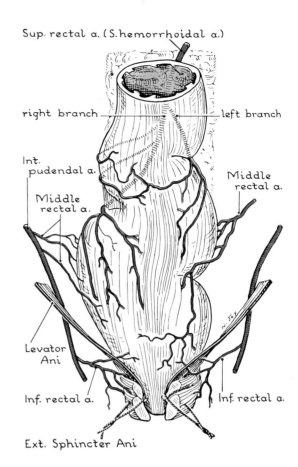

Sup. rectal a. (S. hemorrhoidal a.)

right branch — — left branch

Int. pudendal a.

Middle rectal a.

Middle rectal a.

Levator Ani

Inf. rectal a. — — Inf. rectal a.

Ext. Sphincter Ani

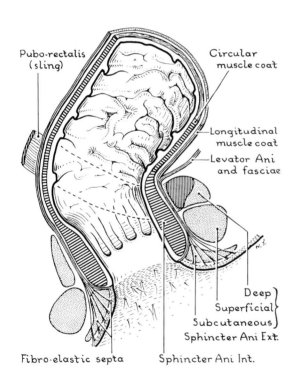

Pubo-rectalis (sling)

Circular muscle coat

Longitudinal muscle coat

Levator Ani and fasciae

Deep } Superficial } Subcutaneous } Sphincter Ani Ext.

Fibro-elastic septa

Sphincter Ani Int.

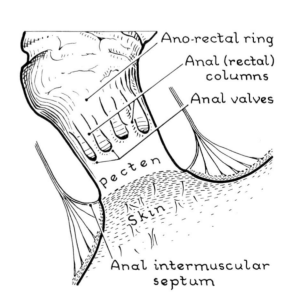

Ano-rectal ring

Anal (rectal) columns

Anal valves

Pecten

Skin

Anal intermuscular septum

196 and 196.1   Anal Canal, on median section, semidiagrammatic

(partly after Wilde)

(See text of fig. 194.)

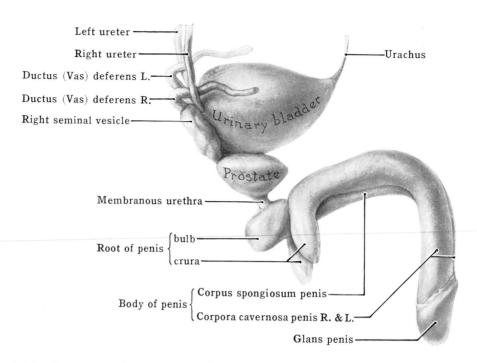

Left ureter

Right ureter

Ductus (Vas) deferens L.

Ductus (Vas) deferens R.

Right seminal vesicle

Urachus

Urinary bladder

Prostate

Membranous urethra

Root of penis { bulb
crura

Body of penis { Corpus spongiosum penis
Corpora cavernosa penis R. & L.

Glans penis

197   Lower Parts of the Genital and Urinary Tracts in the Male

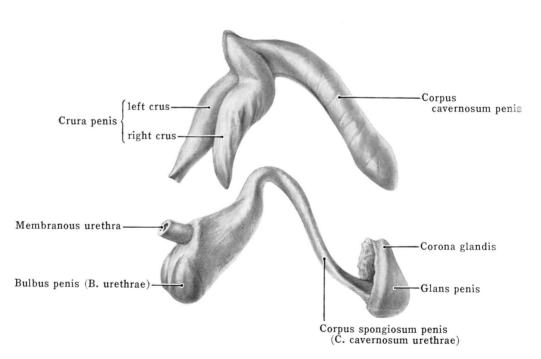

Crura penis { left crus
right crus

Corpus cavernosum penis

Membranous urethra

Corona glandis

Bulbus penis (B. urethrae)

Glans penis

Corpus spongiosum penis
(C. cavernosum urethrae)

198   Dissection of the Penis

The urethra is cut across below the perineal membrane and, with its enveloping erectile tissue, is separated from the corpora cavernosa penis. The natural flexures are preserved.

Observe:

1. The corpora cavernosa penis bent where that organ is slung by the suspensory ligament of the penis, and grooved by encircling vessels.
2. The corpus spongiosum penis massed (a) below the urethra posteriorly to form the bulb of the penis, and (b) above the urethra anteriorly to form the glans which fits like a cap on the blunt ends of the corpora cavernosa penis.

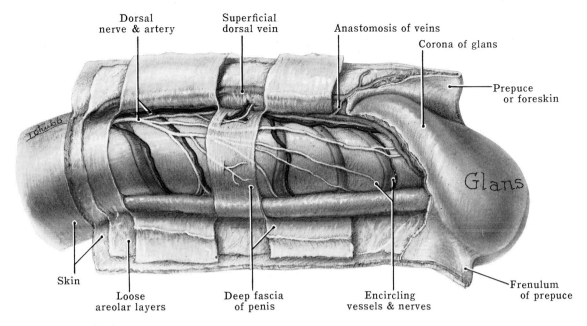

Dorsal nerve & artery — Superficial dorsal vein — Anastomosis of veins — Corona of glans — Prepuce or foreskin — Glans — Skin — Loose areolar layers — Deep fascia of penis — Encircling vessels & nerves — Frenulum of prepuce

199 Penis, side view

The three tubular envelopes of the penis are reflected, so also is the prepuce.

Observe:

1. The skin carried forward as the prepuce.
2. The loose, laminated, subcutaneous, areolar tissue (Dartos and Colles' fascia), called the superficial fascia of the penis, carried forward into the prepuce, and containing the superficial dorsal vein. This vein begins in the prepuce, anastomoses with the deep dorsal vein from the glans, and ends in the superficial inguinal veins.
3. The deep fascia penis (Buck's fascia). It ends at the glans penis.
4. Large encircling tributaries of the deep dorsal vein; thread-like companion arteries; numerous oblique nerves.
5. The vessels and nerves at the neck plunging into the glans penis.

199.1 Interior of the Spongy Urethra

A longitudinal incision was made on the urethral surface of the penis and carried through the floor of the urethra; so, the view is of the dorsal surface of the interior of the urethra. The prepuce is retracted.

External urethral orifice — Fossa navicularis — Septum of glans — Glans penis — Valvule of navicular fossa — Lacuna magna — Other lacunae and orifices of mucous glands in rows — Corpus spongiosum — Skin

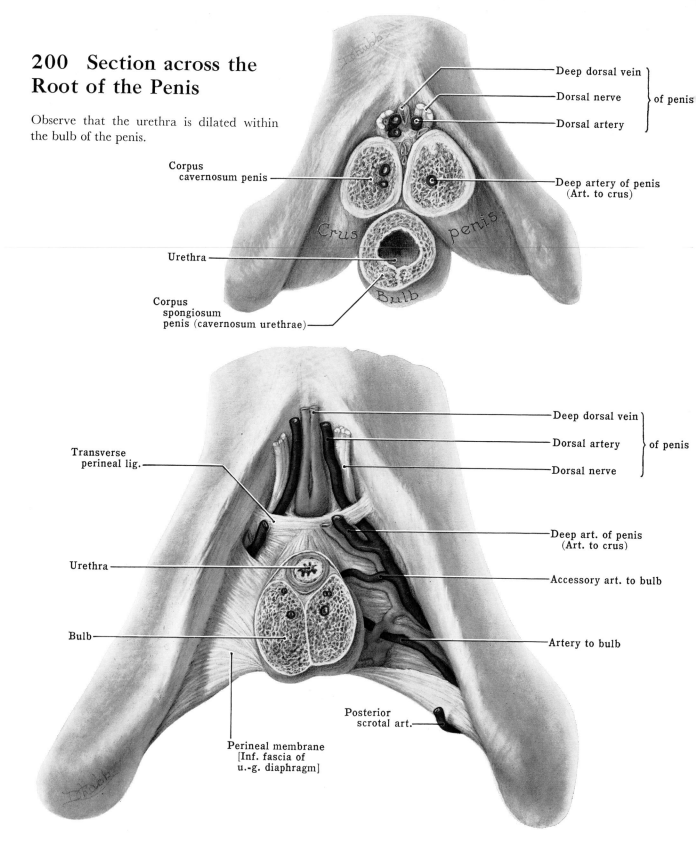

200 Section across the Root of the Penis

Observe that the urethra is dilated within the bulb of the penis.

Deep dorsal vein
Dorsal nerve } of penis
Dorsal artery

Corpus cavernosum penis

Deep artery of penis (Art. to crus)

Urethra

Crus penis

Bulb

Corpus spongiosum penis (cavernosum urethrae)

Transverse perineal lig.

Deep dorsal vein
Dorsal artery } of penis
Dorsal nerve

Urethra

Deep art. of penis (Art. to crus)

Accessory art. to bulb

Bulb

Artery to bulb

Posterior scrotal art.

Perineal membrane [Inf. fascia of u.-g. diaphragm]

201 Vessels of the Penis: The Perineal Membrane

The crura are removed and the bulb is cut shorter than in figure 200 and viewed more from below. The perineal membrane [inf. fascia of the uro-genital diaphragm] is partly removed on the left side.

Observe:

1. The fibres of the perineal membrane converging on the bulb and mooring it to the pubic arch.
2. The urethra, still membranous and bound to the dorsum of the bulb.
3. The septum in the bulb indicating its bilateral origin.
4. The artery to the bulb (here double); the artery to the crus, called the deep artery; and the dorsal artery which ends in the glans penis. The deep dorsal vein, originally double, which ends in the prostatic plexus.

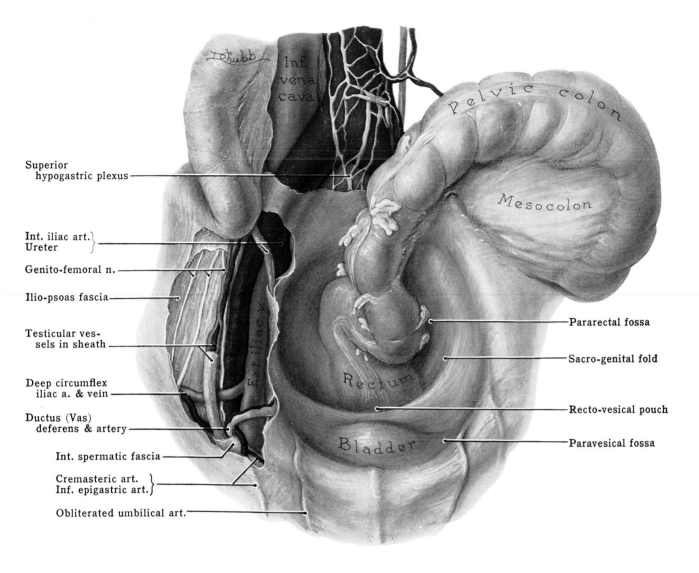

Superior
  hypogastric plexus

Int. iliac art.
Ureter

Genito-femoral n.

Ilio-psoas fascia

Testicular ves-
  sels in sheath

Deep circumflex
  iliac a. & vein

Ductus (Vas)
  deferens & artery

Int. spermatic fascia

Cremasteric art.
Inf. epigastric art.

Obliterated umbilical art.

Inf.
vena
cava

Pelvic colon

Mesocolon

Ext. iliac v.

Rectum

Bladder

Pararectal fossa

Sacro-genital fold

Recto-vesical pouch

Paravesical fossa

202   Male Pelvis Minor and Surroundings, antero-superior view

Observe:

1. One limb of the inverted V-shaped root of the sigmoid (pelvic) mesocolon ascending near the external iliac vessels; the
other descending to the third piece of the sacrum. At the
apex is the mouth of the intersigmoid recess, and behind the
mouth lies the left ureter.

2. The taeniae coli forming two wide bands; one in front of the
rectum, the other behind.

3. The crescentic fold of peritoneum called the sacro-genital
fold.

4. The superior hypogastric plexus (presacral nerve) lying in
the fork of the aorta and in front of the left common iliac vein.

5. The ureter adhering to the peritoneum, crossing the external
iliac vessels, and descending in front of the internal iliac
artery. The ductus deferens and its artery also adhering to
peritoneum, crossing the external iliac vessels, and then hooking round the inferior epigastric artery to join the other constituents of the spermatic cord.

6. The genito-femoral nerve on the Psoas fascia, on a deeper
plane than the testicular vessels. Its two lateral (femoral)
branches become cutaneous; its medial (genital) branch
supplies Cremaster and becomes cutaneous.

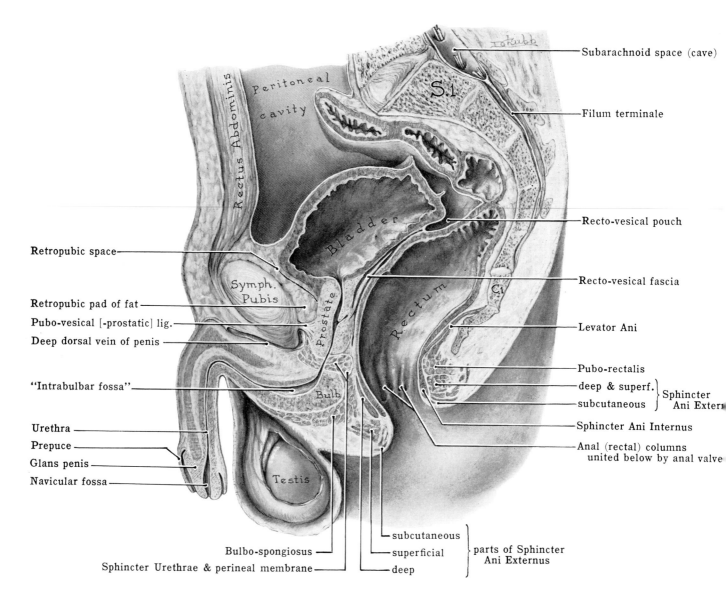

Subarachnoid space (cave)

Filum terminale

Recto-vesical pouch

Recto-vesical fascia

Levator Ani

Pubo-rectalis

deep & superf. ⎫
subcutaneous ⎬ Sphincter
              ⎭ Ani Extern

Sphincter Ani Internus

Anal (rectal) columns
united below by anal valve

Retropubic space

Retropubic pad of fat

Pubo-vesical [-prostatic] lig.

Deep dorsal vein of penis

"Intrabulbar fossa"

Urethra

Prepuce

Glans penis

Navicular fossa

Peritoneal cavity

Rectus Abdominis

Symph. Pubis

Prostate

Bulb

Bladder

Rectum

S.1

Testis

subcutaneous ⎫
superficial ⎬ parts of Sphincter
deep   ⎭ Ani Externus

Bulbo-spongiosus

Sphincter Urethrae & perineal membrane

203 Male Pelvis, in median section

Observe:

1. The urinary bladder slightly distended and resting on the rectum; the prostatic urethra descending vertically through a somewhat elongated prostate and showing the prostatic utricle opening on to its posterior wall; the short membranous urethra passing through the deep perineal pouch; the spongy or penile urethra with a low lying dilatation in the bulb and another in the glans; and the Bulbo-spongiosus which by contracting empties the urethra.

2. The involuntary Sphincter Ani Internus not descending so far as the voluntary Sphincter Ani Externus, and separated from it by an areolar layer.

3. The two layers of recto-vesical fascia in the median plane between bladder and rectum. On each side it contains the deferent duct, seminal vesicle, and vesical vessels (figs. 204, 205).

4. The peritoneum passing from the abdominal wall above the symphysis to the distended bladder, over the bladder to the bottom of the recto-vesical pouch, and up the anterior aspect of the rectum.

5. The tunica vaginalis, opened in order to expose the testis, which here happens to be rotated so that the epididymis is to the front.

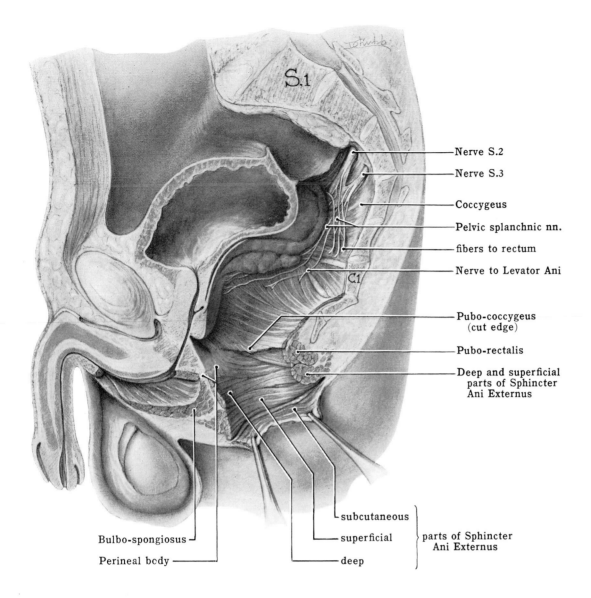

Nerve S.2

Nerve S.3

Coccygeus

Pelvic splanchnic nn.

fibers to rectum

Nerve to Levator Ani

Pubo-coccygeus (cut edge)

Pubo-rectalis

Deep and superficial parts of Sphincter Ani Externus

subcutaneous

superficial

deep

} parts of Sphincter Ani Externus

Bulbo-spongiosus

Perineal body

204   Sphincter Ani Externus and Levator Ani

This is figure 203 from which the rectum, anal canal, and bulb of the penis are removed.

Observe:

1. The subcutaneous fibres of Sphincter Ani Externus held reflected with forceps; the superficial fibres mingling posteriorly with deep fibres; and deep fibres mingling posteriorly with Pubo-rectalis (inferior fibres of Pubo-coccygeus) which forms a sling that occupies the angle between the rectum and the anal canal (fig. 194).

2. Pubo-coccygeus divided to allow of the removal of the anal canal to which it is in part attached (fig. 209).

3. The ampulla of the deferent duct and the seminal vesicle curving to fit the cylindrical rectum.

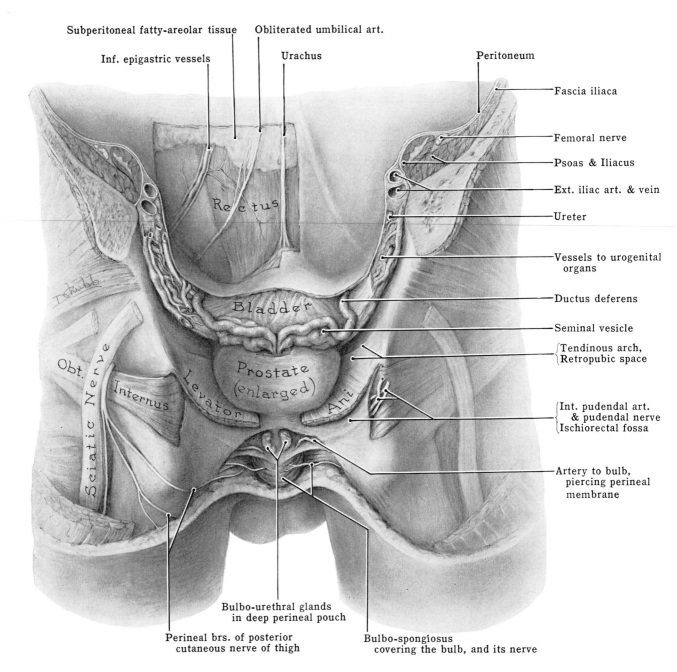

Subperitoneal fatty-areolar tissue   Obliterated umbilical art.

Inf. epigastric vessels   Urachus   Peritoneum

Fascia iliaca

Femoral nerve

Psoas & Iliacus

Ext. iliac art. & vein

Ureter

Vessels to urogenital organs

Ductus deferens

Seminal vesicle

Tendinous arch, Retropubic space

Int. pudendal art. & pudendal nerve
Ischiorectal fossa

Artery to bulb, piercing perineal membrane

Rectus

Ischium

Bladder

Obt. Nerve

Internus

Levator

Prostate (enlarged)

Ani

Sciatic Nerve

Bulbo-urethral glands in deep perineal pouch

Perineal brs. of posterior cutaneous nerve of thigh

Bulbo-spongiosus covering the bulb, and its nerve

205 Coronal Section of the Male Pelvis, just in front of the rectum. View of the anterior portion from behind

Observe:

1. The inferior epigastric artery and venae comitantes entering the Rectus sheath, whilst the obliterated umbilical artery and the urachus, like the bladder, remain in subperitoneal fatty-areolar tissue.

2. The femoral nerve lying between Psoas and Iliacus outside the Psoas fascia, which is attached to the pelvic brim, whilst the external iliac art. and vein lie inside.

3. The ductus deferens and ureter, both subperitoneal. Near the

bladder, the ureter accompanying a leash of vesical vessels enclosed in recto-vesical fascia.

4. Levator Ani and its fascial coverings separating the retro-pubic (prevesical) space from the ischio-rectal fossa.

5. The free, anterior borders of Levatores Ani. They are the width of the handle of a scalpel apart.

6. The bulbo-urethral glands (Cowper's) and the artery to the bulb lying above the perineal membrane [inf. fascia of the urogenital diaphragm], i.e. in the deep perineal pouch.

7. Obturator Internus making a right-angled turn as it escapes from its osseo-fascial packet (fig. 281).

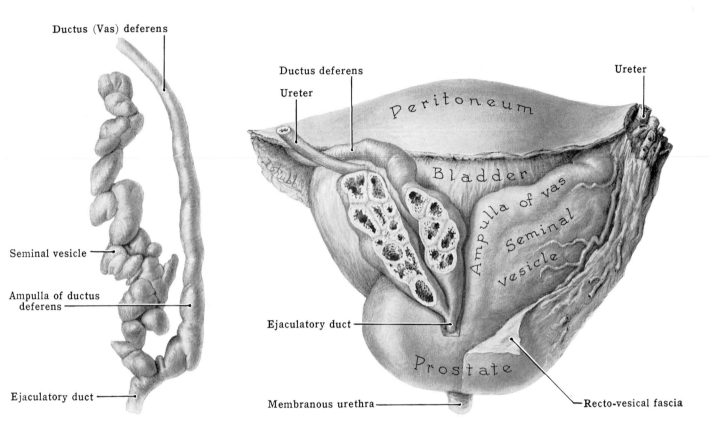

Ductus (Vas) deferens

Seminal vesicle

Ampulla of ductus deferens

Ejaculatory duct

Ductus deferens

Ureter

Peritoneum

Bladder

Ampulla of vas

Seminal vesicle

Ureter

Ejaculatory duct

Prostate

Membranous urethra

Recto-vesical fascia

06 Seminal Vesicle, unravelled

he vesicle is a tortuous tube with numerous out-
chings. The lower end of the ampulla of the ductus
erens has outpouchings of minor degree.

207 Bladder, Deferent Ducts, Seminal Vesicles, and Prostate, from behind

The left vesicle and ampulla are dissected free and
sliced open, and part of the prostate is cut away in
order to expose the left ejaculatory duct. The posterior
part of the prostatic fascia is the thickened lower part
of the rectovesical fascia.

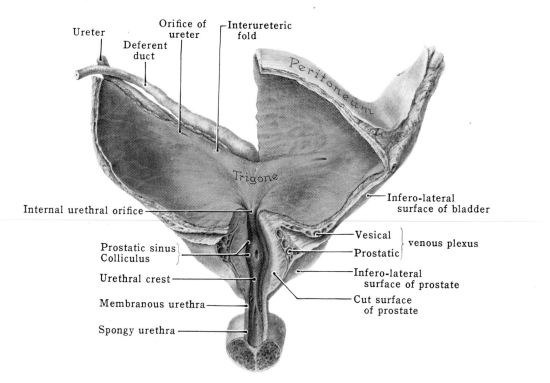

208 Interior of the Male Urinary Bladder and Prostatic Urethra

The anterior walls of the bladder, prostate and urethra were cut away. The knife was then carried through the posterior wall of the bladder, at the upper border of the right ureter, in order to expose the course of the ureter in the bladder wall. Parts of the posterior and superior walls of the bladder were removed.

Observe:

1. The right ureter not joining the bladder wall but traversing it obliquely and, beyond the slit-like ureteral orifice, joined by the interureteric fold or plica.
2. The mucous membrane, smooth over the trigone, but rugose elsewhere—especially when the bladder is empty.
3. The slight fulness behind the internal urethral orifice, which, when exaggerated, becomes the uvula vesicae.
4. The mouth of the prostatic utricle (not labelled) at the summit of the colliculus, on the urethral crest, and the orifice of an ejaculatory duct on each side of the utricle.
5. The urethral crest extending rather higher than usual and bifurcating rather lower than usual.
6. The prostatic fascia enclosing a venous plexus.

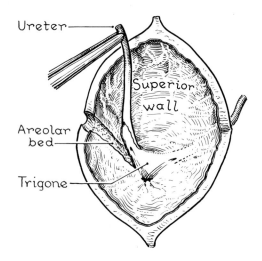

208.1

Sketch of the ureter being raised from its areolar bed as it passes obliquely through the muscular coat of the bladder to blend with the trigonal muscle.

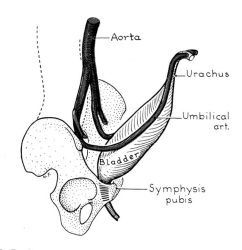

208.2

At birth the bladder is abdominal in position and fusiform in shape and the two umbilical arteries lie along its sides.

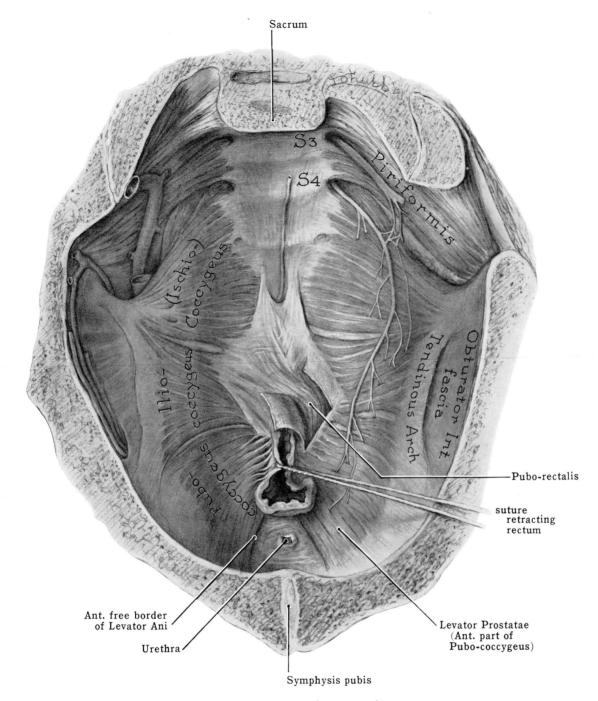

Sacrum

S3

S4

Piriformis

(Ischio-) Coccygeus

Obturator Int. fascia Tendinous Arch

Ilio- coccygeus

Pubo-coccygeus

Pubo-rectalis

suture retracting rectum

Ant. free border of Levator Ani

Urethra

Symphysis pubis

Levator Prostatae (Ant. part of Pubo-coccygeus)

209 Levatores Ani and Coccygei, from above

The pelvic viscera are removed and the bony pelvis is sawn through transversely.

Observe:

1. Pubo-coccygeus arising mainly from the pubic bone, Ischio-coccygeus from the ischial spine, and Ilio-coccygeus from the tendinous arch in between.   Pubo-coccygeus is strong (fig. 216); Ilio-coccygeus is weak; Ischio-coccygeus is largely transformed into the sacrospinous ligament (fig. 217). Pubo- and Ilio-coccygei together constitute Levator Ani.

2. The anterior free border of Pubo-coccygeus; the posterior free border of Ischio-coccygeus; the clefts at the borders of Ilio-coccygeus closed by areolar membranes.

3. The urethra passing between the anterior borders of Pubo-coccygei.   The rectum perforating Pubo-coccygei, thus: (a) the anterior fibres of the muscles of opposite sides meet and

unite in the central tendon of the perineum (perineal body) in front of the rectum; (b) the posterior fibres unite behind the rectum in an aponeurosis that extends backwards to the anterior sacro-coccygeal ligament; (c) the middle fibres blend with the outer wall of the anal canal and pass between Internal and External Sphincters of the anus (fig. 194); (d) on the left side, this aponeurosis is reflected to show Pubo-rectalis; i.e., the lower fibres of Pubo-coccygeus uniting behind the rectum with those of the opposite side form a pubo-rectal sling at the ano-rectal junction (fig. 204).

4. Branches of S.3 & 4 supplying Levator Ani and Coccygeus. (The pudendal nerve, via its perineal branch, fig. 215, also supplies Levator Ani.)

(For perineal aspect of Levatores Ani see figure 194.)

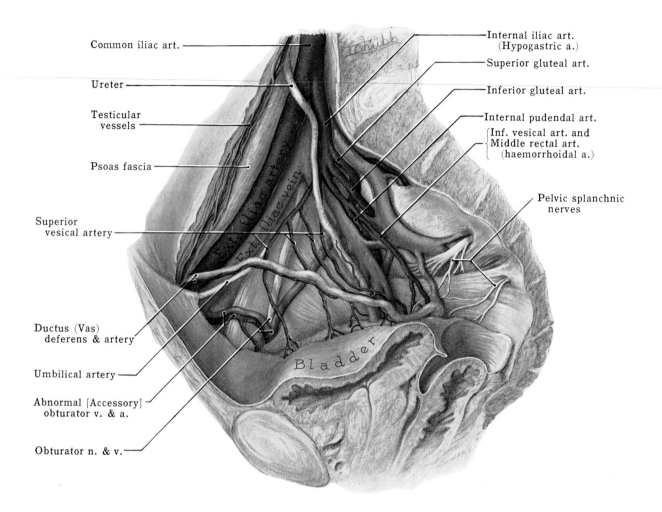

Common iliac art.

Internal iliac art.
(Hypogastric a.)

Superior gluteal art.

Ureter

Inferior gluteal art.

Testicular
vessels

Internal pudendal art.

Inf. vesical art. and
Middle rectal art.
(haemorrhoidal a.)

Psoas fascia

Pelvic splanchnic
nerves

Superior
vesical artery

Ductus (Vas)
deferens & artery

Umbilical artery

Bladder

Abnormal [Accessory]
obturator v. & a.

Obturator n. & v.

210 Side Wall of the Male Pelvis Minor

Observe:

1. The ureter and ductus deferens running a subperitoneal course across the external iliac vessels, umbilical artery, obturator nerve and vessels, and each receiving a branch from a vesical artery.

2. The umbilical artery, obliterated beyond the origin of the last superior vesical artery and creating a peritoneal fold.

3. The obturator artery here springing from the inferior epigastric artery, i.e., the artery is "abnormal". There are here both a normal and an "abnormal" obturator vein.

4. The veins forming an open network through which the arteries are threaded.

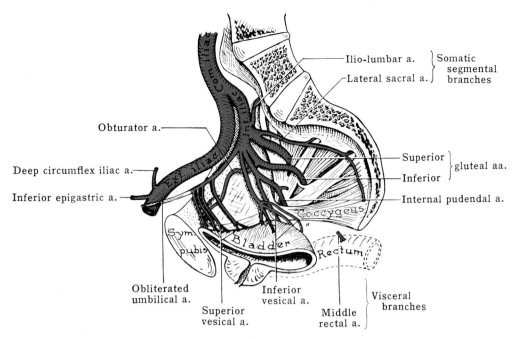

Ilio-lumbar a. } Somatic segmental branches

Lateral sacral a.

Obturator a.

Deep circumflex iliac a.

Inferior epigastric a.

Superior } gluteal aa.

Inferior

Internal pudendal a.

Coccygeus

Sym. pubis

Bladder

Rectum

Obliterated umbilical a.

Superior vesical a.

Inferior vesical a.

Middle rectal a.

Visceral branches

211 Iliac Arteries and their Branches, side view

Observe:

1. The common iliac artery having two terminal branches, but no collateral branches.
2. The external iliac artery having two collateral branches, and ending as the femoral artery.
3. The internal iliac (hypogastric) artery ending as an anterior and a posterior division. From these, branches arise variably. Commonly, as here the ilio-lumbar a., lateral sacral a., and

superior gluteal a. spring from the posterior division; the others spring from the anterior division.

4. Of the 10 branches of the internal iliac artery, the obliterated umbilical, which in the fetus passed to the placenta, and 3 others are visceral; 2 supply the 5th lumbar and the sacral segments and are somatic segmental; 3 enter the gluteal region; and one passes to the front of the thigh.

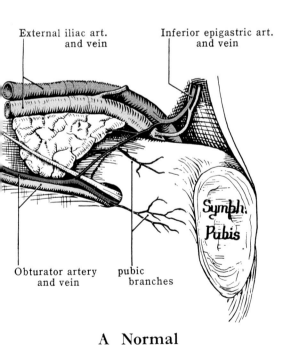

External iliac art. and vein

Inferior epigastric art. and vein

Inferior epigastric art.

External iliac art. and vein

pubic branch

Symph. Pubis

Symph. pubis

Obturator artery and vein

pubic branches

pubic branch

Obturator art. and vein

A Normal

B Abnormal [Accessory]

212 Normal and Abnormal [Accessory] Obturator Arteries

A. The pubic branch of the obturator artery anastomoses behind the body of the pubis with the pubic branch of the inferior epigastric artery.

B. The obturator artery sprang from the internal iliac

artery in 70.0% of 283 limbs; from the inferior epigastric via the pubic anastomoses in 25.4%; and nearly equally from both internal iliac and inferior epigastric in 4.6%. (J.C.B.G.)

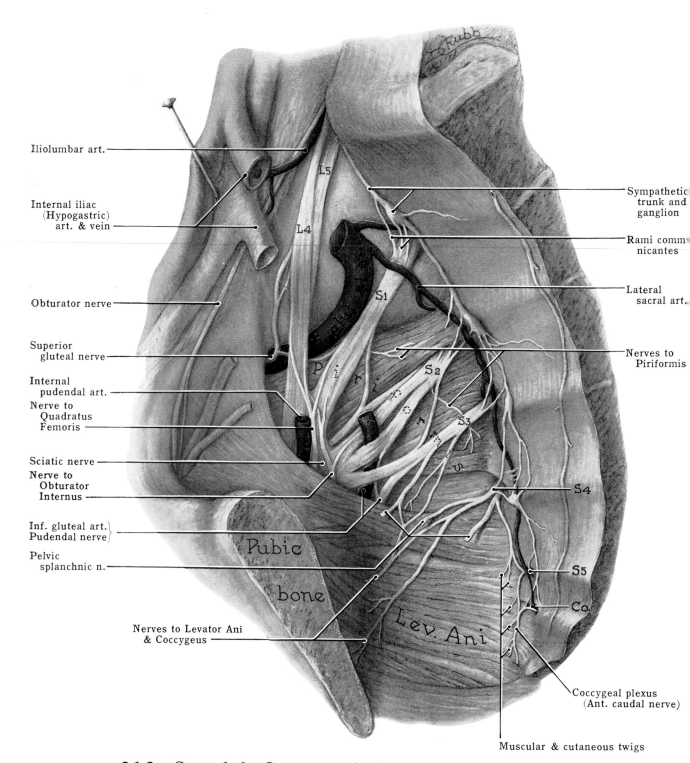

Iliolumbar art.

Internal iliac (Hypogastric) art. & vein

Obturator nerve

Superior gluteal nerve

Internal pudendal art.

Nerve to Quadratus Femoris

Sciatic nerve

Nerve to Obturator Internus

Inf. gluteal art. Pudendal nerve

Pelvic splanchnic n.

Nerves to Levator Ani & Coccygeus

Sympathetic trunk and ganglion

Rami communicantes

Lateral sacral art.

Nerves to Piriformis

S4

S5

Co.

Coccygeal plexus (Ant. caudal nerve)

Muscular & cutaneous twigs

L5

L4

S1

S2

S3

Pubic bone

Lev. Ani

213   Sacral & Coccygeal Nerve Plexuses, antero-median view

Observe:

1. Either the sympathetic trunk or its ganglia sending gray rami communicantes to each sacral nerve and the coccygeal nerve.

2. The branch from L.4 joining L.5 to form the lumbo-sacral trunk.

3. The roots of S.1, 2 supplying Piriformis; S.3, 4 supplying Coccygeus and Levator Ani; S.(2), 3, 4 each contributing a branch to the formation of the pelvic splanchnic nerve.

4. The sciatic nerve springing from segments L.4, 5, S.1, 2, 3; the pudendal nerve from S.2, 3, (4); the coccygeal plexus from S.4, 5, Co.

5. The ilio-lumbar artery accompanying nerve L.5; the branches of the lateral sacral artery accompanying the sacral nerves; the superior gluteal artery passing backwards between L.5 and S.1—its position is not constant.

6. In this specimen the inferior gluteal artery splitting S.2.

214 Diagram of the Nerve Supply to the Bladder and Urethra

(Broken lines indicate afferent fibres.)

Parasympathetic: The pelvic splanchnic nerves (nervi erigentes; S.2, 3, 4) are the motor nerves to the bladder; when they are stimulated the bladder empties, the blood vessels dilate, and the penis becomes erect. They are also the sensory nerves of the bladder.

Sympathetic, through the superior hypogastric plexus (presacral nerve; Th. lower, L. 1, 2, 3) is motor to a continuous muscle sheet comprising the ureteric musculature, the trigonal muscle, and the muscle of the urethral crest. It also supplies the muscle of the epididymis, ductus deferens, seminal vesicle, and prostate. When the plexus is stimulated, the seminal fluid is ejaculated into the urethra but is hindered from entering the bladder perhaps by the muscle sheet which is drawn towards the internal urethral orifice. The sympathetic is also vaso-contrictor and to some slight extent it is sensory to the trigonal region.

The pudendal nerve is motor to the sphincter urethrae and sensory to the glans penis and the urethra.

It would seem that the sympathetic supply to the bladder has a vaso-constrictor and a sexual effect and that as regards micturition it is not antagonistic to the parasympathetic supply. (Learmonth; Langworthy; and Mitchell.)

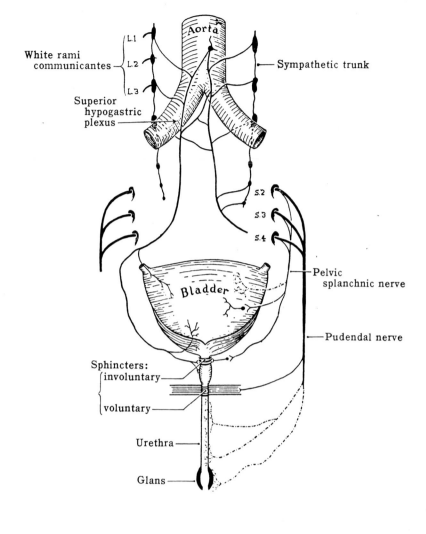

215 Diagram of the Pudendal Nerve

Note:

1) the 5 regions in which it runs, and
2) the 3 divisions into which it divides.

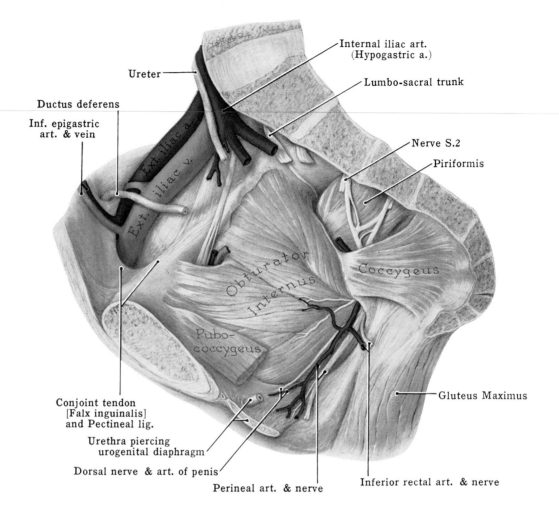

Ureter

Ductus deferens

Inf. epigastric
art. & vein

Internal iliac art.
(Hypogastric a.)

Lumbo-sacral trunk

Nerve S.2

Piriformis

Ext. iliac a.

Ext. iliac v.

Obturator Internus

Coccygeus

Pubo-coccygeus

Gluteus Maximus

Conjoint tendon
[Falx inguinalis]
and Pectineal lig.

Urethra piercing
urogenital diaphragm

Dorsal nerve & art. of penis

Perineal art. & nerve

Inferior rectal art. & nerve

216 Muscles of the Pelvis Minor (male specimen)

Observe:

1. Obturator Internus padding the side wall of the pelvis and escaping through the lesser sciatic foramen; its nerve is seen. Piriformis padding the posterior wall and escaping through the greater sciatic foramen. Coccygeus concealing the sacro-spinous lig. Pubococcygeus, which is the chief and strongest part of Levator Ani, springing from the body of the pubis.

2. The obturator nerve, artery and vein escaping through the obturator foramen. The internal pudendal artery and the pudendal nerve making an exit through the greater foramen, and a re-entry through the lesser foramen, and taking a forward course (in the pudendal canal) within the Obturator Internus fascia to the urogenital diaphragm.

3. In the pelvis major, the deferent duct and the ureter descending across the external iliac artery and vein, the Psoas fascia, and the pelvic brim to enter the pelvis minor or true pelvis.

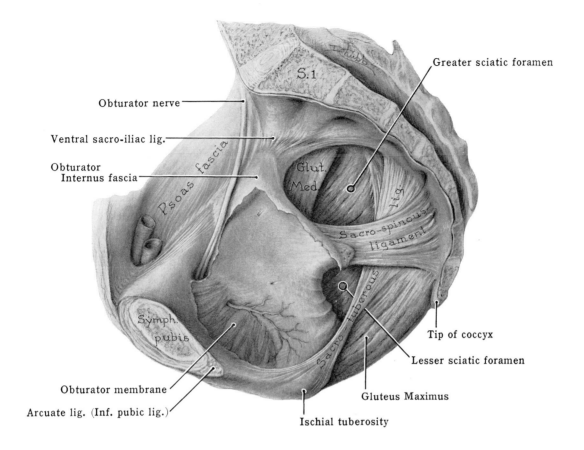

Greater sciatic foramen

Obturator nerve

Ventral sacro-iliac lig.

Obturator
Internus fascia

S.1

Glut.
Med

Sacro-spinous
ligament

Psoas fascia

Symph.
pubis

Obturator membrane

Arcuate lig. (Inf. pubic lig.)

Tip of coccyx

Lesser sciatic foramen

Gluteus Maximus

Ischial tuberosity

217 Bony and Ligamentous Walls of the Pelvis Minor (female specimen)

In front is the pubis; behind are the sacrum and coccyx. Postero-laterally, the coccyx and lower part of the sacrum are fastened to the ischial tuberosity by the sacro-tuberous lig. and to the ischial spine by the sacro-spinous lig., whilst the upper part of the sacrum is joined to the ilium by the ventral sacro-iliac lig. Anterior to the sacro-tuberous lig. are the greater and lesser sciatic foramina, the one being above, and the other below, the sacro-spinous lig.

Antero-laterally, the fascia covering Obturator Internus is snipped away and Obturator Internus removed from its osseo-fascial pocket, thereby exposing the ischium and obturator membrane. The mouth of this pocket is the lesser sciatic foramen. Through it Obturator Internus escapes from the pelvis, and the grooves made by its tendon are conspicuous.

Obturator Internus fascia is attached along the line of the obturator nerve above; to the sacro-tuberous lig. below; and to the posterior border of the body of the ischium behind.

(For interosseous lig. see fig. 223.1, dorsal ligs. fig. 273, and ilio-lumbar lig. fig. 190.)

218   Male Pelvis, from the front

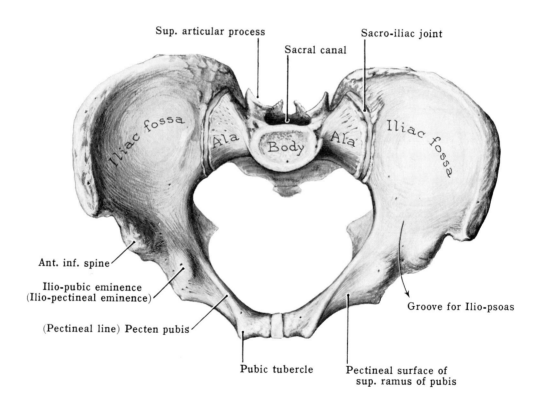

Sup. articular process

Sacral canal

Sacro-iliac joint

Iliac fossa

Ala

Body

Ala

Iliac fossa

Ant. inf. spine

Ilio-pubic eminence
(Ilio-pectineal eminence)

(Pectineal line) Pecten pubis

Groove for Ilio-psoas

Pubic tubercle

Pectineal surface of
sup. ramus of pubis

219   Male Pelvis, from above

The iliac fossae and the alae (of the base) of the sacrum constitute the false or
greater pelvis. The groove between the anterior inferior iliac spine and the ilio-
pubic eminence conducts Ilio-psoas from the false pelvis to the thigh. The pectineal
(anterior) surface of the superior ramus of the pubis is part of the thigh. It gives
origin to Pectineus and is limited behind by the pecten pubis.

220 Female Pelvis, from the front

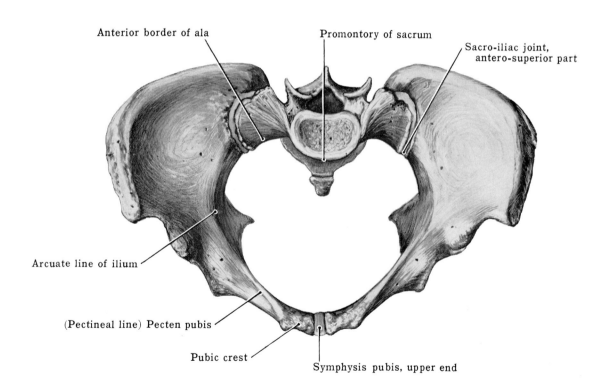

Anterior border of ala   Promontory of sacrum   Sacro-iliac joint, antero-superior part

Arcuate line of ilium

(Pectineal line) Pecten pubis

Pubic crest

Symphysis pubis, upper end

221 Female Pelvis, from above

Three bones separated by three joints share in the formation of the pelvic brim. The bones are: the sacrum and the two hip bones. The joints are: the symphysis pubis and the two sacro-iliac joints.

The parts labelled are the component parts of the pelvic brim.

Iliac crest

Ant. sup. spine

Ant. inf. spine

Ilio-pubic (-pectineal) eminence

Pecten pubis

Sup. ramus of pubis

Body of pubis

Inf. ramus of pubis

(Spiral) Margin of obturator foramen

Iliac fossa

Tuberosity

Auricular surface

Body of Ischium

Post. sup. spine

Post. inf. spine

Preauricular sulcus

Greater sciatic notch

Ischial spine

Lesser sciatic notch

Falciform crest

Ischial tuberosity

Ramus of ischium

Sup. articular process

Lat. sacral crest

Body

Tuberosity

Auricular surface

Cornua of sacrum & coccyx

Transverse process of coc

Tip of coccyx

222   Hip Bone, medial aspect: Sacrum and Coccyx, lateral aspect

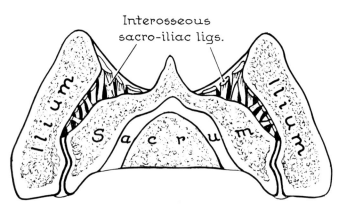

Interosseous sacro-iliac ligs.

Ilium   *Ilium*

Sacrum

223   Sacro-iliac Joint, transvers section

(For dorsal sacro-iliac ligs. see fig. 273, sacro-tuberous sacro-spinous ligs. figs. 217 & 273, and ilio-lumbar lig. 190.)

Incipient stage

223.1   Synostosis of the Sacro-iliac Joint

Synostosis of this joint was found in 14 of 182 half pe (91 dissecting room subjects); 5 times on the right s only, 3 times on the left side only, and 3 times on b sides. One subject was a female (aged 64 years); others were males, (aged 30 to 84 years). The ossificat commonly begins, as here, (red) in the ventral sac iliac ligament and is associated with bony overgro elsewhere, e.g., acetabular margin, lumbo-sacral jo and iliac crest (yellow). *(J.C.B.G.)*

224 Clitoris

This miniature penis comprises two corpora cavernosa which are bent, suspended by a suspensory ligament, and capped by a glans as in the male (fig. 198).

The male bulb and body of the corpus spongiosum (corpus cavernosum urethrae) are represented in the female by the bulbs of the vestibule and the commissure of the bulbs (pars intermedia). These, however, are not regarded as part of the clitoris and are not traversed by the urethra.

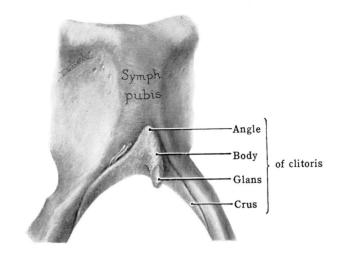

Symph. pubis

Angle ⎫
Body ⎪ of clitoris
Glans ⎬
Crus ⎭

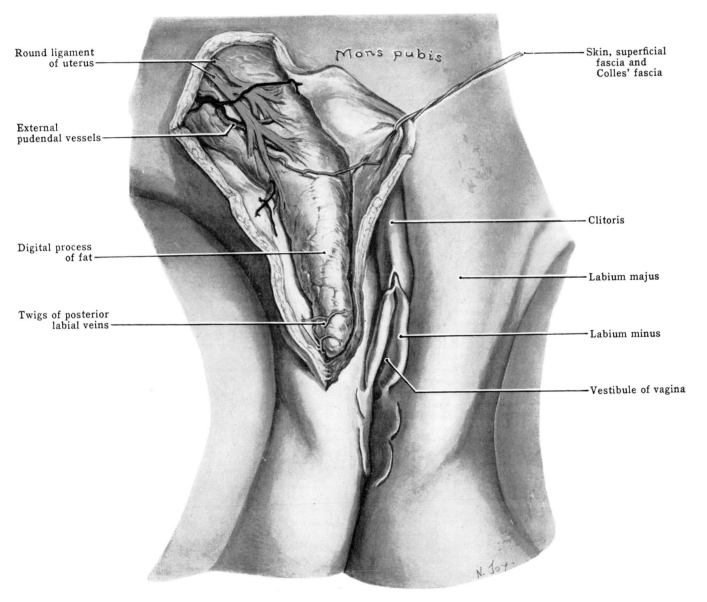

Round ligament of uterus

Mons pubis

Skin, superficial fascia and Colles' fascia

External pudendal vessels

Clitoris

Labium majus

Digital process of fat

Twigs of posterior labial veins

Labium minus

Vestibule of vagina

225 Female Perineum—I

Observe:

1. A long digital, or finger-like, process of fat lying deep to the subcutaneous fatty tissue and descending far into the labium majus.

2. The thin transparent veil of areolar tissue that encloses the process and through which its lobulated nature is apparent.

3. The round ligament of the uterus (lig. teres uteri) ending as a branching band of fascia which spreads out in front of the digital process; and the (superficial) external pudendal vessels crossing the process.

4. The vestibule of the vagina, as the region between the labia minora and external to the hymen.

Mons pubis

Skin and subcutaneous tiss[ue]

External pudendal vessels

Ilio-inguinal nerve

Digital process of fat

Ext. pudendal vessels

Anastomosis between ext.
and int. pudendal vessels

Perineal br. of posterior
cutaneous nerve of thigh

Labium majus,
cut surface

Posterior labial
vessels and nerves

Transverse perineal vesse[l]

Anus

Ischio-rectal fossa

226 Female Perineum—II

Observe:

1. On the right side, the lobulated digital process of fat opened up, and anastomotic vessels, which unite the external to the internal pudendal vessels, running through its long axis like a core.

2. On the left side, the digital process of fat is largely removed. The posterior labial vessels and nerves (S.2, 3), joined by the perineal branch of the posterior cutaneous nerve of the thigh (S.1, 2, 3) running forwards almost to the mons pubis, the vessels there anastomosing with the external pudendal vessels, and the nerves meeting the ilio-inguinal nerve (L.1).

3. Note that there is here a hiatus in the numerical sequence of the nerve segments, accounted for by the fact that L.2, 3, 4, 5 and S.1 are drawn down into the lower limb with the result that L.1 is succeeded by S.2 (cf. the similar hiatus in the pectoral region between C.3 & 4 and T.2. See figs. 13 & 665).

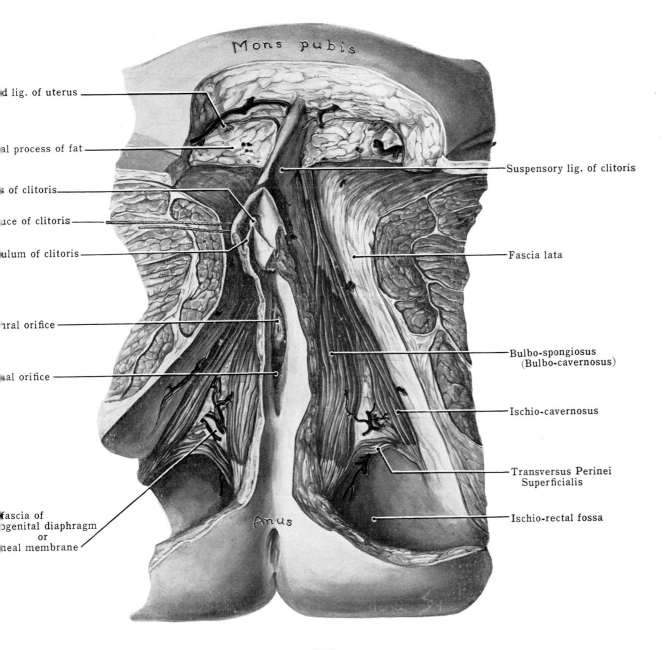

Mons pubis

d lig. of uterus

al process of fat

s of clitoris

ice of clitoris

ulum of clitoris

ıral orifice

ıal orifice

fascia of
ogenital diaphragm
or
ıeal membrane

Suspensory lig. of clitoris

Fascia lata

Bulbo-spongiosus
(Bulbo-cavernosus)

Ischio-cavernosus

Transversus Perinei
Superficialis

Ischio-rectal fossa

Anus

227   Female Perineum—III

Observe:

1. The thickness of the superficial fatty tissue at the mons and the encapsuled digital process of fat deep to this. The suspensory ligament of the clitoris descending from the linea alba and symphysis pubis.

2. The prepuce of the clitoris, thrown like a hood over the clitoris, and the anterior ends of the labia minora uniting to form the frenulum of the clitoris.

3. The 3 muscles on each side: Bulbo-spongiosus, Ischio-cavernosus, and Transversus Perinei Superficialis, which when slightly separated reveal the perineal membrane. The Bulbo-spongiosus overlies the bulb of the vestibule. In the male, the muscles of the two sides are united by a median raphe (fig. 192); in the female, the orifice of the vagina separates the two.

4. The pin-point orifices of the right and the left paraurethral duct below the urethral orifice.

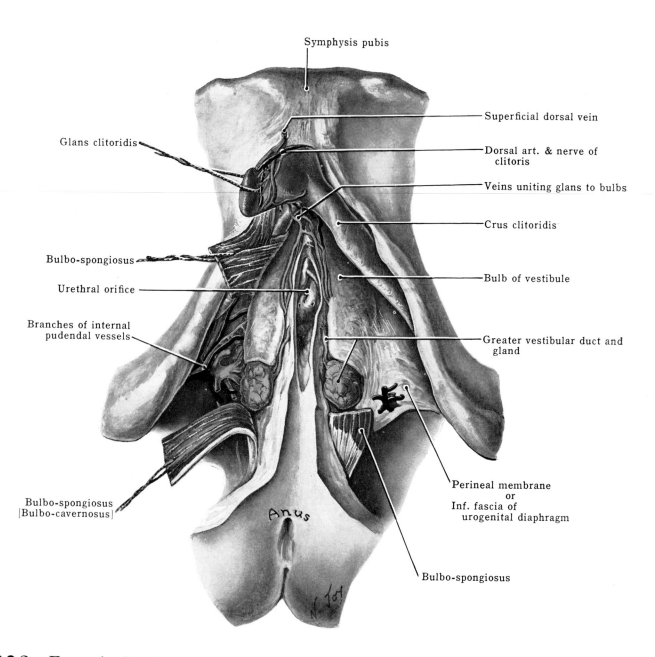

Symphysis pubis

Glans clitoridis

Bulbo-spongiosus

Urethral orifice

Branches of internal
pudendal vessels

Bulbo-spongiosus
[Bulbo-cavernosus]

Anus

Superficial dorsal vein

Dorsal art. & nerve of
clitoris

Veins uniting glans to bulbs

Crus clitoridis

Bulb of vestibule

Greater vestibular duct and
gland

Perineal membrane
or
Inf. fascia of
urogenital diaphragm

Bulbo-spongiosus

228 Female Perineum—IV

On the right side the perineal membrane is removed.

Observe:

1. The paired Bulbo-spongiosus, divided and reflected on the
   right side, and largely excised on the left side.
2. The glans clitoridis, pulled over to the right side and the
   dorsal vessels and nerve of the clitoris running to it, as in the
   male (fig. 199).
3. The bulb of the vestibule (paired, right and left) one on
   each side of the vestibule of the vagina and therein differing
   from the bulb of the penis which is unpaired (fig. 200).

4. Veins (pars intermedia) connecting the bulbs of the vestibule
   to the glans of the clitoris.
5. The greater vestibular gland situated at the posterior blunt
   end of the bulb and like it covered with Bulbo-spongiosus,
   and having a long duct (about $\frac{3}{4}''$) which opens into the
   vestibule (cf., the bulbo-urethral glands and ducts).
6. The perineal membrane to which the bulb is seen to be
   fastened on the left side. On the right side the membrane is
   cut away thereby revealing the vessels of the bulb and the
   dorsal nerve and vessels of the clitoris.

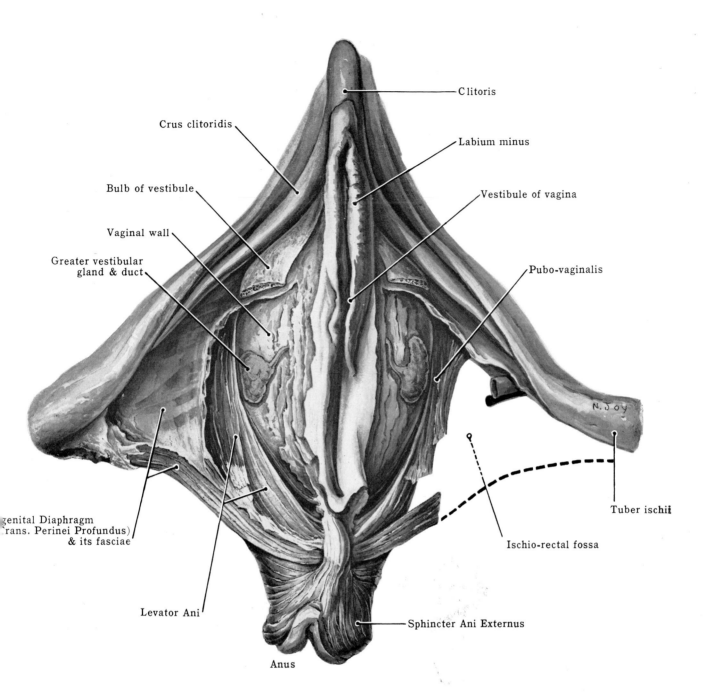

Clitoris

Crus clitoridis

Labium minus

Bulb of vestibule

Vestibule of vagina

Vaginal wall

Greater vestibular
gland & duct

Pubo-vaginalis

genital Diaphragm
rans. Perinei Profundus)
& its fasciae

Tuber ischii

Ischio-rectal fossa

Levator Ani

Sphincter Ani Externus

Anus

29 Female Perineum: The Urogenital Diaphragm—V

Observe:

The bulbs of the vestibule cut short. The urogenital diaphragm and its fasciae partly cut away on the right side and
extensively cut away on the left.

The urogenital diaphragm—a sheet of striated muscle,
mainly Deep Transversus Perinei, placed between a superior
and an inferior sheet of fascia, and having 2 parts: (a) a posterior which is a strong fleshy band that meets its fellow in the
central point of the perineum and (b) an anterior which is
more areolar than fleshy.

Medially, the diaphragm and its fasciae have been raised
from the sloping inferior surface of Levator Ani and detached
from the sloping outer wall of vagina with which it fuses.

4. The anterior parts of the Levatores Ani (Pubo-vaginales)
meeting behind the vaginal orifice. The greater vestibular
glands and the bulbs of the vestibule applied to the sides of
the vagina, medial to the anterior borders of the Levatores
Ani.

5. The laminated nature of this part of the wall of the vagina.
It is laminated because several layers of fascia fuse with it
and lose their identity in it, namely the superficial perineal
fascia, the diaphragm and its fasciae, and the fasciae of the
Levatores Ani.

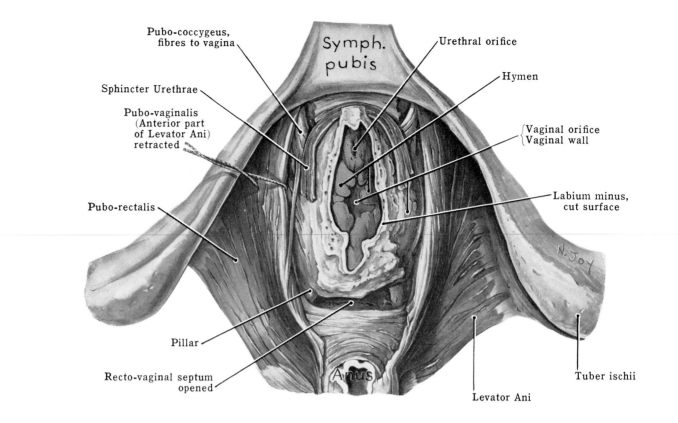

Pubo-coccygeus, fibres to vagina

Sphincter Urethrae

Pubo-vaginalis (Anterior part of Levator Ani) retracted

Pubo-rectalis

Symph. pubis

Urethral orifice

Hymen

Vaginal orifice
Vaginal wall

Labium minus, cut surface

N. Joy

Pillar

Recto-vaginal septum opened

Anus

Levator Ani

Tuber ischii

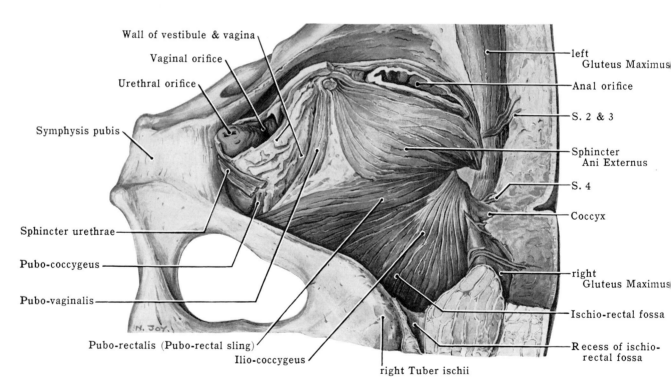

Wall of vestibule & vagina

Vaginal orifice

Urethral orifice

Symphysis pubis

Sphincter urethrae

Pubo-coccygeus

Pubo-vaginalis

N. Joy.

Pubo-rectalis (Pubo-rectal sling)

Ilio-coccygeus

right Tuber ischii

left Gluteus Maximus

Anal orifice

S. 2 & 3

Sphincter Ani Externus

S. 4

Coccyx

right Gluteus Maximus

Ischio-rectal fossa

Recess of ischio-rectal fossa

230, 230.1 Female Perineum: The Levator Ani—VI

(The front view and the oblique side view are of different specimens.)

Observe:

1. The Sphincter Urethrae, of striated muscle, like a saddle, resting on the urethra and straddling the vagina.

2. The labia minora, cut short, bounding the vestibule of the vagina, and the hymen, separating the vestibule from the cavity of the vagina.

Continued on facing page

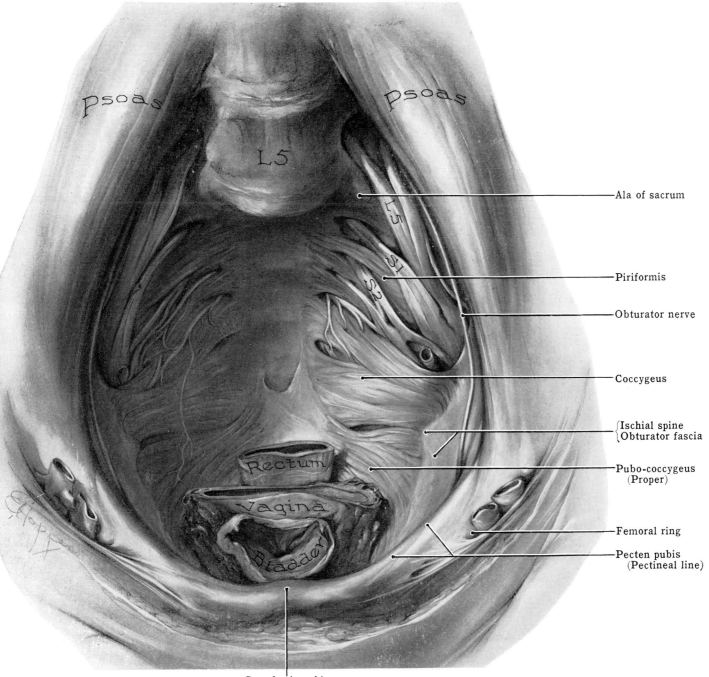

Psoas

Psoas

L5

L5

S1

S2

Ala of sacrum

Piriformis

Obturator nerve

Coccygeus

Ischial spine
Obturator fascia

Pubo-coccygeus
(Proper)

Femoral ring

Pecten pubis
(Pectineal line)

Rectum

Vagina

Bladder

Symphysis pubis

231 Floor of the Female Pelvis, from above, showing the relative positions of the bladder, vagina and rectum

Continued from facing page

3. The subdivisions of Levator Ani:

    A. Pubo-coccygeus { Pubo-coccygeus Proper
                               Pubo-vaginalis
                               Pubo-rectalis
    B. Ilio-coccygeus

4. The recto-vaginal (areolar) septum easily converted into a space, and limited on each side by a "fascial pillar" between rectal and vaginal fasciae.

5. The thick anterior pillar of Pubo-coccygeus Proper extending backwards to the vagina. Pubo-vaginal fibres of opposite sides meeting behind the vaginal orifice. Pubo-rectal fibres of opposite sides meeting in the ano-rectal junction to form the "pubo-rectal sling". Ilio-coccygeus meeting its fellow in an aponeurosis between rectum and coccyx.

6. The vaginal wall laminated, as in figure 229.

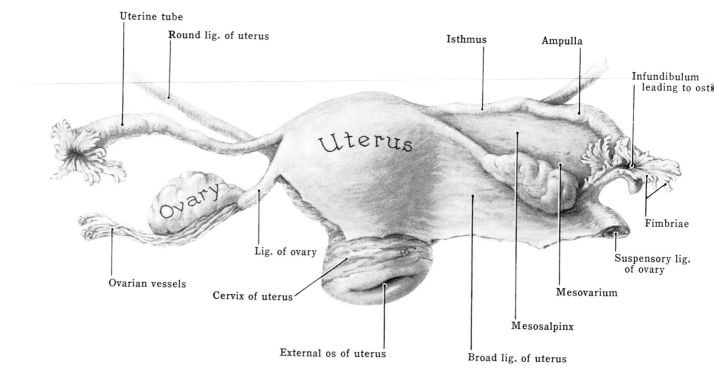

Uterine tube
Round lig. of uterus
Isthmus
Ampulla
Infundibulum leading to osti
Uterus
Ovary
Lig. of ovary
Fimbriae
Ovarian vessels
Cervix of uterus
Suspensory lig. of ovary
Mesovarium
External os of uterus
Mesosalpinx
Broad lig. of uterus

232 Uterus and its Appurtenances, from behind

On the left side, the broad ligament of the uterus is removed, thereby setting free the uterine tube, the round ligament of the uterus, and the ligament of the ovary. These three are attached to the side of the uterus close together, at the junction of its fundus and body.

On the right side is the "mesentery" of the uterus and tube, called the broad ligament. The ovary is attached (a) to the broad ligament by a "mesentery" of its own, called the mesovarium; (b) to the uterus by the ligament of the ovary; and (c) to the false pelvis by the suspensory ligament of the ovary (infundibulo-pelvic lig.), which transmits the ovarian vessels. The part of the broad ligament above the level of the mesovarium is called the mesosalpinx.

Epithelia: The areolar membrane, called the peritoneum, is lined with mesothelium; the ovary is covered with cubical epithelium; the infundibulum and fimbriae of the uterine tube with ciliated columnar epithelium; and the cervix of the uterus with stratified squamous epithelium.

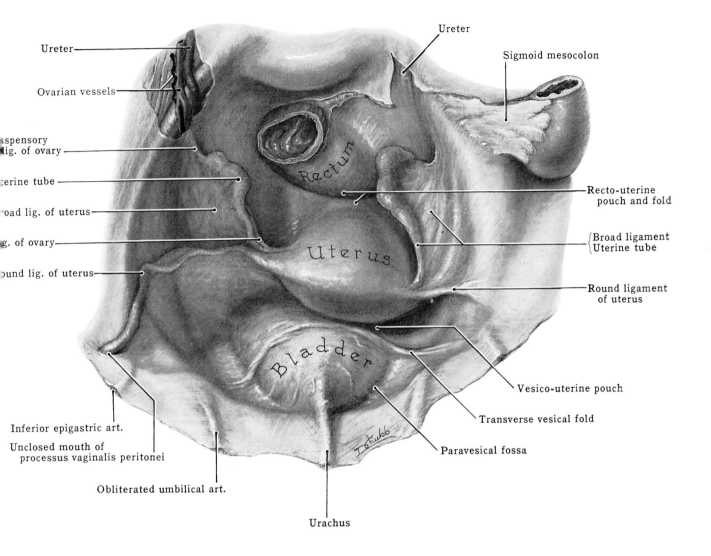

Ureter

Ovarian vessels

spensory
lig. of ovary

erine tube

oad lig. of uterus

g. of ovary

ound lig. of uterus

Inferior epigastric art.

Unclosed mouth of
processus vaginalis peritonei

Obliterated umbilical art.

Urachus

Ureter

Sigmoid mesocolon

Rectum

Uterus

Bladder

Recto-uterine
pouch and fold

Broad ligament
Uterine tube

Round ligament
of uterus

Vesico-uterine pouch

Transverse vesical fold

Paravesical fossa

233 Female True Pelvis, from above

Observe:

1. The uterus asymmetrically placed, as usual; here leaning to the left.

2. The right round ligament of the uterus; here longer than the left one, and having an acquired "mesentery"

3. The free edge of the medial $\frac{4}{5}$ of the broad ligament of the uterus occupied by the uterine tube (Fallopian tube). The lateral $\frac{1}{5}$, occupied by the ovarian vessels, is the suspensory lig. of the ovary (infundibulo-pelvic lig.).

4. The ovarian vessels crossing the external iliac vessels close to ($\frac{1}{4}"-1"$) the ureter; the left ureter crossing at the apex of the inverted V-shaped root of the sigmoid mesocolon.

5. The ovaries lie behind a veil—the broad ligaments.

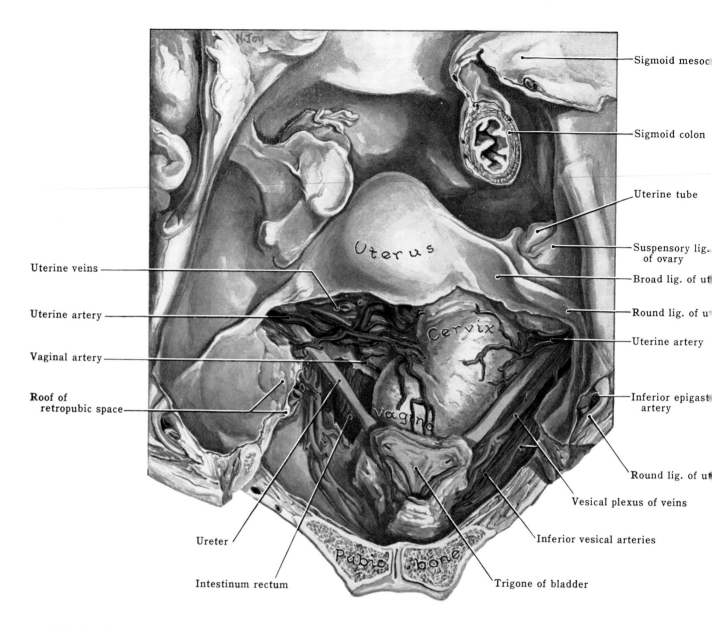

Labels on figure:
- Sigmoid mesoc[olon]
- Sigmoid colon
- Uterine tube
- Suspensory lig. of ovary
- Broad lig. of ut[erus]
- Round lig. of u[terus]
- Uterine artery
- Inferior epigast[ric] artery
- Round lig. of ut[erus]
- Vesical plexus of veins
- Inferior vesical arteries
- Trigone of bladder
- Intestinum rectum
- Ureter
- Roof of retropubic space
- Vaginal artery
- Uterine artery
- Uterine veins

Figure text: N. Joy · Uterus · Cervix · Vagina · Pubic bone

234 Female Genital Organs, from the front—I

Part of the pubic bones and the whole of the bladder, excepting the trigone, are removed, and with them parts of the broad ligaments.

Observe:

1. The uterus asymmetrically placed, which is usual, and also the vagina.

2. As a result, one ureter—in this instance the left one—crosses the lateral fornix of the vagina and is close to the cervix of the uterus, whereas the other ureter is correspondingly far away.

3. The uterine artery, lying with its veins in the base of the broad ligament and running up the side of the uterus.

4. A large vaginal artery, a branch of the uterine artery, supplying the cervix and the anterior surface of the vagina. The vaginal artery arising from the internal iliac artery and supplying the posterior surface of the vagina.

5. The rectal fascia (not labelled) intervening between the foregoing arteries and the rectum.

6. The round ligament of the uterus curving round the inferior epigastric vessels at the deep inguinal ring and passing through the inguinal canal (cf. the ductus deferens in the male, fig. 216).

7. The superior vesical vessels (not labelled) in the roof of the retropubic space.

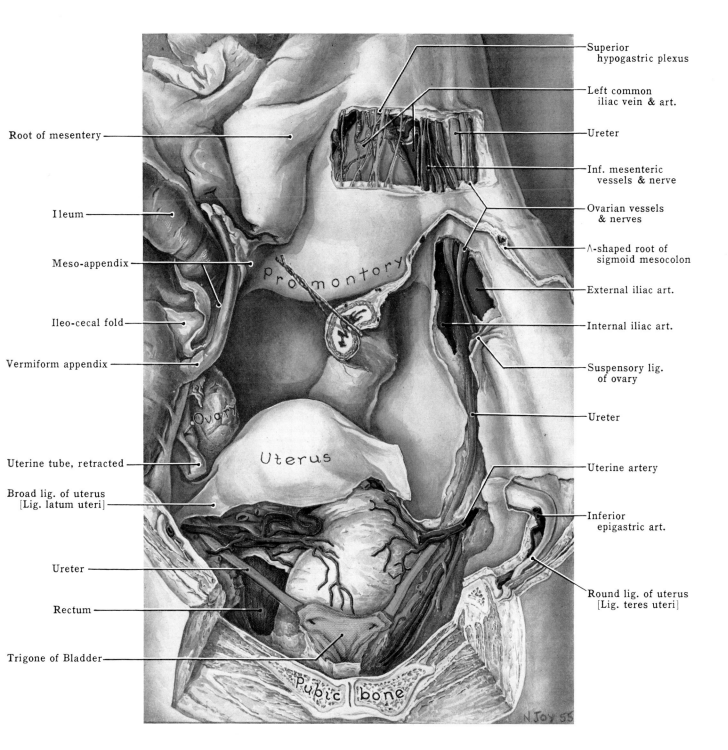

Root of mesentery

Ileum

Meso-appendix

Ileo-cecal fold

Vermiform appendix

Uterine tube, retracted

Broad lig. of uterus
[Lig. latum uteri]

Ureter

Rectum

Trigone of Bladder

Superior
hypogastric plexus

Left common
iliac vein & art.

Ureter

Inf. mesenteric
vessels & nerve

Ovarian vessels
& nerves

Λ-shaped root of
sigmoid mesocolon

External iliac art.

Internal iliac art.

Suspensory lig.
of ovary

Ureter

Uterine artery

Inferior
epigastric art.

Round lig. of uterus
[Lig. teres uteri]

Promontory · Ovary · Uterus · Pubic bone · N Joy 55

235   Female Ureter in its Pelvic Course—II

Observe:

1. The superior hypogastric plexus and some lymph vessels anterior to the left common iliac vein.

2. The left ureter, which has just been crossed by the ovarian vessels and nerves, and which is about to be crossed by sigmoid branches of the inferior mesenteric vessels.

   The apex of the Λ-shaped root of the sigmoid mesocolon situated in front of the left ureter, and acting as a guide to it.

The ureter, crossing the external iliac artery—at the bifurcation of the common iliac artery and close behind the ovarian vessels—and descending in front of the internal iliac artery. Its subperitoneal course from where it enters the pelvis to where it passes deep to the broad ligament and is there crossed by the uterine artery.

3. The vermiform appendix in one of its rarer positions—post-ileal. The ileocecal fold extending from the end of the ileum to the meso-appendix.

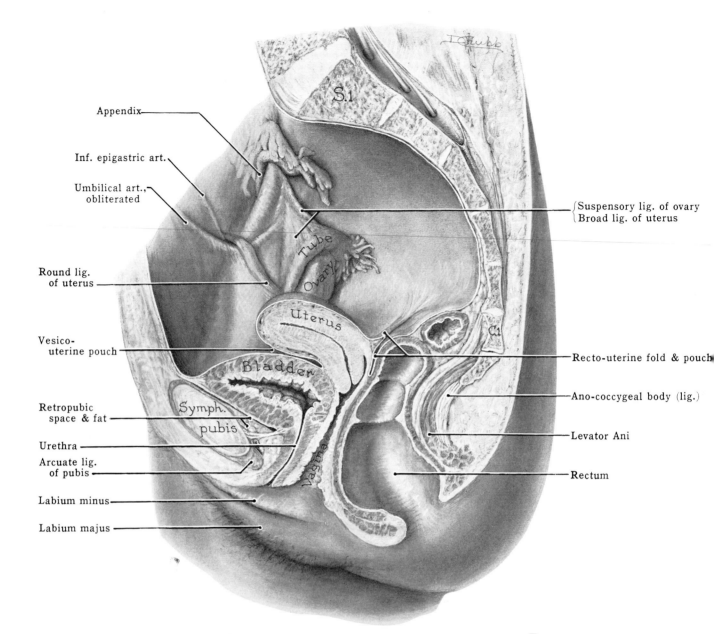

Appendix

Inf. epigastric art.

Umbilical art., obliterated

Round lig. of uterus

Vesico- uterine pouch

Retropubic space & fat

Urethra

Arcuate lig. of pubis

Labium minus

Labium majus

Suspensory lig. of ovary
Broad lig. of uterus

Recto-uterine fold & pouch

Ano-coccygeal body (lig.)

Levator Ani

Rectum

236 Female True Pelvis, in median section

Plugs of cotton wool in the lower parts of the rectum and vagina had slightly distorted these parts. The uterus was sectioned in its own median plane and depicted as though this coincided with the median plane of the body—which is seldom the case.

Observe:

1. The uterine tube and the ovary, in their virginal positions on the side wall of the pelvis, i.e., in the angle between the ureter and the umbilical artery, and medial to the obturator nerve and vessels (fig. 210).

2. The uterus, bent on itself at the junction of body and cervix. The cervix, opening on the anterior wall of the vagina, and having a short, round, anterior lip and a long, thinner, posterior lip.

3. The external os of the uterus, at the level of the upper end of the symphysis pubis.

4. The anterior fornix of the vagina, $\frac{1}{2}''$ or more from the vesico-uterine pouch. The posterior fornix covered with $\frac{1}{2}''$ or more of the recto-uterine pouch, which is the lowest part of the peritoneal cavity, when the subject is erect.

5. The urethra ($1\frac{1}{4}''$ long), the vagina, and the rectum parallel to one another and to the pelvic brim. The uterus, nearly at right angles to them, when the bladder is empty.

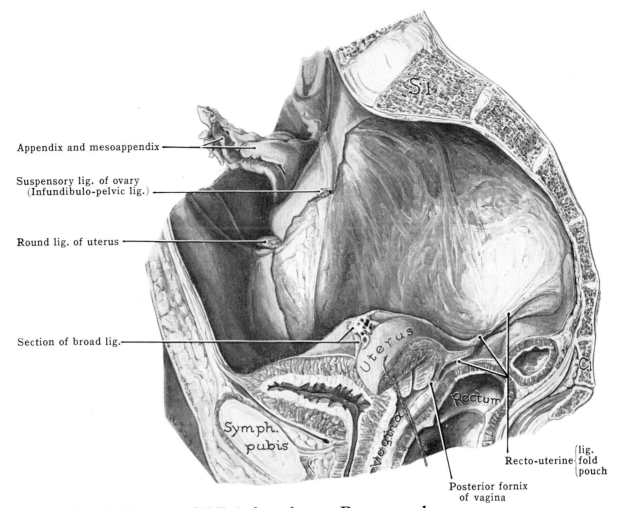

Appendix and mesoappendix

Suspensory lig. of ovary
(Infundibulo-pelvic lig.)

Round lig. of uterus

Section of broad lig.

S.1

Uterus

Symph.
pubis

Vagina

Rectum

Recto-uterine {lig.
{fold
{pouch

Posterior fornix
of vagina

237   Bed from which Figure 237.1 has been Removed

Observe:

. Divided at the pelvic brim are: the round lig. and the suspensory lig. with the contained
ovarian vessels and nerves.

. Divided at the side of the uterus are: the broad lig. with the uterine tube in its free margin
the round lig. anteriorly, the lig. of the ovary posteriorly, and several branches of the uterine
vessels.

. The structures shown in figure 237.1, thus set free, peeled off the side wall of the pelvis
leaving the subperitoneal fatty-areolar tissue (tela subserosa) exposed.

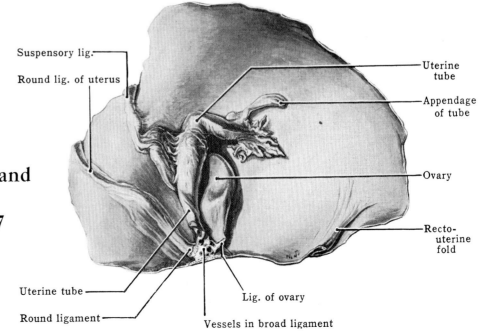

**237.1   Broad Ligament and
its Related Structures,
removed from figure 237**

Suspensory lig.

Round lig. of uterus

Uterine
tube

Appendage
of tube

Ovary

Recto-
uterine
fold

Uterine tube

Round ligament

Lig. of ovary

Vessels in broad ligament

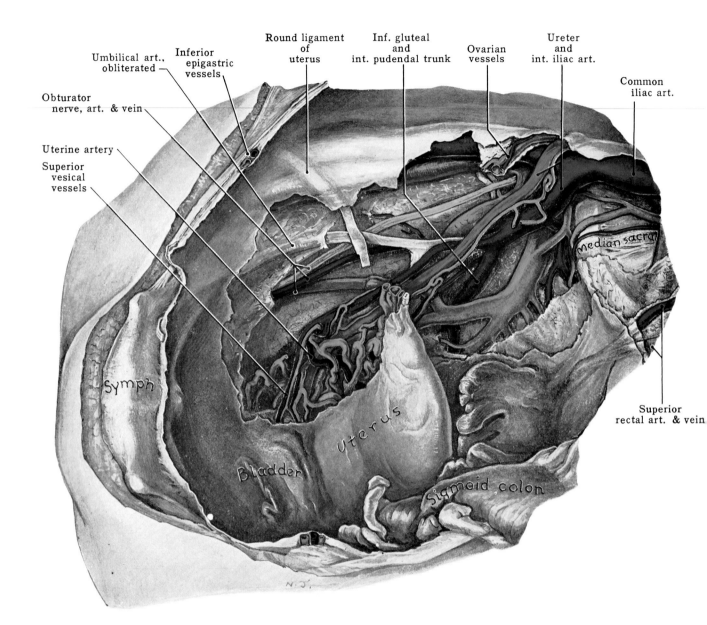

Obturator nerve, art. & vein

Umbilical art., obliterated

Inferior epigastric vessels

Round ligament of uterus

Inf. gluteal and int. pudendal trunk

Ovarian vessels

Ureter and int. iliac art.

Common iliac art.

Uterine artery

Superior vesical vessels

median sacral

Symph

Bladder

Uterus

Sigmoid colon

Superior rectal art. & vein

N.J.

238 Blood Vessels on the side wall of the Female Pelvis, viewed from the left side of a supine cadaver

In this older subject the uterus is retroverted. The inferior gluteal and internal pudendal arteries here spring from a common trunk, not separately as in figure 210.

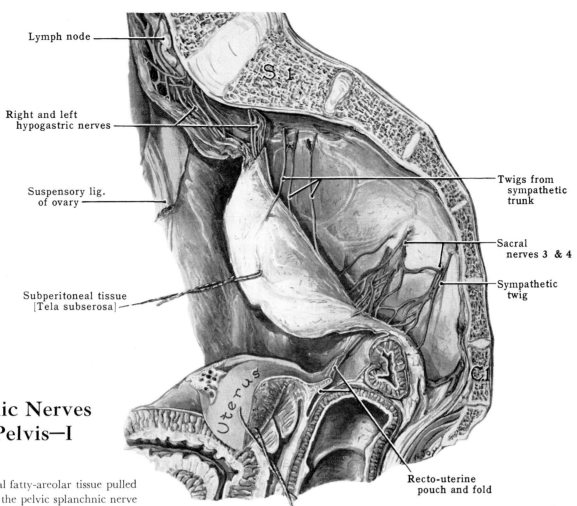

Lymph node

Right and left
hypogastric nerves

Suspensory lig.
of ovary

Subperitoneal tissue
[Tela subserosa]

S. 1

Twigs from
sympathetic
trunk

Sacral
nerves 3 & 4

Sympathetic
twig

C1

Uterus

Recto-uterine
pouch and fold

9 Autonomic Nerves
the Female Pelvis—I

erve:

rectum and subperitoneal fatty-areolar tissue pulled
ards thus rendering taut the pelvic splanchnic nerve
n S. 3 & 4), sympathetic twigs, and the right hypo-
ric nerve.

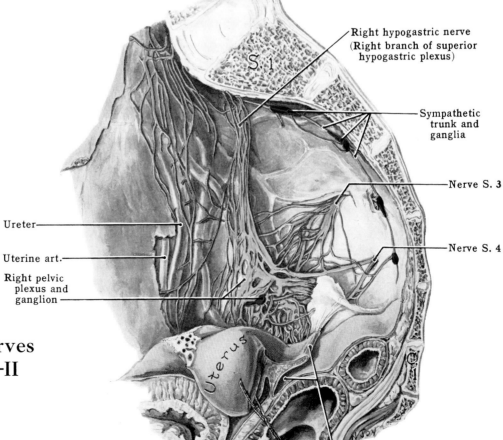

S. 1

Right hypogastric nerve
(Right branch of superior
hypogastric plexus)

Sympathetic
trunk and
ganglia

Nerve S. 3

Nerve S. 4

Ureter

Uterine art.

Right pelvic
plexus and
ganglion

C1

Uterus

40 Autonomic Nerves
the Female Pelvis—II

's is a later stage of figure 239.

Recto-uterine pouch and fold

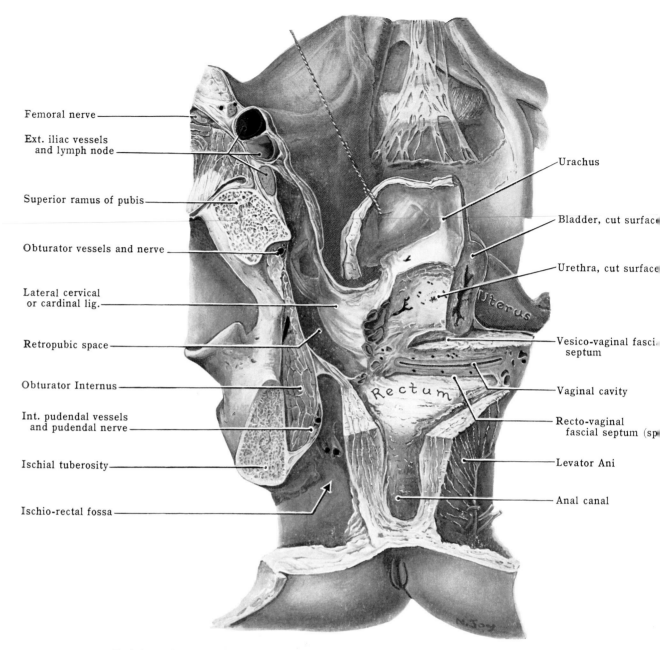

Femoral nerve

Ext. iliac vessels and lymph node

Superior ramus of pubis

Obturator vessels and nerve

Lateral cervical or cardinal lig.

Retropubic space

Obturator Internus

Int. pudendal vessels and pudendal nerve

Ischial tuberosity

Ischio-rectal fossa

Urachus

Bladder, cut surface

Urethra, cut surface

Vesico-vaginal fascial septum

Vaginal cavity

Recto-vaginal fascial septum (sp

Levator Ani

Anal canal

Uterus

Rectum

241   Suspensory and the Supporting Mechanism of the Vagina

This is approximately a coronal section of the pelvis. The neck of the bladder and the vagina are cut across transversely; the bladder is divided sagittally and is rotated backwards.

Observe:

1. The partition that separates the retropubic space from the ischiorectal fossa to be formed merely by the thin origin of Levator Ani from the Obturator Internus fascia, and its areolar coverings.

2. The rectum supporting the posterior wall of the vagina; the posterior wall supporting the anterior wall; and the anterior wall supporting the bladder.

3. The dense areolar tissue within which the vesico-vaginal plexus of veins passes postero-superiorly to join the internal iliac veins. This acts as a suspensory ligament for the cervix and vagina. It is called the cardinal ligament.

4. The cardinal ligament blending with the fascia that encapsules the vagina and with adjacent fasciae.

5. Anteriorly, the fascia encapsuling the vagina blending with the vesical fascia and intimately adherent to the urethra; and posteriorly, loosely attached to the rectal fascia.

The Lower Limb

Iliac crest

Tubercle of crest

Ant. sup. spine

Ant. inf. spine

Head of femur

Greater trochanter

Intertrochanteric line

Lesser trochanter

FEMUR

PATELLA

Lateral epicondyle

Lateral condyle

Apex of head

Head

Neck

FIBULA

Iliac fossa

Ilio-pubic (-pectineal)
eminence

Superior ramus of pubis

Tubercle of pubis

Crest of pubis

Pecten pubis (Pectineal line)

Body of pubis

Pubic arch, left half

Symphysis pubis

Obturator foramen

Ischial tuberosity

Adductor tubercle

Medial epicondyle

Medial condyle

Med. & lat. condyles

Tuberosity (Tubercle)

TIBIA

242 Bones of the Lower Limb, front view

(For Bones of Leg, see fig. 303. For Bones of Foot, dorsal aspect, see figs. 311–313 and 343.)

Iliac crest

Dorsum Ilii

Post. sup. spine —   Tubercle of crest

Post. inf. spine —

Greater sciatic notch —

Ischial spine —   Neck of femur

Dorsum Ischii

Lesser sciatic notch —   Greater trochanter

Intertrochanteric crest

Ischial tuberosity —   Lesser trochanter

Gluteal tuberosity

Spiral line —

Linea aspera —

FEMUR

Med. supracondylar line —   Lat. supracondylar line

Adductor tubercle —   Popliteal surface

Intercondylar line —   Intercondylar notch

Medial condyle —   Lateral condyle

Medial condyle —   Lateral condyle

Apex of head (Styloid process)

Head of fibula

Neck

Soleal (Popliteal) line —

TIBIA —   FIBULA

243   Bones of the Lower Limb, posterior view

(For Bones of Leg, posterior view, see fig. 315. For Bones of Foot, plantar aspect, see fig. 314.)

Inferior epigastric a.

Superficial epigastric a.

Deep circumflex iliac a.

Superficial circumflex iliac a.

Profunda femoris a.

Lateral femoral circumflex a.

Perforating aa.

descending br.

POPLITEAL ART.

Superior lateral genicular a.

Inferior lateral genicular a.

Perforating br. of peroneal a.

Lateral malleolar a.

Lateral tarsal a.

Arcuate a.

Perforating aa.

Dorsal metatarsal aa.

Dorsal digital aa.

ABDOMINAL AORTA

COMMON ILIAC ART.

INTERNAL ILIAC ART.

EXTERNAL ILIAC ART.

(Superficial) External pudendal a.

Obturator a.

Medial femoral circumflex a.

FEMORAL ART.

Unnamed muscular br.

Descending genicular a.

articular br.

Superior medial genicular a.

saphenous br.

Inferior medial genicular a.

Anterior tibial recurrent a.

ANTERIOR TIBIAL ART.

Medial malleolar a.

Dorsalis pedis a.

Medial tarsal aa.

Deep plantar br.

1st Dorsal metatarsal a.

Superficial br.

superior ra

inferior ra

Deep branch

Superior gluteal a.

Inferior gluteal a.

Medial femoral circumflex a.

Profunda femoris a.

FEMORAL ART.

Hiatus in Adductor Magnus

Superior medial genicular a.

Inferior medial genicular a.

POSTERIOR TIBIAL ART.

Tuber calcanei

Medial calcanean brs.

MEDIAL PLANTAR ART.

Deep plantar br. of dorsalis pedis a.

transverse b of Lat. femoral circumflex

Perforating brs

Superior lateral genicular a.

POPLITEAL A

Inferior lateral genicular a.

ANTERIOR TIBIAL ART.

Peroneal a. [Fibular a.]

Perforating br.

Communicating

Lateral calcanea

LATERAL PLANTAR AR

3 Perforating brs

PLANTAR ARCH

Plantar metatarsal aa.

Plantar digital aa

Anterior View

Posterior View

244   A Diagram of the Arteries of the Lower Limb

List of the Named Arteries of the Lower Limb

Internal iliac artery
  Obturator a.
    acetabular br.
    anterior br.
    posterior br.
  Superior gluteal a.
    Superficial br.
    Deep br.
      superior br.
      inferior br.
  Inferior gluteal a.
    branch to sciatic nerve

External iliac artery

Femoral artery
  Superficial epigastric a.
  Superficial circumflex iliac a.
  (Superficial) external pudendal a.
    Anterior scrotal [or labial] brs.
    Inguinal brs.
  Profunda femoris a.
    Medial femoral circumflex a.
      acetabular br.
      ascending br.
      transverse br.
    Lateral femoral circumflex a.
      ascending br.
      transverse br.
      descending br.
    Perforating branches
  Descending genicular a.
    (A. genu suprema)
      articular br.
      saphenous br.

Popliteal artery
  Superior lateral genicular a.
  Superior medial genicular a.
  Middle genicular a.
  Sural aa.
  Inferior lateral genicular a.
  Inferior medial genicular a.

Anterior tibial artery
  Anterior tibial recurrent a.
  Lateral malleolar a.
  Medial malleolar a.

Dorsalis pedis artery
  Lateral tarsal a.
  Medial tarsal aa.
  Arcuate a.
    Dorsal metatarsal aa.
    Dorsal digital aa.
  Deep plantar br.
  1st dorsal metatarsal a.

Posterior tibial artery
  Circumflex fibular br.
  Peroneal [Fibular] art.
    Perforating br.
    Communicating br.
    Lateral malleolar a.
    Lateral calcanean a.
  Medial malleolar a.
  Medial calcanean brs.

Medial plantar artery

Lateral plantar artery
  Plantar arch
    Plantar metatarsal aa.
    Perforating branches
    Plantar digital aa.

245 Superficial Veins of Lower Limb, antero-medial view

The arrows indicate where anastomotic veins perforate the deep fascia and bring the superficial and deep veins into communication with each other.

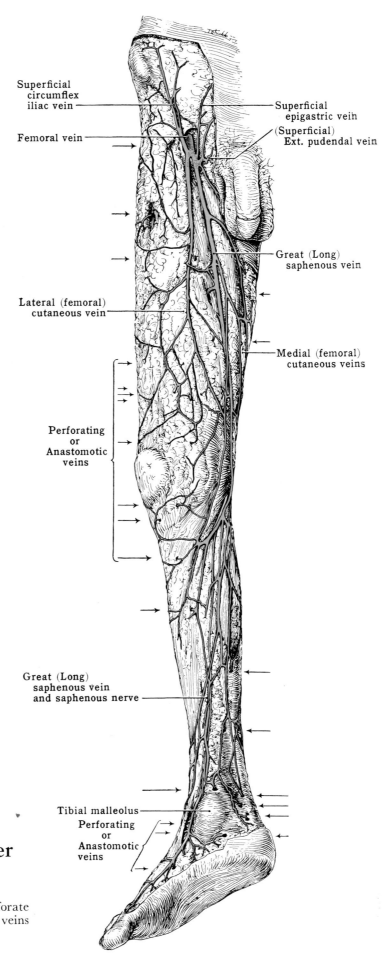

Superficial circumflex iliac vein

Femoral vein

Lateral (femoral) cutaneous vein

Perforating or Anastomotic veins

Great (Long) saphenous vein and saphenous nerve

Tibial malleolus

Perforating or Anastomotic veins

Superficial epigastric vein

(Superficial) Ext. pudendal vein

Great (Long) saphenous vein

Medial (femoral) cutaneous veins

Great (Long) saphenous vein

Common peroneal nerve (Lat. popliteal n.)

Posterior cutaneous nerve of thigh

Small (Short) saphenous vein

Perforating or Anastomotic veins

Small (Short) saphenous vein

Sural nerve

Perforating or Anastomotic veins

Perforating vein

Fibular malleolus

246 Superficial Veins of the Leg, posterior view

The arrows indicate where anastomotic veins perfor the deep fascia and bring the superficial and deep ve into communication with each other.

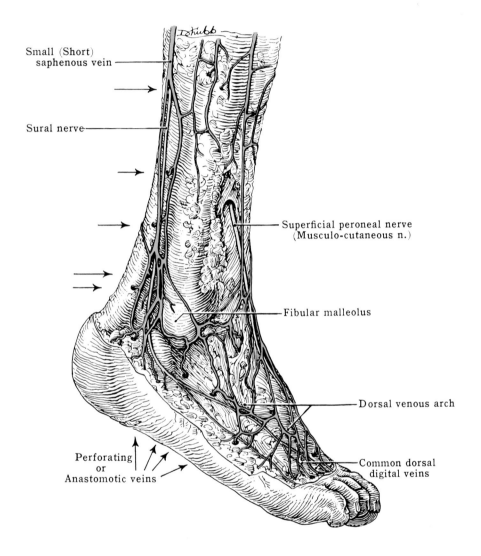

Small (Short)
saphenous vein

Sural nerve

Superficial peroneal nerve
(Musculo-cutaneous n.)

Fibular malleolus

Dorsal venous arch

Perforating
or
Anastomotic veins

Common dorsal
digital veins

247   Superficial Veins of the Ankle and
Dorsum of the Foot, antero-lateral view

Lateral cutaneous branch
of subcostal nerve (T.12)

Lateral cutaneous nerve
of thigh, post. branch

Lateral cutaneous nerve
of thigh, ant. branch

Intermediate
cutaneous n. of thigh

Infrapatellar branch
of saphenous nerve

Cutaneous branches
of (lateral popliteal n.)
common peroneal nerve

(Musculo-cutaneous n.)
Superficial peroneal nerve
becoming dorsal digital
nerves

Dorsal lateral cutaneous
nerve of foot

Femoral brs. of genito-femoral nerve
(Lumbo-inguinal n.)

Genital br. of genito-femoral nerve
(Ext. spermatic n.)

Ilio-inguinal nerve

Cutaneous branch
of obturator nerve

Medial cutaneous nerve
of thigh, ant. branch

Saphenous nerve

Deep peroneal nerve
(Anterior tibial n.)

248 Cutaneous Nerves of the Lower Limb, front view

Cutaneous branches of dorsal rami {L.1 L.2 L.3}

Lat. cutaneous branch of iliohypogastric nerve

Cutaneous branches of dorsal rami {S.1 S.2 S.3}

Lat. cutaneous nerve of thigh, post. branches

Perforating cutaneous n. (S.2, 3)

Post. cutaneous n. of thigh, perineal branch

Post. cutaneous n. of thigh, gluteal branches

Posterior cutaneous nerve of thigh

Cutaneous br. of obturator nerve

Lat. cutaneous n. of thigh

Medial cutaneous nerve of thigh, post. branch

Post. cutaneous n. of thigh, end branch

Lat. sural cutaneous nerve (Cutan. br. of lat. popliteal n.)

Branch of saphenous nerve

Med. sural cutaneous nerve (Cutan. br. of med. popliteal n.)

Branch of saphenous nerve

Medial calcanean nerve

Dorsal lateral cutaneous nerve of foot-termination of the sural nerve

249 Cutaneous Nerves of the Lower Limb, back view

Note:

Sura is Latin for the calf. The medial sural cutaneous nerve is here joined close above the ankle by a communicating branch (not labelled) of the lateral sural cutaneous nerve to form the sural nerve. The level of the junction is variable, being here very low, in figure 286 very high, and in figure 246 in between.

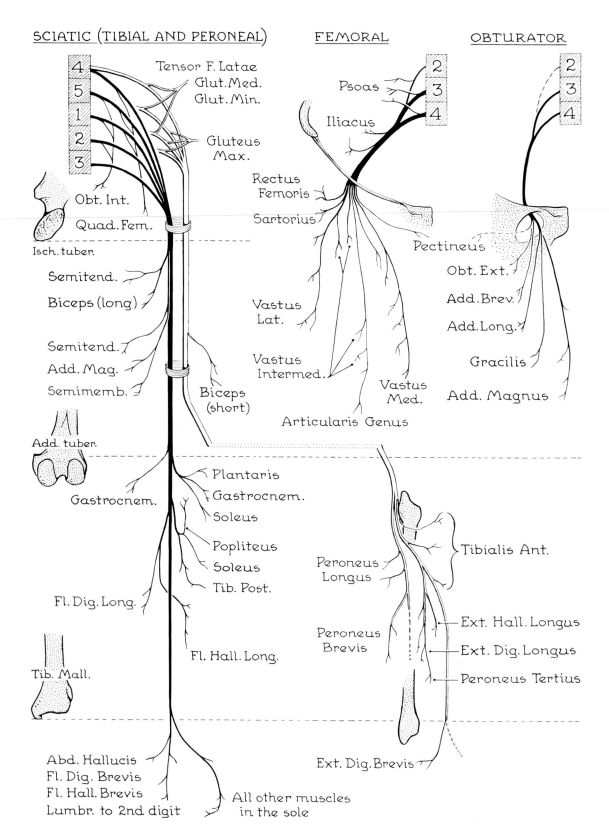

SCIATIC (TIBIAL AND PERONEAL)   FEMORAL   OBTURATOR

4
5
1
2
3

Tensor F. Latae
Glut. Med.
Glut. Min.

Gluteus
Max.

Obt. Int.
Quad. Fem.

Isch. tuber.

Semitend.
Biceps (long)

Semitend.
Add. Mag.
Semimemb.

Add. tuber.

Gastrocnem.

Fl. Dig. Long.

Tib. Mall.

Abd. Hallucis
Fl. Dig. Brevis
Fl. Hall. Brevis
Lumbr. to 2nd digit

Biceps
(short)

Plantaris
Gastrocnem.
Soleus

Popliteus
Soleus
Tib. Post.

Fl. Hall. Long.

All other muscles
in the sole

2
3
4

Psoas

Iliacus

Rectus
Femoris
Sartorius

Vastus
Lat.

Vastus
Intermed.

Vastus
Med.

Articularis Genus

2
3
4

Pectineus

Obt. Ext.
Add. Brev.
Add. Long.

Gracilis

Add. Magnus

Tibialis Ant.

Peroneus
Longus

Peroneus
Brevis

Ext. Hall. Longus
Ext. Dig. Longus
Peroneus Tertius

Ext. Dig. Brevis

250 Scheme of the Motor Distribution of the Nerves of the Lower Limb

The average levels at which the motor branches leave the stems of the main nerves are shown with reference to the ischial tuberosity, adductor tubercle, and tibial malleolus.

250.1 A List of the Muscles of the Lower Limb

Ilio-psoas
  Iliacus
  Psoas Major
Psoas Minor
Gluteus Maximus
Gluteus Medius
Gluteus Minimus
Tensor Fasciae Latae
Piriformis
Obturator Internus
Gemellus Superior
Gemellus Inferior
Quadratus Femoris
Sartorius
Quadriceps Femoris
  Rectus Femoris
  Vastus Lateralis
  Vastus Intermedius
  Vastus Medialis
Articularis Genus
Pectineus
Gracilis
Adductor Longus
Adductor Brevis
Adductor Magnus
Obturator Externus
Biceps Femoris
  long head
  short head
Semitendinosus
Semimembranosus
Tibialis Anterior
Extensor Digitorum Longus
Peroneus Tertius
Extensor Hallucis Longus
Peroneus Brevis
Peroneus Longus
Gastrocnemius
  lateral head
  medial head
Soleus
Plantaris
Popliteus
Tibialis Posterior
Flexor Digitorum Longus
Flexor Hallucis Longus
Extensor Hallucis Brevis
Extensor Digitorum Brevis
Abductor Hallucis
Flexor Hallucis Brevis
Adductor Hallucis
  oblique head
  transverse head
Abductor Digiti Minimi (V)
(Abductor Ossis Metatarsi Quinti)
Flexor Digiti Minimi Brevis
Flexor Digitorum Brevis
Flexor Digitorum Accessorius
Lumbricales
Interossei
  Dorsal
  Plantar

Great saphenous vein

251   Inguinal Lymph Nodes

Observe:

1. The arrangement of the nodes: (a) a proximal chain parallel to the inguinal ligament (superficial inguinal nodes); (b) a distal chain on the sides of the great saphenous vein (superficial subinguinal nodes); and above this, a chain of two or three nodes on the medial side of the femoral vein (deep inguinal nodes), one being below the femoral canal and one or two within it.

    These nodes receive the superficial and deep lymph vessels of the lower limb; the superficial vessels of the lower part of the abdominal wall; the vessels of the penis, including the glans penis and spongy urethra, and of the scrotum (but not of the testis or ovary); the vessels of the vulva, lower part of the vagina, and some vessels from the uterus that run with the round ligament; and vessels of the lower part of the anal canal.

2. The free anastomosis between the lymph vessels.

    About two dozen efferent vessels leave these nodes and, passing deep to the inguinal ligament, enter the external iliac nodes. Of these, less than half traverse the femoral canal; the others ascend alongside the femoral artery and vein, some being inside the femoral sheath and some outside it.

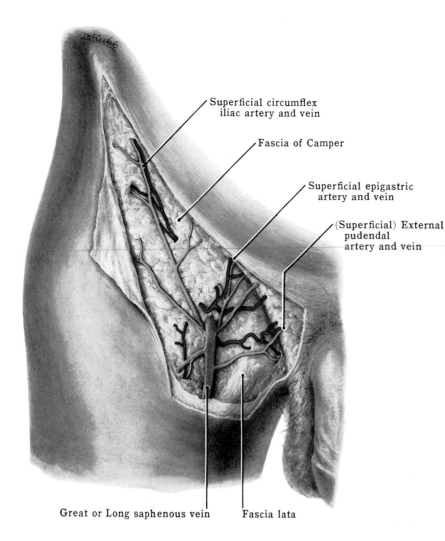

Superficial circumflex
iliac artery and vein

Fascia of Camper

Superficial epigastric
artery and vein

(Superficial) External
pudendal
artery and vein

Great or Long saphenous vein   Fascia lata

252 Superficial Inguinal Arteries and Veins—I

The arteries are branches of the femoral artery but the veins are tributaries of the great saphenous vein.

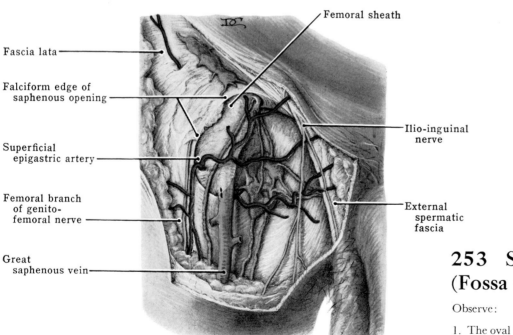

Femoral sheath

Fascia lata

Falciform edge of
saphenous opening

Superficial
epigastric artery

Femoral branch
of genito-
femoral nerve

Great
saphenous vein

Ilio-inguinal
nerve

External
spermatic
fascia

253 Saphenous Opening (Fossa Ovalis)—II

Observe:

1. The oval shape of the hiatus in the fascia lata through which the great saphenous vein passes to join the femoral vein, which lies within the femoral sheath.

2. The sharp superior and inferior free margins, or cornua, of the opening and the less sharply definable lateral margin or falciform edge.

3. The great saphenous vein hooking over the inferior cornu. Occasionally it joins the femoral vein 1 or even 2 cm. above this cornu.

254 Three Compartments of the Femoral Sheath, opened—III

Observe:

1. The falciform edge of the saphenous opening (fossa ovalis) cut away.

2. The superior cornu of the opening passing towards the pubic tubercle and blending with the inguinal ligament and, in this specimen, with the lacunar ligament also.

3. The medial border of the opening formed by the fascia covering Pectineus and as such passing laterally behind the femoral sheath.

4. The 3 compartments of the sheath: (a) the lateral one for the artery, (b) the middle one for vein, and (c) the medial one, called the femoral canal, for lymph vessels.

5. The proximal end of the femoral canal, called the femoral ring, bounded medially by the lacunar ligament, anteriorly by the inguinal ligament, posteriorly by the pectineal fascia, and laterally by the femoral vein.

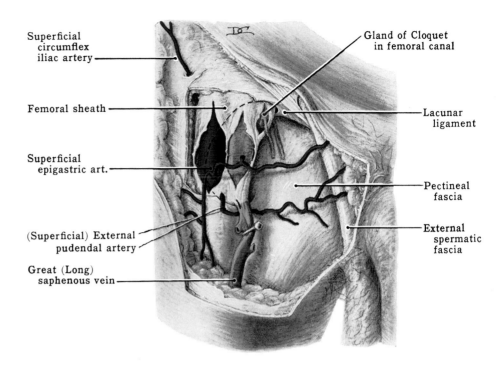

Superficial circumflex iliac artery

Femoral sheath

Superficial epigastric art.

(Superficial) External pudendal artery

Great (Long) saphenous vein

Gland of Cloquet in femoral canal

Lacunar ligament

Pectineal fascia

External spermatic fascia

Femoral vein

Great saphenous vein

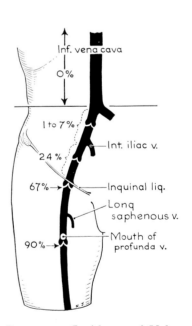

Inf. vena cava

0%

1 to 7%

Int. iliac v.

24%

67% → Inguinal lig.

Long saphenous v.

90% → Mouth of profunda v.

Percentage Incidence of Valves

255 Valves of the Proximal Ends of the Femoral and Great Saphenous Veins—IV

Between the mouth of the great saphenous vein and the heart there were no valves in 21% of 506 limbs, 1 valve in 71%, 2 in 7%, and 3 in 1%.

Valves in the common iliac vein are rarely competent, but $\frac{2}{3}$ of those in the external iliac vein are competent.

(Data collected and summarized by Dr. J. V. Basmajian.)

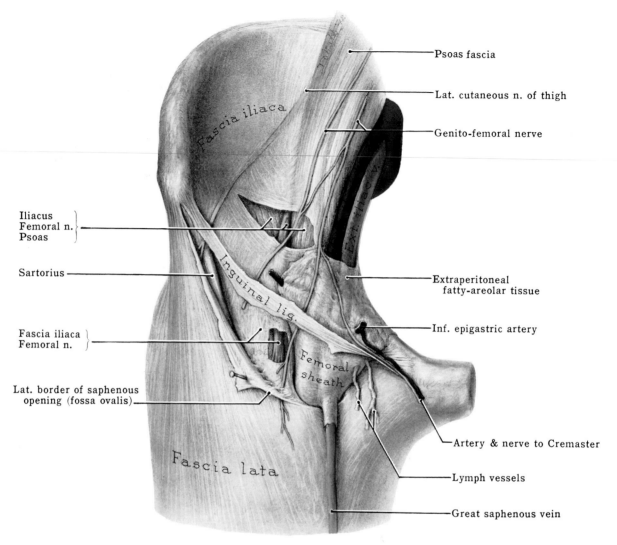

Psoas fascia

Lat. cutaneous n. of thigh

Genito-femoral nerve

Iliacus
Femoral n.
Psoas

Sartorius

Fascia iliaca
Femoral n.

Lat. border of saphenous
opening (fossa ovalis)

Fascia iliaca

Inguinal lig.

Ext. iliaca

Femoral sheath

Fascia lata

Extraperitoneal
fatty-areolar tissue

Inf. epigastric artery

Artery & nerve to Cremaster

Lymph vessels

Great saphenous vein

256 Femoral Sheath

The aponeurosis of Obliquus Externus is cut away
from the upper border of the inguinal ligament, and
the fascia lata from the lower border. The falciform
margin of the saphenous opening or hiatus in the fascia
lata is cut and reflected.

Observe:

1. The fascia iliaca, continuous medially with the Psoas fascia
   and carried downwards in front of Iliacus into the thigh. As
   it passes behind the inguinal ligament it adheres to it.

2. The extraperitoneal fatty-areolar tissue that lines the abdominal cavity and in which the external iliac vessels run,
   carried downwards around these vessels into the thigh as a
   delicate funnel-shaped sac called the femoral sheath. This is
   loosely adherent to the inguinal ligament in front and to the

pecten pubis behind.

3. The femoral sheath containing the femoral artery, vein, and
   lymph vessels; the femoral nerve, being behind the fascia
   iliaca, is *outside* the sheath.

4. The falciform margin of the saphenous opening (part of the
   fascia lata) lying in front of the femoral sheath. Medially the
   fascia passes behind the sheath as the pectineal fascia.

5. The genito-femoral nerve pierces the Psoas fascia high up in
   one or two branches; the lateral cutaneous nerve of the thigh
   pierces the fascia iliaca at a variable point, commonly, as
   here, low down near the anterior superior iliac spine.

Note: The inferior epigastric artery is pulled medially; the
deep circumflex iliac artery is not labelled.

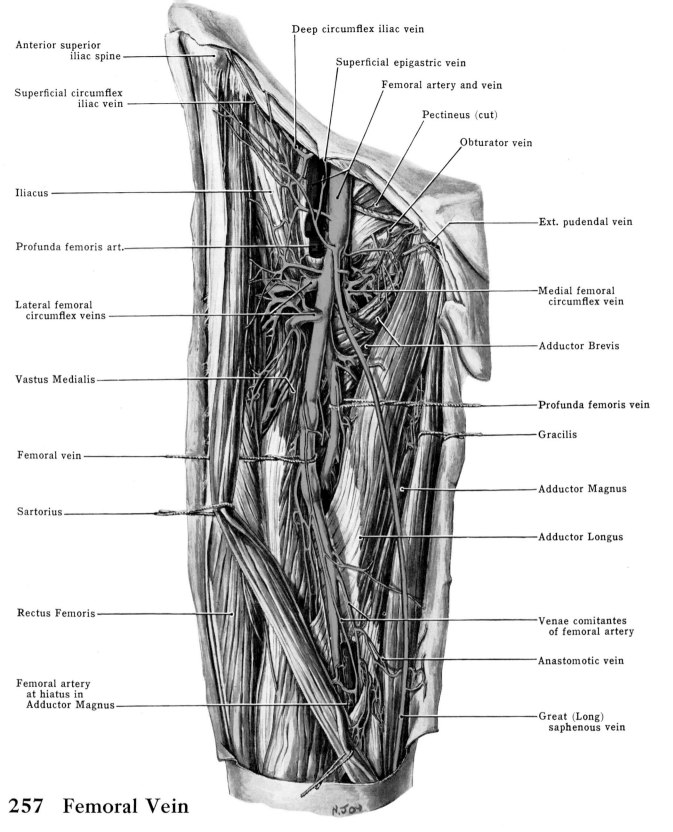

Anterior superior iliac spine

Superficial circumflex iliac vein

Iliacus

Profunda femoris art.

Lateral femoral circumflex veins

Vastus Medialis

Femoral vein

Sartorius

Rectus Femoris

Femoral artery at hiatus in Adductor Magnus

Deep circumflex iliac vein

Superficial epigastric vein

Femoral artery and vein

Pectineus (cut)

Obturator vein

Ext. pudendal vein

Medial femoral circumflex vein

Adductor Brevis

Profunda femoris vein

Gracilis

Adductor Magnus

Adductor Longus

Venae comitantes of femoral artery

Anastomotic vein

Great (Long) saphenous vein

N. Joy

257 Femoral Vein

The veins are injected with latex. Only the stumps of the arteries remain. (The limb is rotated laterally at the hip joint through the force of gravity.)

Observe:

1. The profunda femoris artery arising from the femoral artery about 1½″ below the inguinal ligament. The profunda femoris vein joining the femoral vein twice that distance below the ligament; indeed, in 90 limbs the average distance below the inguinal ligament (actually, below a straight line joining the anterior superior spine to the pubic tubercle) at which the profunda artery sprang from the femoral artery was 5.2 cm. (ranging from 1.0 cm. to 8.5 cm.); whereas the average distance below this line at which the profunda vein

joined the femoral vein was 8.4 cm. (ranging from 4.6 cm. to 12.2 cm.). (J. F. R. Fleming and L. F. Levy.)

2. The large size of the lateral femoral circumflex vein, here double and, like the medial femoral circumflex, ending in the femoral vein.

3. The many long, slender, paired venae comitantes that accompany the various arteries.

4. The superficial circumflex iliac vein, in this specimen receiving the superficial epigastric vein, communicating with the veins proximal and distal to it, and ending both in the great saphenous and in the femoral vein.

5. The great saphenous vein communicating with a vena comitans of the femoral artery. The medial femoral circumflex vein communicating with the obturator vein.

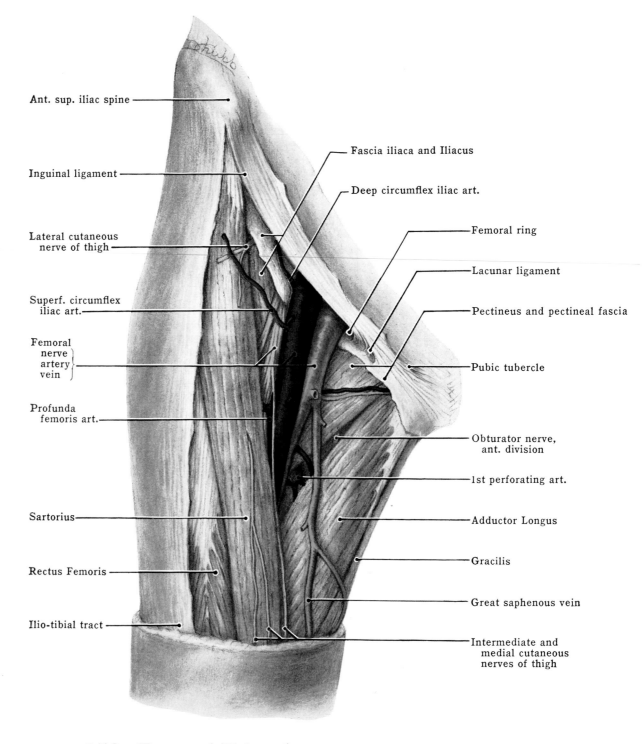

Ant. sup. iliac spine

Inguinal ligament

Lateral cutaneous
nerve of thigh

Superf. circumflex
iliac art.

Femoral
nerve
artery
vein

Profunda
femoris art.

Sartorius

Rectus Femoris

Ilio-tibial tract

Fascia iliaca and Iliacus

Deep circumflex iliac art.

Femoral ring

Lacunar ligament

Pectineus and pectineal fascia

Pubic tubercle

Obturator nerve,
ant. division

1st perforating art.

Adductor Longus

Gracilis

Great saphenous vein

Intermediate and
medial cutaneous
nerves of thigh

258　Femoral Triangle

Observe:

1. The boundaries of the triangle: The inguinal ligament, which curves gently from ant. sup. spine to pubic tubercle, being the base; the medial border of Sartorius being the lateral side; the lateral border of Adductor Longus being the medial side; and the point where the two converging sides meet below being the apex. (Some authors regard the medial border of Add. Longus as the medial side of the triangle.)

2. The femoral artery and vein lying in front of the fascia covering Ilio-psoas and Pectineus, and the femoral nerve lying behind.

3. The artery appearing midway between the anterior superior spine and the pubic tubercle, and disappearing where the medial border of Sartorius crosses the lateral border of Adductor Longus—in short, from the mid point of the base of the triangle to the apex.

4. That when the adjacent borders of Pectineus and Adductor Longus are not contiguous, as here a glimpse is had of the anterior branch of the obturator nerve lying in front of Adductor Brevis.

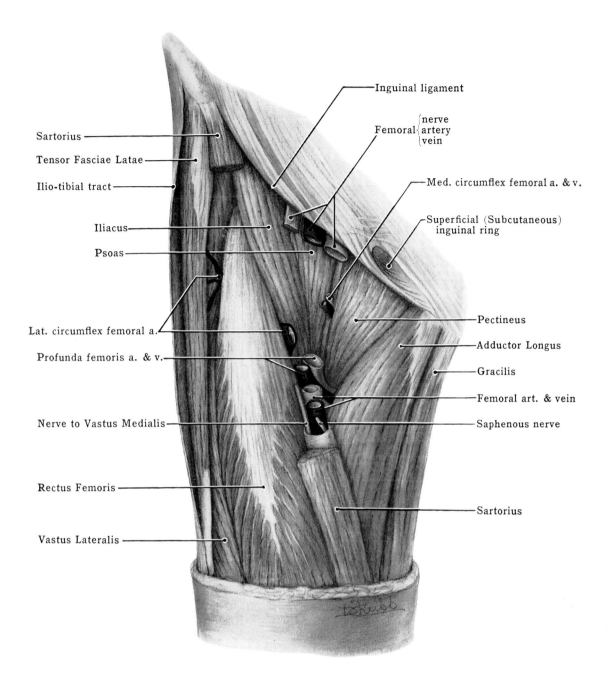

Sartorius

Tensor Fasciae Latae

Ilio-tibial tract

Iliacus

Psoas

Lat. circumflex femoral a.

Profunda femoris a. & v.

Nerve to Vastus Medialis

Rectus Femoris

Vastus Lateralis

Inguinal ligament

Femoral {nerve / artery / vein}

Med. circumflex femoral a. & v.

Superficial (Subcutaneous) inguinal ring

Pectineus

Adductor Longus

Gracilis

Femoral art. & vein

Saphenous nerve

Sartorius

259 Floor of the Femoral Triangle

Sections are removed from Sartorius and from the femoral vessels and nerve.

Observe:

1. The floor of the triangle to be a trough with sloping lateral and medial walls. This is notably so, if Adductor Longus is included with Pectineus in the medial wall; Ilio-psoas and the border of Rectus Femoris form the lateral wall.

2. The trough to be shallow at the base and deep at the apex.

3. At the apex four vessels, one in front of the other, and two nerves pass into the adductor canal of Hunter (subsartorial canal).

Iliacus
Ant. sup. spine
Psoas Minor
Psoas Major
Iliacus
Psoas (Major)
Fascia lata
Tensor Fasciae Latae
Tensor Fasciae Latae
Rectus Femoris (cut)
Pubic tubercle
Pectineus
Gluteus Minimus
Adductor Longus (c
Adductor Brevis
Sartorius
Pectineus (cu
Adductor Longus
Ilio-tibial tract
Adductor Longus (cu
Rectus Femoris
Gracilis
Gracilis
Ilio-tibial tract
Vastus Intermedius
Vastus Lateralis
Adductor Magnus
Patella
Vastus Lateralis
Vastus Medialis
Vastus Medialis
Sartorius
Rectus Femoris (cut)
Sartorius
Medial meniscus
Ligamentum patellae
Sartorius

260 Muscles of the Front of the Thigh—I

261 Muscles of the Front of the Thigh—II

Sections of Sartorius, Rectus Femoris, Pectineus and Adductor Longus are excised.

Ext. iliac art. & vein

Psoas

Obturator Internus

Adductor Longus

Adductor Magnus

Rectus Femoris

Sartorius

Vastus Medialis

GRACILIS

5

1

Piriformis

Sacrospinous lig.

Coccygeus

Int. pudendal art.

Gluteus Maximus

Semitendinosus

Semimembranosus

Biceps Femoris

Semitendinosus

Gastrocnemius, med. head

Soleus

**262 Muscles of the Medial Side
of the Thigh—III**

Ant. sup. iliac spine

Iliacus

Femoral nerve artery vein

Sartorius

Rectus Femoris

Descending br. of lat. circumflex a.

Vastus Lateralis

Vastus Intermedius

Rectus Femoris

Vastus Medialis

Obliquus Abdominis Internus

Ilio-hypogastric nerve

Ilio-inguinal nerve

Med. circumflex art. Pectineus

Adductor Longus

Gracilis

Profunda femoris art. Adductor Brevis

Cutaneous br. of obturator nerve

N. to Vastus Medialis Saphenous nerve Femoral artery

Adductor Magnus

Sartorius

Saphenous { nerve vein artery

Great saphenous vein

Add. Long.

263 Dissection of Front of Thigh and Adductor Region

(The limb is rotated laterally)

Observe:

1. The femoral nerve breaking up into a leash of nerves on entering the thigh.

2. The femoral artery lying between two motor territories, namely that of the obturator nerve which is medial, and that of the femoral nerve which is lateral. No motor nerve crosses in front of the femoral artery, but the twig to Pectineus is seen crossing behind it.

3. The nerve to Vastus Medialis and the saphenous nerve accompanying the femoral artery into the adductor canal. The saphenous nerve and artery and their companion anastomotic vein emerging from the lower end of the canal. They become superficial between Sartorius and Gracilis.

4. The profunda femoris artery arising $1\frac{1}{2}''$ below the inguinal ligament, lying behind the femoral artery, and disappearing behind Adductor Longus.

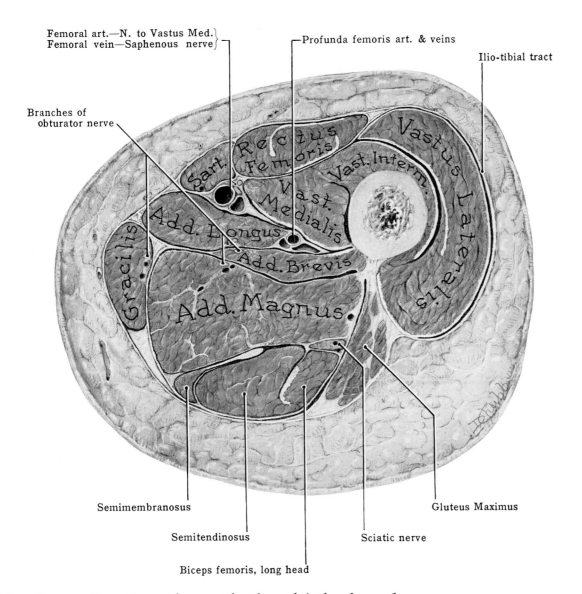

Femoral art.—N. to Vastus Med.\
Femoral vein—Saphenous nerve⟩

Profunda femoris art. & veins

Ilio-tibial tract

Branches of
obturator nerve

Sart. *Rectus Femoris*

Vast. Interm.

Vastus Lateralis

Vast. Medialis

Gracilis

Add. Longus

Add. Brevis

Vastus Lateralis

Add. Magnus

Semimembranosus

Semitendinosus

Biceps femoris, long head

Sciatic nerve

Gluteus Maximus

264 Cross Section through the thigh, female

Observe:

1. The level of the section—(a) through the insertion of Gluteus Maximus and therefore above that of short head of Biceps; (b) below insertion of Pectineus, above that of Adductor Longus and therefore, through that of Adductor Brevis; (c) through the adductor canal and therefore below the apex of the femoral triangle—say 4″–6″ down the femur.

2. Gracilis abutting against the free, medial borders of the Adductor muscles.

3. Adductor Longus intervening between the femoral and the profunda femoris vessels.

4. Adductor Brevis intervening between the anterior and the posterior division of the obturator nerve.

5. Aponeurosis of semimembranosus not dissimilar from the sciatic nerve and mistakable for it.

6. Vastus Intermedius arising from the anterior and lateral surfaces of the shaft of the femur; Vastus Medialis covering the medial surface but not arising from it. That is to say, Vastus Intermedius alone arises from the surfaces, the other muscles are relegated to the linea aspera or to its upward and downward extensions.

7. The considerable amount of subcutaneous fat present in the female.

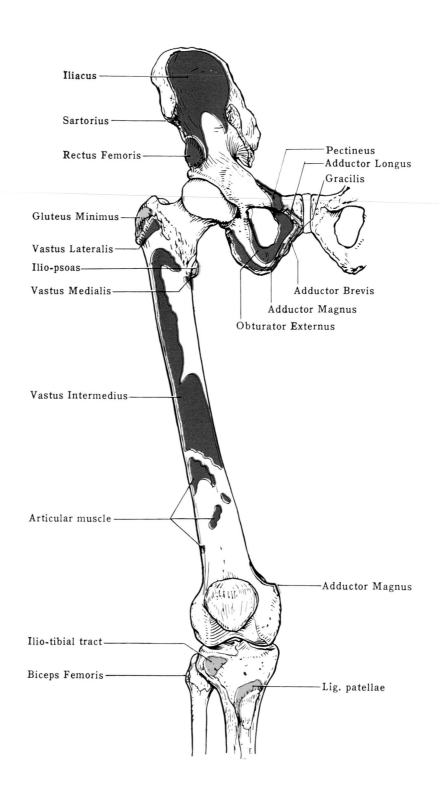

Iliacus

Sartorius

Rectus Femoris

Pectineus

Adductor Longus

Gracilis

Gluteus Minimus

Vastus Lateralis

Ilio-psoas

Vastus Medialis

Adductor Brevis

Adductor Magnus

Obturator Externus

Vastus Intermedius

Articular muscle

Adductor Magnus

Ilio-tibial tract

Biceps Femoris

Lig. patellae

**265   Bones of the Lower Limb showing
Attachments of Muscles, anterior view**

(For Tibia and Fibula, see fig. 303; Bones of Foot, dorsal aspect, see figs. 311, 312 & 313.)

Gluteus Maximus

Gluteus Medius

Gluteus Minimus

Tensor Fasciae Latae

Sartorius

Rectus Femoris

Gluteus Medius

Gemelli

Quadratus Femoris

Biceps, long head

Vastus Lateralis

Semitendinosus

Adductor Magnus

Gluteus Maximus

Semimembranosus

Adductor Magnus

Ilio-psoas

Pectineus

Adductor Brevis

Adductor Longus

Vastus Intermedius

Vastus Lateralis

Vastus Medialis

Biceps, short head

Adductor Magnus

Plantaris

Gastrocnemius, med. head

Gastrocnemius, lat. head

Semimembranosus

Popliteus

Soleus

266   Bones of the Lower Limb showing Attachments of Muscles, posterior view

(For Tibia and Fibula, posterior aspect, see fig. 316; Bones of Foot, plantar aspect, see fig. 314.)

Gluteus Medius

Gluteus Maximus

Adductor Magnus

Semitendinosus

Semimembranosus

Gracilis

Gastrocnemius,
med. head

Ilio-tibial tract

long head

short head

Biceps
Femoris

Plantaris

Gastrocnemius,
lat. head

Gluteus Mediu

Piriformis

Obturator Inte.
& Gemelli

Quadratus Femoris

Adductor Magnus

Gluteus Maxim

Ilio-tibial tract

3 Ham Muscles:
Biceps Femoris

Semitendinosus

Semimembranosus

Plantaris

Popliteus

Soleus

Gastrocnemius,
medial head

Gastrocnemius,
lateral head

**267 Muscles of the Gluteal
Region and Back of the Thigh**

268 Ham Muscles

Gluteus Minimus

Tensor Fasciae Latae

Gluteus Medius (cut)

Piriformis

Obturator Internus
and Gemelli

Quadratus
Femoris

Hams (cut)

Gluteus Maximus

Adductor Magnus

Ilio-tibial tract

Biceps Femoris,
short head

Vastus Medialis

Biceps Femoris,
long head (cut)

Semimembranosus

Plantaris

Oblique
popliteal lig.

Popliteus

Soleus

269 Adductor Magnus, from behind

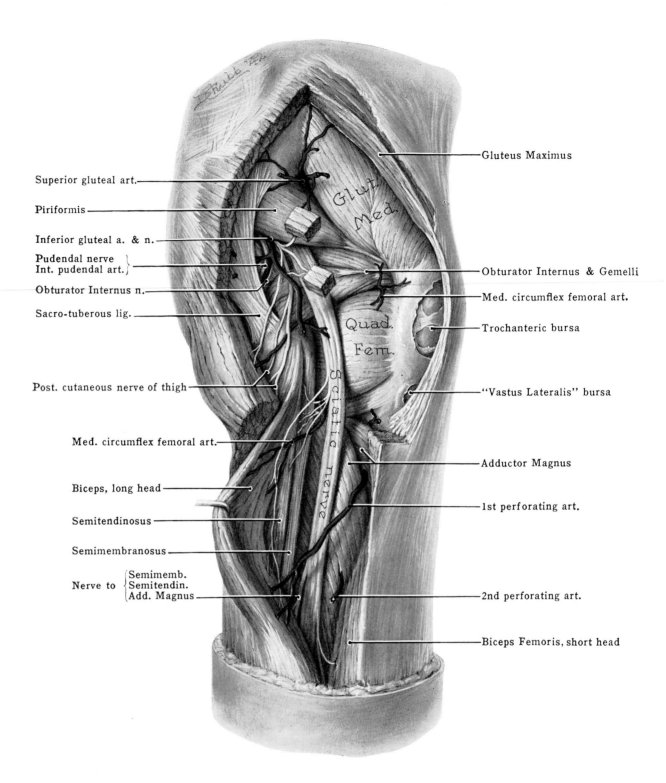

Superior gluteal art.—

Piriformis—

Inferior gluteal a. & n.—

Pudendal nerve
Int. pudendal art.

Obturator Internus n.—

Sacro-tuberous lig.—

Post. cutaneous nerve of thigh—

Med. circumflex femoral art.—

Biceps, long head—

Semitendinosus—

Semimembranosus—

Nerve to {Semimemb.
Semitendin.
Add. Magnus—

Gluteus Maximus

Glut.
Med.

Quad.
Fem.

Sciatic nerve

Obturator Internus & Gemelli

Med. circumflex femoral art.

Trochanteric bursa

"Vastus Lateralis" bursa

Adductor Magnus

1st perforating art.

2nd perforating art.

Biceps Femoris, short head

270 Gluteal Region and the Back of the Thigh—I

Gluteus Maximus is split, both above and below, in the direction of its fibres, and the middle part is then excised, but two cubes remain to identify its nerve. The long head of Biceps is pulled medially.

Observe:

1. Gluteus Maximus is the only muscle to cover the greater trochanter. It is aponeurotic where it plays on the trochanter and the aponeurosis of Vastus Lateralis, and has underlying bursae.

2. The nerve (inf. gluteal n.) enters Gluteus Maximus in two chief branches near its centre.

3. Above Piriformis are Gluteus Medius and Gluteus Minimus. Between Piriformis and Quadratus Femoris are Obturator Internus and Gemelli. Below Quadratus Femoris is Adductor Magnus.

4. The sciatic nerve appears below Piriformis and crosses in turn: dorsum ischii, Obturator Internus and Gemelli, Quadratus Femoris, and Adductor Magnus. Its branches spring from its medial side at variable levels to supply the hams and part of Adductor Magnus. Only the branch to Biceps (short head) springs from its lateral side, which, therefore, is the safer side to dissect on.

5. Semimembranosus, in the upper part of the thigh, is readily mistaken for the sciatic nerve.

Posterior superior iliac spine

Superior gluteal a. & n.

Sacro-tuberous lig.

Pudendal nerve
Int. pudendal art.

Obturator Internus n.

Tip of coccyx

Inferior gluteal n. & a.
Post. cutaneous
n. of thigh

Perineal branch

Biceps, long head

Semitendinosus

Semimembranosus

Adductor Magnus

Gracilis

Semimembranosus

Semitendinosus

Biceps, long head

Gluteus Minimus

Gluteus Medius

Obturator Internus & Gemelli

Greater trochanter
Obturator Externus

Med. circumflex femoral art.

Gluteus Maximus

Post. cutaneous n. of thigh

1st perforating art.

Intermuscular septum

2nd perforating art.

Biceps, short head

Piriformis

Sciatic

Quad. Fem.

Nerve

271   Gluteal Region and the Back of the Thigh—II

The upper three quarters of Gluteus Maximus is re-flected, and parts of Gluteus Medius and the three ham muscles are excised.

Observe:

1. The superior gluteal vessels and nerve appearing above Piri-formis; all other vessels and nerves appearing below it.

2. There are no nerves and no vessels of importance lateral to the sciatic nerve.

3. The horizontal groove (the natal fold) crossing the lower border of Gluteus Maximus indicates the upper limit of the sleeve-like deep fascia of the thigh.

4. Gluteus Maximus consisting of bundles of parallel fibres. It is rhomboidal and the deep fascia covering it is thin. Gluteus Medius arising in part from the covering deep fascia which, therefore, is strong and thick. It is fan-shaped.

5. The sciatic nerve is accessible deep in the angle between the lower border of Gluteus Maximus and the lateral border of the long head of Biceps.

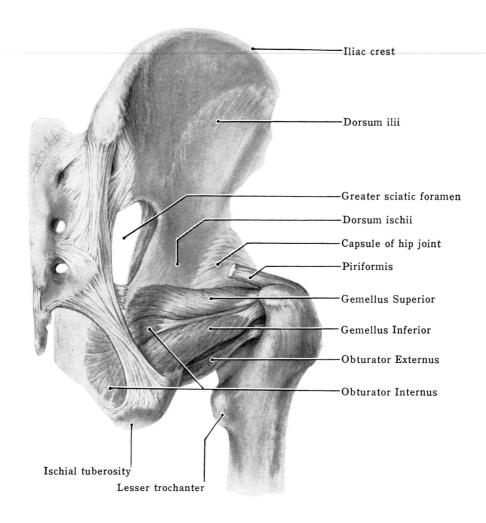

Iliac crest

Dorsum ilii

Greater sciatic foramen

Dorsum ischii

Capsule of hip joint

Piriformis

Gemellus Superior

Gemellus Inferior

Obturator Externus

Obturator Internus

Ischial tuberosity

Lesser trochanter

272   Obturator Muscles, from behind

Obturator Internus and Gemelli fill the gap between Piriformis above and Quadratus Femoris below.

Note that the lower end of the ischial tuberosity is on the level of the lesser trochanter.

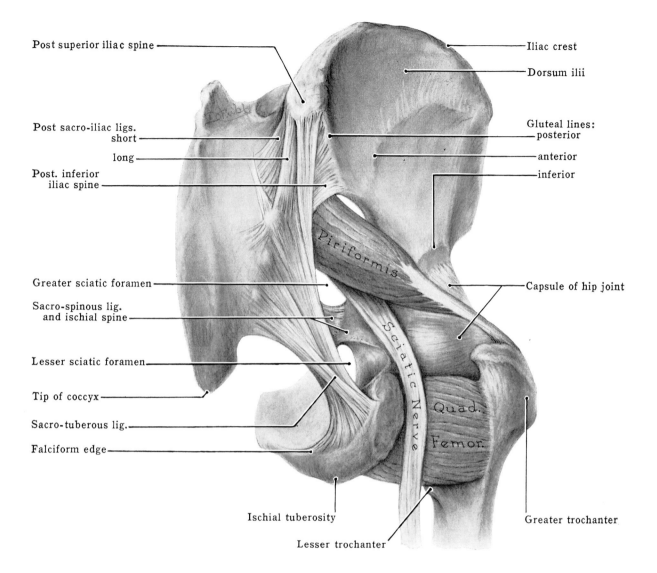

Post superior iliac spine

Post sacro-iliac ligs.
short

long

Post. inferior
iliac spine

Greater sciatic foramen

Sacro-spinous lig.
and ischial spine

Lesser sciatic foramen

Tip of coccyx

Sacro-tuberous lig.

Falciform edge

Iliac crest

Dorsum ilii

Gluteal lines:
posterior

anterior

inferior

Capsule of hip joint

Piriformis

Sciatic Nerve

Quad.

Femor.

Ischial tuberosity

Lesser trochanter

Greater trochanter

273   Bony and Ligamentous Parts of Gluteal Region: Certain Landmarks

Observe:

1. The tip of the coccyx lies above the level of the ischial tuberosity and below that of the ischial spine.

2. The lower border of Piriformis is defined by joining the midpoint between the tip of the coccyx and the posterior superior iliac spine to the top of the greater trochanter.

3. The lower border of Quadratus Femoris is level with the lower end of the ischial tuberosity and it crosses the lesser trochanter.

4. The lateral border of the sciatic nerve lies midway between the lateral surface of the greater trochanter and the medial surface of the ischial tuberosity, provided the body is in the anatomical posture—toes pointing forward.

Ant. sup. iliac spine

Ant. inf. iliac spine

Rectus Femoris

Ilio-femoral lig.

Greater trochanter

Intertrochanteric line

Lesser trochanter

Acetabular labrum
(Glenoid labrum)

Head of femur

Pectineus
Pectineal fascia

Pectineal lig.

Pubic tubercle

Obturator Externus

Obturator nerve,
ant. & post. divisions

274 Hip Joint, from the front

Observe:

1. The head of the femur exposed just medial to the ilio-femoral lig. and facing not only upwards and medially, but also forwards. Here, at the site of the Psoas bursa, the capsule is weak or, as in this specimen, partially deficient, but it is guarded by the Psoas tendon.

2. The ilio-femoral lig., shaped like an inverted Y, attached above deep to Rectus Femoris, and so directed as to become taut on medial rotation of the femur.

3. Obturator Externus crossing obliquely below the neck of the femur (see fig. 272).

4. The thinness of Pectineus; and its fascia blending with the pectineal ligament (Cooper's lig.) along the pecten pubis (pectineal line).

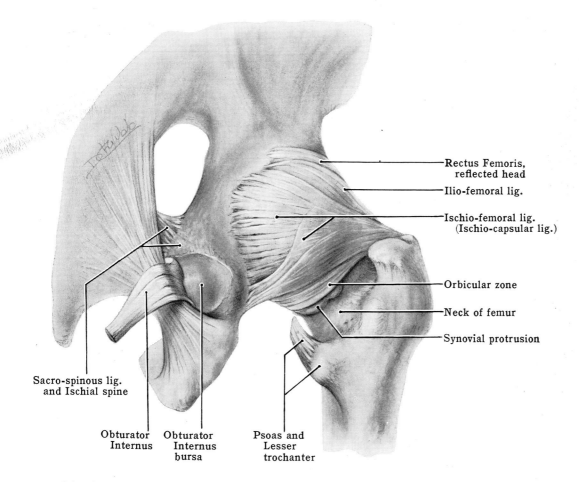

Rectus Femoris,
reflected head

Ilio-femoral lig.

Ischio-femoral lig.
(Ischio-capsular lig.)

Orbicular zone

Neck of femur

Synovial protrusion

Sacro-spinous lig.
and Ischial spine

Obturator
Internus

Obturator
Internus
bursa

Psoas and
Lesser
trochanter

275 Hip Joint, from behind

Observe:

1. The fibres of the capsule so directed spirally as to become taut during extension and medial rotation of the femur.

2. The fibres crossing the neck posteriorly, but not attached to it; indeed, the synovial membrane protrudes below the fibrous capsule and there forms a bursa for the tendon of Obturator Externus.

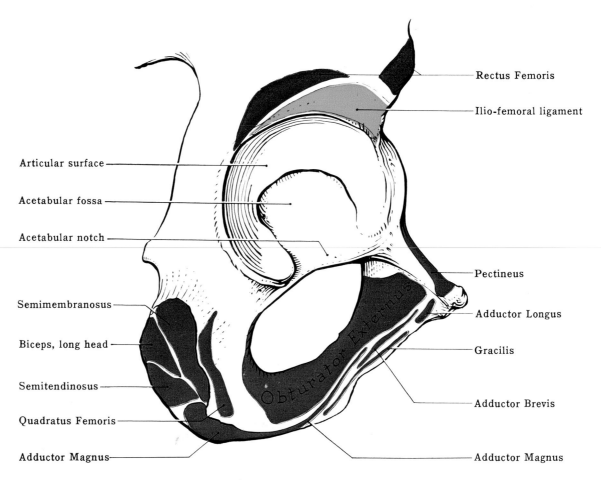

Rectus Femoris

Ilio-femoral ligament

Articular surface

Acetabular fossa

Acetabular notch

Pectineus

Adductor Longus

Semimembranosus

Gracilis

Biceps, long head

Semitendinosus

Adductor Brevis

Quadratus Femoris

Obturator Externus

Adductor Magnus

Adductor Magnus

276   Acetabulum and the Surrounding Parts, showing Attachment of Muscles

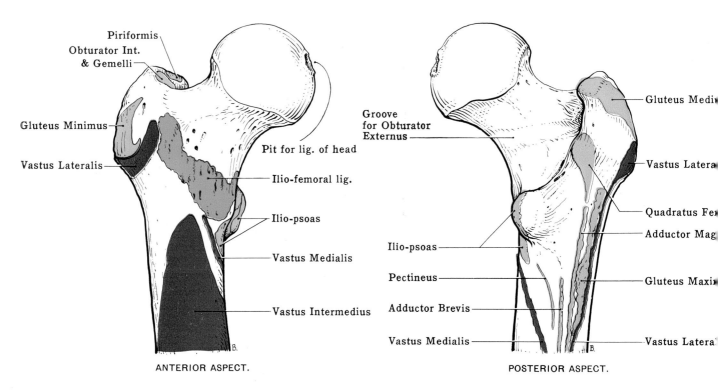

Piriformis

Obturator Int. & Gemelli

Gluteus Minimus

Gluteus Medi▸

Vastus Lateralis

Pit for lig. of head

Groove for Obturator Externus

Vastus Latera▸

Ilio-femoral lig.

Ilio-psoas

Quadratus Fe▸

Adductor Mag▸

Vastus Medialis

Ilio-psoas

Vastus Intermedius

Pectineus

Gluteus Maxi▸

Adductor Brevis

Vastus Medialis

Vastus Latera▸

ANTERIOR ASPECT.

POSTERIOR ASPECT.

276.1   Upper End of Femur showing Attachments of Muscles

77 Hip Bone in Youth, external aspect

The three elements of the hip bone meet in the acetabulum at a tri-radiate synchondrosis. Of these, the pubis contributes least to the acetabulum, the ilium next least, and the ischium most, including the non-articular part.

Secondary centres of ossification appear along the whole length of the iliac crest (attachment of the 3 flat abdominal muscles), at the anterior inferior spine (origin of Rectus Femoris), at the ischial tuberosity (origin of the ham muscles), and also at the symphysis pubis, hence the wavy surfaces. These appear about puberty. Fusion may start as early as the 17th or 18th year; complete fusion is never delayed beyond the 23rd year (McK. & S.).

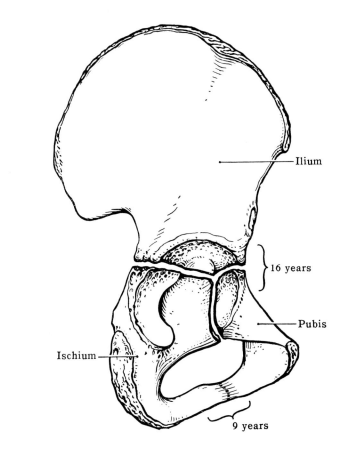

78 Consolidation of the Acetabulum: The Os Acetabuli

One or more centres of ossification appear in the triradiate cartilage of the acetabulum about the 12th year. One of these, the os acetabuli, extends widely over the acetabular surface of the pubic bone.

From lat. femoral circumflex art.

Lig. of head

ANTERIOR VIEW

From med. femoral circumflex art.

POSTERO-SUPERIOR VIEW

From med. femoral circumflex art.

POSTERO-INFERIOR VIEW

Inferior gluteal art.

Internal pudendal art.

To Piriformis

To Gluteus Maximus

Perforating arteries

1st

2nd

3rd

4th

POPLITEAL

Tibial division (Med. popliteal n.)

Peroneal division (Lat. popliteal n.)

280 Blood Supply to the Sciatic Nerve

(Dissected, traced from an enlarged photograph, and drawn by W. R. Mitchell.)

Note the continuous anastomotic chain of arteries. Compare this with the blood supply to the ureter (fig. 184) and to the oesophagus (fig. 454).

279 Blood Supply to the Head of the Femur

Note:—

The head receives 3 sets of arteries: (a) the never-failing and main set of 3 or 4 ascends in the synovial retinacula on the postero-superior and postero-inferior parts of the neck, to perforate just distal to the head, bend at 45° towards its centre, and anastomose freely with (b) terminal branches of the medullary artery of the shaft, and in 80% of cases with (c) the artery of the lig. of the head. This last artery enters the head only when the centre of ossification has extended to the pit for the lig. of the head (12th to 14th year). This anastomosis persists even in advanced age; but in 20% it is never established. (Wolcott.)

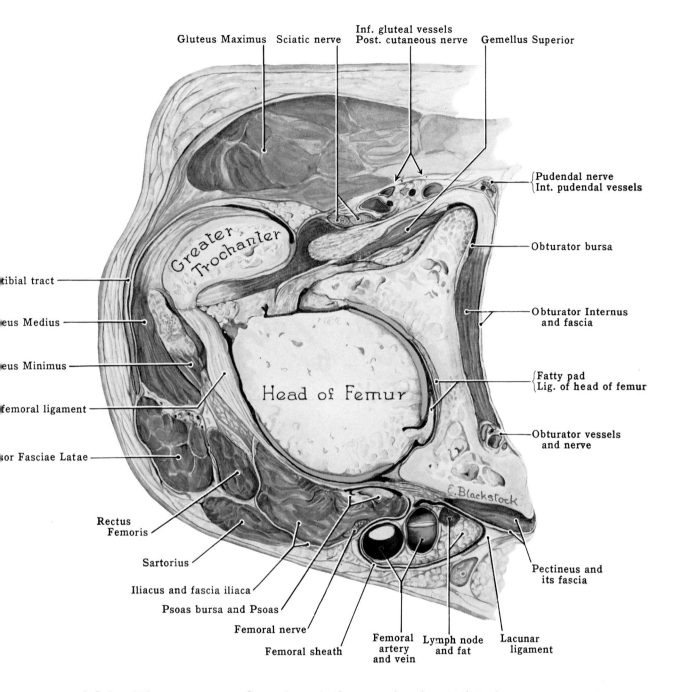

Gluteus Maximus Sciatic nerve Inf. gluteal vessels Post. cutaneous nerve Gemellus Superior

Pudendal nerve
Int. pudendal vessels

Obturator bursa

Obturator Internus
and fascia

Fatty pad
Lig. of head of femur

Obturator vessels
and nerve

Pectineus and
its fascia

Greater Trochanter

Head of Femur

E. Blackstock

tibial tract

eus Medius

eus Minimus

femoral ligament

or Fasciae Latae

Rectus
Femoris

Sartorius

Iliacus and fascia iliaca

Psoas bursa and Psoas

Femoral nerve

Femoral sheath

Femoral
artery
and vein

Lymph node
and fat

Lacunar
ligament

281 Transverse Section Through the Thigh at the Level of the Hip Joint

Observe:

1. The articular cartilage spread unevenly over the head of the femur.

2. The fibrous capsule of the joint to be very thick where forming the ilio-femoral ligament, and thin dorsal to the Psoas tendon, the Psoas bursa here intervening.

3. The femoral sheath, which encloses the femoral artery, vein, lymph node, lymph vessels and fat, to be free except posteriorly where, between Psoas and Pectineus, it is attached to the capsule of the hip joint.

4. The femoral artery separated from the joint by the tough Psoas tendon; the vein at the interval between Psoas and Pectineus; the lymph node anterior to Pectineus. The femoral nerve lying between Iliacus and fascia Iliaca.

5. The two cusps of the valve in the femoral vein so placed that pressure on the skin surface tends to close the valve.

6. The sciatic nerve descending between Gluteus Maximus and the short lateral rotators of the femur.

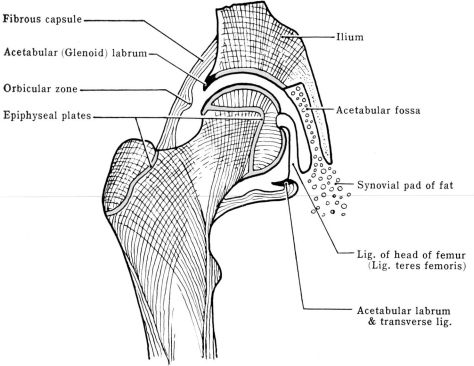

Fibrous capsule

Acetabular (Glenoid) labrum

Orbicular zone

Epiphyseal plates

Ilium

Acetabular fossa

Synovial pad of fat

Lig. of head of femur
(Lig. teres femoris)

Acetabular labrum
& transverse lig.

282 Hip Joint on Coronal Section, partly schematic

Observe:

1. The bony trabeculae of the ilium proj
   into the head of the femur as lines of
   sure and the trabeculae that cross the
   lines of tension.

2. The epiphysis of the head of the femur
   tirely within the capsule of the joint.

3. The lig. of the head of the femur,
   synovial tube that is fixed above at th
   (fovea) on the head of the femur and
   below at the acetabular foramen where
   continuous with the synovial memb
   covering the fat in the acetabular fossa
   also with the synovial membrane cove
   the transverse ligament (fig. 284).

4. The ligament of the head, obviously
   comes taut during adduction of the
   joint, as when crossing the legs.

5. The fluid fat below the joint can be su
   into the acetabular fossa during flex

Lig. of head
of femur

283 Blood Vessels of the Acetabular Fossa

Prepared by Dr. K. O. McCuaig.

The acetabular branches (an artery
a vein) of the posterior division of
obturator vessels pass through the
tabular foramen and enter the acetab
fossa where they ramify in the fatty-are
tissue. The branches, mostly in pairs
artery and a vein) radiate to the ma
of the fossa where they enter nutr
foramina. One pair runs through
ligament of the head of the femur to
head. Twigs supply the fat.

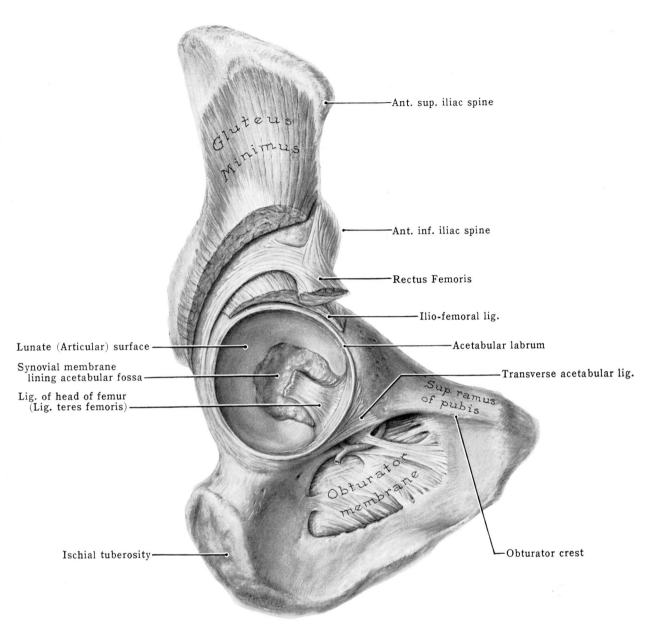

Ant. sup. iliac spine

Gluteus Minimus

Ant. inf. iliac spine

Rectus Femoris

Ilio-femoral lig.

Lunate (Articular) surface

Acetabular labrum

Synovial membrane
lining acetabular fossa

Transverse acetabular lig.

Lig. of head of femur
(Lig. teres femoris)

Sup. ramus of pubis

Obturator membrane

Ischial tuberosity

Obturator crest

284   Socket for the Head of the Femur

Observe:

1. The transverse acetabular ligament (whose fibres decussate like the limbs of a St. Andrew's cross) converting the acetabular notch into the acetabular foramen.

2. The acetabular labrum, attached to the acetabular rim and to the transverse ligament. It forms a complete ring around the head of the femur beyond its equator.

3. The articular or lunate surface.

4. The synovial membrane attached to the margin of the articular cartilage and covering the pad of fat and the vessels in the acetabular fossa.

5. The ligament of the head of the femur, which is a hollow cone of synovial membrane compressed between the head of

the femur and its socket. It resembles a collapsed bell tent. It envelopes ligamentous fibres; these are attached above to the pit on the head of the femur, and below to the transverse ligament and the margins of the acetabular notch. Through it passes the artery to the head of the femur; this is a branch of the posterior division of the obturator artery, not labelled but seen passing through the acetabular foramen.

6. Gluteus Minimus which, being a medial rotator as well as an abductor of the hip joint, is thickest in front. It covers the two heads of Rectus femoris which in turn cover, and are nearly co-extensive with, the attachment of the iliofemoral ligament.

Semimembranosus

Branch communicating
with inf. gluteal vein

Sartorius

Gracilis

Semitendinosus

Small saphenous vein

Medial sural
cutaneous nerve

Gastrocnemius, med. head

Biceps Femoris

Tibial nerve
(Med. popliteal n.)

Popliteal vein

Popliteal artery

Common peroneal nerve
(Lat. popliteal n.)

Lateral sural
cutaneous nerve

Communicating peroneal nerve

Gastrocnemius, lat. head

Soleus

285 Superficial Dissection of the Popliteal Fossa

Observe:

1. The two heads of Gastrocnemius, embraced on the medial side by Semimembranosus, which is overlaid by Semitendinosus, and on the lateral side by Biceps. The result is the lozenge-shaped popliteal fossa.

2. The small saphenous vein running between the two heads of Gastrocnemius. Deep to this vein is the medial sural cutaneous nerve which, followed proximally, leads to the tibial nerve. This latter nerve is superficial to the popliteal vein, which in turn is superficial to the popliteal artery.

3. The common peroneal nerve following the posterior border of Biceps, and here giving off two cutaneous branches. (See cutaneous nerves, fig. 249).

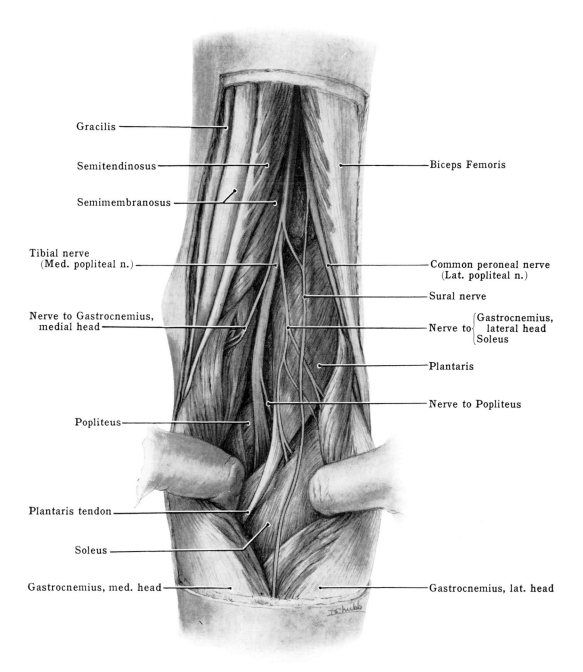

Gracilis

Semitendinosus

Semimembranosus

Tibial nerve
(Med. popliteal n.)

Nerve to Gastrocnemius,
medial head

Popliteus

Plantaris tendon

Soleus

Gastrocnemius, med. head

Biceps Femoris

Common peroneal nerve
(Lat. popliteal n.)

Sural nerve

Nerve to { Gastrocnemius,
lateral head
Soleus

Plantaris

Nerve to Popliteus

Gastrocnemius, lat. head

286 Nerves of the Popliteal Fossa

The two heads of Gastrocnemius are pulled forcibly apart.

Observe:

1. A cutaneous branch of the tibial nerve joining a cutaneous branch of the common peroneal nerve to form the sural nerve. Here the junction is very high—usually it is two or three inches above the ankle.

2. All motor branches in this region springing from the tibial nerve, one branch coming from its medial side, the others from its lateral side. Hence, it is safer to dissect on the medial side.

Gracilis

Semitendinosus

Semimembranosus

Popliteal art.
Popliteal vein
Tibial nerve
(Med. poplit. n.)

Sup. medial genicular a.

Semitendinosus

Semimembranosus

Bursa

Gastrocnemius

Inf. medial genicular a.

Popliteus fascia

Biceps, long head

Biceps, short head

Lat. intermuscular septum

Common peroneal nerve
(Lat. popliteal n.)

Biceps Femoris

Sup. lateral genicular a.

Plantaris

Gastrocnemius

Inf. lateral genicular a.

Popliteus

Nerve to Popliteus

Soleus

Plantaris

Gastrocnemius

287 Step Dissection of the Popliteal Fossa

Observe:

1. The thickness of the various muscles.

2. The popliteal artery lying on the floor of the fossa (i.e. femur, capsule of joint, Popliteus fascia), giving off genicular branches which also lie on the floor, and ending by bifurcating into the anterior and the posterior tibial artery at the upper border of Soleus.

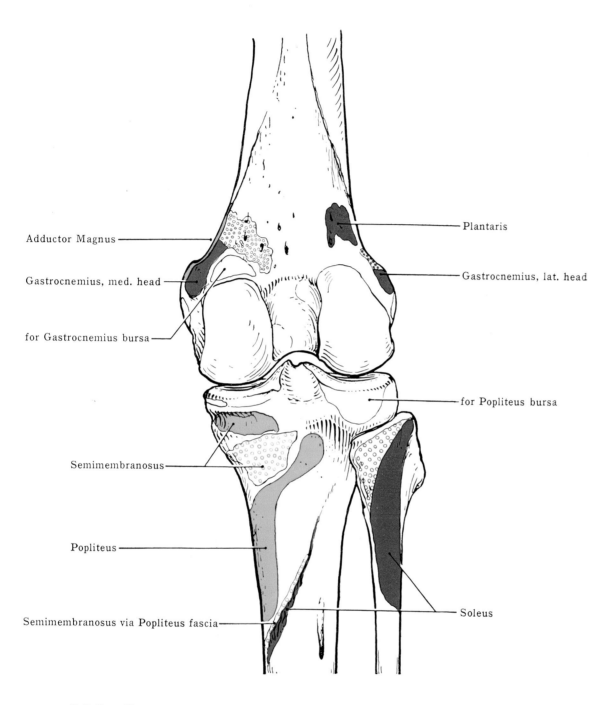

Adductor Magnus

Gastrocnemius, med. head

for Gastrocnemius bursa

Semimembranosus

Popliteus

Semimembranosus via Popliteus fascia

Plantaris

Gastrocnemius, lat. head

for Popliteus bursa

Soleus

**288 Bones of the Knee Joint showing
Attachments of Muscles, from behind—IV**

Adductor Magnus

Popliteal artery

Superior medial
genicular art.

Superior lateral
genicular art.

Semimembranosus

Inferior lateral
genicular art.

Popliteus

Inferior medial
genicular art.

Anterior tibial art.

Posterior tibial art.

Soleus

Nancy Joy

289 Anastomoses around the Knee, posterior view

Latex injection. *Dissection by Dr. J. S. Simpson.*

Observe:

1. The popliteal artery throughout its course, from the hiatus in Adductor Magnus proximally to the lower border of Popliteus distally (or, if you prefer, to the upper border of Soleus), where it bifurcates into the anterior and posterior tibial arteries.

2. The 3 ventral relations of the artery: the femur (fat intervening), the capsule of the joint, and the Popliteus (covered with popliteus fascia).

3. The 4 named genicular branches that hug the skeletal plane, nothing intervening except the popliteus tendon which the inferior lateral genicular artery must cross. (The median genicular art. is not in view.)

4. An unnamed genicular artery arising on each side.

Adductor Magnus

Vastus Medialis

Descending genicular art.
(Art. genu suprema)

Superior medial
genicular art.

Tibial
collateral lig.

Synovial
capsule

Medial
meniscus

Coronary
lig.

—Inferior
medial
genicular art.

—Tibial
collateral lig.

atellae—

Synovial
capsule

Superior lateral
genicular art.—

Biceps
Cruris—

Tibial
collateral lig.—

Inferior lateral
genicular art.—

Lat. meniscus ⎫
Coronary lig. ⎬

Anterior
recurrent
tibial art.—

—Lig.
patellae

290 Antero-medial view   291 Antero-lateral view

Anastomoses around the Knee

Observe:

1. Two named genicular branches of the popliteal artery, on each side—a superior and an inferior.

2. Two supplementary arteries, viz., the descending genicular artery, which is a branch of the femoral artery, supero-medially; the anterior recurrent branch of the anterior tibial artery, inferolaterally.

3. The inferior lateral genicular artery running along the lateral meniscus; an unnamed artery running similarly along the medial meniscus.

292 Cruciate Ligaments

In each illustration one half of the femur is removed with the proximal part of the corresponding cruciate ligament.

Observe:

1. The posterior cruciate ligament, which prevents forward sliding of the femur, particularly when the knee is flexed.

2. The anterior cruciate ligament, which prevents backward sliding of the femur and hyperextension of the knee, and limits medial rotation of the femur when the foot is on the ground—i.e., when the leg is fixed.

293   Ligaments of the Knee Joint, from behind

Observe:

1. The bandlike medial ligament attached to the medial meniscus (semilunar cartilage). The cordlike lateral ligament separated from the lateral meniscus by the width of the Popliteus tendon (removed).

2. The posterior cruciate ligament joined by a cord from the lateral meniscus and passing to the fore part of the medial condyle of the femur. The anterior cruciate ligament attached to the hinder part of the lateral condyle.

Anterior intercondylar area

Med. intercondylar tubercle

Articular surface
of medial condyle

Lat. intercondylar tubercle

Articular surface
of lateral condyle

Fibular facet

Posterior intercondylar area

Superior Aspect of the Proximal End of the Tibia

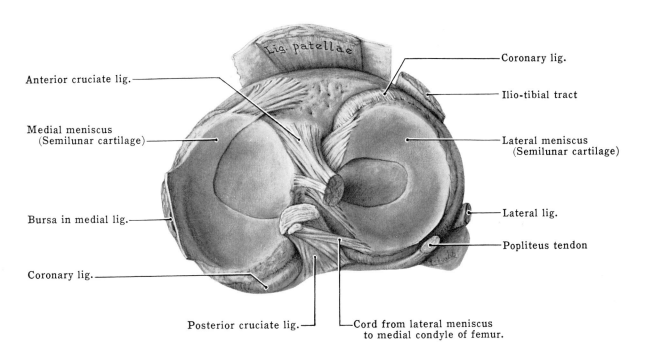

Lig. patellae

Anterior cruciate lig.

Medial meniscus
(Semilunar cartilage)

Bursa in medial lig.

Coronary lig.

Coronary lig.

Ilio-tibial tract

Lateral meniscus
(Semilunar cartilage)

Lateral lig.

Popliteus tendon

Posterior cruciate lig.

Cord from lateral meniscus
to medial condyle of femur.

294 Cruciate Ligaments and the Menisci (Semilunar Cartilages)

The sites of attachment of the cruciate ligaments are coloured yellow; those of the medial meniscus, blue; and those of the lateral meniscus, red.

Of the tibial condyles, the lateral is flatter, shorter from front to back, and more circular; the medial is concave, longer from front to back, and more oval.

The menisci are cartilaginous and tough where compressed between femur and tibia, but ligamentous and pliable at their attachments—as is the case with other intra-articular fibro-cartilages.

The menisci conform to the shapes of the surfaces on which they rest. Since the horns of the lateral meniscus are attached close together and its coronary ligament is slack, this meniscus can slide forwards and backwards on the (flat) condyle; since the horns of the medial meniscus are attached far apart, its movements on the (concave) condyle are restricted.

Note the bursa between the long and short parts of the medial ligament of the knee.

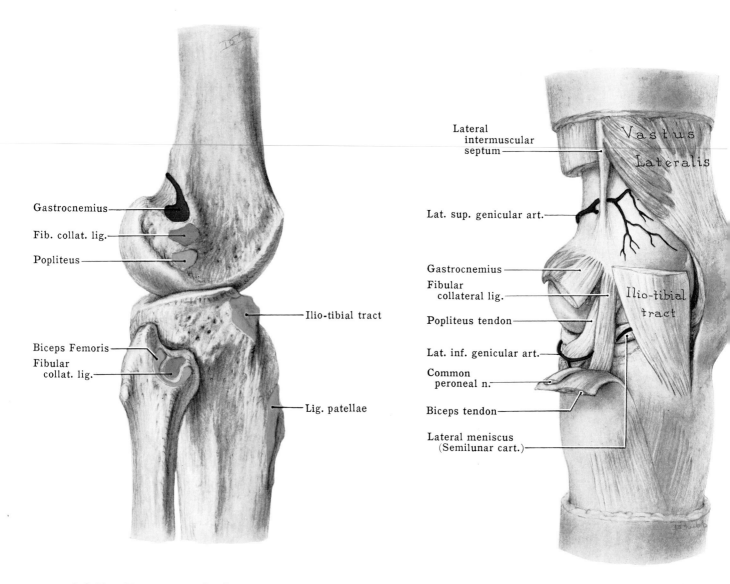

Gastrocnemius

Fib. collat. lig.

Popliteus

Biceps Femoris

Fibular
collat. lig.

Ilio-tibial tract

Lig. patellae

Lateral
intermuscular
septum

Vastus

Lateralis

Lat. sup. genicular art.

Gastrocnemius

Fibular
collateral lig.

Popliteus tendon

Lat. inf. genicular art.

Common
peroneal n.

Biceps tendon

Lateral meniscus
(Semilunar cart.)

Ilio-tibial
tract

295   Bones of the Knee Joint showing Muscle Attachments, lateral view

296   Dissection of the Knee, lateral aspect

Observe:

1. The ilio-tibial tract intervening between the skin and the synovial membrane and which, by virtue of its toughness, protects this exposed aspect of the joint.

2. The 3 structures that arise from the lateral epicondyle and that are uncovered by reflecting Biceps. Of these, Gastrocnemius is postero-superior; Popliteus is antero-inferior; the fibular collateral lig. is in between, and it crosses superficial to Popliteus.

3. The lateral inferior genicular artery coursing along the lateral meniscus.

Adductor Magnus

Gastrocnemius

Tibial
collateral lig.

Tibial collat. lig.

Semimembranosus

atellae

rius

lis

tendinosus

Tibial
collateral lig.

Vastus
Medialis

Adductor Magnus

Med. sup.
genicular art.

Gastrocnemius

Semimembranosus

Meniscus

Tibial collat. lig.

Coronary lig.
(cut edge)

Med. inf.
genicular art.

Gracilis

Semitendinosus

Sartorius

Popliteus fascia

297 Bones of the Knee Joint
showing Muscle Attachments,
medial view

298 Dissection of the Knee,
medial aspect

Note: The band-like part of the tibial collateral ligament of the knee: attached to the medial
epicondyle; almost in line with Adductor Magnus tendon; crossing the insertion of Semimembranosus; crossing the medial inferior genicular artery; and crossed by the tendons of 3 medial
rotators (Sartorius, Gracilis, Semitendinosus), each of which is supplied by a different nerve
(femoral, obturator, sciatic).

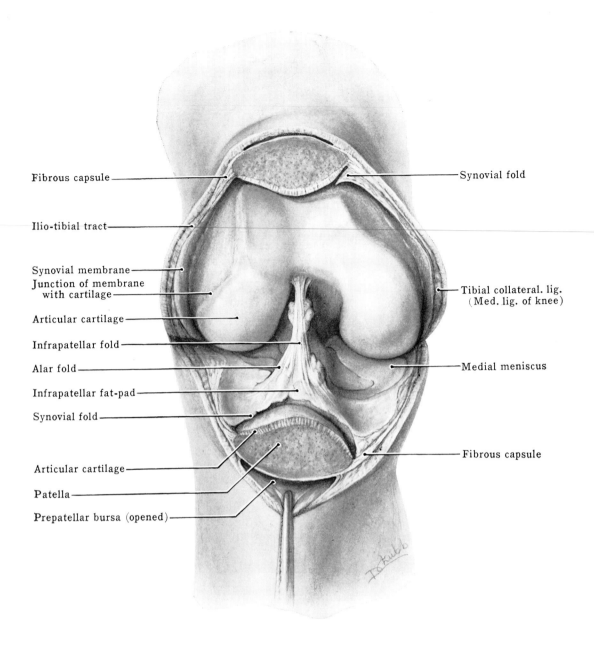

Fibrous capsule

Ilio-tibial tract

Synovial membrane
Junction of membrane
with cartilage

Articular cartilage

Infrapatellar fold

Alar fold

Infrapatellar fat-pad

Synovial fold

Articular cartilage

Patella

Prepatellar bursa (opened)

Synovial fold

Tibial collateral. lig.
(Med. lig. of knee)

Medial meniscus

Fibrous capsule

299 Knee Joint, opened from the front

The patella is sawn through; the skin and joint capsule are cut through; and the joint is flexed.

Observe:

1. The articular cartilage of the patella, not of uniform thickness but spread unevenly, as on other bones.

2. The infrapatellar synovial fold resembling a partially collapsed bell-tent whose apex is attached to the intercondylar notch and whose base is below the patella (cf. lig. of the head of femur, fig. 282). The infrapatellar pad of fat is continued into the tent.

3. A fracture of the patella would bring the prepatellar bursa into communication with the joint cavity.

4. Articular cartilage and synovial membrane continuous with each other on the side of the condyle, as in other joints.

Patellar surface

Indentation for
lateral meniscus
during extension

Popliteus tendon

Lateral meniscus

Coronary lig. (cut edge)

Fibular collateral lig.

Biceps extension to
deep fascia of leg

(1) Lower facets

(2) Middle facets

(3) Upper facets

Indentation for
medial meniscus
during extension

Notch for anterior
cruciate lig.

Posterior cruciate lig.

Anterior cruciate lig.

Medial meniscus

Coronary lig. (cut edge)

Tibial collateral lig.

Sartorius

Lig. patellae

Apex of patella

Nonarticular area

(4) Medial vertical facet

Base of patella

Quadriceps tendon

300 Ligaments of the Knee Joint, front view

The patella is thrown down and the joint is flexed.

Observe:

1. The indentations on the sides of the femoral condyles at the junction of the patellar and tibial articular areas. The lateral tibial articular area, shorter than the medial one.

2. The subsidiary notch, at the antero-lateral part of the intercondylar notch, for the reception of the anterior cruciate ligament on full extension.

3. The three paired facets on the posterior surface of the patella for articulation with the patellar surface of the femur successively during (1) extension, (2) slight flexion, (3) flexion; and the most medial facet on the patella (4) for articulation during full flexion with the crescentic facet that skirts the medial margin of the intercondylar notch of the femur.

Quadriceps Femoris

Quadriceps bursa

Prepatellar bursa

Patella

Lateral meniscus
(Lat. semilunar cart.)

Lig. patellae

Ilio-tibial tract,
turned down

Gastrocnemius,
lat. head,
turned up

Fibular
collateral lig.

Popliteus

Biceps
Femoris,
turned down

Femur

Fib.   Tibia

301   Distended Knee Joint, lateral view

Latex is injected into the joint cavity and fixed with acetic acid; the distended synovial capsule is exposed and cleaned. Gastrocnemius is thrown up; Biceps and the ilio-tibial tract are thrown down. The latex, in this specimen, has flowed into the proximal tibio-fibular joint cavity.

Observe:

1. The extent of the synovial capsule:—
    (a) Superiorly, it rises about two fingers' breadth above the patella and here rests on a layer of fat which allows it to glide freely in movements of the joint. This upper part, called the suprapatellar (Quadriceps Femoris) bursa, is obviously not a frictional bursa.
    (b) Posteriorly, it rises as high as the origin of Gastrocnemius.
    (c) Laterally, it curves below the lateral femoral epicondyle where popliteus tendon and the fibular collateral ligament are attached.
    (d) Inferiorly, it bulges below the lateral meniscus, overlapping about $\frac{1}{3}''$ of the tibia. The coronary ligament is removed to show this.
2. Biceps and ilio-tibial tract protecting the joint laterally.
3. The prepatellar bursa, here more extensive than usual, more than covering the patella.

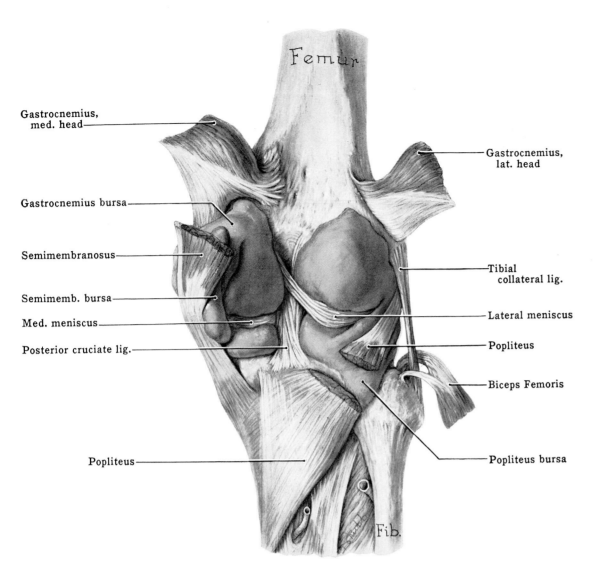

Gastrocnemius, med. head

Gastrocnemius bursa

Semimembranosus

Semimemb. bursa

Med. meniscus

Posterior cruciate lig.

Popliteus

Femur

Gastrocnemius, lat. head

Tibial collateral lig.

Lateral meniscus

Popliteus

Biceps Femoris

Popliteus bursa

Fib.

302 Distended Knee Joint, posterior view

The heads of Gastrocnemius are thrown up; Biceps is thrown down; and a section is removed from Popliteus.

Observe:

1. The posterior cruciate ligament exposed from behind without opening the synovial capsule or joint cavity.
2. The origins of Gastrocnemius limiting the extent to which the synovial membrane can rise·
3. The Semimembranosus bursa here communicating with the Gastrocnemius bursa, which in turn communicates with the joint cavity (fig. 287).
4. The Popliteus tendon separated from the lateral meniscus, the upper end of the tibia, and the proximal tibio-fibular joint by an elongated bursa. This bursa communicates with the cavity of the knee joint both above and below the meniscus, and in this specimen it also communicates with the proximal tibio-fibular joint cavity as revealed by figure 301.

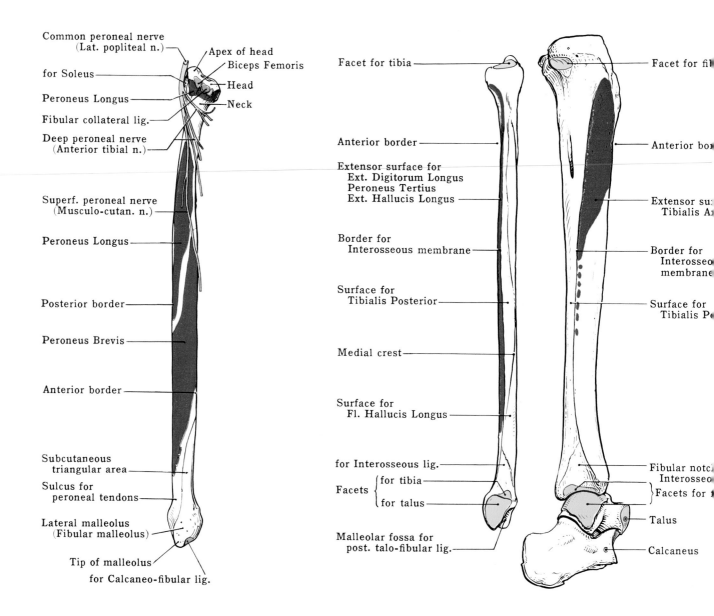

Common peroneal nerve
(Lat. popliteal n.)
Apex of head
Biceps Femoris
for Soleus
Head
Peroneus Longus
Neck
Fibular collateral lig.
Deep peroneal nerve
(Anterior tibial n.)

Superf. peroneal nerve
(Musculo-cutan. n.)

Peroneus Longus

Posterior border

Peroneus Brevis

Anterior border

Subcutaneous
triangular area
Sulcus for
peroneal tendons
Lateral malleolus
(Fibular malleolus)
Tip of malleolus
for Calcaneo-fibular lig.

Facet for tibia
Facet for fi[bula]

Anterior border
Anterior bo[rder]

Extensor surface for
Ext. Digitorum Longus
Peroneus Tertius
Ext. Hallucis Longus
Extensor su[rface]
Tibialis A[nterior]

Border for
Interosseous membrane
Border for
Interosseo[us]
membrane

Surface for
Tibialis Posterior
Surface for
Tibialis P[osterior]

Medial crest

Surface for
Fl. Hallucis Longus

for Interosseous lig.
Fibular notc[h]
Interosseo[us]
Facets { for tibia
Facets for [tibia]
for talus
Talus

Malleolar fossa for
post. talo-fibular lig.
Calcaneus

303 Lateral Surface of Fibula

Tibia and Fibula, opposed asp[ect]

Observe:

1. The lateral (or peroneal) surface of the fibula describing a quarter of a spiral, its distal end being grooved and facing posteriorly. This allows the lateral malleolus to act as a pulley for the long and short peroneal tendons.

2. The common peroneal nerve and its terminal branches having long contact with the fibula.

3. On the fibula, 2 small articular facets for the tibia; one proximally and one distally. Below the latter a large tri-

angular facet for articulation with almost the entire dept[h] of the lateral surface of the body of the talus.

4. Interosseous borders of the tibia and fibula, for the attach[-]ment of the interosseous membrane, separating the anterio[r] or extensor surface from the posterior or flexor surface[.] Each of these borders widening below into a triangular are[a] for the interosseous ligament.

5. The extensor surface of the fibula narrow below and almos[t] linear above.

Biceps tendon

Common peroneal nerve

Gastrocnemius

Peroneus Longus

Soleus

Superficial
peroneal nerve

Peroneus Brevis

Tendo calcaneus

Peroneus Longus

Peroneus Brevis

Peroneus Tertius

Ilio-tibial tract

Patella

Fibular collateral lig.,
uncovered by retracting
fascia

Deep fascia

Tibialis Anterior

Ext. Digitorum Longus

Ext. Hallucis Longus

Peroneus Tertius

Ext. Hallucis Brevis

Ext. Digitorum Brevis

Ext. Digitorum Longus

304   Muscles of the Leg and Foot, side view

Lig. patellae

Deep peroneal nerve
(Ant. tibial n.)

Anterior tibial art.

Deep fascia

Vascular twig of nerve

Ext. Digitorum Longus

Tibialis Anterior

Peroneus Tertius

Ext. Hallucis Longus

Vascular twig of nerve

Perforating branch
of peroneal artery

Inf. extensor retinaculum
(Cruciate crural lig.)

Lateral branch to:
Articulations and
Ext. Digitorum Brevis

Medial branch to:
Articulations and
1st & 2nd digits

305 Front of the Leg

The muscles are separated in order to display the artery and nerve.

Observe:

1. Tibialis Anterior, arising in part from the deep fascia which, therefore, is strong, has longitudinal fibres, and makes sharp the upper part of the anterior border of the tibia.

2. Peroneus Tertius is merely the lower part of Ext. Digitorum Longus. Ext. Hallucis Longus
   extends farther proximally than usual. These three muscles are unipennate and arise from
   the fibula.

3. The arterial and articular branches of the deep peroneal nerve.

Ilio-tibial tract

Head of fibula

Common peroneal nerve
(Lat. popliteal n.)

Peroneus Longus

Superf. peroneal nerve
(Musculo-cutaneous n.)

Peroneus Brevis

Perforating branch of
peroneal artery

Peroneus Longus

Lateral malleolar art

Inf. peroneal retinaculum

Ext. Digitorum Brevis

Peroneus Brevis

Peroneus Digiti V
Perforating branches of
metatarsal arteries

Dorsal digital aa.

Lig. patellae

Anterior recurrent
tibial nerve & art.

Tuberosity of tibia

Anterior border (Crest)
of tibia

Lateral surface of tibia

Interosseous membrane

Anterior [Extensor] surface
of fibula

Deep peroneal nerve
(Ant. tibial n.)

Anterior tibial artery

Superior extensor retinaculum
(Transverse crural lig.)

Medial malleolar art.

Lateral tarsal art.

Dorsalis pedis art.

Arcuate artery

Dorsal metatarsal aa.

306 Arteries and Nerves of the Front of Leg and Dorsum of Foot

The anterior crural muscles are removed and Peroneus Longus is excised.

Observe:

1. The artery entering the region in contact with the medial side of the neck of the fibula; the nerve in contact with the lateral side. Hence, the nerve approaches the artery from the lateral side.

2. The artery and nerve and their named branches lying on the skeletal plane and undisturbed by the removal of the muscles.

3. The superficial peroneal nerve following the anterior border of Peroneus Brevis which guides it to the surface a variable distance above the triangular subcutaneous area of the fibula.

4. The fibres of the interosseous membrane, so directed as to allow the fibula to be forced upwards but not pulled downwards.

Sup. extensor retinaculum
(Transverse crural lig.)

Ext. Digitorum Longus

Peroneus Tertius

Inf. extensor retinaculum
(Cruciate crural lig.)

Ext. Hallucis Brevis

Ext. Digitorum Brevis

Extensor expansion
(Dorsal aponeurosis)

Ext. Hallucis Longus

Tibialis Anterior

Deep peroneal nerve
(Ant. tibial n.)

Dorsalis pedis art.

1st Dorsal Interosseous

Extensor expansion

307 Dorsum of the Foot, front view

The vessels and nerves are cut short.

Observe:

1. At the ankle, the vessels and nerve lying midway between the malleoli and having two tendons on each side.

2. On the dorsum of the foot, the artery crossed by Ext. Hallucis Brevis and disappearing between the two heads of the 1st Dorsal Interosseous (cf. the radial artery on the dorsum of the hand, figs. 78 & 79).

3. The inferior extensor retinaculum restraining the tendons from bowstringing forwards and also from bowstringing medially; i.e. it restrains them in two planes.

ankle, subtalar, and calcaneo-
id joints are exposed in order to
l their positions.

ve:

e calcaneo-fibular ligament at-
:hed to the fibular malleolus in
nt of its tip, thereby allowing the
to overlap the Peronei tendons
d so prevent them from slipping
wards.

e inferior peroneal retinaculum
ached to the lateral surface of the
caneus, and in line with the in-
ior extensor retinaculum which is
ached to the superior surface.

{ Small saphenous vein
{ Sural nerve

Tendo calcaneus

Ant. inf. tibio-fibular lig.
(Ant. lig. of lat. malleolus)

Anterior talo-fibular lig.

Inf. extensor retinaculum

Ext. Digitorum Longus

Ext. Digitorum Brevis

Peroneus Tertius

Sup. peroneal retinaculum
Calcaneo-fibular lig.

Peroneus Brevis   Abductor Digiti Quinti

Calcaneo-cuboid joint

Peroneus Longus

Inf. peroneal retinaculum   Subtalar joint (Post. talo-calcanean joint)

9 Synovial Sheaths
the Tendons at the
kle, antero-lateral
W

e tendons of Peroneus Longus and
eus Brevis are enclosed in a com-
synovial sheath behind the fibular
olus and this sheath splits into two,
r each tendon, behind the peroneal
lea.

e tendon of Peroneus Longus has a
d sheath (not in view) which ac-
anies it across the sole of the foot.

46.6 per cent of 131 feet, the two
ns of the Longus were demonstrated
jection to be in continuity on their
or frictional, surface—though not
eir superficial surface (R. K. G.).

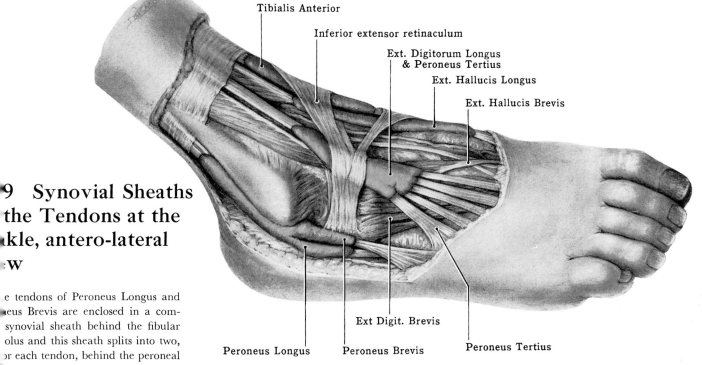

Tibialis Anterior

Inferior extensor retinaculum

Ext. Digitorum Longus
& Peroneus Tertius

Ext. Hallucis Longus

Ext. Hallucis Brevis

Ext Digit. Brevis

Peroneus Longus   Peroneus Brevis   Peroneus Tertius

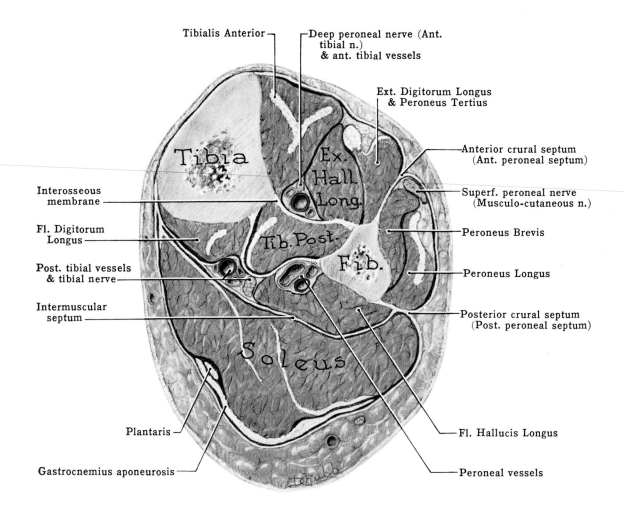

Tibialis Anterior

Deep peroneal nerve (Ant. tibial n.) & ant. tibial vessels

Ext. Digitorum Longus & Peroneus Tertius

Anterior crural septum (Ant. peroneal septum)

Superf. peroneal nerve (Musculo-cutaneous n.)

Interosseous membrane

Fl. Digitorum Longus

Post. tibial vessels & tibial nerve

Intermuscular septum

Peroneus Brevis

Peroneus Longus

Posterior crural septum (Post. peroneal septum)

Plantaris

Fl. Hallucis Longus

Gastrocnemius aponeurosis

Peroneal vessels

Tibia — *Ex. Hall. Long.* — *Tib. Post.* — *Fib.* — *Soleus*

310 Cross Section through the Leg, male

Observe:

1. The level of the section—(a) Extensor and Flexor Hallucis Longus are both present and Tibialis Anterior has ceased to arise from the deep fascia, therefore the section is below the upper $\frac{1}{3}$rd of the leg; (b) the anterior tibial artery has not yet moved on to the front of the tibia, therefore it is above the lower $\frac{1}{3}$rd; (c) Peronei Longus et Brevis are both arising from the fibula, therefore it is in the middle $\frac{1}{3}$rd. (d) Gastrocnemius is aponeurotic, therefore, it is in the lower $\frac{1}{2}$—say through the lower part of the middle $\frac{1}{3}$rd.

2. The anterior tibio-fibular compartment, bounded by tibia, interosseous membrane, fibula, anterior intermuscular crural septum and deep fascia, and containing the anterior tibial vessels and deep peroneal nerve. (*Peroneal* is Greek for *fibular*, which is Latin.)

3. The peroneal or fibular compartment bounded by fibula, anterior and posterior intermuscular crural septa and the deep fascia, and containing the superficial peroneal nerve.

4. The posterior tibio-fibular compartment bounded by tibia, interosseous membrane, fibula, posterior intermuscular crural septum and deep fascia. This compartment is subdivided by two coronal septa into three subcompartments:—1st, or deepest, contains Tibialis Posterior; the 2nd, or intermediate, contains Flexor Hallucis Longus, Flexor Digitorum Longus and posterior tibial vessels and tibial nerve; and the 3rd, or most superficial, contains Soleus, Gastrocnemius and Plantaris.

311 Bones of the Foot, medial aspect

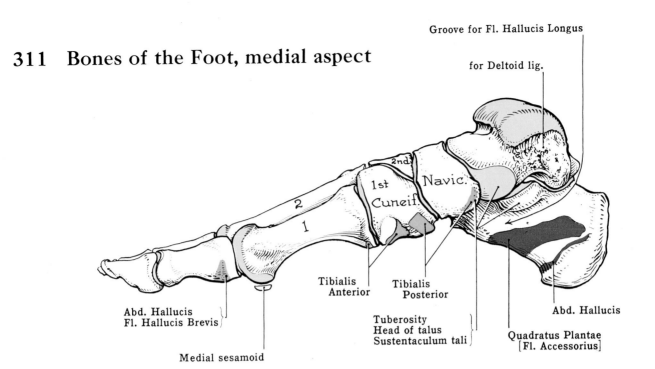

Groove for Fl. Hallucis Longus

for Deltoid lig.

2nd

1st Cuneif.

Navic.

2

1

Abd. Hallucis
Fl. Hallucis Brevis

Medial sesamoid

Tibialis
Anterior

Tibialis
Posterior

Tuberosity
Head of talus
Sustentaculum tali

Abd. Hallucis

Quadratus Plantae
[Fl. Accessorius]

312 Bones of the Foot, lateral aspect

The trochlea of the talus is the part of the body of the talus that articulates with the ankle socket. It has an upper, a medial malleolar, and a lateral malleolar part.

Neck & head of talus

Body

Cuneiforms

Metatarsals

Phalanges

Lateral
tubercle

2nd

Navic

3rd

2

Cuboid

3

Calcaneum

4

5

for Calcaneo-
fibular lig.

Peroneal trochlea (tubercle)

Groove for Peroneus Longus

Base

Tuberosity

Shaft

Head

Tubercle

Ext. Hallucis Longus

Ext. Hallucis Brevis

5 Metatarsals

3 Cuneiforms

Tuberosity

for Tibial malleolus

for Tibia

Medial tubercle

Groove for Fl. Hallucis Longus

1

2

3

4

5

1st

2nd

3rd

Navicular

Talus

Cuboid

Peroneus Tertius

Peroneus Brevis

Tuberosity

Groove for Peroneus Longus

Ext. Digitorum Brevis

for Fibular malleolus

for Transverse tibio-fibular lig.

Lateral tubercle
(Post. tubercle)

Tuber calcanei (Post. surface)

313 Bones of the Foot, dorsal aspect

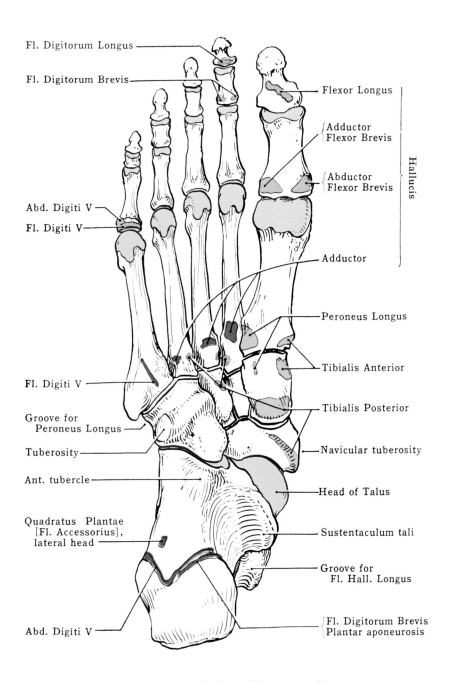

Fl. Digitorum Longus

Fl. Digitorum Brevis

Flexor Longus

{ Adductor
  Flexor Brevis

{ Abductor
  Flexor Brevis

Hallucis

Abd. Digiti V

Fl. Digiti V

Adductor

Peroneus Longus

Tibialis Anterior

Fl. Digiti V

Tibialis Posterior

Groove for
Peroneus Longus

Navicular tuberosity

Tuberosity

Ant. tubercle

Head of Talus

Quadratus Plantae
[Fl. Accessorius],
lateral head

Sustentaculum tali

Groove for
Fl. Hall. Longus

Abd. Digiti V

{ Fl. Digitorum Brevis
  Plantar aponeurosis

314   Bones of the Foot, plantar aspect

Adductor tercle

Groove & rough area
for Semimembranosus

Popliteal area

Soleal (Popliteal) line

Vertical line

TIBIA

Groove for:
Tibialis Posterior }
Fl. Digit. Longus }

Medial malleolus

Medial tubercle of talus

Sustentaculum tali

Groove for Fl. Hallucis Longus

Medial process

Apex of head (Styloid process)
Head of fibula
Neck of fibula

FIBULA

Peroneal surface

Groove for:
{Peroneus Brevis
{Peroneus Longus

Lateral malleolus

Lateral tubercle of talus

for bursa

for Tendo calcaneus

Subcutaneous area

Lateral process

315 Bones of the Leg, posterior view

(For anterior view, see fig. 303; for os coxae and femur, see figs. 242 & 243.)

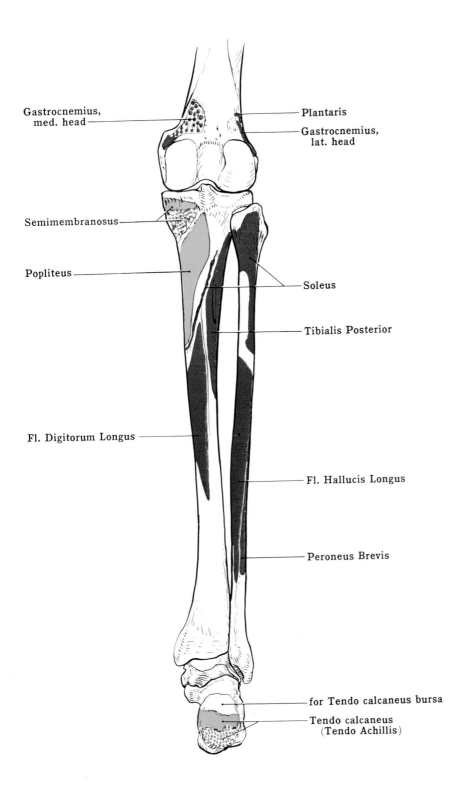

Gastrocnemius, med. head

Plantaris

Gastrocnemius, lat. head

Semimembranosus

Popliteus

Soleus

Tibialis Posterior

Fl. Digitorum Longus

Fl. Hallucis Longus

Peroneus Brevis

for Tendo calcaneus bursa

Tendo calcaneus (Tendo Achillis)

316 Bones of the Leg showing Attachments of Muscles, posterior view

(For Os coxae and Femur, posterior aspect, see fig. 266; Bones of Foot, plantar aspect, see fig. 314.)

Semitendinosus

Semimembranous

Gracilis

Vastus Medialis

Sartorius

Gastrocnemius, med. head

Biceps Femoris

Tibial nerve

Common peroneal nerve

Medial sural cutaneous nerve

Gastrocnemius, lat. head

Soleus

Peroneus Longus

Peroneus Brevis

Fl. Digitorum Longus

Tendo calcaneus

Tibialis Posterior

Flexor retinaculum

Superior peroneal retinaculum

317 Muscles of the Leg, posterior view—I

Semitendinosus

Semimembranosus

Gastrocnemius, med. head

Med. inferior genicular vessels

Gastrocnemius

Fl. Digitorum Longus

Tibialis Posterior

Biceps Femoris

Popliteal vein

Tibial nerve

Gastrocnemius, lat. head

Common peroneal nerve

Soleus

Peroneus Longus

Peroneus Brevis

Fl. Hallucis Longus

318 Muscles of the Leg, posterior view—II

The fleshy bellies of Gastrocnemius are largely excised, and the origin of Soleus is thereby exposed. Plantaris is absent from this specimen.

Semimembranosus

Popliteus fascia

Fl. Digitorum Longus
Post. tibial artery
(Post.) Tibial nerve

Flex.
Hall.
Long.

Tibial nerve
(Med. popliteal n.)
Popliteus
Common peroneal nerve
(Lat. popliteal n.)
Soleus

Fibula
Tibialis Posterior
Peroneal artery

Investing deep fascia

Intermuscular fascial septum

Flexor retinaculum
(Laciniate lig.)
Tibialis Posterior
Fl. Digitorum Longus

Tendo calcaneus (Tendo Achillis)

Med. plantar nerve & art.
Lat. plantar nerve & art.

319 Back of the Leg, deep structures undisturbed

The tendo calcaneus is divided; Gastrocnemius and a horseshoe-shaped section of Soleus are removed.

Observe:

1. The bipennate structure of the large Flexor Hallucis Longus and of the smaller Flexor Digitorum Longus.

2. The posterior tibial artery and the tibial nerve descending between these two muscles, on a layer of fascia that covers Tibialis Posterior.

3. The tough, intermuscular fascial septum deep to Soleus and tendo calcaneus that acts as a restraining anklet at the ankle and there blends medially with the weaker investing deep fascia to form the flexor retinaculum.

Semimembranosus

Popliteal artery & vein

{ Biceps
Common peroneal nerve

Popliteus and nerve

Sartorius

Gracilis

Soleus

Semitendinosus

Ant. tibial art. & vein

Post. crural septum
(Post. peroneal septum)

Soleus

Tibialis Posterior
and nerve

(Post.) Tibial nerve

Peroneal artery

Fl. Digitorum Longus

Fl. Hallucis Longus

Tibialis Posterior

Post. tibial artery
& venae comitantes

Intermuscular
fascial septum

Flexor retinaculum
(Laciniate lig.)

Tendo calcaneus
(Tendon of Achilles)

320 Back of the Leg, deep structures displayed

Soleus is largely cut away; the two long digitial flexors are pulled apart; the posterior
tibial artery is excised.

Observe:

1. The bipennate Tibialis Posterior lying deep to the long digital flexors.

2. The peroneal artery overlapped by Fl. Hallucis Longus.

3. The nerve to Tibialis Posterior here arising in conjunction with the nerve to Popliteus, and
   the nerve to Fl. Digitorum Longus arising in conjunction with the nerve to Fl. Hallucis
   Longus.

4. In the popliteal fossa the nerve is superficial to the artery: at the ankle the artery is superficial to the nerve.

Saphenous nerve

Great saphenous vein

Investing deep fascia

Intermuscular
fascial septum

Fl. Hallucis Longus

Posterior tibial art.
(Posterior) Tibial nerve

Fl. Digitorum Longus

Tibialis Posterior

Flexor retinaculum

Abductor Hallucis and nerve

Medial plantar art. & nerve

Lateral plantar nerve & art.

Medial calcanean branches

Nerve to Fl. Digitorum Brevis

321   Medial Side of the Ankle and Heel

The skin and fasciae are removed and part of Abductor Hallucis is excised.

Observe:

1. The posterior tibial artery and the tibial nerve lying between Fl. Digitorum Longus and Fl. Hallucis Longus; separated from the tibial malleolus by the width of two tendons (Tibialis Posterior and Fl. Digitorum Longus); and dividing into medial and lateral plantar branches on the surface of the osseo-fibrous tunnel of Fl. Hallucis Longus (figs. 322 & 333).

2. Tibialis Posterior and Fl. Digitorum Longus occupying separate and individual osseo-fibrous tunnels.

3. The medial and lateral plantar nerves lying within the fork of the medial and lateral plantar arteries.

Posterior tibial vessels & (post.) tibial nerve

Fl. Digitorum Longus

Tibialis Posterior

Fl. Hall. Long.

Deltoid lig.

Tibialis Posterior

Fl. Digitorum Longus

Abductor Hallucis

Plantar vessels & nerves

Quadratus Plantae [Fl. Accessorius]

Tendo calcaneus

Peroneus Brevis

Peroneus Longus

Post. inf. tibio-fibular lig.

Transverse tibio-fibular lig.

Post. talo-fibular lig.

Calcaneo-fibular lig.

Tendo calcaneus (Tendo Achillis)

322 Ankle Joint, posterior view

Observe:

1. Fl. Hallucis Longus placed midway between the two malleoli; and having the two tendons (Fl. Digitorum Longus and Tibialis Posterior) that groove the tibial malleolus medial to it and the two tendons (Peronei Longus et Brevis) that groove the fibular malleolus lateral to it.

2. The entrance to the sole "porta pedis" lying deep to Abd. Hallucis. The plantar vessels and nerves, the two long digital flexors, and part of Tibialis Posterior enter here. Quadratus Plantae serves as a soft pad for the vessels and nerves.

3. The posterior tibial artery and the tibial nerve lying medial to Fl. Hallucis Longus above and, after bifurcating, postero-lateral to it below. The crossing takes place where the long flexor is within its osseo-fibrous tunnel.

4. The strongest parts of the ligaments of the ankle are those that prevent forward displacement of the leg bones, viz. posterior part of the deltoid (posterior tibio-talar), posterior talo-fibular, tibio-calcanean, and calcaneo-fibular.

A

The Relationship of the Sciatic Nerve to Piriformis. (a) In 87.3% of 640 limbs both the tibial and the peroneal division of the sciatic nerve passed below Piriformis; (b) in 12.2% the peroneal division passed through Piriformis; and (c) in 0.5% it passed above. (*J. C. B. G.*)

C

Bipartite Patella, posterior view. Occasionally th supero-lateral angle of the patella ossifies independentl and remains discrete.

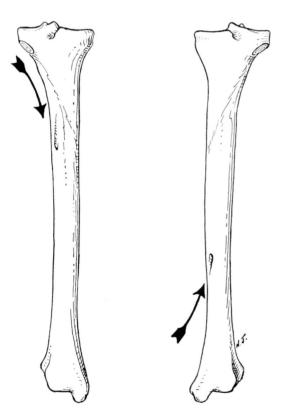

B

The Nutrient Canals of Long Bones are directed away from the more actively growing ends of the bones, but in this pair of tibiae (taken from the same subject) they take opposite directions.

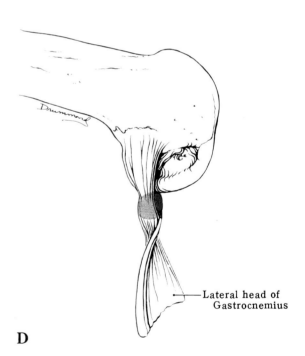

—Lateral head of Gastrocnemius

D

A Sesamoid Bone (Fabella) in the Lateral Head Gastrocnemius was present in 21.6% of 116 limb (*J. C. B. G.*)

323   Variations and Anomalies

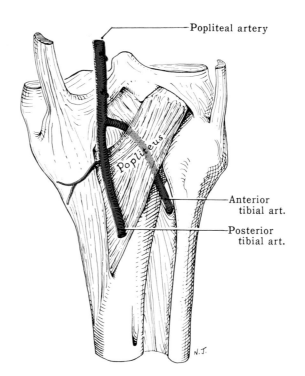

High Division of Popliteal Artery with the anterior tibial artery descending anterior to Popliteus occurred in 1.8% of 218 limbs (Quain).

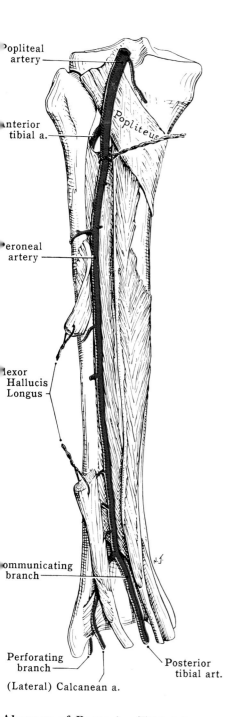

Absence of Posterior Tibial Artery (left side), with compensatory enlargement of the peroneal artery. This occurred in 5.2% of 211 limbs (Quain).

The reverse condition, i.e., absence of peroneal artery with enlargement of the posterior tibial artery probably never occurs (Senior)

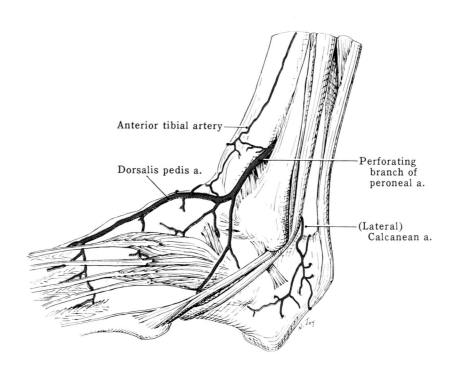

The Dorsalis Pedis Artery (left side) as a continuation of the perforating branch of the peroneal artery. When this occurs (3.7% of 592 limbs) the anterior tibial artery either fails to reach the ankle or is a very slender vessel. (*J. C. B. G.*)

324 Variations and Anomalies

Fl. Digitorum Longus

Fibrous digital sheaths

Superficial transverse
metatarsal lig.

Plantar apon.

Plantar fascia

Cutaneous branches of
lateral plantar
nerve & artery

Heel pad of fat

Fl. Hallucis Longus

Plantar digital nn. & aa.

Plantar fascia

Cutaneous branches of
medial plantar
nerve & artery

Medial calcanean
nerve & artery

Plantar digital
arteries

Plantar
metatarsal aa.

Perforating art.
(Deep art.)

Plantar arch
"Superf. arch"

Medial plantar a.

Lateral plantar a.

Post. tibial art.

Calcanean br.

325 Superficial Dissection of the Sole of the Foot

The plantar aponeurosis, the medial and lateral parts of the plantar fascia, and the digital vessels and nerves should be compared and contrasted with the corresponding structures in the palm (figs. 59, 67, & 68).

326 Diagram of the Arteries of the Sole of the Foot

Plantar digital nn. & aa.

Fl. Hallucis Longus

Plantar digital nn.

Br. connecting lat. & med. plantar nn.

1st Lumbrical

Fl. Digiti Quinti (V)

Fl. Hallucis Brevis

Abd. Digiti Quinti (V)

Abductor Hallucis

Fl. Digitorum Brevis

Plantar aponeurosis, reflected

327 The First Layer of Muscles of the Sole: Digital Nerves and Arteries

The plantar aponeurosis and fascia are reflected or removed, and a section is taken from Fl. Digitorum Brevis in order to show the fibrous box encasing it.

The muscles of the first layer are: Abd. Digiti Quinti, Fl. Digitorum Brevis, Abd. Hallucis.

The lateral and medial plantar digital nerves, like the corresponding palmar digital branches of the ulnar and median nerves, supply $1\frac{1}{2}$ and $3\frac{1}{2}$ digits respectively and are united by a connecting (communicating) branch (cf. fig. 68).

The lateral nerve to the little toe is here thickened. Fl. Digitorum Brevis here, as commonly, fails to send a tendon to the little toe.

Soleus

Gastrocnemius tendon

Tendo calcaneus

Fl. Hallucis Longus

Fl. Digitorum Longus

Tibialis Posterior

Tibialis Anterior

Tuberosity of navicular

Peroneus Longus

Peroneus Brevis

Quadratus Plantae
[Fl. Accessorius]

Fl. Digitorum Longus

Slip from Fl. Hallucis

Fl. Hallucis Longus

Lumbricales

328 Second Layer of Muscles of the Sole

These are: Fl. Hallucis Longus, Fl. Digitorum Longus, Four Lumbricales, and Quadratus Plantae.

Observe:

1. Fl. Digitorum Longus crossing superficial to Tibialis Posterior behind the medial malleolus and superficial to Fl. Hallucis Longus abreast of the tuberosity of the navicular bone.

2. The four Lumbricals passing to the hallux side of the toes just as, in the hand, they pass to the pollex side of the fingers (fig. 61).

3. Fl. Hallucis Longus sending a strong tendinous slip to Fl. Digitorum Longus.

Fl. Hallucis Longus

Fl. Digitorum Longus

Tibialis Posterior

Tendo calcaneus
[Tendo Achillis]

Tibialis Anterior

Tibialis Posterior

Quadratus Plantae

Fl. Digitorum Longus

Fl. Hallucis Longus

1st Lumbrical

Fl. Hallucis Brevis

Sesamoid bone

329 Foot Raised as in Walking, medial view

Observe:

1. The heel raised, and the toes remaining applied to the ground.

2. The sesamoid bones in Fl. Hallucis Brevis tendons acting as a foot-stool for the first metatarsal and giving it increased height.

3. Quadratus Plantae lining the concave medial surface of the calcaneus between Fl. Hallucis
Longus tendon and the heel.

Plantar lig. (plate)

Deep transverse
metatarsal lig.

Add. Hallucis Transversus

Fl. Digiti Quinti (V)

Deep br. of
lateral plantar a. & n.

Lateral plantar a. & n.

Abd. Digiti Quinti (V)

Fl. Digitorum Brevis ⎫
Plantar aponeurosis ⎭

Fibrous digital sheath

Add. Hallucis Obliquus

lat. head ⎫ Flexor
           ⎬ Hallucis
med. head ⎭ Brevis

Fl. Hallucis Longus
Fl. Digitorum Longus

Medial plantar nerve

Abductor Hallucis

Quadratus Plantae

330 Third Layer of Muscles of the Sole

Of the 1st layer, Abd. Digiti V and Abd. Hallucis are pulled aside and Fl. Digitorum Brevis is cut short. Of the 2nd layer, Fl. Digitorum Longus and Lumbricales are excised and Quadratus Plantae is cut long.

The 3rd layer comprises: Fl. Digiti V, Add. Hallucis Transversus, and Fl. Hallucis Brevis, which form three sides of a square in the anterior half of the sole, largely filled by a fourth muscle, namely, Add. Hallucis Obliquus.

The lateral Interossei are seen in the floor of the square.

The lateral plantar nerve and artery course laterally between muscles of the 1st and 2nd layers; their deep branches then course medially between muscles of the 3rd and 4th layers.

Fl. Digitorum Longus

Fl. Digitorum Brevis

Fl. Digiti Quinti Brevis

Lateral "cord" of plantar aponeurosis

Peroneus Longus

Abd. Digiti Quinti

Fl. Hallucis Longus

Sesamoids

Plantar lig. (plate)

medial head
lateral head
tendon of origin

} Flexor Hallucis Brevis

Tibialis Posterior

Plantar calcaneo-cuboid lig. (Short plantar lig.)

Long plantar lig.

Abd. Hallucis

{ Fl. Digitorum Brevis
Plantar aponeurosis

331 Fourth Layer of Muscles of the Sole

Of the first three layers, Abductor and Flexor Brevis of the fifth toe and Abductor and Flexor Brevis of the big toe remain for purposes of orientation.

The muscles of the 4th layer are: (a) three Plantar and four Dorsal Interossei in the anterior half of the foot and (b) the tendon of Peroneus Longus and of Tibialis Posterior in the posterior half.

Note: The Plantar Interossei adduct the three lateral toes towards an axial line that passes through the 2nd metatarsal bone and second toe; whereas the Dorsal Interossei abduct from this line.

Peroneus Brevis

Anterior (Extensor) surface

Interosseous membrane

Subcutaneous triangular area above lateral malleolus

Ant. inf. tibio-fibular lig. (Lig. of lat. malleolus)

Ant. talo-fibular lig.

Interosseous talo-calcanean lig.

Bifurcated lig.

Cuboid bone

3rd Cuneiform bone

Dorsal intermetatarsal ligs.

Tibialis Anterior

Medial malleolus

Deltoid ligament [Med. lig. of ankle]

(Dorsal) Talo-navicular lig.

Navicular bone

Dorsal cuneo-navicular ligs.

1st cuneiform bone

Dorsal tarso-metatarsal ligs.

1st metatarsal bone.

332 Ankle Joint and the Joints of the Foot, dorsal view

The foot is extended and the anterior capsular fibers of the ankle joint are removed.

Observe:

1. The fibers of the membrane and ligaments uniting the fibula to the tibia are so directed as to allow the fibula to be forced upwards but not pulled downwards.
2. The anterior talo-fibular ligament is but a weak band.
3. The dorsal ligaments of the foot resist the same thrusts as the plantar ligaments, and, therefore, are identically disposed, as reference to figure 342 shows. The plantar ligaments, however, act also as tie-beams for the arches of the foot and, therefore, are stronger.
4. Tibialis Anterior clinging to the skeleton throughout.

333 Horizontal Section through the Ankle Joint

Observe:

1. The body of the talus on section wedge-shaped and grasped by the malleoli, which are bound to it by the deltoid and the posterior talo-fibular ligament and are thereby prevented from sliding forward.

2. Several synovial folds projecting into the joint.

3. Flexor Hallucis Longus within its fibro-osseous sheath and lying between the medial and lateral tubercles of the talus; 2 tendons each within a separate sheath (fibrous and synovial) behind the medial malleolus, and 2 within a common sheath behind the lateral malleolus.

4. Because of the intervening fibrous sheath, the posterior tibial vessels and the tibial nerve are not disturbed by the excursions of Flexor Hallucis Longus.

5. The small inconstant bursa superficial to tendo Achillis and the large constant bursa deep to it and containing a long synovial fold.

6. The anterior tibial artery and its companion nerve at the mid-point of the front of the ankle, with 2 tendons medial to it and 2 lateral to it (Peroneus Tertius being partly fleshy).

7. The intermuscular fascial septum shown and described in fig. 319.

334 Vertical Section through the Region of the Ankle

Observe:

1. The tibia resting on the talus and the talus resting on the calcaneus, and between the calcaneus and the skin several large and many small encapuled cushions of fat.

2. The malleolus of the fibula descending much farther than that of the tibia. The weak interosseous tibio-fibular ligament.

3. The interosseous band between talus and calcaneus separating the subtalar or posterior talo-calcanean joint from the talo-calcaneo-navicular joint. (For clarification see fig. 337.)

4. Sustentaculum tali acting as a pulley for Flexor Hallucis Longus and giving attachment to the calcaneo-tibial band of the deltoid ligament. Tibialis Posterior rubbing on the band and Flexor Digitorum Longus on the sustentaculum.

5. The plantar vessels and nerves separated from calcaneus by Quadratus Plantae and the sheath of Flexor Hallucis Longus.

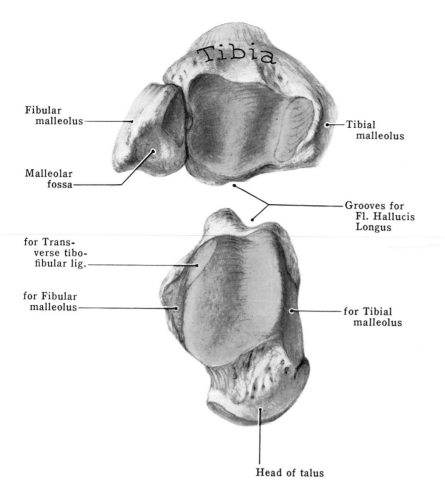

Fibular malleolus

Tibia

Tibial malleolus

Malleolar fossa

Grooves for Fl. Hallucis Longus

for Transverse tibo-fibular lig.

for Fibular malleolus

for Tibial malleolus

Head of talus

335 Articular Surfaces of the Ankle Joint

Note:

The superior articular surface of the talus is broader in front than behind; hence the tibial and fibular malleoli which grasp the sides of the talus tend, in dorsiflexion, to be forced apart. The virtue of the inferior tibio-fibular joint, on which the brunt of the strain then falls, is in the resilience it gives to the ankle joint.

336 Joints of Inversion and Eversion

The ankle joint has been immobil by nailing together tibia, fibula talus, thereby making a single rigid of these 3 bones. The remaining bone the foot—all but talus—have been w together into another unit. Movem between these 2 units constitute inver and eversion of the foot.

The talus takes part in 3 joints:

1. The "*supratalar joint*", i.e., the a joint.

2. the "*infratalar joints*"

   posterior talo-
      calcanean or
      subtalar joint
   anterior talo-
      calcanean joint

   talo-calcar

3. The "*pretalar joint*",   navicula
   i.e., the talo-   joint.
   navicular joint

At the supratalar joint only moveme of flexion and extension are norm permitted—they are here eliminated k nail.

At the infratalar and pretalar jo movements of inversion and eversion t place.

The 2 parts of the infratalar joint separated from each other by the sul tali and the sulcus calcanei, which, w the talus and calcaneus are in articu tion, become the tarsal sinus or tunn

The convex posterior talar facet of calcaneus, the concave middle and ar rior talar facets, and the concave ta facet of the navicular all have th counterparts on the talus. The star (* at the site of the spring ligament. T middle talar facet is the cartilage-cove upper surface of the sustentaculum t

The calcaneo-cuboid joint is access to the foregoing joints.

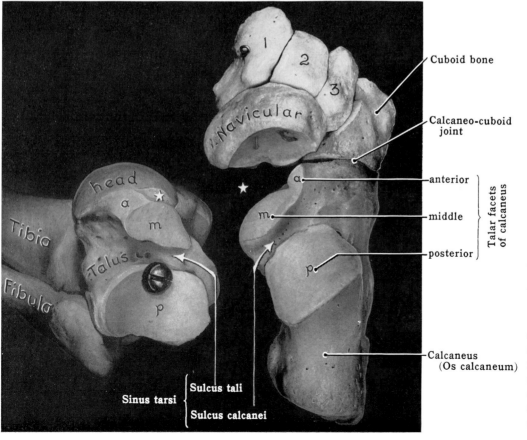

Cuboid bone

Calcaneo-cuboid joint

anterior

middle

posterior

Talar facets of calcaneus

Calcaneus (Os calcaneum)

Sinus tarsi

Sulcus tali

Sulcus calcanei

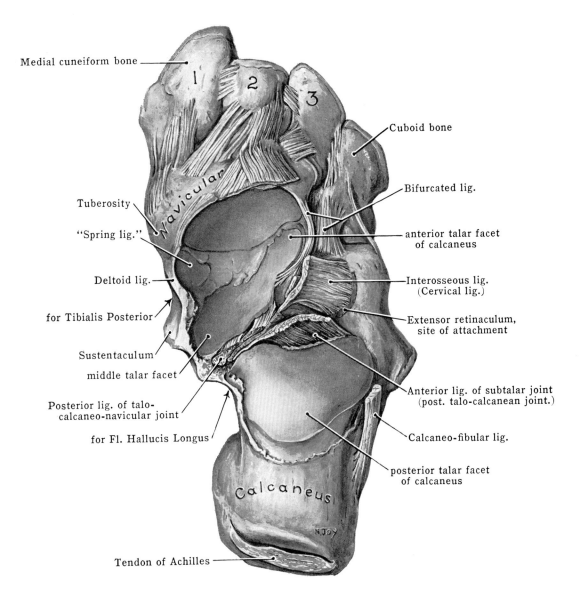

Medial cuneiform bone

Cuboid bone

Bifurcated lig.

Navicular

Tuberosity

"Spring lig."

anterior talar facet
of calcaneus

Deltoid lig.

Interosseous lig.
(Cervical lig.)

for Tibialis Posterior

Extensor retinaculum,
site of attachment

Sustentaculum

middle talar facet

Posterior lig. of talo-
calcaneo-navicular joint

Anterior lig. of subtalar joint
(post. talo-calcanean joint.)

for Fl. Hallucis Longus

Calcaneo-fibular lig.

posterior talar facet
of calcaneus

Calcaneus

Tendon of Achilles

337 Joints of Inversion (Supination) and Eversion (Pronation)

This specimen was prepared by sawing through the body of the talus and, after discarding it, by nibbling away the neck and head of the talus, thereby fully exposing the structures in the tarsal sinus. (Prepared by Dr. J. E. Anderson.)

Observe:

1. The convex, posterior talar facet separated from the concave, middle and anterior facets by the ligamentous structures within the tarsal sinus.

2. At the wide lateral end of the sinus: (a) the strong interosseous talo-calcanean ligament; and (b) in blue, the attachments of the extensor retinaculum, which extends medially between the posterior lig. of the anterior talo-calcanean joint and the anterior lig. of the posterior talo-calcanean, or subtalar, joint.

3. The subtalar joint has a synovial cavity to itself; whereas the talo-navicular joint and the anterior talo-calcanean

joint share a common synovial cavity, hence the collective title—talo-calcaneo-navicular joint.

4. The angular space between the navicular bone and the middle talar facet, on the sustentaculum tali, to be bridged by the plantar calcaneo-navicular, or spring, lig., the central part of which is fibro-cartilaginous.

5. The socket for the head of the talus to be deepened medially by the part of the deltoid lig. that is attached to the spring lig., and laterally by the calcaneo-navicular part of the bifurcated lig.

6. Various synovial folds overlying the margins of the articular cartilage; some of these containing fat.

Tibialis Anterior

Tendo calcaneus

Synovial fold

Ant. inferior tibio-fibular lig.

(Dorsal) Talo-navicular lig.

Navicular bone
Head of talus
Bifurcated lig.

Anterior talo-fibular lig.

Bursa

Cuneiform bones

Calcaneo-fibular lig.

Interosseous talo-calcanean lig.

Peronei Longus et Brevis

Dorsal calcaneo- cuboid lig.
Calcaneus and cuboid

338   Ankle Joint and the Joints of Inversion and Eversion, lateral view

The joints of inversion and eversion are (1) the subtalar (i.e., posterior talo-calcanean) joint, (2) the talo-calcaneo-navicular (i.e., combined anterior talo-calcanean and talo-navicular) joint, and (3) the transverse tarsal (i.e., combined calcaneo-cuboid and talo-navicular) joint. Hence, the talo-navicular joint is twice involved.

The foot has been inverted in order to demonstrate (a) the areas of articular surface uncovered, and (b) the ligaments rendered taut, on inverting the foot.

Observe:

1. The uncovered parts of the posterior talar facet of the calcaneus, anterior surface of the calcaneus, and head of the talus, all of which are palpable. Since inversion of the foot is commonly associated with plantar flexion of the ankle joint, the upper and side parts of the trochlea of the talus are commonly uncovered too.

2. The ligaments that resist further inversion.

3. The anterior talo-fibular lig. and the dorsal calcaneo-cuboid lig. are weak. The strong calcaneo-fibular lig. not attached to the tip of the malleolus but to a facet in front of the tip. Hence, this projecting flange helps to retain the peroneal tendons.

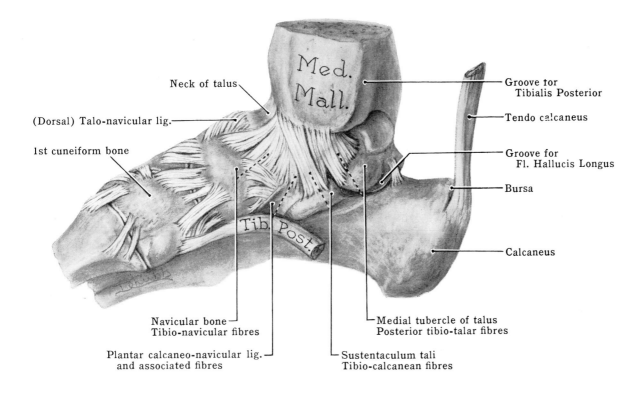

Neck of talus

(Dorsal) Talo-navicular lig.

1st cuneiform bone

Med. Mall.

Tib. Post.

Groove for Tibialis Posterior

Tendo calcaneus

Groove for Fl. Hallucis Longus

Bursa

Calcaneus

Navicular bone
Tibio-navicular fibres

Plantar calcaneo-navicular lig.
and associated fibres

Medial tubercle of talus
Posterior tibio-talar fibres

Sustentaculum tali
Tibio-calcanean fibres

339 Ligaments of the Ankle Joint and Foot, medial view

Observe:

1. Tibialis Posterior displaced from its bed—malleolus, deltoid lig., and plantar calcaneo-navicular, or spring, lig.
2. The bed of Fl. Hallucis Longus—the groove between the two tubercles of the talus and the continuation of that groove beneath the sustentaculum tali.

3. The chief parts of the deltoid lig. passing downwards and backwards and thereby preventing forward displacement of the bones of the leg. The parts of the deltoid lig. are: tibio-navicular, tibio-(spring lig.), ant. tibio-talar, tibio-calcanean, and post. tibio-talar.

Posterior inferior tibio-fibular ligament

Anterior inferior tibio-fibular ligament

Calcaneo-fibular lig.
Talo-calcanean lig.

Head of talus

Interosseous lig.
(Cervical lig.)

Anterior talo-fibular lig.

340 A Distended Ankle Joint

Observe:

1. The far forward extension of the synovial cavity on the neck of the talus.
2. Posteriorly and laterally, the closeness of the synovial cavity to the subtalar joint (posterior talo-calcanean joint).

Plantar inter-
metatarsal ligs.

Plantar tarso-
metatarsal ligs.

Cuboid bone

(Short plantar lig.)
Plantar calcaneo-
cuboid lig.

Long plantar lig.

Calcaneus

Metatarsal bone

Plantar tarso-
metatarsal ligs.

1st cuneiform bone

Tibialis Anterior

Navicular bone

Plantar calcaneo-
navicular lig.

Sustentaculum tali

Medial malleolus

Tibialis Posterior

Groove for Fl. Hallucis Longus

341 Ligaments of the Sole: The Insertions of the Tendons—I

Observe:

1. The tendon of Peroneus Longus crossing the sole in the groove in front of the ridge of the cuboid; bridged by some fibres of the long plantar ligament; and inserted into the base of the 1st metatarsal. Usually, like Tibialis Anterior, it is also inserted into the 1st cuneiform. It is an evertor (pronator) of the foot.

2. Slips of the tendon of Tibialis Posterior extending like the fingers of an open hand to grasp the bones anterior to the transverse tarsal joint (i.e. the five small tarsal bones and several metatarsal bones). It is an invertor (supinator) of the foot.

Plantar inter-
metatarsal ligs.

Plantar cuneo-
cuboid lig.

Plantar cubo-
navicular lig.

Plantar calcaneo-cuboid lig.
(Short plantar lig.)

Anterior tubercle
of calcaneus

Metatarsal bone

Plantar tarso-
metatarsal ligs.

1st cuneiform bone

Plantar cuneo-
navicular ligs.

Navicular bone

Plantar calcaneo-navicular
lig. (Spring lig.)

Sustentaculum tali

Calcaneus
(Os calcaneum)

342 Ligaments of the Sole—II

The plantar calcaneo-cuboid or short plantar lig. and the plantar calcaneo-navicular or spring lig. are the inferior ligaments of the transverse tarsal joint. Having a common purpose, they have a common direction.

The ligaments in the fore part of the foot diverge backwards from each side of the long axis of the 3rd metatarsal and 3rd cuneiform. Hence a backward thrust to the 1st metatarsal, as when rising on the big toe in walking, is transmitted directly to the navicular and talus by the 1st cuneiform, and indirectly by the 2nd metatarsal and 2nd cuneiform and also by the 3rd metatarsal and 3rd cuneiform.

A backward thrust to the 4th and 5th metatarsals is transmitted directly to the cuboid and calcaneus. That these four bones (i.e., the bones of the lateral longitudinal arch of the foot) are not displaced backwards is to the credit of the adjoining ligaments.

Distal (3rd) phalanges

Middle (2nd) phalanges

Proximal (1st) phalanges

Metatarsal bones

LONG BONES OF
ANTERIOR HALF
OF THE FOOT

Medial (1st) cuneiform bone

Middle (2nd) cuneiform bone

Lateral (3rd) cuneiform bone

Navicular bone

Cuboid bone

5 SMALL TARSAL BONES

Talus

2 LARGE TARSAL BONES

Calcaneus
(Os calcaneum)

343 Bones of the Foot, upper or dorsal aspect

The bones are divisible, at the transverse tarsal and tarso-metatarsal joints, into three sections—anterior, middle, and posterior.

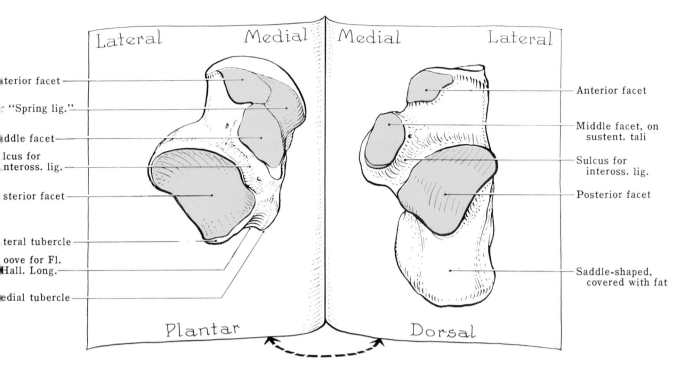

Lateral   Medial   Medial   Lateral

nterior facet —

r "Spring lig."

iddle facet —

lcus for
nteross. lig. —

sterior facet —

teral tubercle —

oove for Fl.
Hall. Long. —

edial tubercle —

— Anterior facet

— Middle facet, on
    sustent. tali

— Sulcus for
    inteross. lig.

— Posterior facet

— Saddle-shaped,
    covered with fat

Plantar   Dorsal

344   Bony Surfaces of the Talo-calcanean Joints

The under or plantar surface of the talus and the upper or dorsal surface of the calcaneus are displayed.

The joints are gliding joints, hence apposed or corresponding facets are not exact counterparts of each other, one being more extensive than the other.

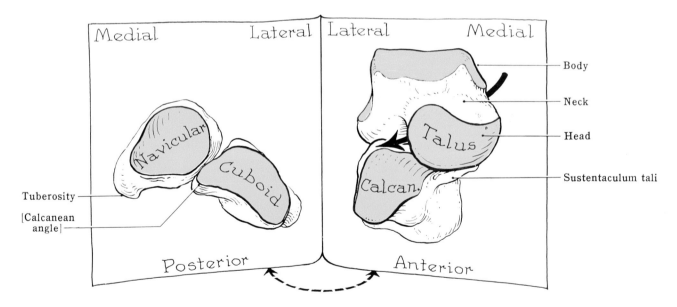

Medial   Lateral   Lateral   Medial

Navicular

Cuboid

Talus

Calcan.

Tuberosity —

[Calcanean
angle] —

— Body

— Neck

— Head

— Sustentaculum tali

Posterior   Anterior

345   Bony Surfaces of the Transverse Tarsal Joint (talo-navicular and calcaneo-cuboid)

The posterior surfaces of the navicular and cuboid bones, and the anterior surfaces of the talus and calcaneus are displayed. The black arrow traverses the tarsal sinus (tunnel), which lodges the interosseous talo-calcanean ligament.

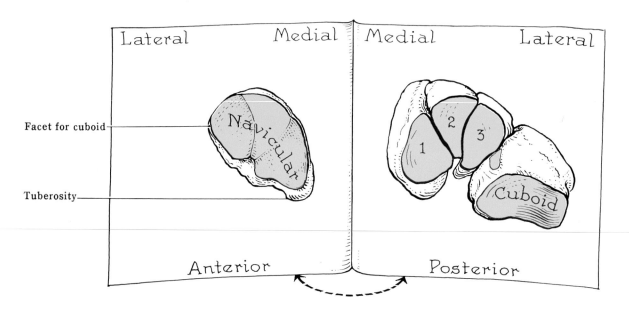

Facet for cuboid

Tuberosity

346   Bony Surfaces of the Cuneo-navicular and Cubo-navicular Joints

The anterior surface of the navicular bone, the posterior surfaces of the three cuneiform bones, and the medial and posterior surfaces of the cuboid bone are displayed.

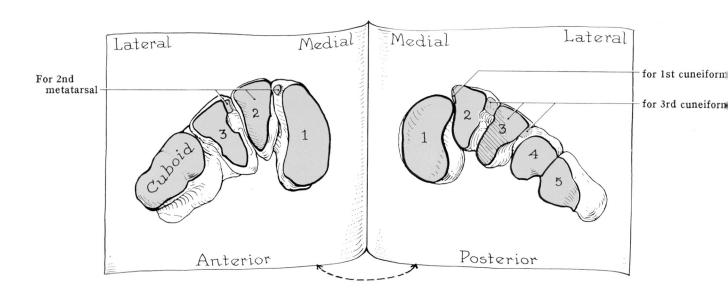

For 2nd metatarsal

for 1st cuneiform

for 3rd cuneiform

347   Bony Surfaces of the Tarso-metatarsal Joints

The anterior surfaces of the cuboid and 3 cuneiform bones, and the posterior surfaces of the bases of the 5 metatarsal bones are displayed.

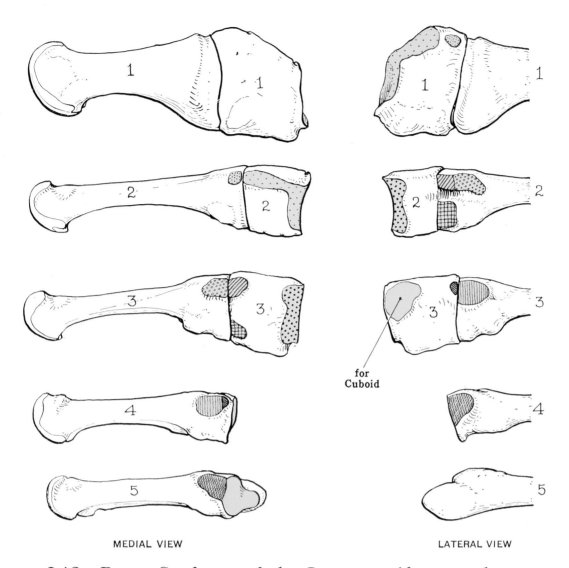

MEDIAL VIEW   LATERAL VIEW

348 Bony Surfaces of the Intercuneiform and Intermetatarsal Joints

The medial and lateral surfaces of the 3 cuneiform and 5 metatarsal bones are displayed.

The joints are gliding joints, hence apposed or corresponding facets are not exact counterparts of each other, one being more extensive than the other.

For purposes of identification, corresponding facets have been marked with corresponding designs.

a   b   c   d

349 Long and Short 1st Metatarsal Bones

The extent of the forward projection of the 1st, 2nd, and 3rd metatarsal bones varies: In (a) the 1st and 2nd metatarsals project equally far; in (b) the 2nd projects much farther than either the 1st or 3rd; in (c) the 1st is the most projecting; and in (d) the 2nd and 3rd project equally far.

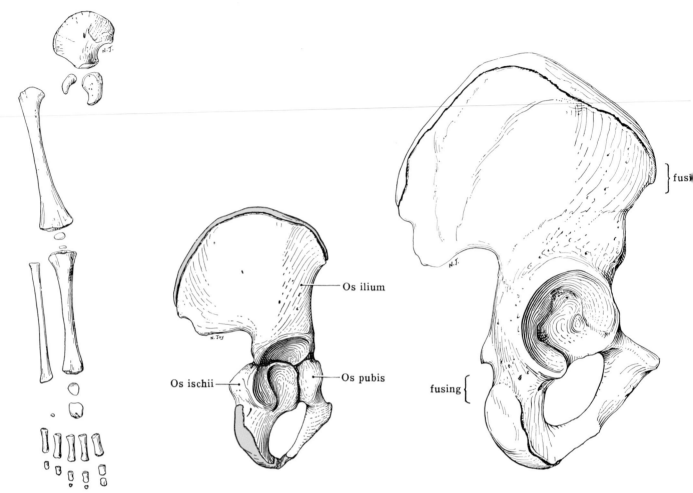

350 Bones of Lower Limb at Birth

The hip bone is in 3 primary parts—ilium, ischium, and pubis. The diaphyses of the long bones are well ossified. Certain epiphyses and certain tarsal bones have started to ossify, namely, the distal epiphysis of the femur and perhaps the proximal epiphysis of the tibia; the calcaneus, talus, and perhaps the cuboid.

351 Epiphyses of the Hip Bone

Os ilium

Os ischii

Os pubis

fusing {

} fusi

Hip Bone, aged about 5 years

The triradiate cartilage in the acetabulum is ossified and fused before the end of the 16th year. A bar of cartilage that unites the pubic and ischial rami ossifies about the 9th year. There is a cartilaginous epiphysis along the whole length of the iliac crest and one on the ischial tuberosity and ramus.

(*All ages given in figures 350—356 are for males.*)

Hip Bone, aged about 19 years

The acetabulum and the pubic arch now consolidated. The epiphysis along iliac crest and that on the ischial tubero are ossified and fusion is beginning—in one, anteriorly; in the other, superio Fusion starts in many cases before the 1 year: most (80%) crests are partly fused 18th year and most tuberosities by the 19 Complete fusion is never delayed beyond 23rd year (*T. W. McKern & T. D. Stewa* (*See also figures 277 & 278.*)

OSSIFICATION—EPIPHYSES

ANTERIOR VIEW

Head

Greater
trochanter

POSTERIOR VIEW

EPIPHYSES DETACHED, POSTERIOR VIEW.

352   Epiphyses at the Proximal End of the Femur

The epiphysis of the head fits like a cap on to the slightly conical end of the diaphysis. The apposed surfaces are billowy—pitted and ridged—as at other epiphyses. The articular cartilage of the head is carried for a few mm. on to the inferior aspect of the neck, compare the humerus (fig. 101). The epiphysis of the greater trochanter lies above the site of confluence of the shaft and neck. That of the lesser trochanter is a thick scale.

The epiphysis of the head begins to ossify during the 1st year; that of the greater trochanter before the 5th year; and that of the lesser trochanter before the 14th year. These have in most cases fused completely with the shaft before the end of the 18th year, and in all cases by the 20th (*McK. & S.*).

OSSIFICATION—EPIPHYSES

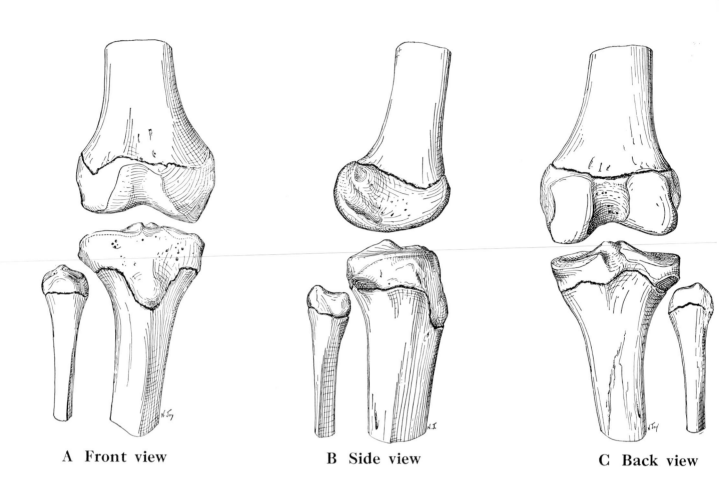

A Front view   **B Side view**   **C Back view**

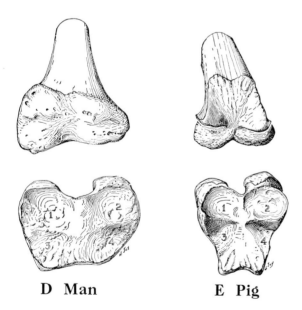

D Man   **E Pig**

353 Epiphyses in the Region of the Knee Joint

A, B, C.—The epiphyseal plate splits the adductor tubercle, skims above the patellar trochlea, shaves the cartilage of the lateral condyle, and follows along the intercondylar line.

The proximal epiphyseal plate of the tibia shaves the fibular facet and passes below the groove for the Semi-membranosus tendon. Anteriorly, it dips down like a tongue to include the tuberosity. The epiphyseal plate of the fibula lies well above the neck.

The distal epiphysis of the femur begins to ossify before birth; that of the tibia soon follows it; that of the fibula begins to ossify before the 5th year. These 3 epiphyses at the knee have usually completely fused with their respective diaphyses before the end of the 19th year, and always by the 22nd—that of the tibia may be the 23rd (*McK. & S.*). A separate centre for the tibial tuberosity may appear before puberty.

D, E.—A quadruped walks with bent knees and the distal epiphysis of its femur has 4 deep pits into which 4 prongs project. In man, who walks erect, these are replaced by shallow impressions and slight bosses.

OSSIFICATION—EPIPHYSES

Epiphyseal plate

Synovial folds

Epiphysis

1st metatarsal

Nancy Joy

Epiphyseal plate

Synovial folds

2nd metatarsal bone

Epiphysis

Nancy Joy

Epiphysis of calcaneus

ANTERIOR VIEW

EDIAL VIEW

54 Distal Epiphyses the Tibia and Fibula

he epiphyseal plate of the fibula lies at
level of the ankle joint, and, therefore,
essarily below the level of the epiphyseal
te of the tibia. The tibial epiphysis starts
ossify during the 1st year; the fibular
ing the 1st or 2nd year (*C. C. Francis*
l.). Fusion is usually complete by the
h or 18th year, and in all cases by the
h (*McK. & S.*).

355 Longitudinal Sections through the Feet of Children aged about 4 and 10 years

Observe:

1. From the younger foot, that epiphyses of long bones (e.g., tibia, metatarsals, and phalanges) ossify like short bones (i.e., carpal and tarsal bones)—the ossific centres being
   enveloped in cartilage; and that ossification has already extended to the surface of the
   larger tarsal bones.

2. From the older foot, that ossification has spread to the dorsal and plantar surfaces of all
   the tarsal bones in view; and that cartilage persists on the articular surfaces only.

3. The traction epiphysis of the calcaneus for the tendo Achillis and plantar aponeurosis.
   This starts to ossify between the ages of 6 and 10 years (C. C. Francis).

4. That the 1st metatarsal bone behaves as a phalanx in that its epiphysis is at its base and
   not at its head like the 2nd and other metatarsal bones (c.f. the hand, fig. 104).

5. The synovial folds projecting between the articular cartilages where they are liable to be
   pinched.

OSSIFICATION—EPIPHYSES

A Sesamoid Bone in Tibialis Posterior Tendon was found in 80 or 23% of 348 adult feet; 42 were paired and 38 unpaired (C. E. Storton).

Accessory Navicular Bone (Tibiale Externum). The tuberosity of the navicular bone, to which Tibialis Posterior is largely inserted, appeared as an independent bone in 4.1% of 3619 men examined by X-ray (R. I. Harris and T. Beath).

Os Trigonum. The lateral (posterior) tubercle of the talus has a separate centre of ossification, which appears between the ages of 7 and 13 years. Half (50%) of these fuse at the age of 12 years. (*C. C. F.*) When this fails to fuse with the body of the talus, as in the left bone of this pair, it is called an os trigonum. It was found in 43 or 7.7% of 558 adult feet; 22 were paired, 21 were unpaired. (*C. E. S.*)

Tendon of
Peroneus
Longus

A Sesamoid Bone in Peroneus Longus Tendon was found in 26% of 92 feet. In this specimen it is bipartite, and Peroneus Longus has an additional attachment to the 5th metatarsal bone. (*C.E.S.*)

A Bipartite Medial Cuneiform Bone, in dorsal and plantar halves, is not common.

356   Anomalies of the Tarsal Bones

*The Vertebrae and
the Vertebral Column*

FUNCTIONS: PARTS:

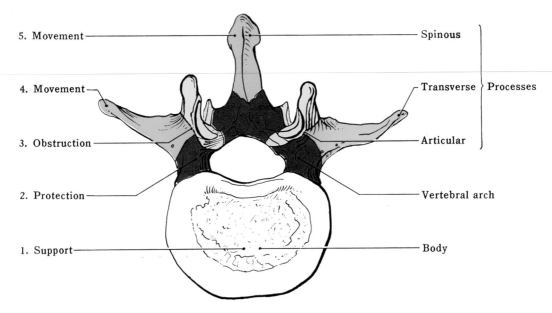

5. Movement———————————————————— Spinous

4. Movement——— ———————————— Transverse ⎫ Processes

3. Obstruction——— ——————————— Articular

2. Protection——— ——————————— Vertebral arch

1. Support——————————————————— Body

357   Functions of Constituent Parts of a Vertebra

A typical vertebra comprises the following parts:

1. A columnar body, situated anteriorly or ventrally. Its function, like that of the femur and
   tibia, is to support weight. Like them and other long bones, it is narrow about its middle
   and expanded at both ends. These ends also are articular and during growth have epiphyses
   (fig. 361.)

2. A vertebral arch, placed behind the body. With the body this arch encloses a foramen,
   called the vertebral foramen. Collectively, the vertebral foramina constitute the vertebral
   canal wherein lodges the spinal cord. The function of a vertebral arch is to afford protection
   to the cord much as the bones of the vault of the skull afford protection to the brain.

3. Three processes—2 transverse and 1 spinous. These project from the vertebral arch like
   spokes from a capstan. They afford attachment to muscles. Indeed, they are the levers
   that help to move the vertebrae.

4. Four articular processes—2 superior and 2 inferior. These project upwards and downwards
   respectively from the arch and come into apposition with the corresponding processes of
   the vertebrae above and below. Their function is to restrict movements to certain directions,
   or at least to decree in what directions movements may be permitted, and they prevent
   the vertebrae from slipping forwards. When one rises from the flexed position, they bear
   weight temporarily. The lower articular processes of the 5th lumbar vertebra bear weight
   even in the erect posture (fig. 383).

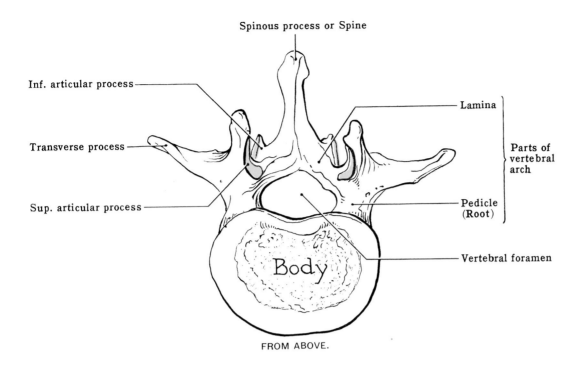

Spinous process or Spine

Inf. articular process

Transverse process

Sup. articular process

Lamina

Parts of vertebral arch

Pedicle (Root)

Vertebral foramen

Body

FROM ABOVE.

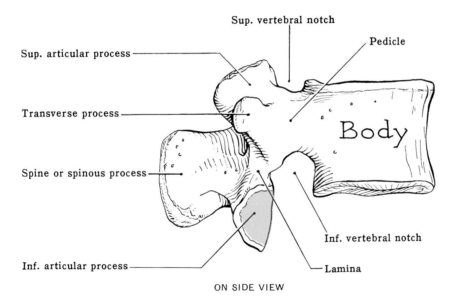

Sup. vertebral notch

Pedicle

Sup. articular process

Transverse process

Spine or spinous process

Inf. articular process

Body

Inf. vertebral notch

Lamina

ON SIDE VIEW

358 A Vertebra

(Second lumbar vertebra.)

Observe:

1. The vertebral arch. It consists of two stout, rounded pedicles, one on each side, which spring from the body and which are united posteriorly by two flat plates or laminae.

2. A small notch above the pedicle and a larger one below it, called the superior and the inferior vertebral notch. When two vertebrae are in articulation, the two adjacent vertebral notches become an intervertebral foramen for the transmission of a spinal nerve and its accompanying intervertebral vessels.

3. Obviously, each articular process has an articular facet—the two terms are not synonymous.

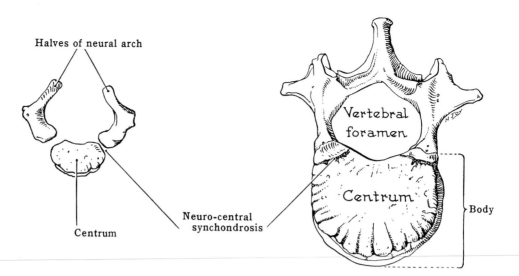

Halves of neural arch

Centrum

Neuro-central
synchondrosis

Vertebral
foramen

Centrum

Body

359 A Vertebra at Birth

360 A Vertebra in Childhoo

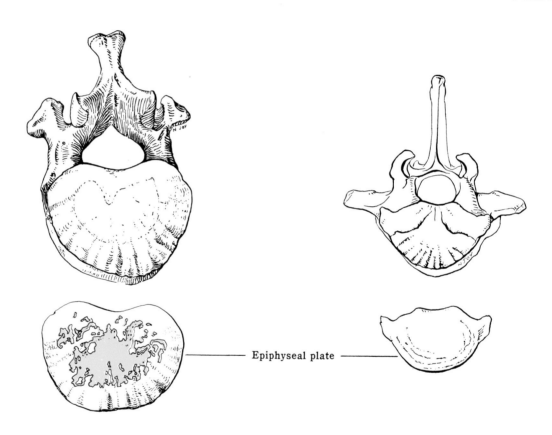

Epiphyseal plate

361 A Vertebra in Adolescence

362 A Vertebra of a sheep

Observe:

1. At birth each typical vertebra consists of three bony parts, united by hyaline cartilage
   (fig. 359).

2. The synchondrosis between the two halves of the neural arch undergoes synostosis before
   the neuro-central synchondroses (fig. 360).

3. The body of a vertebra, being the upper and lower epiphyseal plates and the part of the
   vertebra between them, includes the entire centrum and the anterior ends of the neural
   arch. The rest of the neural arch is the vertebral arch.

4. The epiphyseal plate is a plate of hyaline cartilage and a circumferential bony ring—that
   is, in man (fig. 361). In other mammals it is a complete bony plate (fig. 362).

5. The apposed surfaces of the plate and centrum are corrugated. Their interlocking acts as a
   nonslipping device.

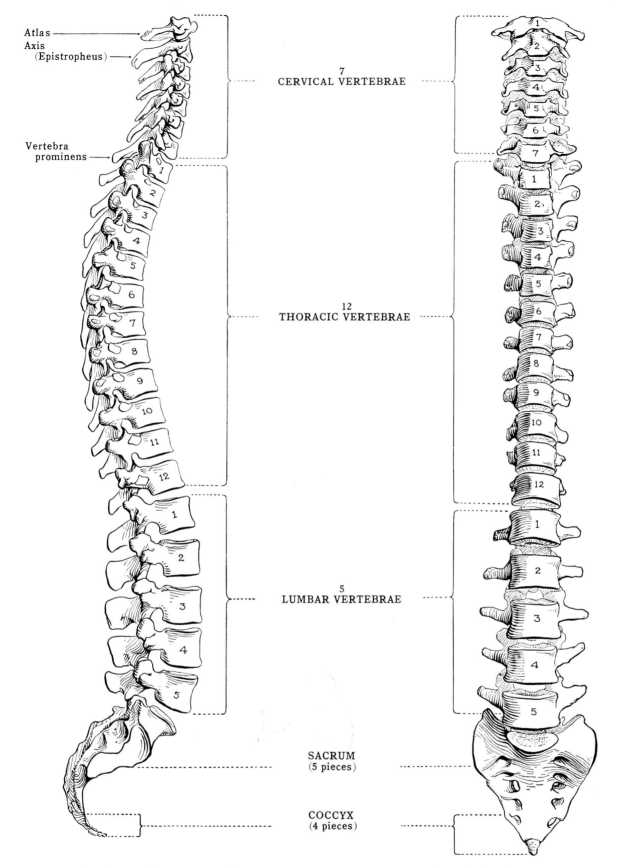

Atlas

Axis
(Epistropheus)

7
CERVICAL VERTEBRAE

Vertebra
prominens

12
THORACIC VERTEBRAE

5
LUMBAR VERTEBRAE

SACRUM
(5 pieces)

COCCYX
(4 pieces)

363   Vertebral Column, side view   **364   Vertebral Column, front view**

Observe:

The vertebral column comprises 24 true or pre-sacral
vertebrae and 2 composite vertebrae—the sacrum and the
coccyx. Of the 24 pre-sacral vertebrae, 12 (50 percent)
support ribs and therefore are thoracic; of the other 12, 7
are in the neck and 5 are in the lumbar region.

Vertebrae lying behind bony cavities (the thoracic vertebrae
behind the thoracic cavity, and the sacrum and coccyx

behind the pelvic cavity) are concave forwards; but elsewhere (in the cervical and lumbar regions), by way of compensation, they are convex forwards.

3. The transverse processes of the atlas spread widely; those of
C. 7 spread almost as far; those of C. 2 to C. 6 much less. The
spread diminishes progressively from T. 1 to T. 12. In the
lumbar region it is greatest at L. 3.

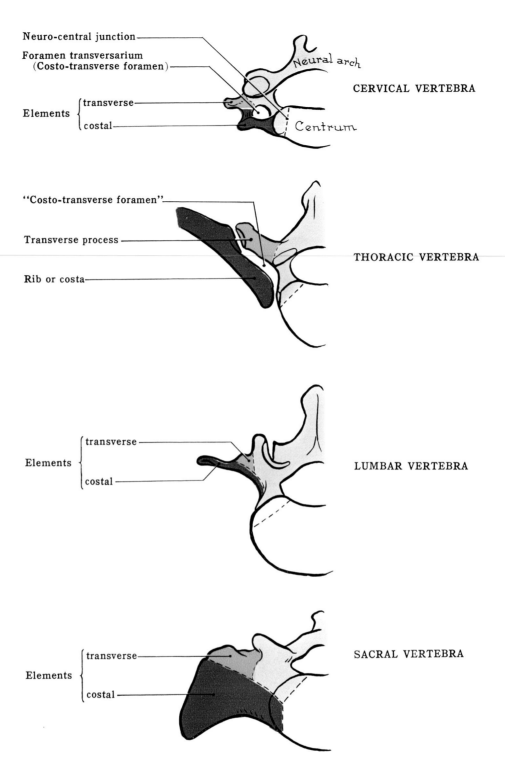

Neuro-central junction

Foramen transversarium
(Costo-transverse foramen)

Elements { transverse
            costal

Neural arch

CERVICAL VERTEBRA

Centrum

"Costo-transverse foramen"

Transverse process

Rib or costa

THORACIC VERTEBRA

Elements { transverse
            costal

LUMBAR VERTEBRA

Elements { transverse
            costal

SACRAL VERTEBRA

365   Diagram of the Homologous Parts of the Vertebrae

Red = rib or costal element; blue = neural arch
    and its processes; uncoloured = centrum.

Note:

1. A rib or costa is a free element in the thoracic region. In the cervical region it is represented
   by the anterior part of a transverse process; in the lumbar region likewise by the anterior
   part of a transverse process; and in the sacrum by the anterior part of the pars lateralis
   (lateral mass, fig. 373).

2. The heads of the ribs (thoracic region) articulate with the sides of the bodies of the vertebrae posterior to the neuro-central junctions, i.e., not with the centra, but with the neural
   arches.

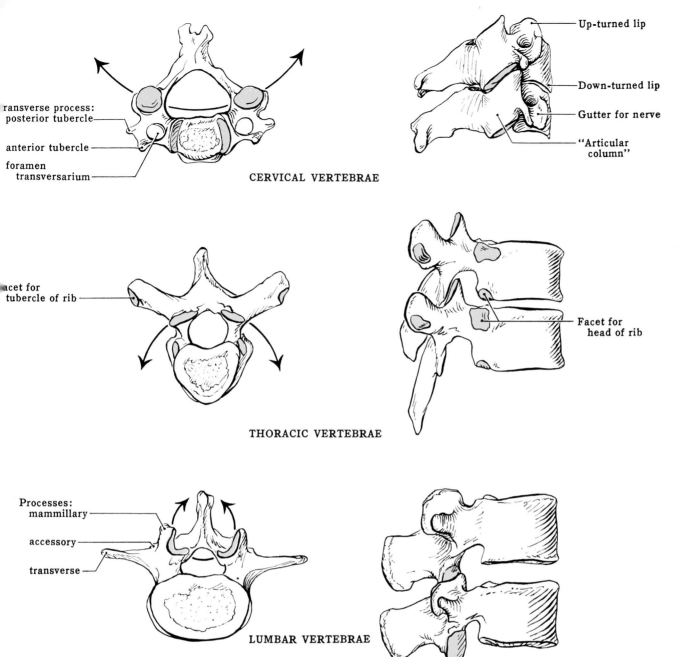

CERVICAL VERTEBRAE

transverse process:
posterior tubercle

anterior tubercle

foramen
transversarium

Up-turned lip

Down-turned lip

Gutter for nerve

"Articular
column"

THORACIC VERTEBRAE

Facet for
tubercle of rib

Facet for
head of rib

LUMBAR VERTEBRAE

Processes:
mammillary

accessory

transverse

366 Distinguishing Features and the Movements of the Free Vertebrae

Distinctive Features:

Foramina transversaria are distinctive of all cervical verte-brae; facets for the heads of ribs are distinctive of all thoracic vertebrae; the absence of these proclaims a vertebra to be lumbar.

Typical Features:

1. The *Bodies* of cervical and lumbar vertebrae are greater in the transverse diameter than in the antero-posterior, and the vertebral foramina are triangular. In thoracic vertebrae the two diameters are about equal and the foramen is circular. Further, the superior surface of the body of a cervical vertebra ends at each side in an up-turned lip, hence it is concave from side to side. The inferior surface ends anteriorly in a down-turned lip. The superior and inferior surfaces of thoracic and lumbar bodies are flat.

2. A *Transverse Process* in the cervical region points laterally, downwards and forwards, and ends in two tubercles with a gutter between them. In the thoracic region it points

laterally, backwards and upwards, has a facet for the tubercle of a rib, and is stout. In the lumbar region it points laterally, and is long and slender.

3. *Spinous Processes* are bifid if cervical, spine-like if thoracic, and oblong if lumbar.

4. *Articular Processes* in the cervical region collectively form a cylinder which is in part weight-bearing; it is cut obliquely into segments. In the thoracic and lumbar regions, the superior articular facets lie behind the pedicles, and the inferior facets are in front of the laminae.

Superior Articular Facets in the cervical region face mainly upwards; in the thoracic region mainly backwards; in the lumbar region mainly medially. The change in direction is gradual from cervical to thoracic, but from thoracic to lumbar it is abrupt.

Movements: In all three regions the articular processes permit flexion and extension and side to side movement. Cervical verte-brae allow one to look sideways up. Thoracic vertebrae allow of medial and lateral rotation, but lumbar vertebrae do not.

Posterior arch:
posterior tubercle

groove for vertebral a.

Anterior arch:
facet for dens

anterior tubercle

Lateral mass:
tubercle for transverse lig.

superior articular process

foramen transversarium

transverse process

Atlas

Inferior articular process

Transverse process

Superior articular facet

Dens (Odontoid process)

Axis

Transverse process:
posterior tubercle

costo-transverse bar

anterior tubercle

C3

Foramen transversarium

C4

Spine

Lip

Body

C5

Articular process:
inferior

superior

Carotid tubercle

C6

"Vestigial
anterior tubercle"

C7

367 Cervical Vertebrae, from above

367, 368 Cervical Vertebrae

Observe:

Numbers 3, 4, 5 and 6 are typical; 1, 2 and 7 are peculiar

1. The body, transversely elongated. It is of equal depth in front and behind. Its upper surface, resembling a seat with up-turned side arms, which bear facets, and rounded front but no back. The absence of a body for the atlas—the missing body having joined the axis as the dens,—and the presence of an anterior arch which lies in front of the dens

2. The vertebral foramen, in this most mobile section of the column, large and triangular. It is largest in the atlas

3. The superior and inferior vertebral notches, nearly equal in depth.

4. The spinous process, short and bifid, except that of the atlas which is reduced to a tubercle, and that of C. 7 (vertebra prominens) which is long and nonbifid. That of the axis is massive.

5. The vertebral arch, also massive in the axis but, as the posterior arch, slender in the atlas.

6. The transverse processes, short, perforated and ending laterally in anterior and posterior tubercles with a gutter between them. Those of the atlas and of C. 7 are longer and have but one (posterior) tubercle; so has the axis, but it is short.

7. Three paired articular facets, viz., the superior facets of the axis and the inferior and superior facets of the atlas are in series with the facets at the sides of the upper and lower surfaces of the bodies.

anterior arch

anterior tubercle

(Odontoid process) Dens

Axis

transverse process:
anterior tubercle

costo-transverse bar

posterior tubercle

3

gutter for nerve

4

Lip

5

Lip

carotid tubercle

6

7

N.JOY

FRONT VIEW

for Vertebral art.

Posterior
tubercle

Anterior
tubercle
of atlas

Axis

Spinous
processes
or spines

Column of
articular
processes

Anterior
tubercles of
transverse
processes
of vertebrae
C. 3, 4, 5 & 6

Lamina

Carotid
tubercle

Spinous
processes

C. 7

JOY

SIDE VIEW

368   Cervical Vertebrae

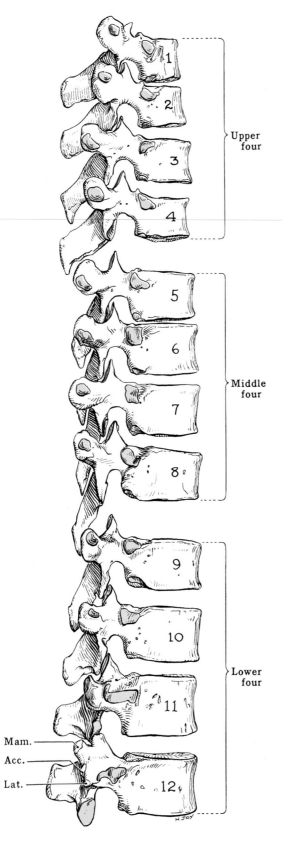

369 Thoracic Vertebrae, side view

369, 370 Thoracic Vertebrae

Observe:

1. The middle 4 are typical; those at the ends have cervical and lumbar features respectively.

2. The body, deeper dorsally than ventrally; with flat upper and lower surfaces; the surface area (weight-bearing surface) increasing from T.1 to T.12. (Indeed, from C.3 to L.5.) The triangular shape of the middle 4 (i.e., equal antero-posterior and transverse diameters), the transverse diameter increasing towards the cervical and lumbar ends of the series.

3. The rib facet at the upper postero-lateral angle of the body encroaching on the lower postero-lateral angle of the body above; except the facets of (T.10), 11 and 12 which are on the pedicles.

4. The superior vertebral notch, present on T.1 only.

5. The vertebral foramen, circular and smaller than a finger-ring, and becoming triangular towards the cervical and lumbar ends.

6. The spines of the middle 4, which are long, overlapping and nearly vertical. Those of 1, 2 and 11, 12 which are nearly horizontal; and those of 3, 4 and 9, 10 which are oblique.

7. The stretch of the transverse processes diminishing progressively from T.1 to T.12. T.1 to T.10 having rib facets on the transverse processes. These are concave and placed anteriorly on T.1 to T.7; flat and superiorly placed on T.8 to T.10.

8. The cervical features of T.1—possession of superior vertebral notches, and upturned side lips on the body.

9. The lumbar features of T.12—the lateral direction of the inferior articular processes; possession of mamillary, accessory and lateral tubercles.

369.1 Demonstrating the small size of a vertebral foramen.

Upper four   Middle four   Lower four

370   **Thoracic Vertebrae, from above**

Mamillary ⎫
Accessory ⎬ Processes
Transverse ⎭

371, 372   Lumbar Vertebrae

Observe:

1. The kidney-shaped bodies, greater in transverse diameter than in antero-posterior. Bodies L.1 and L.2 deeper behind; L.4 and L.5 deeper in front; L.3 transitional, being sometimes deeper behind and sometimes deeper in front.

2. The vertebral foramina, small and triangular, and having pinched lateral angles in L.5.

3. The slight superior vertebral notches.

4. The large, oblong, and horizontal spinous processes.

5. The long, slender, horizontal transverse processes. That of L.3 projecting furthest; that of L.5 spreading forward on to the body, being conical and its apex having an upward tilt. The mamillary process (for origin of Multifidus) on the superior articular process. The accessory process (for insertion of Longissimus) on the transverse process.

6. The superior articular processes, facing each other and grasping the inferior processes of the vertebra above. The inferior articular processes, close together in L.1, but far apart in L.5 and facing more anteriorly.

371   Lumbar Vertebrae, from above

Mam.

Acc.

Trans.

Superior
articular
process

Inferior
articular
process

Superior
articular
process

Inferior
articular
process

FROM BEHIND

FROM THE SIDE

372 Lumbar Vertebrae

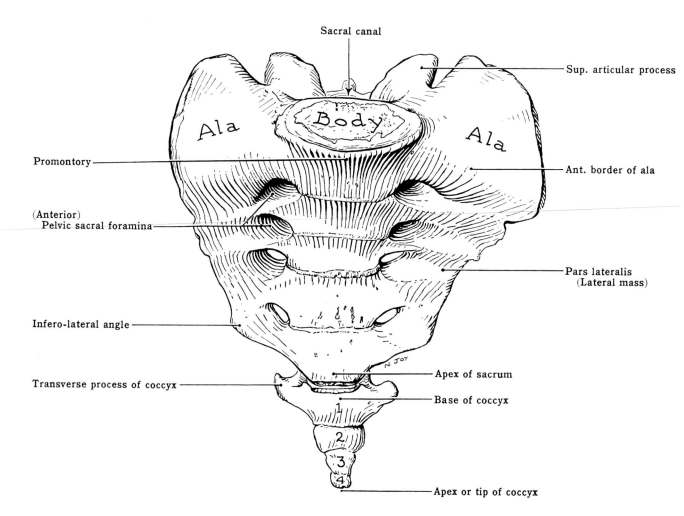

Sacral canal

Sup. articular process

Ala · Body · Ala

Promontory

Ant. border of ala

(Anterior)
Pelvic sacral foramina

Pars lateralis
(Lateral mass)

Infero-lateral angle

Transverse process of coccyx

Apex of sacrum

Base of coccyx

Apex or tip of coccyx

373   Sacrum and Coccyx, pelvic surface and base

373.1   Sacrum in Youth

The costal elements (fig. 365) begin to fuse with each other about puberty. The bodies begin to fuse with each other from below upwards about the 17th–18th year, fusion being complete by the 23rd year. A gap, however, may persist between the 3rd and 2nd bodies until the 24th year, and between the 2nd and 1st until the 33rd year. (McKern & Stewart.)

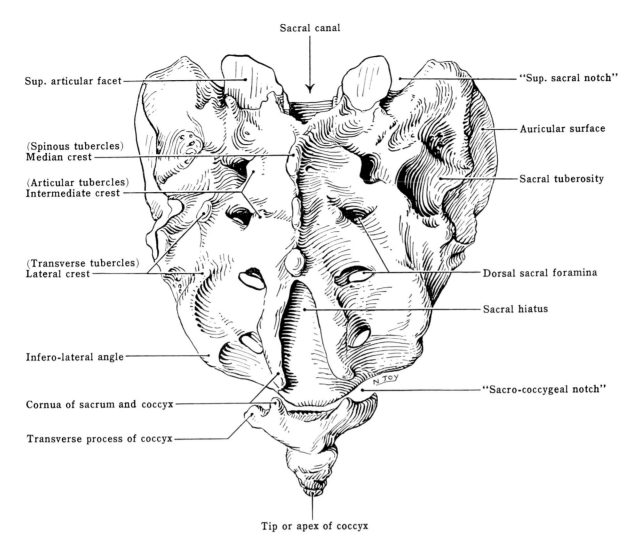

Sacral canal

Sup. articular facet

"Sup. sacral notch"

Auricular surface

(Spinous tubercles)
Median crest

(Articular tubercles)
Intermediate crest

Sacral tuberosity

(Transverse tubercles)
Lateral crest

Dorsal sacral foramina

Sacral hiatus

Infero-lateral angle

"Sacro-coccygeal notch"

Cornua of sacrum and coccyx

Transverse process of coccyx

Tip or apex of coccyx

374   Sacrum and Coccyx, dorsal surface

Observe, on *Anterior View* (fig. 373):

1. The 5 sacral bodies, demarcated by 4 transverse lines which end laterally in 4 pairs of pelvic (anterior) sacral foramina.

2. The foramina of the two sides, approximately equidistant throughout. Their margins rounded laterally, but sharp elsewhere, indicating the courses of the emerging nerves.

3. The coccyx having 4 pieces. The 1st piece having a pair of transverse processes and a pair of cornua; the other 3 pieces being nodular.

Observe, on *Posterior View* (fig. 374):

4. The absence of the 4th and 5th sacral spines and laminae.

5. The superior articular processes, the intermediate crest, and the sacral and coccygeal cornua are serially homologous;

6. so, likewise, are the "superior sacral notch", the 4 dorsal sacral foramina, and the "sacro-coccygeal notch";

7. and, likewise, the postero-superior angle of the ala, the lateral crest, the inferolateral angle, and the transverse process of the coccyx.

8. A straight probe can be passed through a lower dorsal foramen, across the sacral canal, and through a pelvic foramen. Side view see figure 222.

375 A Half Vertebra

The entire right half of the 3rd thoracic vertebra and the corresponding rib are absent. The left lamina and the spine are fused throughout with those of T.4, and the left intervertebral foramen is reduced in size. Observe the associated scoliosis (lateral curvature). (From the Anatomy Department, University of Manitoba, courtesy of Professor I. Maclaren Thompson.)

376 Instance of Failure of Two Halves of a Vertebral Arch to undergo Synostosis

377 Congenital Synostosis of Axis and 3rd Cervical Vertebra

It is not very rare for the laminae and articular processes of these two bones to be fused together.

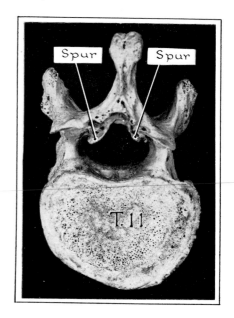

378 Ossifying Ligamenta Flava

Sharp, bony spurs commonly grow from the laminae caudally into the ligg. flava thereby reducing the lengths of these elastic bands. Hence, when the vertebral column is flexed, they are likely to be torn. Restricted to the thoracic and lumbar regions, commonest and largest on T. 11, they diminish in size and frequency cranially to T. 1 and caudally to L. 5 (*G. T. Ho*).

379 "Kissing Spines"

In macerated vertebral columns contact facets, either horizontal or obliquely overlapping, between lumbar spines (1 & 2), 2 & 3, 3 & 4, and 4 & 5 are commonly found (fig. 386). (*J.C.B.G.*)

ANOMALIES OF THE VERTEBRAE

380   A Transitional Lumbo-sacral Vertebra

In this instance, the 1st sacral vertebra is partly free (lumbarized). Not uncommonly the 5th lumbar vertebra is partly fused to the sacrum (sacralized).

381   Maldevelopment of the Sacrum

The left side of the sacrum is imperfectly developed.

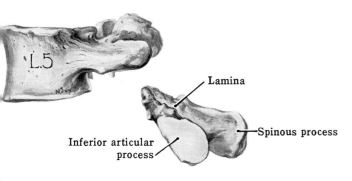

Lamina

Spinous process

Inferior articular process

SIDE VIEW

DORSAL VIEW

382   A Bipartite Fifth Lumbar Vertebra

383   Spondylolisthesis

382, 383. Commonly (in 5% of vertebral columns) the 5th lumbar vertebra is in two pieces, the inferior articular processes, the laminae, and the spine forming a separate unit. Hence, the body and the superimposed vertebrae tend to slide forwards (spondylolisthesis). Less often the 4th lumbar vertebra is bipartite. (*See T. D. Stewart.*)

ANOMALIES OF THE VERTEBRAE

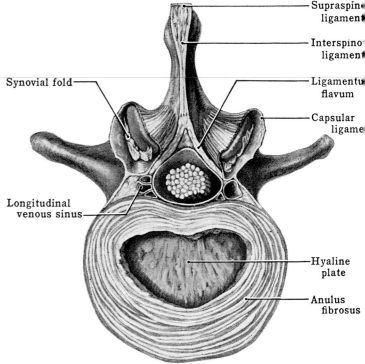

384   Diagram of an Intervertebral Disc (Fibro-cartilage)

To illustrate the cushioning value of the nucleus pulposus and the presence of a thin, hyaline epiphyseal plate.

385   An Intervertebral Disc and Ligaments, on cross section

The nucleus pulposus has been scooped out and the cartilaginous epiphyseal plate exposed.

Observe:

1. The rings of the anulus fibrosus, least numerous behind.
2. The continuity of the following ligaments—capsular, flavum, interspinous, and supraspinous.
3. The synovial fold, containing a pad of fat, such as is present in all synovial joints.
4. The longitudinal vertebral venous sinuses which extend extradurally throughout the length of the vertebral canal (fig. 390).
5. The cauda equina of the spinal cord (not labelled) lying free within the subarachnoid space.

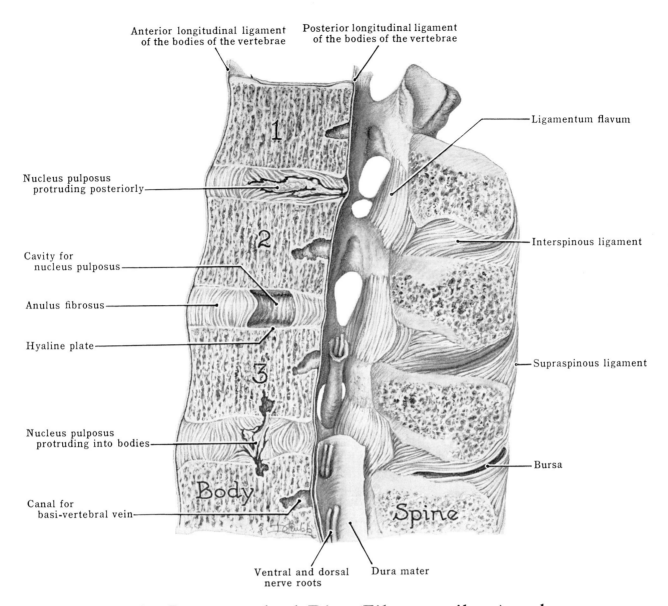

Anterior longitudinal ligament
of the bodies of the vertebrae

Posterior longitudinal ligament
of the bodies of the vertebrae

Ligamentum flavum

Nucleus pulposus
protruding posteriorly

Interspinous ligament

Cavity for
nucleus pulposus

Anulus fibrosus

Hyaline plate

Supraspinous ligament

Nucleus pulposus
protruding into bodies

Bursa

Canal for
basi-vertebral vein

Ventral and dorsal
nerve roots

Dura mater

386   An Intervertebral Disc (Fibro-cartilage) and Ligaments, on median section

Observe:

1. The nucleus pulposus of the normal disc between the 2nd and 3rd vertebrae has been scooped out from the enclosing anulus fibrosus.

2. The ligamentum flavum, extending from the upper border and adjacent part of the posterior aspect of one lamina to the lower border and adjacent part of the anterior aspect of the lamina above, and extending laterally to the intervertebral foramen which it bounds posteriorly.

3. The interspinous ligament, uniting obliquely the upper and lower borders of two adjacent spines.

4. The adventitious bursa between the 3rd and 4th lumbar spines, acquired presumably as the result of habitual hyperextension which brings the lumbar spines into contact, as in fig. 379.

5. Two degenerative changes—(a) The pulp of the disc between the 1st and 2nd vertebrae has herniated backwards through the anulus, and (b) the pulp of the disc between the 3rd and 4th vertebrae has herniated through the cartilaginous epiphyseal plates into the bodies of the vertebrae above and below.

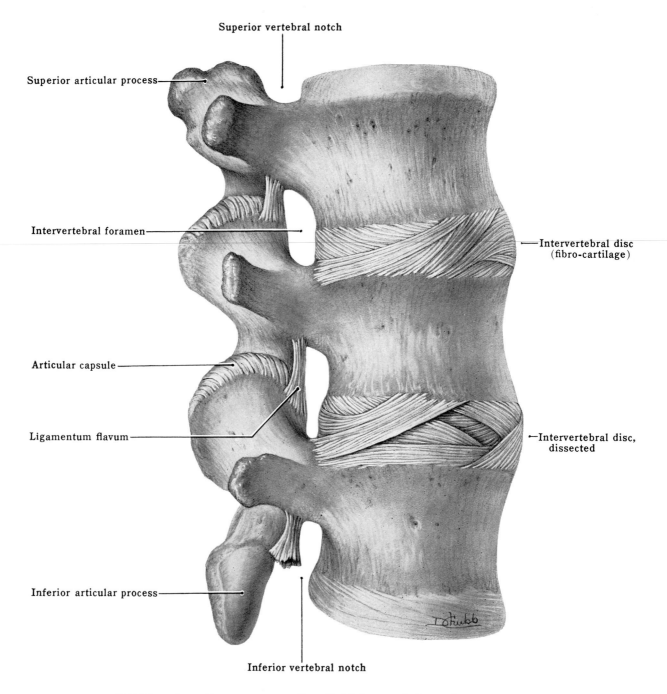

Superior vertebral notch

Superior articular process

Intervertebral foramen

Articular capsule

Ligamentum flavum

Inferior articular process

Intervertebral disc
(fibro-cartilage)

Intervertebral disc,
dissected

Inferior vertebral notch

387 An Intervertebral Disc, side view

Sections have been removed from the superficial layers of the lower disc, in order to show the directions of the fibres.

Observe:

1. The anulus fibrosus, resembling the flat muscles of the abdominal wall in being arranged in layers of parallel fibres which criss-cross those of the next layer.

2. An intervertebral foramen, resulting from the apposition of a superior and an inferior vertebral notch, bounded above and below by pedicles, in front by an intervertebral disc and parts of the two bodies united by that disc, and behind by a capsular ligament and parts of the two articular processes united by that capsular ligament. Further, the anterior part of the capsule is strengthened by the lateral border of the ligamentum flavum.

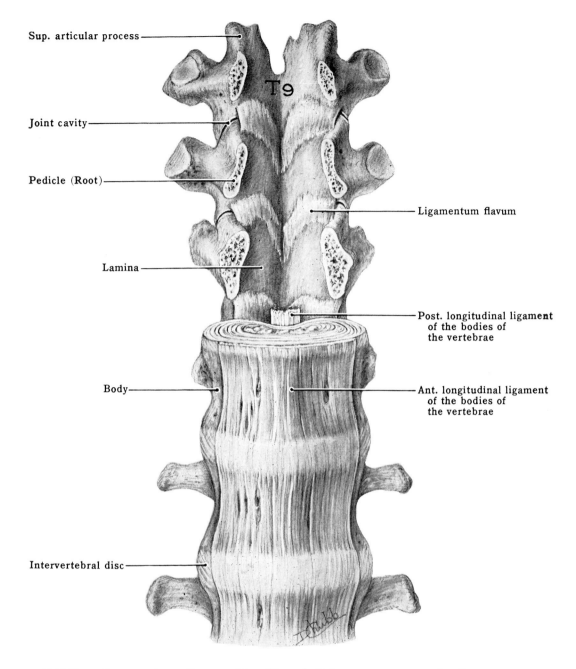

Sup. articular process

Joint cavity

Pedicle (Root)

Lamina

Body

Intervertebral disc

T9

Ligamentum flavum

Post. longitudinal ligament
of the bodies of
the vertebrae

Ant. longitudinal ligament
of the bodies of
the vertebrae

388 Anterior Longitudinal Ligament and the Ligamenta Flava, anterior view

The pedicles of the 9th, 10th, and 11th thoracic vertebrae have been sawn through and their bodies discarded.

Note:

1. The anterior and posterior longitudinal ligaments are ligaments of the bodies; the ligamenta flava are ligaments of the vertebral arches.

2. The anterior longitudinal ligaments are broad, strong, fibrous bands. They are attached to the intervertebral discs and to the adjacent parts of the fronts of the bodies. They have foramina for veins and arteries passing from and to the bodies.

3. The ligamenta flava, composed of yellow or elastic fibres, extend between adjacent laminae. Those of opposite sides meet and blend in the median plane. They extend laterally to the articular processes where they blend with the anterior fibres of the capsule of the joint. Being elastic, they tend, at all times, to restore the vertebral column to the extended or erect position. Above, they are in series with the posterior atlanto-axial and posterior atlanto-occipital membranes.

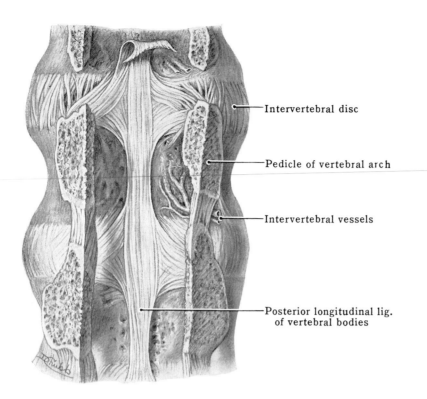

———Intervertebral disc

———Pedicle of vertebral arch

———Intervertebral vessels

———Posterior longitudinal lig.
of vertebral bodies

389 Posterior Longitudina[l]
Ligament, posterior view

The vertebral arches have been sawn thro[ugh]
and largely removed.

Observe:

1. This taut but somewhat flimsy band passing [from]
   disc to disc, spanning the posterior surfaces of [the]
   bodies of the vertebrae, and rendering smooth [the]
   anterior wall of the vertebral canal.

2. The diamond shape taken by the ligament be[hind]
   each disc, where it both gives and receives fibers[.]

3. Between the ligament and a vertebral body [a]
   plexus of veins which receives the basiverte[bral]
   vein from the body (fig. 386), communicates [with]
   the longitudinal vertebral venous sinus on e[ach]
   side, and drains by way of the intervertebral ve[in.]

The ligament extends to the sacrum below [and]
becomes the strong membrana tectoria above [(fig.]
565).

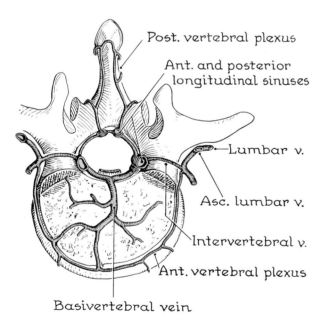

Post. vertebral plexus

Ant. and posterior
longitudinal sinuses

———Lumbar v.

———Asc. lumbar v.

———Intervertebral v.

———Ant. vertebral plexus

Basivertebral vein

390 Diagram of the Vertebral
Venous Plexuses

The Internal Plexus: The vertebral canal contains a plexus of [thin-]
walled, valveless veins which surround like a basket-work the [dura]
mater of the spinal cord and also the posterior longitudinal ligam[ent.]
Anterior and posterior longitudinal channels (ant. and post. lo[ngi-]
tudinal venous sinuses) can be discerned in this plexus. Above, [the]
plexus communicates through the foramen magnum with the [occi-]
pital and basilar sinuses. At each spinal segment the plexus rec[eives]
veins from the spinal cord and a basivertebral vein from the [body]
of a vertebra. The plexus in turn is drained by intervertebral v[eins]
which pass through the intervertebral and sacral foramina to [the]
vertebral, intercostal, lumbar, and lateral sacral veins.

The External Plexus: Through the body of each vertebra c[ome]
veins which form a meagre anterior vertebral plexus, and thr[ough]
the ligamenta flava pass veins which form a well marked post[erior]
vertebral plexus.

In the cervical region, these plexuses communicate freely [with]
the occipital and profunda cervicis veins which receive from [the]
sigmoid sinus the mastoid and condyloid emissary veins. In [the]
thoracic, lumbar, and pelvic regions the azygos (or hemiazy[gos),]
the ascending lumbar, and the lateral sacral veins respecti[vely]
further link segment to segment. (*See Batson, O. V.*)

The Thorax

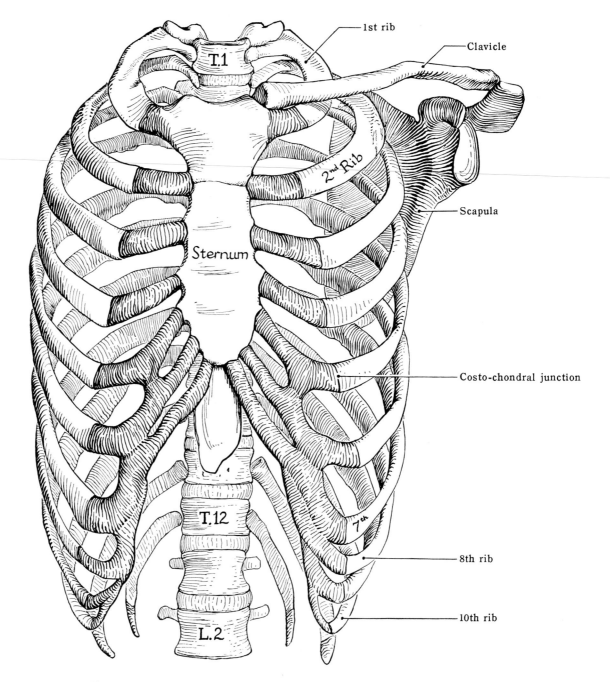

391 Bony Thorax, anterior aspect

Observe from figures 391 and 392:

1. The component parts of the bony thorax—12 vertebrae, 12 pairs of ribs and cartilages, and the sternum.

2. Each rib articulating posteriorly with the vertebral column.

3. The cartilages of the upper seven pairs of ribs articulating directly with the sternum. (The eighth pair may do so, as in fig. 406.) The 8th, 9th and 10th cartilages articulating with the cartilages next above; the 11th and 12th cartilages being free or floating anteriorly.

4. The downward inclination of all ribs. The cartilages of the upper two and of the lower two pairs of ribs, continuing this downward inclination (the 2nd cartilages, however, may be horizontal); the cartilages of the 3rd to 10th ribs inclining upwards.

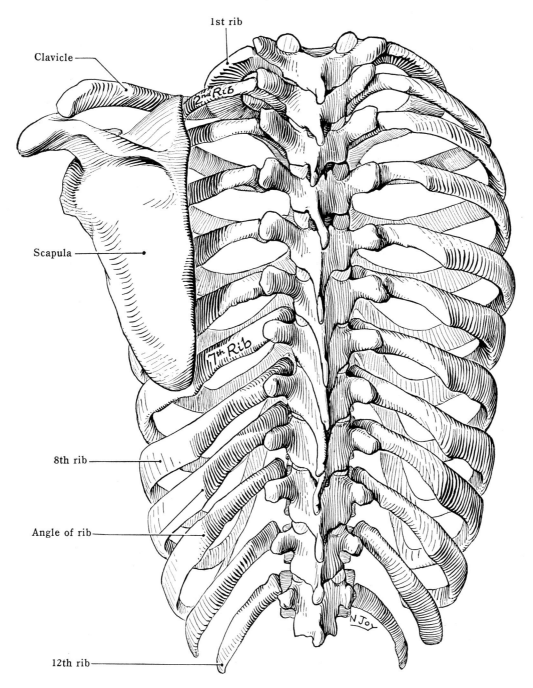

1st rib

Clavicle

2nd Rib

Scapula

7th Rib

8th rib

Angle of rib

12th rib

N JOY

392 Bony Thorax, posterior aspect

5. The progressive increase in length of the first seven ribs and of the first seven cartilages. The seventh rib is the longest rib, but the eighth and ninth are more oblique.

6. The sternal end of the first costal cartilage, being about $1\frac{1}{2}$ inches below the level of the head of its rib. The tip of the twelfth costal cartilage, being at the level of the second lumbar vertebra.

7. The tenth ribs and cartilages, being the lowest ribs and cartilages to appear at the front.

8. The clavicle, thrusting the scapula laterally and backwards. The scapula crossing 50 per cent of the twelve ribs, namely, 2nd–7th inclusive.

9. The distance between the spines of the vertebrae and the angles of the ribs diminishing from the eighth rib upwards.

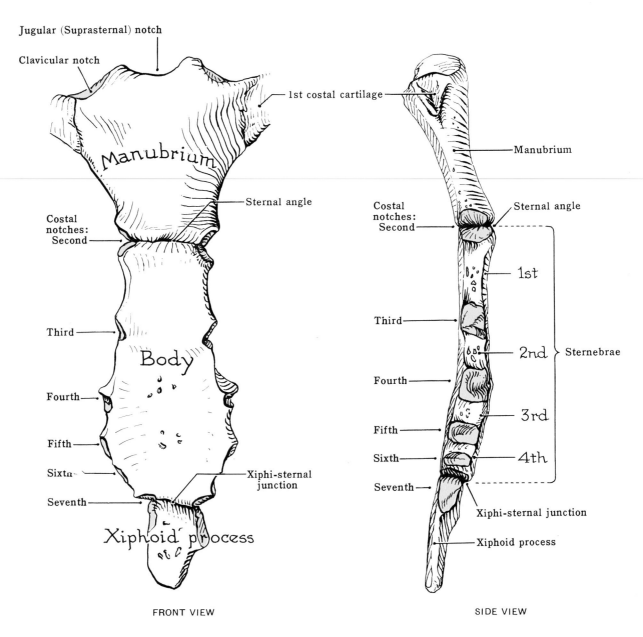

Jugular (Suprasternal) notch

Clavicular notch

1st costal cartilage

Manubrium

Sternal angle

Costal notches:
Second

Third

Body

Fourth

Fifth

Sixth

Seventh

Xiphi-sternal junction

Xiphoid process

FRONT VIEW

Manubrium

Sternal angle

Costal notches:
Second

1st

Third

2nd ⎱ Sternebrae

Fourth

3rd

Fifth

Sixth

4th

Seventh

Xiphi-sternal junction

Xiphoid process

SIDE VIEW

393 Sternum

Observe:

1. The great thickness of the upper third of the manubrium, between the clavicular notches.

2. The thin and tapering tip and sides of the xiphoid process, which give attachment to the linea alba and to the Transversus Abdominis aponeurosis.

3. Two landmarks—(a) The sternal angle at the junction of the manubrium and body, at the level of the 2nd costal cartilages; and (b) the sharp lower edge of the body, at the xiphi-sternal junction.

4. Seven pairs of costal cartilages articulating with the sternum; the 1st by synchondrosis; the 6th at the sides of the 4th sternebra; the other 5, at the angles between two pieces of the sternum. Of these, the 7th lies in front of the xiphoid process. Commonly, the 8th costal cartilages articulate with the sternum as in figure 406.

394 Young Sterum

Times of synostosis are shown. The four sternebrae fuse together from below upwards. Numbers, 4, 3 and 2 are usually fused together not later than the 17th or 18th year, and 2 to 1 not later than the 23rd year. They may, however, be delayed. (McK. & Stewart.) Synostosis of manubrium and body was found in about 10% of adults, aged 30 to 80 years. It is apparently unrelated to age. (Trotter, M.)

395 Common Form of Sternum

The manubrium is 2″ long and the body 4″ +. It is a variant of figure 393.

396 Sternal Foramen

This defect of ossification, suggestive of a bullet wound is common. Note synostosis of xiphisternal joint.

397 Low Sternal Angle

This, at the level of the 3rd costal cartilages, is usual in the gibbon; rare in man.

[From the Anatomy Department, University of Manitoba, courtesy of Professor I. Maclaren Thompson.]

OSSIFICATION—VARIATIONS

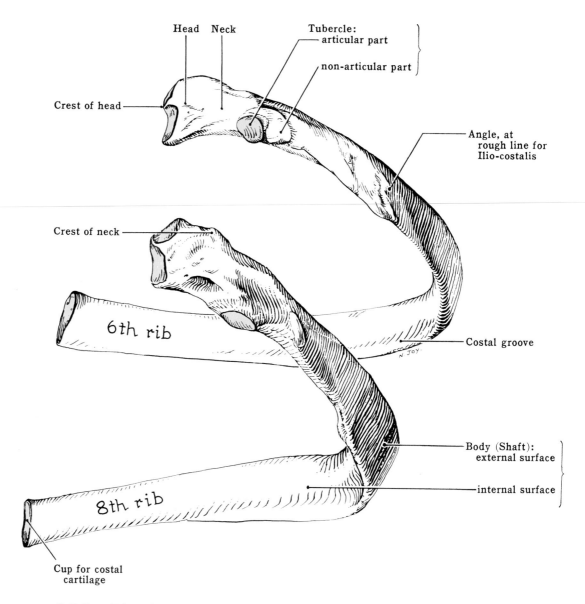

Head   Neck

Tubercle:
— articular part

non-articular part

Crest of head —

Angle, at
rough line for
Ilio-costalis

Crest of neck —

6th rib

Costal groove

Body (Shaft):
external surface

8th rib

internal surface

Cup for costal
cartilage

398   Typical Ribs, seen from behind

Observe:

1. The wedge-shaped head, with a larger lower facet for its own vertebra (6th or 8th) and a smaller facet for the vertebra above.

2. The crest of the head, which is joined to the intervertebral disc by an intra-articular ligament.

3. The posterior surface of the neck, rough for the costo-transverse ligament (lig. of the neck).

4. The crest of the neck, sharp for the superior costo-transverse ligament.

5. The non-articular part of the tubercle, for the lateral costo-transverse ligament (lig. of the tubercle).

6. The articular part of the tubercle, convex and on the posterior aspect of the upper seven (vertebro-sternal) ribs, but flat and on the inferior aspect of the 8th, 9th and 10th (vertebro-chondral) ribs. Indeed, on the 7th it is transitional, being either convex or flat.

7. The posterior part of the shaft is round on cross-section; the anterior part is flattened. The anterior end, being articular, is slightly enlarged.

8. The rough line for the attachment of Ilio-costalis where the rib takes not only a bend but also a twist, on which account it will not lie flat on a table.

9. The costal groove, which lodges the intercostal vein, artery and nerve.

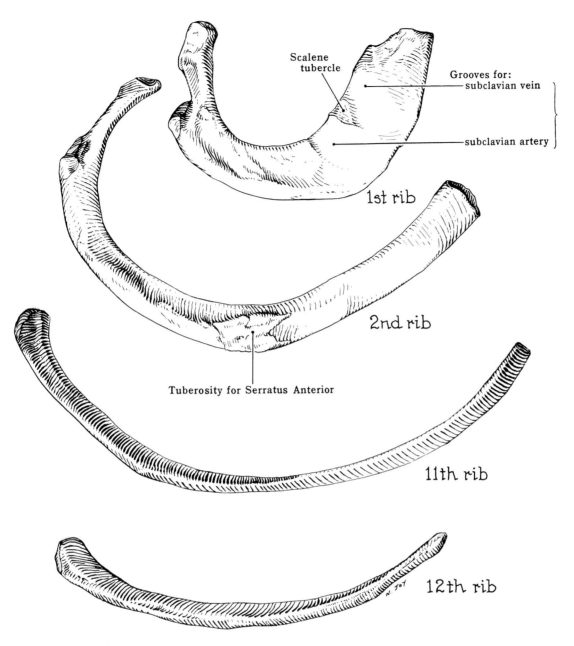

Scalene tubercle

Grooves for:
subclavian vein

subclavian artery

1st rib

2nd rib

Tuberosity for Serratus Anterior

11th rib

12th rib

399 Peculiar or Atypical Ribs—1st, 2nd, 11th and 12th—viewed from above

Observe:

These ribs have but faint angles, if any, and can lie flat on the table.

The 1st is superlative in being the highest, shortest, broadest, strongest, and most curved. Its head and neck are directed medially and downwards—not medially and upwards—and the head has a single facet. Its tubercle is the most prominent of all, for here tubercle and angle coincide. The tubercle for Scalenus Anterior on the upper (external) surface of the shaft separates the groove for the subclavian vein in front from the groove for the subclavian artery and lowest trunk of the brachial plexus behind.

The 2nd rib is marked by the tuberosity for Serratus Anterior. The 11th and 12th ribs, or floating ribs, have each a single facet on the head, no tubercle, and a tapering end.

400 Cervical Ribs

A cervical rib is an enlarged costal element (fig. 365) of the 7th cervical vertebra. The subclavian artery and the lowest root of the brachial plexus arch over such ribs. Radiologically, they occur in 5.6 patients per 1000; twice as often in females as in males; and 50% occur bilaterally (Adson). [From the Anatomy Department, University of Manitoba, by the courtesy of Professor I. Maclaren Thompson.]

401 Bicipital Rib

This was occasioned by the partial fusion of the 1st and 2nd thoracic ribs. A similar condition results from the partial fusion of a cervical rib and the 1st thoracic rib. [Courtesy of Dr. H. A. Cates.]

402 Bifid Rib

The upper limb of this 3rd rib is supernumerary. It articulated with the side of the 1st sternebra of the body of the sternum; the lower limb articulated in the normal situation for a 3rd rib, i.e., at the junction of the 1st and 2nd sternebrae. The condition is not uncommon.

403 Lateral Costal Artery

This branch of the int. thoracic artery, which descends near the midlateral line, was found in 31 (about 25%) of 112 cadavera. It was bilateral in six. Of these 37 arteries, 14 reached the 1st or 2nd intercostal space; 8 the 3rd space; 10 the 4th; and 5 the 5th or 6th. (Kropp, B. N.)

VARIATIONS—ANOMALIES

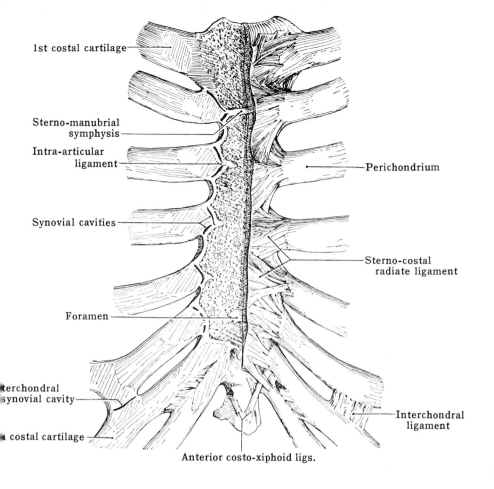

1st costal cartilage

Sterno-manubrial symphysis

Intra-articular ligament

Synovial cavities

Foramen

terchondral synovial cavity

costal cartilage

Anterior costo-xiphoid ligs.

Perichondrium

Sterno-costal radiate ligament

Interchondral ligament

404 Sterno-costal and Interchondral Joints, anterior view

The cortex of the right half of the sternum and of the right costal cartilages has been shaved away.

Observe:

1. The fibres of the perichondrium, parallel to the long axes of the costal cartilages and therefore acting as ligaments which end as radiate ligaments.
2. The joint between the 1st costal cartilage and the manubrium is a synchondrosis, so, in this instance is the joint between the 7th costal cartilage and the sternum.
   The sterno-manubrial joint is a symphysis.
   The other sterno-costal joints and the interchondral joints are synovial joints with or without intra-articular ligaments.

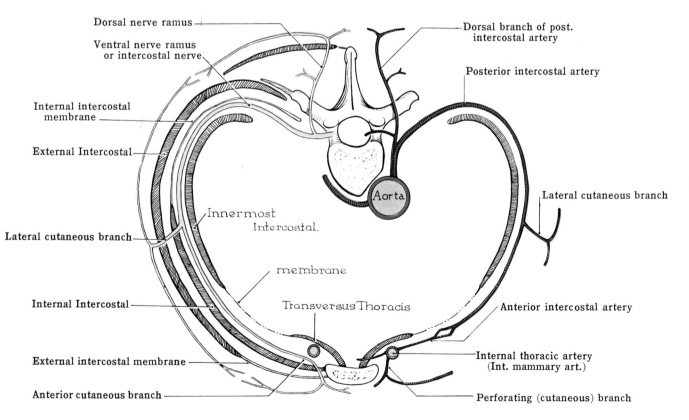

Dorsal nerve ramus

Ventral nerve ramus or intercostal nerve

Internal intercostal membrane

External Intercostal

Innermost Intercostal.

membrane

Lateral cutaneous branch

Internal Intercostal

Transversus Thoracis

External intercostal membrane

Anterior cutaneous branch

Dorsal branch of post. intercostal artery

Posterior intercostal artery

Aorta

Lateral cutaneous branch

Anterior intercostal artery

Internal thoracic artery (Int. mammary art.)

Perforating (cutaneous) branch

405   Diagram of an Intercostal Space

Observe:

1. Three layers: (a) External Intercostal muscle and membrane, (b) Internal Intercostal muscle and membrane, and (c) Innermost Intercostal and Transversus Thoracis muscles and the membrane connecting them.

2. The intercostal vessels and nerves running in the plane between the middle and innermost layers of muscles. Subsequently, the lower intercostal vessels and nerves occupy the corresponding morphological plane in the abdominal wall (figs. 106 and 408).

Scaleni:
Posterior
Medius
Anterior
Subclavian vein
Sterno-thyroid
Sterno-hyoid
1st intercostal nerve
Internal thoracic (Int. mammary) vein and artery
External Intercostal
Internal Intercostal
Transversus Thoracis

Sterno-mastoid

Brachial plexus
Subclavian artery
Subclavian vein

Subclavius

Pectoralis Minor

Pectoralis Major

Cor.-brach. and Biceps

3rd

4th

Pectoralis Major

Rectus Abdominis

8th costal cartilage

External Oblique

Serratus Anterior

406 Anterior Wall of the Thorax

Observe:

1. The muscles to be removed before dissection is begun: External Oblique, Rectus Abdominis, Pectoralis Major, Pectoralis Minor, Subclavius, sternal head of Sternomastoid, and Scalenus Posterior at the front; Serratus Anterior and Latissimus Dorsi at the sides (figs. 23 & 24); Serrati Posteriores, Longissimus, and Ilio-costalis at the back (fig. 409).

2. Pulling the arm backwards and downwards forces the clavicle, padded with Subclavius, to compress the subclavian vessels against the 1st rib and thus arrest the blood flow.

3. The 11th and 12th ribs are too short to be seen from the front.

4. The 7th costal cartilages are usually the last to reach the sternum, although not uncommonly, as here, the 8th also do so.

5. The H-shaped cut made through the perichondrium of the 3rd and 4th cartilages prior to shelling out segments of cartilage.

6. The internal thoracic vessels, crossed anteriorly by the intercostal nerves and associated with parasternal lymph nodes.

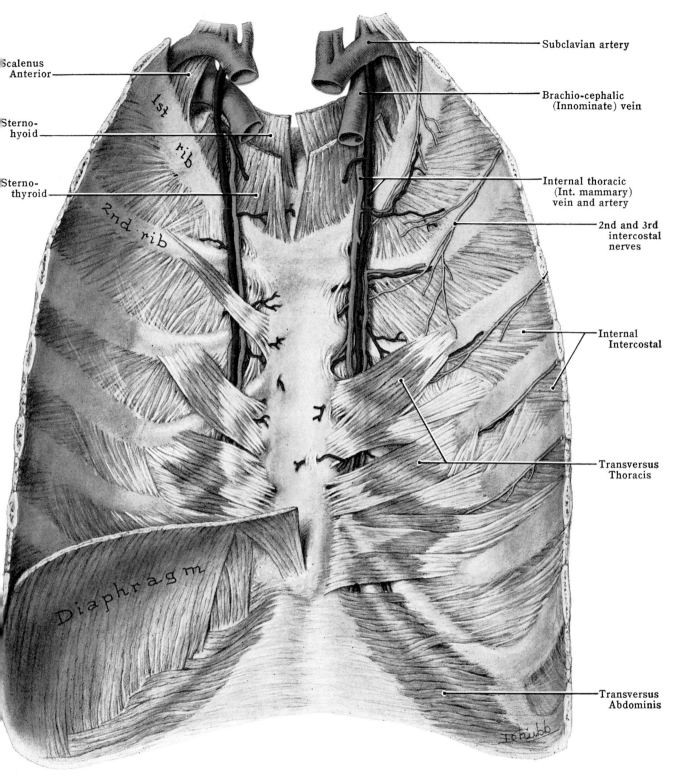

Scalenus Anterior

Sterno-hyoid

Sterno-thyroid

1st rib

2nd rib

Diaphragm

Subclavian artery

Brachio-cephalic (Innominate) vein

Internal thoracic (Int. mammary) vein and artery

2nd and 3rd intercostal nerves

Internal Intercostal

Transversus Thoracis

Transversus Abdominis

407 Anterior Thoracic Wall, from behind

(*Dissection by Dr. S. A. Crooks*)

Observe:

1. The continuity of Transversus Thoracis with Transversus Abdominis, these being the innermost layer of the three muscles of the thoraco-abdominal wall.

2. The internal thoracic artery, arising from the first part of the subclavian artery, accompanied by two veins (venae comitantes) up to the 3rd or 2nd intercostal space and above this by a single vein (internal thoracic vein), which proceeds to the brachio-cephalic vein.

3. The lower portions of the internal thoracic vessels, covered posteriorly with Transversus Thoracis; the upper portions in contact with parietal pleura (removed).

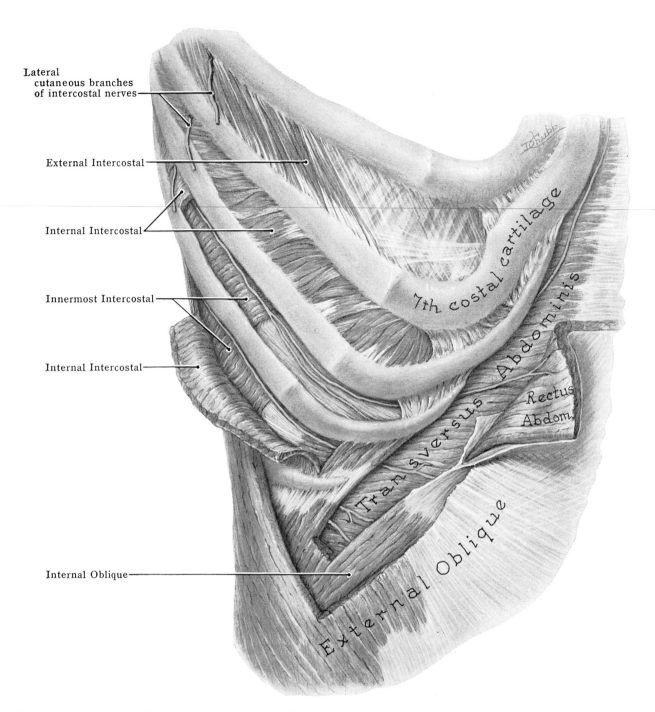

Lateral
cutaneous branches
of intercostal nerves

External Intercostal

Internal Intercostal

Innermost Intercostal

Internal Intercostal

Internal Oblique

7th costal cartilage

Transversus Abdominis

Rectus Abdom.

External Oblique

408   Anterior Ends of Lower Intercostal Spaces, front view

Observe:

1. The common direction of the fibres of the External Intercostal and External Oblique.

2. The continuity of the Internal Intercostal with the Internal Oblique, at the anterior ends of the 9th, 10th, and 11th intercostal spaces.

3. The morphological plane in which an intercostal nerve lies—deep to an Internal Intercostal but superficial to an Innermost Intercostal and either the Transversus Thoracis or the Transversus Abdominis, according to the level.

4. The direction in which an intercostal nerve runs—first, parallel to the ribs immediately above and below, and then, parallel to the costal cartilages. Thus, on gaining the abdominal walls nerves T.7 and T.8 continue upwards, T.9 continues nearly horizontally, and T.10 continue, downwards towards the umbilicus.

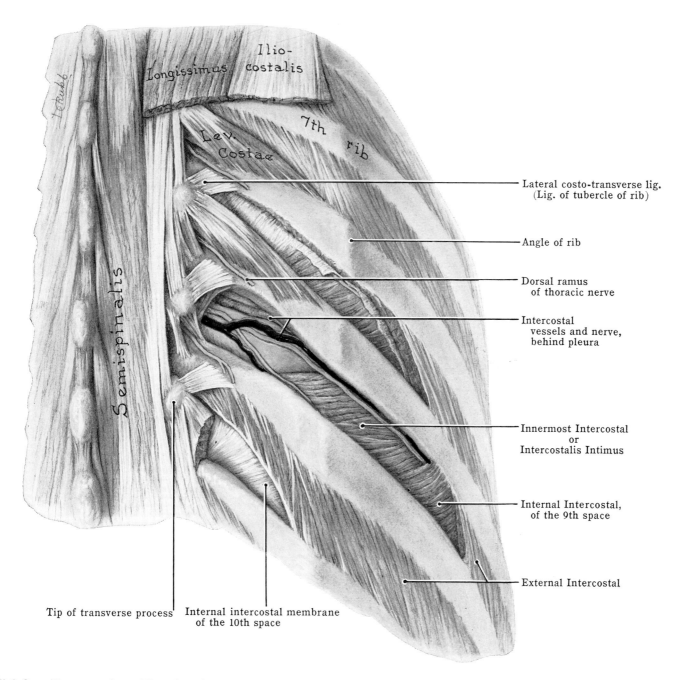

Lateral costo-transverse lig.
(Lig. of tubercle of rib)

Angle of rib

Dorsal ramus
of thoracic nerve

Intercostal
vessels and nerve,
behind pleura

Innermost Intercostal
or
Intercostalis Intimus

Internal Intercostal,
of the 9th space

External Intercostal

Tip of transverse process   Internal intercostal membrane
of the 10th space

109   Posterior End of an Intercostal Space, from behind

Note:

1. Medial to the angles of the ribs, Ilio-costalis and Longissimus have been removed and Levatores Costarum thereby uncovered.

2. Of the five intercostal spaces depicted: the upper two are intact; from the 10th, or lowest, space Levator Costae and the underlying part of the External Intercostal have been removed thereby revealing the internal intercostal membrane; from the 8th space more of the External Intercostal has been removed and the Internal intercostal membrane is seen extending laterally as an areolar sheet; finally, in the 9th space this sheet also has been removed in order to show the intercostal vessels and nerve (a) appearing medially between the superior costo-transverse ligament and the pleura and (b) disappearing laterally between the Internal Intercostal and the Innermost Intercostal.

Transverse process

Superior costo-transverse lig.

External Intercostal

Innermost Intercostal

Subcostalis

Internal intercostal membrane

Intercostal vessels and nerve

Spinal ganglion

Radiate lig. of head of rib

Disc

Anterior longitudinal ligament

Sympathetic trunk

Splanchnic nerve

410 Vertebral End of an Intercostal Space and the Costo-vertebral Ligaments, anterior view

Observe:

1. Portions of the Innermost Intercostal muscle that bridge two intercostal spaces are called Subcostal muscles.

2. An External Intercostal muscle in the uppermost space.

3. An internal intercostal membrane in the middle space, continuous medially with a superior costo-transverse ligament.

4. In the lowest space, the order of the structures—intercostal vein, artery, and nerve and note their collateral branches.

5. The ventral ramus of a thoracic nerve, crossing in front of a superior costo-transverse ligament and a dorsal ramus crossing behind.

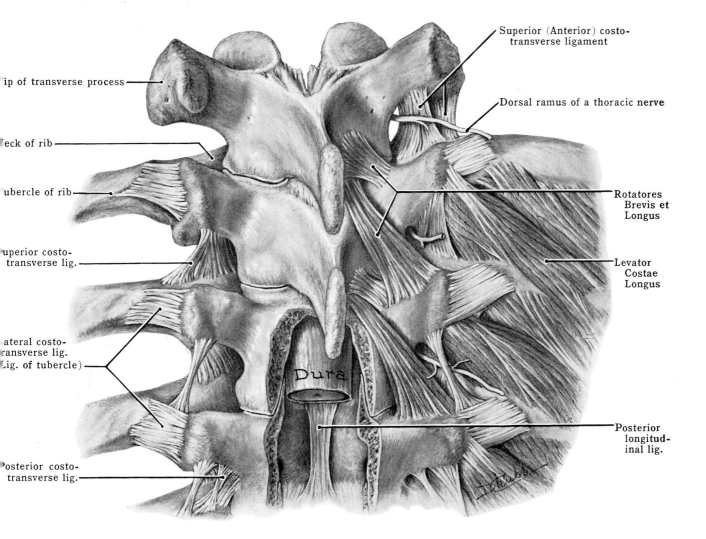

ip of transverse process —

eck of rib ——

ubercle of rib ——

uperior costo-
transverse lig. ——

ateral costo-
ransverse lig.
Lig. of tubercle) ——

Posterior costo-
transverse lig.——

Dura

Superior (Anterior) costo-
transverse ligament

Dorsal ramus of a thoracic **nerve**

Rotatores
Brevis et
Longus

Levator
Costae
Longus

Posterior
longitud-
inal lig.

411   Rotatores and the Costo-transverse Ligaments

Note:

1. Of the 3 layers of Transverso-spinales or oblique muscles of the back—Semispinales, Multi-fidus, Rotatores—the Rotatores are the deepest and shortest. They pass from the root of one transverse process to the junction of the transverse process and lamina of the vertebra next above; but some (Rotatores Longi) pass to the vertebra two above.

2. Similarly, the Levatores Costarum pass from the tip of one transverse process to the rib next below; but some (Levatores Longi) pass to the rib two below.

3. Of the 3 sets of costo-transverse ligaments—superior, lateral, and medial—(a) the superior splits laterally into two sheets between which the medial border of a Levator Costae and of an External Intercostal are received. The dorsal ramus of a thoracic nerve passes behind this ligament and the ventral ramus, or intercostal nerve, passes in front. (b) the lateral ligament is strong and, if there were no joint cavity between transverse process and rib, it would be continuous with (c) the medial ligament (lig. of the neck, fig. 431), which passes between the front of a transverse process and the back of the neck of its own rib. It is called "the" costo-transverse ligament. (A few fibers of little account, lying postero-medial to the superior lig. constitute a posterior costo-transverse lig.)

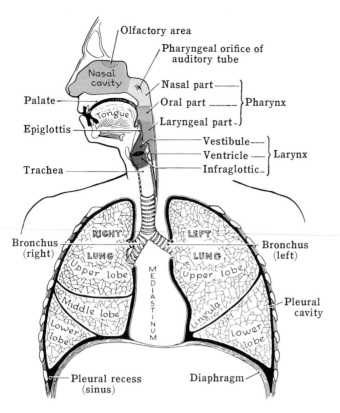

412 **Diagram of Respiratory System**

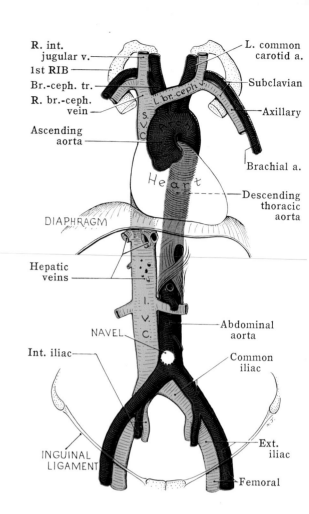

413 **Diagram of Great Arteries and Vei**

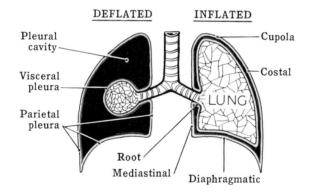

412.1 **Scheme of Pleural Cavity and Pleura**

The parts of the parietal pleura are labelled on the right side.

412.2 **Scheme of Fibrous and Serous Pericardia**

413.1 **Subdivisions of Mediastinun**

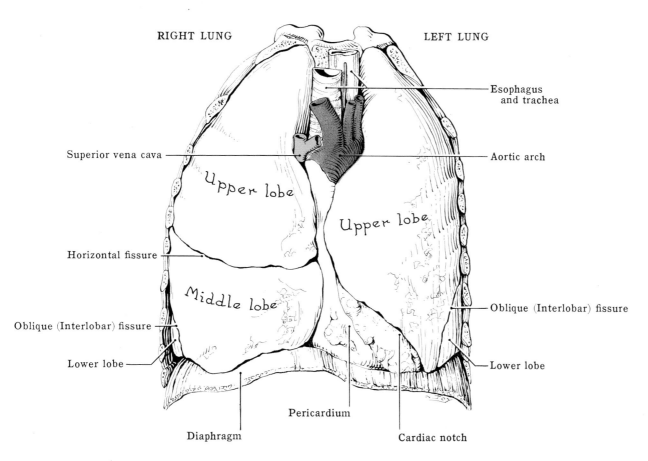

RIGHT LUNG

LEFT LUNG

Esophagus
and trachea

Superior vena cava

Aortic arch

Upper lobe

Upper lobe

Horizontal fissure

Middle lobe

Oblique (Interlobar) fissure

Oblique (Interlobar) fissure

Lower lobe

Lower lobe

Pericardium

Diaphragm

Cardiac notch

414 Lungs and Pericardium, anterior view

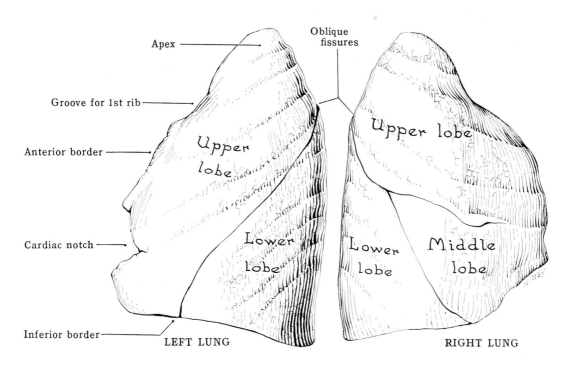

Apex

Oblique
fissures

Groove for 1st rib

Upper
lobe

Upper lobe

Anterior border

Lower
lobe

Lower
lobe

Middle
lobe

Cardiac notch

Inferior border

LEFT LUNG

RIGHT LUNG

414.1 Lungs, lateral views

Observe:

1. The three lobes of the right lung and the two lobes of the left lung.

2. The middle lobe (of the right lung) lying at the front of the thorax; i.e., it is entirely anterior to the midlateral line.

3. The deficiency of the upper lobe of the left lung, called the cardiac notch, allowing the pericardium to appear.

4. A horizontal fissure (of the right lung), complete in figure 414 and incomplete in figure 414.1.

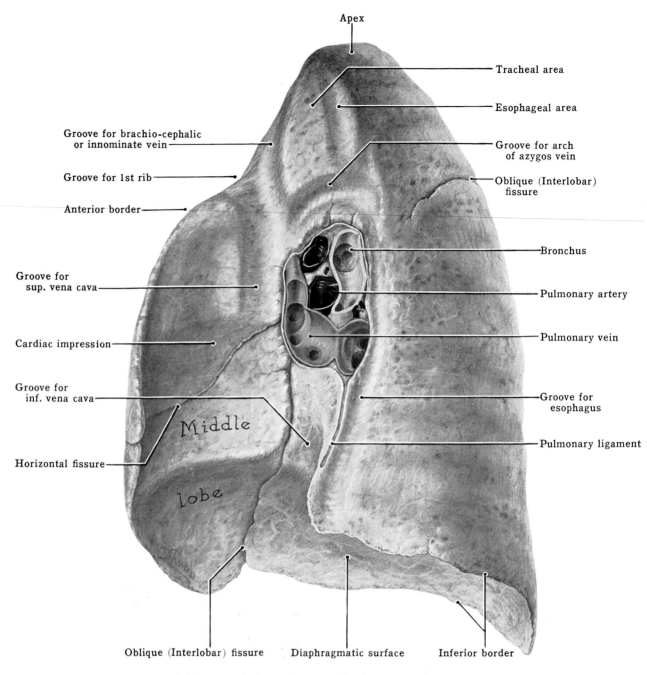

Apex

Tracheal area

Esophageal area

Groove for brachio-cephalic
or innominate vein

Groove for arch
of azygos vein

Groove for 1st rib

Oblique (Interlobar)
fissure

Anterior border

Bronchus

Groove for
sup. vena cava

Pulmonary artery

Cardiac impression

Pulmonary vein

Groove for
inf. vena cava

Groove for
esophagus

Pulmonary ligament

Middle

Horizontal fissure

lobe

Oblique (Interlobar) fissure　　Diaphragmatic surface　　Inferior border

415　Mediastinal Surface of the Right Lung

Observe:

1. The lungs, resembling inflated balloons in that they take the impressions of the structures with which they come into contact. Thus, the base is fashioned by the cupola of the diaphragm; the costal surface bears the impressions of the ribs; distended vessels leave their mark; empty vessels and nerves do not.

2. The somewhat pear-shaped root of the lung near the centre of the mediastinal surface, and the pulmonary ligament descending like a stalk from the root.

3. The groove for (or line of contact with) the esophagus throughout the length of the lung, except where the arch of the azygos vein intervenes. This groove passes behind the root and therefore behind the pulmonary ligament, which separates it from the groove for the l. v. cava.

4. The oblique (interlobar) fissure, here not complete.

5. The two pulmonary veins, here uniting unusually close to the lung.

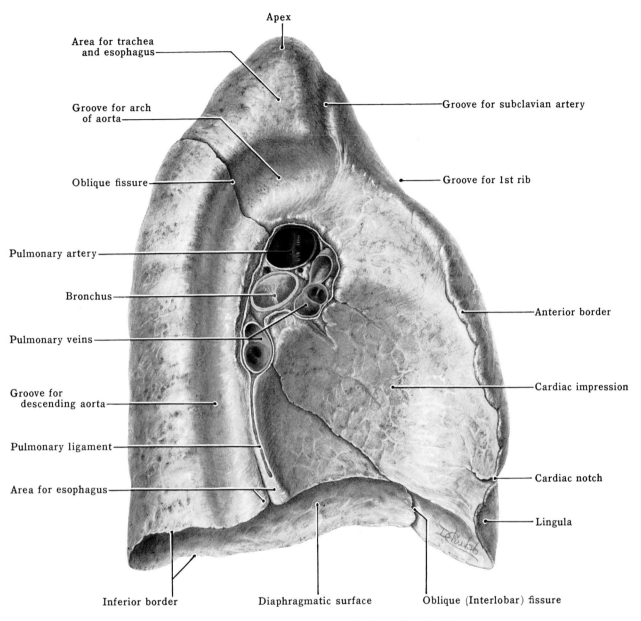

Apex

Area for trachea and esophagus

Groove for subclavian artery

Groove for arch of aorta

Oblique fissure

Groove for 1st rib

Pulmonary artery

Bronchus

Anterior border

Pulmonary veins

Groove for descending aorta

Cardiac impression

Pulmonary ligament

Area for esophagus

Cardiac notch

Lingula

Inferior border

Diaphragmatic surface

Oblique (Interlobar) fissure

416 Mediastinal Surface of the Left Lung

Observe:

1. Near the centre, the root and the pulmonary ligament descending from it.

2. The site of contact with the esophagus, between the aorta and the lower end of the ligament.

3. The oblique (interlobar) fissure, cutting completely through the lung substance.

4. In both the right root and the left—the artery is above; the bronchus is behind; one vein is in front, and the other is below. In the right root, however, a bronchus (eparterial) to the upper lobe is the highest structure.

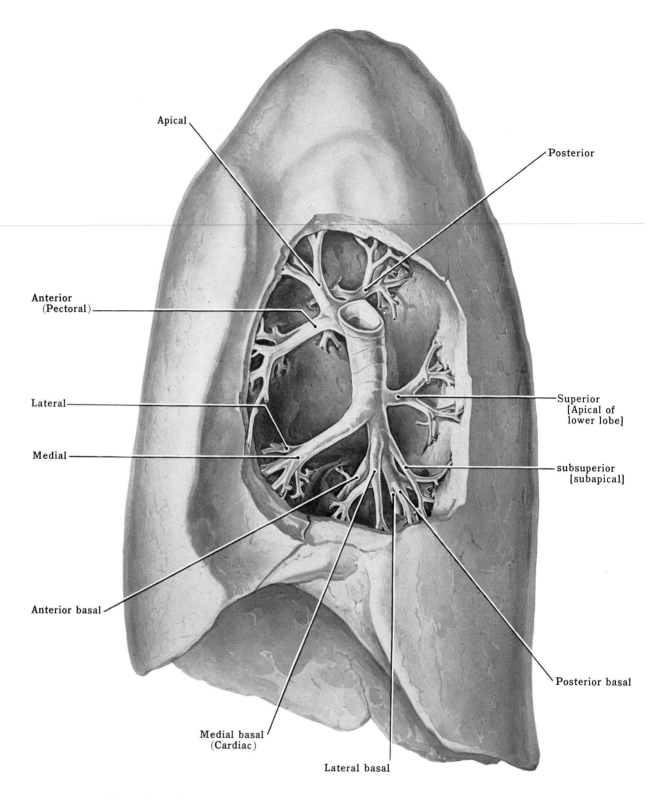

Apical

Posterior

Anterior
(Pectoral)

Lateral

Medial

Superior
[Apical of
lower lobe]

subsuperior
[subapical]

Anterior basal

Posterior basal

Medial basal
(Cardiac)

Lateral basal

417 Right Bronchial Tree

Fresh lungs were kept inflated with air under low pressure until thoroughly dry (about a week) and their natural form thereby assured. The tissues surrounding the bronchi were then moistened and cut away.

Terminology (after Jackson and Huber). There are usually 10 right and 8 left tertiary or segmental bronchi. They are approximately symmetrical in the two lungs. The reduced number in the left lung is accounted for by the fact that the left apical and posterior bronchi arise from a common stem, as do also the left anterior basal and medial basal.

Right Bronchi and
~~mo~~nary Veins

~~__~~ veins of fresh lungs were filled with blue
~~a~~nd the bronchi kept inflated and treated as
~~f~~ure 417. (Dissected by Dr. C. W. Hill.)

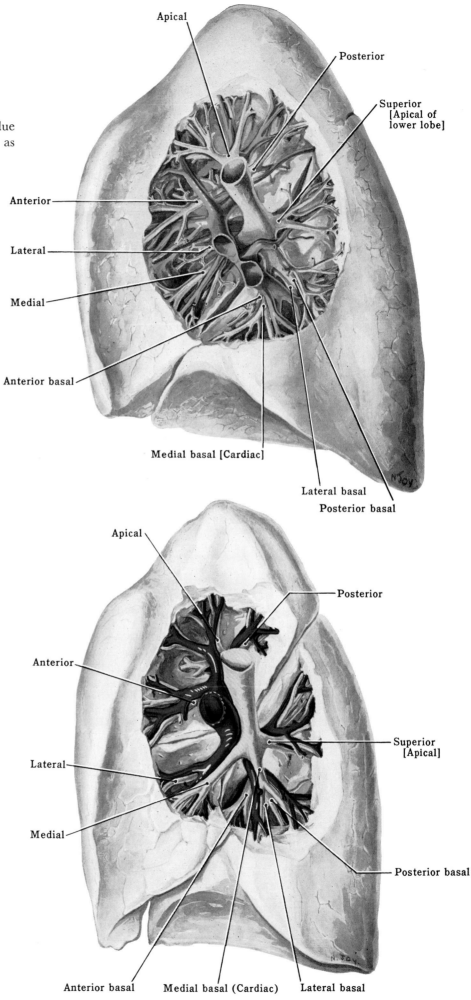

Apical

Posterior

Superior
[Apical of
lower lobe]

Anterior

Lateral

Medial

Anterior basal

Medial basal [Cardiac]

Lateral basal

Posterior basal

Apical

Posterior

Anterior

Superior
[Apical]

Lateral

Medial

9   Right Bronchi and
~~Pu~~lmonary Arteries

~~t~~he arteries of fresh lungs were filled with
~~l~~atex and the bronchi kept inflated and
~~treat~~ed as for figure 417.

Posterior basal

Anterior basal

Medial basal (Cardiac)

Lateral basal

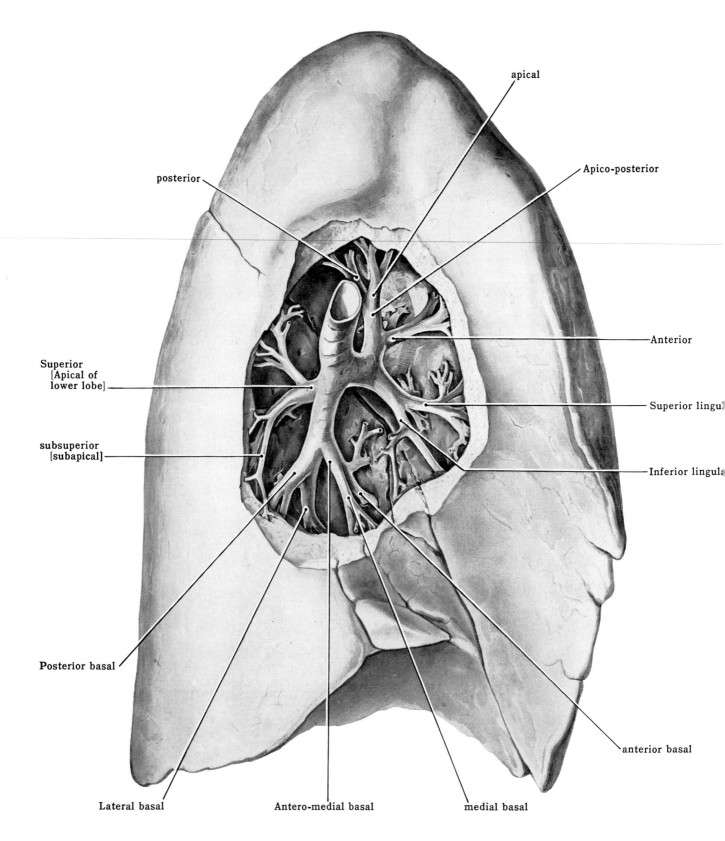

apical

Apico-posterior

posterior

Anterior

Superior
[Apical of
lower lobe]

Superior lingul[a]

subsuperior
[subapical]

Inferior lingula

Posterior basal

anterior basal

Lateral basal   Antero-medial basal   medial basal

420 Left Bronchial Tree

Fresh lungs were kept inflated with air under low pressure until thoroughly dry (about a week) and their natural form thereby assured. The tissues surrounding the bronchi were then moistened and cut away.

Terminology (after Jackson and Huber). There are usually 10 right and 8 left tertiary or segmental bronchi. They are approximately symmetrical in the two lungs. The reduced number in the left lung is accounted for by the fact that the left apical and posterior bronchi arise from a common stem, as do also the left anterior basal and the medial basal.

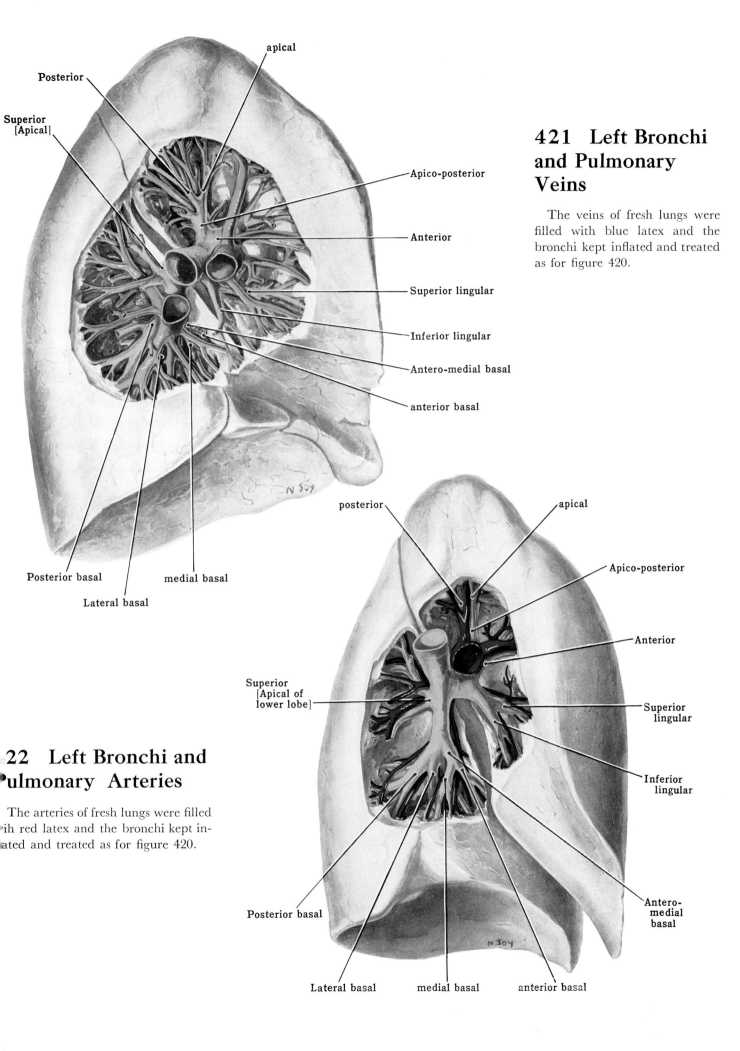

Posterior

Superior
[Apical]

apical

Apico-posterior

Anterior

Superior lingular

Inferior lingular

Antero-medial basal

anterior basal

Posterior basal

Lateral basal

medial basal

421 Left Bronchi and Pulmonary Veins

The veins of fresh lungs were filled with blue latex and the bronchi kept inflated and treated as for figure 420.

22 Left Bronchi and ulmonary Arteries

The arteries of fresh lungs were filled ih red latex and the bronchi kept in- ated and treated as for figure 420.

posterior

apical

Apico-posterior

Anterior

Superior
[Apical of
lower lobe]

Superior
lingular

Inferior
lingular

Antero-
medial
basal

Posterior basal

Lateral basal

medial basal

anterior basal

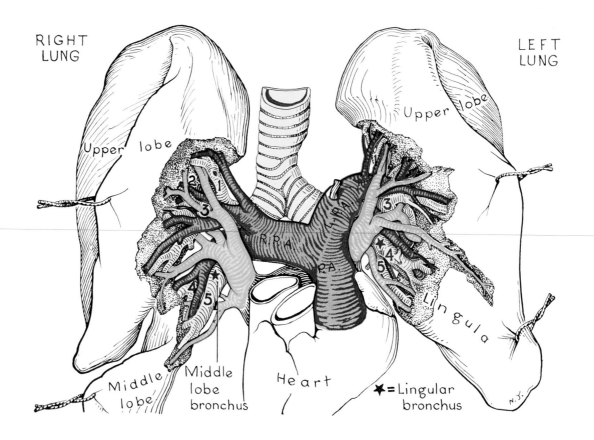

RIGHT
LUNG

LEFT
LUNG

Upper lobe

Upper lobe

R.P.A.

L.P.A.

R.P.A.

R.A.

Lingula

Middle
lobe

Middle
lobe
bronchus

Heart

★ = Lingular
bronchus

423   Dissection of the Hili of the Lungs, from the front

(The bronchi and the pulmonary veins and arteries were injected.)

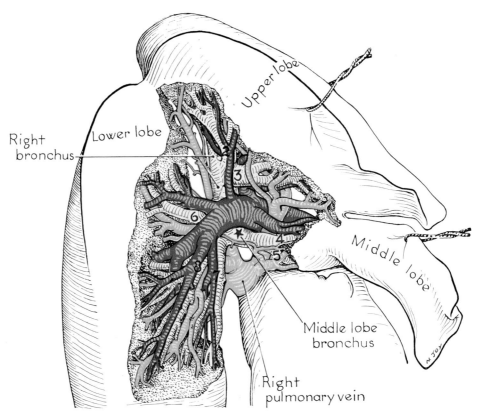

Upper lobe

Right
bronchus

Lower lobe

Middle
lobe

Middle lobe
bronchus

Right
pulmonary vein

**423.1   Dissection of the Hilus of the Right Lung, after
opening the oblique fissure**

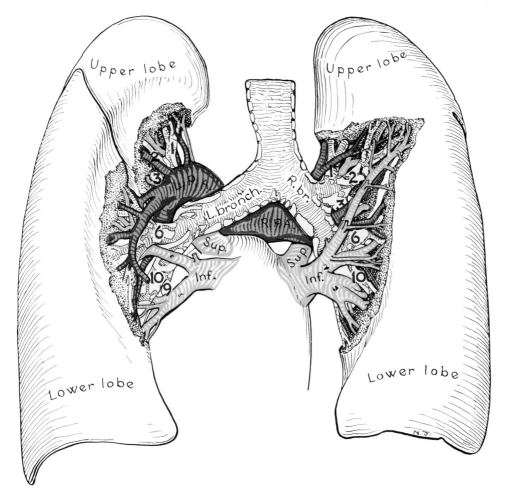

423.2 Dissection of the Hili of the Lungs, from behind

(The bronchi and the pulmonary veins and arteries were injected.)

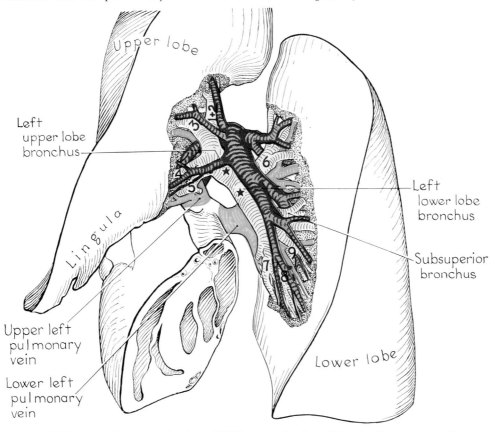

423.3 Dissection of the Hilus of the Left Lung, after opening the oblique fissure

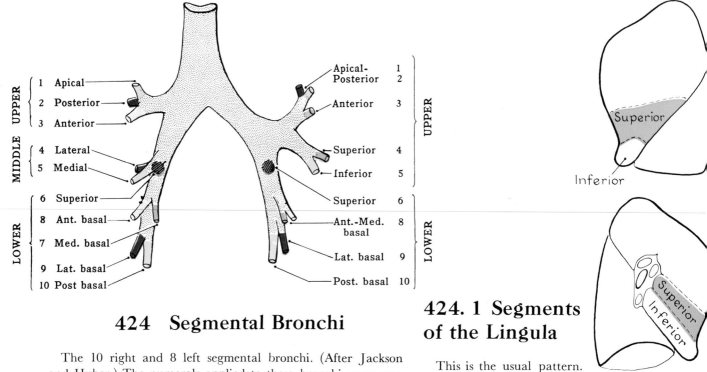

MIDDLE UPPER						UPPER
UPPER	1	Apical	Apical-Posterior	1		
	2	Posterior		2		
	3	Anterior	Anterior	3		
MIDDLE	4	Lateral	Superior	4		
	5	Medial	Inferior	5		
LOWER	6	Superior	Superior	6		LOWER
	8	Ant. basal	Ant.-Med. basal	8		
	7	Med. basal				
	9	Lat. basal	Lat. basal	9		
	10	Post basal	Post. basal	10		

424   Segmental Bronchi

The 10 right and 8 left segmental bronchi. (After Jackson and Huber.) The numerals applied to these bronchi were suggested by the Thoracic Society.

424. 1 Segments of the Lingula

This is the usual pattern. Compare with fig. 427. (After Jackson and Huber.)

Right lung   Left lung

ANTERIOR VIEW

Left lung   Right lung

POSTERIOR VIEW

425   Broncho-pulmonary Segments

(All specimens were prepared by Dr. J. Callaghan, Dr. K. Nancekivell, C. E. Storton.)

The tertiary bronchi of fresh lungs were isolated within the hili of the lungs and injected with latex of various colours. Ten such bronchi may be recognized in each lung. Usually there are ten in the right lung, but in the left lung only eight, due to the fact that the left apical and posterior arise from a single stem, as do the left ante-rior basal and medial basal. Each tertiary or segmental bronchus and the portion of lung it ventilates is called a bronchopulmonary segment. Minor variations in the branching of the bronchi make for variations in the surface pattern.

For detailed information see "Segmental Anatomy of the Lungs" by E. A. Boyden.

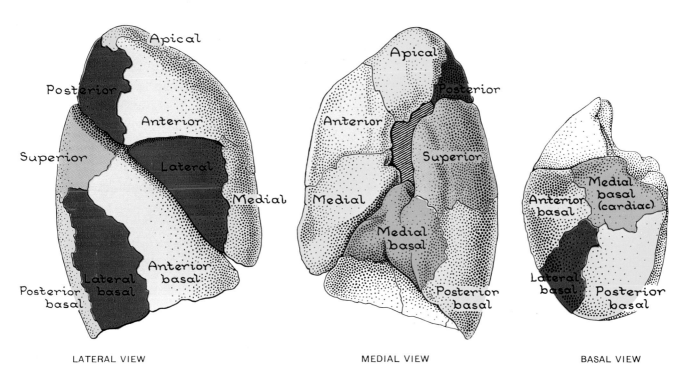

LATERAL VIEW   MEDIAL VIEW   BASAL VIEW

426   Right Broncho-pulmonary Segments

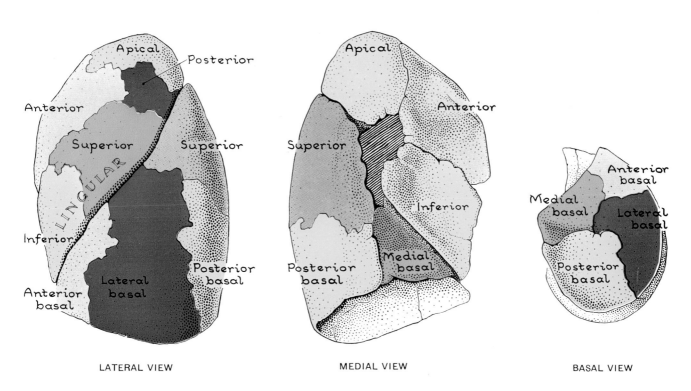

LATERAL VIEW   MEDIAL VIEW   BASAL VIEW

427   Left Broncho-pulmonary Segments

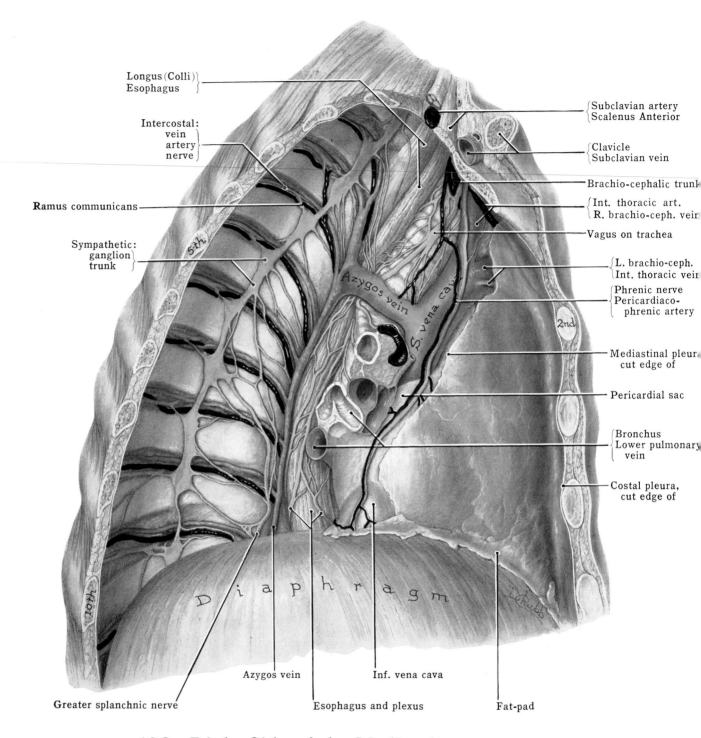

Longus (Colli)
Esophagus

Intercostal:
vein
artery
nerve

Ramus communicans

Sympathetic:
ganglion
trunk

Subclavian artery
Scalenus Anterior

Clavicle
Subclavian vein

Brachio-cephalic trunk

Int. thoracic art.
R. brachio-ceph. vein

Vagus on trachea

L. brachio-ceph.
Int. thoracic vein

Phrenic nerve
Pericardiaco-
phrenic artery

Mediastinal pleura,
cut edge of

Pericardial sac

Bronchus
Lower pulmonary
vein

Costal pleura,
cut edge of

Azygos vein

S. vena cava

2nd

5th

10th

Diaphragm

Greater splanchnic nerve

Azygos vein

Esophagus and plexus

Inf. vena cava

Fat-pad

428 Right Side of the Mediastinum

(From a dissection by Major B. L. Guyatt.)

The costal and mediastinal pleura is largely removed and the underlying structures
are thereby exposed.

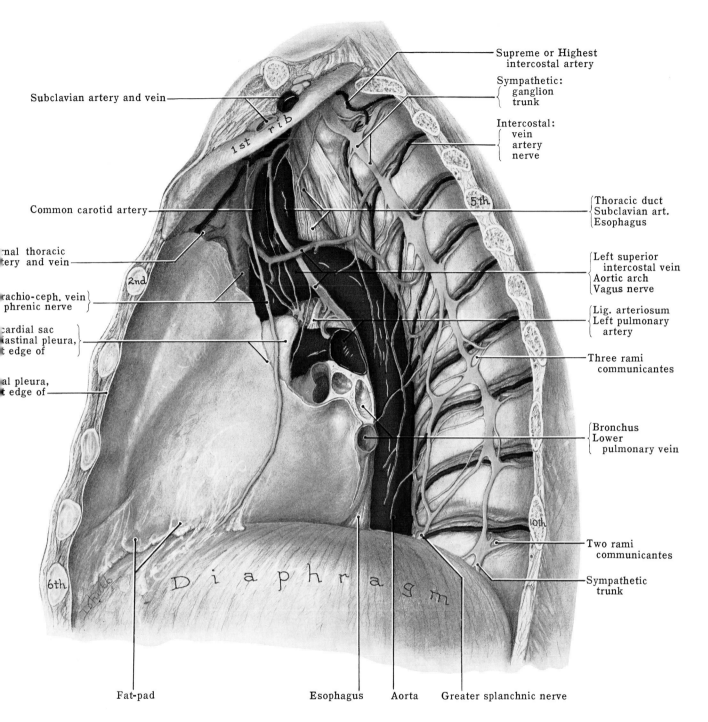

Subclavian artery and vein

Common carotid artery

rnal thoracic
tery and vein

rachio-ceph. vein
phrenic nerve

cardial sac
iastinal pleura,
t edge of

al pleura,
t edge of

Supreme or Highest
intercostal artery

Sympathetic:
ganglion
trunk

Intercostal:
vein
artery
nerve

Thoracic duct
Subclavian art.
Esophagus

Left superior
intercostal vein
Aortic arch
Vagus nerve

Lig. arteriosum
Left pulmonary
artery

Three rami
communicantes

Bronchus
Lower
pulmonary vein

Two rami
communicantes

Sympathetic
trunk

1st rib

2nd

5th

6th

10th

Diaphragm

Fat-pad   Esophagus   Aorta   Greater splanchnic nerve

429   Left Side of the Mediastinum

(From a dissection by Major B. L. Guyatt.)

The costal and mediastinal pleura is largely removed and the
underlying structures are thereby exposed.

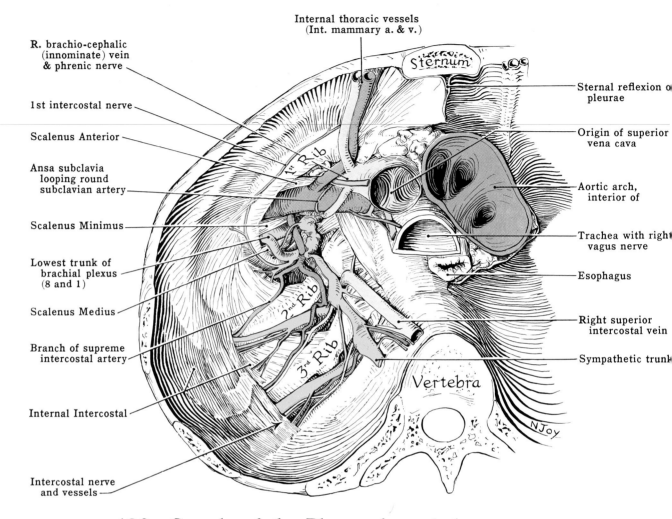

Internal thoracic vessels
(Int. mammary a. & v.)

R. brachio-cephalic
(innominate) vein
& phrenic nerve

1st intercostal nerve

Scalenus Anterior

Ansa subclavia
looping round
subclavian artery

Scalenus Minimus

Lowest trunk of
brachial plexus
(8 and 1)

Scalenus Medius

Branch of supreme
intercostal artery

Internal Intercostal

Intercostal nerve
and vessels

Sternum

Sternal reflexion o
pleurae

Origin of superior
vena cava

Aortic arch,
interior of

Trachea with right
vagus nerve

Esophagus

Right superior
intercostal vein

Sympathetic trunk

Vertebra

NJoy

430   Cupola of the Pleura, from below

The cupola of the pleura (also called the cervical pleura, dome of the pleura, and apical pleura) is removed. It forms, so to speak, both the roof of the pleural cavity and the floor of the root of the neck—see figure 536.

Observe:

1. The first part of the subclavian artery, arching over the cupola and disappearing between Scalenus Anterior and Scalenus Minimus, which is an occasional muscle.

2. The internal thoracic artery and the supreme intercostal branch of the costo-cervical trunk.

3. Two nerves—the ansa subclavia from the sympathetic trunk and the recurrent laryngeal nerve from the vagus—looping round the subclavian artery.

4. The supreme intercostal artery crossing the neck of the 1st rib between the sympathetic trunk, which is on its medial side, and the ventral ramus of T. 1 to the brachial plexus, which is on its lateral side.

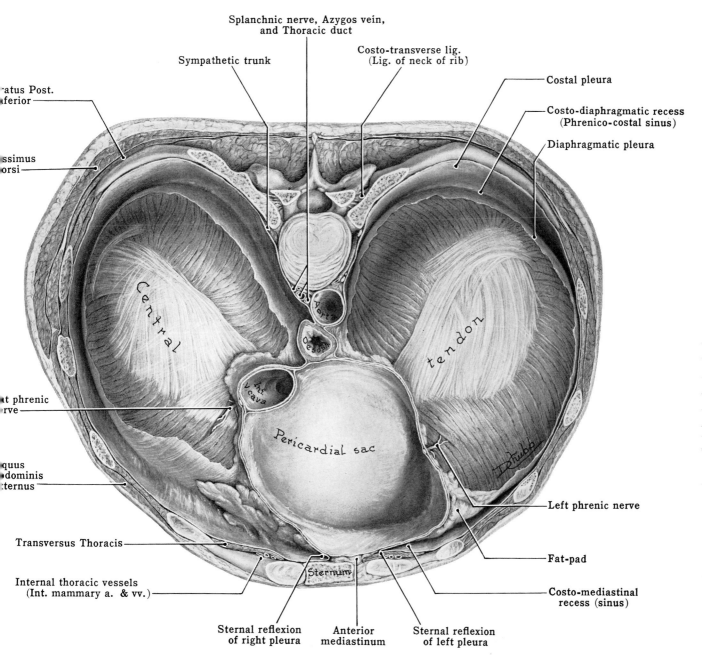

Splanchnic nerve, Azygos vein,
and Thoracic duct

Sympathetic trunk

Costo-transverse lig.
(Lig. of neck of rib)

Costal pleura

Costo-diaphragmatic recess
(Phrenico-costal sinus)

Diaphragmatic pleura

ratus Post.
fterior

ssimus
orsi

Central

tendon

Aorta

Oesoph

Inf
v cava

Pericardial sac

t phrenic
rve

quus
dominis
ternus

Left phrenic nerve

Transversus Thoracis

Fat-pad

Internal thoracic vessels
(Int. mammary a. & vv.)

Sternum

Costo-mediastinal
recess (sinus)

Sternal reflexion
of right pleura

Anterior
mediastinum

Sternal reflexion
of left pleura

431   Diaphragm and the Pericardial Sac, from above

The diaphragmatic pleura is mostly removed.

Observe:

1. The pericardial sac, situated on the anterior half of the diaphragm; one third being to the right of the median plane and two thirds being to the left; the most caudal point being anteriorly and to the left—like the apex of the heart.

2. The mouths of large hepatic veins, opening into the inferior vena cava and directed upwards, towards the heart.

3. The left pleural sac, failing to meet the right sac in the median plane, in front of the pericardium.

4. The right and left pleural sacs almost meeting between esophagus and aorta to form a mesoesophagus.

5. The costa-diaphragmatic recess, deepest about the mid-lateral line.

6. The costal pleura, on reaching the vertebral column inperceptibly becoming the mediastinal pleura.

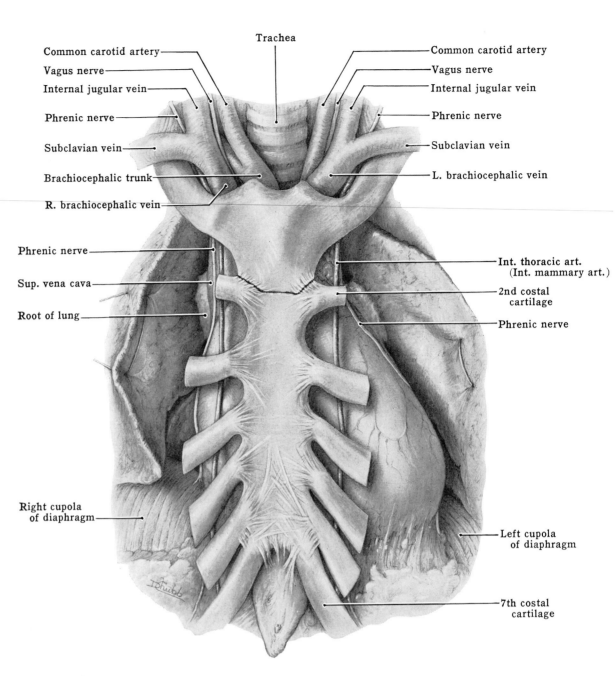

Trachea

Common carotid artery

Vagus nerve

Internal jugular vein

Phrenic nerve

Subclavian vein

Brachiocephalic trunk

R. brachiocephalic vein

Common carotid artery

Vagus nerve

Internal jugular vein

Phrenic nerve

Subclavian vein

L. brachiocephalic vein

Phrenic nerve

Sup. vena cava

Root of lung

Int. thoracic art.
(Int. mammary art.)

2nd costal
cartilage

Phrenic nerve

Right cupola
of diaphragm

Left cupola
of diaphragm

7th costal
cartilage

432 Pericardial Sac in Relation to the Sternum

Observe:

1. The internal thoracic arteries lying a finger's breadth from the borders of the sternum.

2. The pericardial sac, extending in the median plane from just above the level of the sterno-manubrial joint to the level of the xiphi-sternal junction; i.e., practically co-extensive with the body of the sternum, but one third lying to the right of the median plane and two thirds to the left.

3. The right and left phrenic nerves applied to the pericardial sac.

Note, the sterno-manubrial joint was divided preparatory to turning the body of the sternum downwards in order to permit of dissection.

Brachiocephalic trunk

Left common carotid artery

Cardiac branch,
vago-sympathetic

Left vagus nerve

brachiocephalic
(innominate) vein

Left subclavian artery

1st rib

Inferior cardiac branch

Arch of
azygos vein

Aortic arch

Superior
vena
cava

Recurrent nerve and
Lig. arteriosum

Ascending
aorta

Left pulmonary artery

Cut edge of
pericardium

Pulm.
artery

Anterior pulmonary
plexus

Left auricle

ılcus terminalis

Right
atrium

Anterior
interventricular
branch of left
coronary artery
(Ant. descend. br.)

ght coronary art.

Great cardiac
vein

Right ventricle

terior cardiac veins

Left
ventricle

Cut edge of
pericardium

Diaphragm

433 Sternocostal Surface of the Heart and Great Vessels, in situ

Brachiocephalic trunk (Innominate artery)

Right brachiocephalic vein (R. innominate vein)

Left common carotid artery

Left subclavian artery

Left brachiocephalic vein

Ligamentum arteriosum

L. innom. vein

Aortic arch

Superior vena cava

Asc. aorta

Pulm. artery

Left pulmonary artery

Left pulmonary veins

Right pulmonary artery

Right pulmonary veins

auricle

Right atrium

Right border of heart

Coronary sulcus (Atrio-ventricular groove)

Inferior vena cava

Inferior border of heart

Right ventricle

Auricle of left atrium

Coronary sulcus (Atrio-ventricular groove)

Left ventricle

Left border of heart

Ant. interventricular sulcus (Ant. longitudinal groove)

Apex of heart

N·JOY

434 Heart and Great Vessels, hardened in situ and removed en masse, sternocostal aspect

The pericardium is colored yellow.

Observe:

1. In shape and in size the heart resembles a closed right fist, the apex being the proximal interphalangeal joint of the index.

2. The right border, formed by the right atrium, slightly convex and almost in line with the superior and inferior caval veins. The inferior border (margo acutus), formed by the right ventricle and slightly by the left ventricle. The left border, formed by the left ventricle and very slightly by the left auricle.

3. The entire right auricle and much of the right atrium are visible from the front, but only a slight portion of the left auricle is visible. The auricles, like two closing claws, grasping the pulmonary artery and ascending aorta from behind.

4. The anterior interventricular sulcus, about a thumb's breadth from the left border.

5. The pulmonary trunk (artery), bifurcating below the aortic arch into the right and the left pulmonary artery.

6. The ligamentum arteriosum, continuing the direction of the pulmonary trunk (artery), and passing from the root of the left pulmonary artery to the aortic arch beyond the site of origin of the left subclavian artery.

7. The three branches of the aortic arch, crossed anteriorly by the left innominate vein.

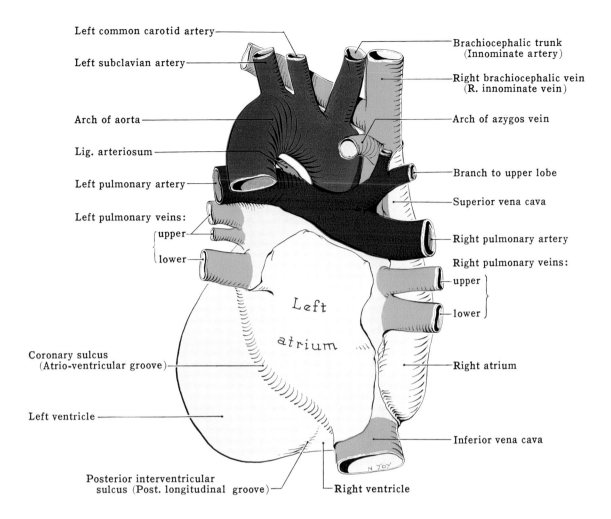

Left common carotid artery

Left subclavian artery

Arch of aorta

Lig. arteriosum

Left pulmonary artery

Left pulmonary veins:
  upper
  lower

Coronary sulcus
(Atrio-ventricular groove)

Left ventricle

Posterior interventricular
sulcus (Post. longitudinal groove)

Brachiocephalic trunk
(Innominate artery)

Right brachiocephalic vein
(R. innominate vein)

Arch of azygos vein

Branch to upper lobe

Superior vena cava

Right pulmonary artery

Right pulmonary veins:
  upper
  lower

Right atrium

Inferior vena cava

Right ventricle

Left atrium

435 Heart and Great Vessels, hardened in situ and removed en masse, posterior aspect

Observe:

1. Visible from behind: most of the left atrium, much of the left ventricle, a little of the right atrium, and almost none of the right ventricle.

2. The right and left pulmonary veins, converging to open into the left atrium. The part of the atrium between them lies to the left of the line of the i. vena cava, occupies the median plane, and forms the anterior wall of the pericardial cul-de-sac called the oblique pericardial sinus, which admits two fingers. Compare this with figures 176 and 136 of the caudate lobe of the liver, which likewise lies to the left of the line of the i. vena cava, occupies the median plane and forms the anterior wall of the peritoneal cul-de-sac called the upper recess of the omental bursa (lesser sac), which admits two fingers.

3. The right and left pulmonary arteries, just above and parallel to the pulmonary veins and inclining from the left side downwards and to the right. Hence, the root of the right lung is lower than that of the left.

4. The aorta, arching over the left pulmonary vessels (and bronchus); the azygos vein arching over the right pulmonary vessels (and bronchus).

5. The aortic arch, arched in two planes: (a) upwards, (b) to the left. The convexity to the left is moulded on the esophagus and trachea.

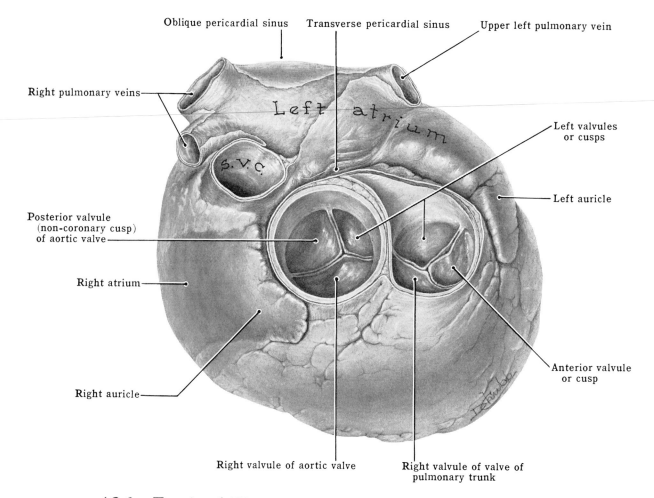

Oblique pericardial sinus　Transverse pericardial sinus　Upper left pulmonary vein

Right pulmonary veins

Left atrium

S.V.C.

Left valvules or cusps

Left auricle

Posterior valvule (non-coronary cusp) of aortic valve

Right atrium

Right auricle

Anterior valvule or cusp

Right valvule of aortic valve　Right valvule of valve of pulmonary trunk

436　Excised Heart, viewed from above

Observe:

1. The anterior position of the ventricles; the posterior position of the atria.

2. The ascending aorta and the pulmonary trunk, which conduct blood from the ventricles, accordingly placed anterior to the atria and to the s. vena cava and pulmonary veins, which conduct blood to the atria.

3. These two stems, enclosed within a common tube of serous pericardium; and partly embraced by the auricles of the atria.

4. The transverse pericardial sinus, curving behind the enclosed stems of the aorta and pulmonary trunk, and in front of the s. vena cava and upper limits of the atria.

Note: (a) The upper border of the atria is also the upper border of the heart.

(b) The names of the semilunar cusps or valvules of the aortic valve and valve of the pulmonary trunk have a developmental origin, as explained in figure 446.3.

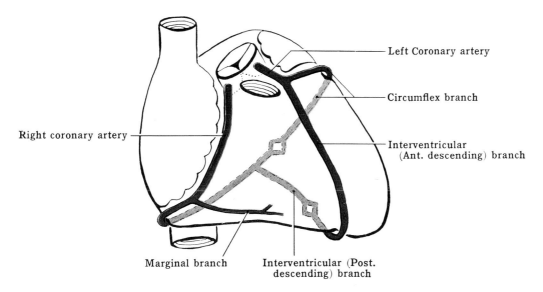

Left Coronary artery

Circumflex branch

Right coronary artery

Interventricular
(Ant. descending) branch

Marginal branch

Interventricular (Post.
descending) branch

437 Diagram of the Coronary (Cardiac) Arteries

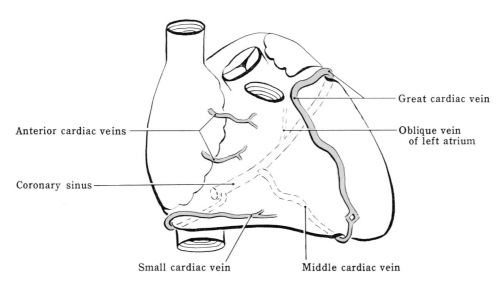

Great cardiac vein

Anterior cardiac veins

Oblique vein
of left atrium

Coronary sinus

Small cardiac vein

Middle cardiac vein

438 Diagram of the Cardiac Veins

A.
Left coronary artery supplying
part of right coronary artery
territory.

B.
A single coronary artery.

C.
Circumflex branch springing
from right aortic sinus.

439 Some Varieties of Coronary Arteries

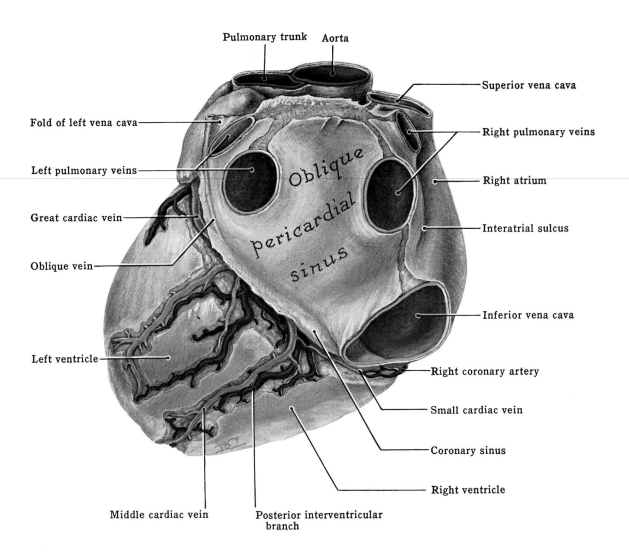

Pulmonary trunk   Aorta

Superior vena cava

Fold of left vena cava

Right pulmonary veins

Left pulmonary veins

Right atrium

Oblique pericardial sinus

Great cardiac vein

Interatrial sulcus

Oblique vein

Inferior vena cava

Left ventricle

Right coronary artery

Small cardiac vein

Coronary sinus

Right ventricle

Middle cardiac vein   Posterior interventricular branch

440 Heart, viewed from behind

This heart was excised from specimen 441, on the opposite page

Observe:

1. The entire base, or posterior surface, and part of the diaphragmatic surface are in view.
2. The slight appearance made by the right atrium.
3. The superior and the much larger inferior caval vein joining the upper and lower limits of the right atrium.
4. The left atrium, forming the greater part of the posterior surface.
5. The coronary arteries, here irregular in that the left one supplies the posterior interventricular branch.
6. Branches of the cardiac veins, when crossing branches of the coronary arteries, mostly do so superficially.
7. The fold of the left caval vein. For its significance consult figure 456.
8. The right pulmonary artery (removed) lay on the bare strip at the upper border of the atria, and therefore intervened between the oblique sinus and the transverse sinus (not labelled).

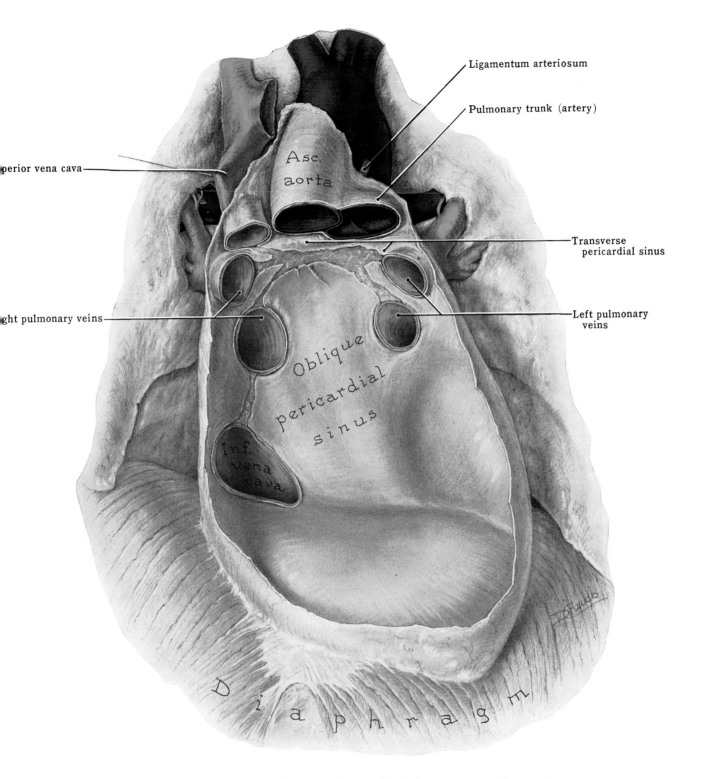

Ligamentum arteriosum

Pulmonary trunk (artery)

Asc. aorta

perior vena cava

Transverse pericardial sinus

ght pulmonary veins

Left pulmonary veins

Oblique pericardial sinus

Inf. vena cava

Diaphragm

441   Interior of the Pericardial Sac, anterior view

Observe:

1. The 8 vessels severed on excising a heart—2 caval veins, 4 pulmonary veins, and 2 arteries.

2. The oblique sinus, circumscribed by 5 veins; open below and to the left; and rising to the level of the right pulmonary artery which separates it from the transverse sinus.

3. The peak of the sac, on the aorta, at, or near, the junction of the ascending part and the arch.

4. The superior vena cava, partly inside and partly outside the pericardium, and the ligamentum arteriosum entirely outside.

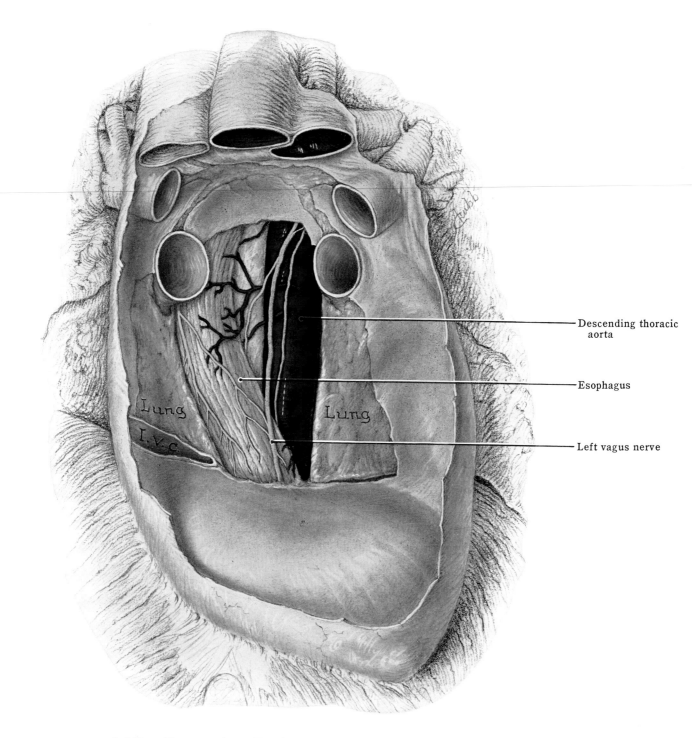

Descending thoracic
aorta

Esophagus

Left vagus nerve

Lung

Lung

I.v.c.

442 Posterior Relations of the Heart and Pericardium

The parietal pericardium (fibrous and serous layers) has been removed behind the oblique sinus and also on each side of it.

Observe:

1. The posterior relations are:—part of the right lung and the esophagus grooving it; part of the left lung and the aorta grooving it; and the vagus nerves forming a plexus on the esophagus.

2. The esophagus is here unduly deflected to the right. It usually lies in contact with the aorta.

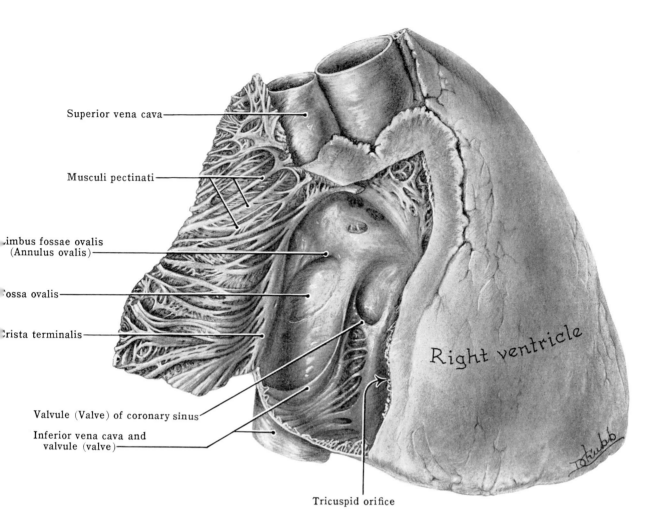

Superior vena cava

Musculi pectinati

Limbus fossae ovalis
(Annulus ovalis)

Fossa ovalis

Crista terminalis

Valvule (Valve) of coronary sinus

Inferior vena cava and
valvule (valve)

Right ventricle

Tricuspid orifice

443 Interior of the Right Atrium, antero-lateral view

Observe:

1. The smooth part of the atrial wall (primitive sinus venarum) and the rough part (primitive atrium).

2. The crista terminalis, the valvule of the i. v. cava, and the valvule of the coronary sinus, separating the smooth from the rough.

3. The 2 caval veins and the coronary sinus opening on to the smooth part.

4. That blunt forceps, passed upwards through the i. v. cava and in contact with its posterior wall, would catch on the limbus fossae ovalis; and, if the foramen ovale were patent (25 per cent), would pass through the interatrial septum into the left atrium.

5. The crista terminalis, descending from the front of the s. v. cava to the front of the i. v. cava; and the musculi pectinati, passing forwards from the crista like teeth from the back of a comb. The crista underlies the sulcus terminalis (fig. 433).

6. The right atrio-ventricular or tricuspid orifice, situated at the anterior aspect of the atrium.

7. The anterior cardiac veins (fig. 433) and the venae minimae (Thebesian veins) not visible, also open into the atrium.

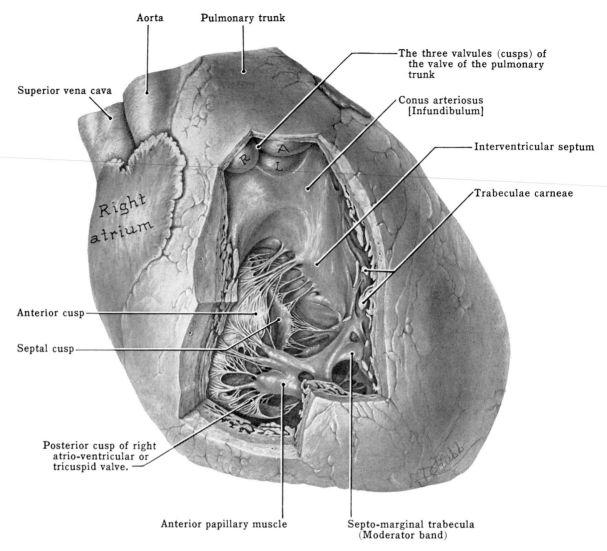

Aorta   Pulmonary trunk

Superior vena cava

The three valvules (cusps) of the valve of the pulmonary trunk

Conus arteriosus [Infundibulum]

Interventricular septum

Trabeculae carneae

Right atrium

R A L

Anterior cusp

Septal cusp

Posterior cusp of right atrio-ventricular or tricuspid valve.

Anterior papillary muscle   Septo-marginal trabecula (Moderator band)

444   Interior of the Right Ventricle

Observe:

1. The entrance to this chamber (right atrio-ventricular or tricuspid orifice), situated behind; the exit (orifice of the pulmonary trunk) situated above.

2. The smooth funnel-shaped wall (conus arteriosus) below the pulmonary orifice; the remainder of the ventricle, rough with fleshy trabeculae.

3. Three types of trabeculae—(a) mere ridges, (b) bridges, attached only at each end, and (c) finger-like projections called papillary muscles. The anterior papillary muscle rising from the anterior wall; the posterior (not labelled) from the posterior wall; and a series of small septal papillae from the septal wall.

4. The septo-marginal trabecula, here very thick, extending from the septum to the base of the anterior papillary muscle. It is a bridge.

5. The chordae tendineae (not labelled), passing from the tips of the papillary muscles to the free margins and ventricular surfaces of the three cusps of the tricuspid valve.

6. Each papillary muscle controlling the adjacent sides of two cusps (fig. 446).

(For names given to valvules or cusps of pulmonary trunk, see fig. 446.3.)

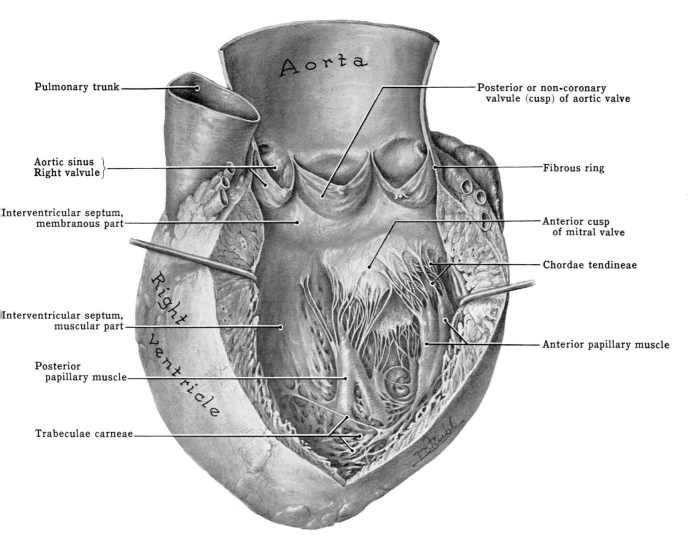

Pulmonary trunk

Aortic sinus }
Right valvule }

Interventricular septum,
membranous part

Interventricular septum,
muscular part

Posterior
papillary muscle

Trabeculae carneae

Aorta

Right Ventricle

Posterior or non-coronary
valvule (cusp) of aortic valve

Fibrous ring

Anterior cusp
of mitral valve

Chordae tendineae

Anterior papillary muscle

445   Interior of the Left Ventricle

Observe:

1. The conical shape of the left chamber.
2. The entrance (left atrio-ventricular, bicuspid, or mitral orifice), situated posteriorly. The exit (aortic orifice), situated superiorly.
3. The wall, thin and muscular near the apex; thick and muscular above; thin and fibrous (nonelastic) at the aortic orifice.
4. Trabeculae carneae, as in the right ventricle, forming ridges,

bridges, and papillary muscles.

5. Two large papillary muscles—the anterior from the anterior wall and the posterior from the posterior wall—each controlling, via chordae tendineae, the adjacent halves of two cusps of the mitral valve.
6. The anterior cusp of the mitral valve intervening between the inlet (mitral orifice) and the outlet (aortic orifice).

Note the structure of the mitral and of the aortic valves (fig. 446).

445.1

Diagram of the impulse conducting system of the heart, after *J. W. A. Duckworth.*

The ventricles have been opened and the tricuspid valve has been removed.

Note the sinu-atrial node (S-A. node) at the upper end of the sulcus terminalis, and the atrio-ventricular node (A-V. node) in the lower part of the interatrial septum becoming the A-V. bundle which divides into a right and a left limb.

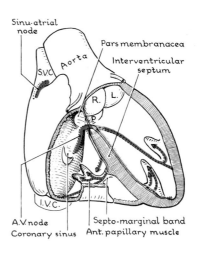

Sinu-atrial
node

Pars membranacea

Interventricular
septum

Aorta

SVC

R. L.
P.

I.V.C.

A.V. node
Coronary sinus

Septo-marginal band
Ant. papillary muscle

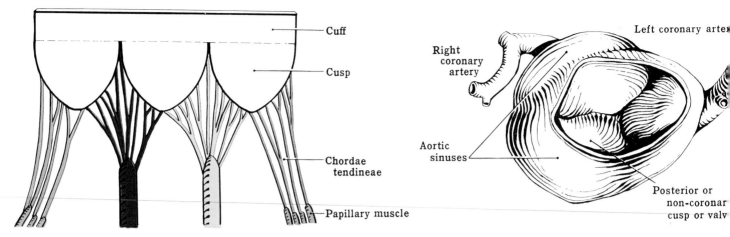

Cuff

Cusp

Chordae
tendineae

Papillary muscle

Left coronary arter

Right
coronary
artery

Aortic
sinuses

Posterior or
non-coronar
cusp or valv

446 Diagram of Right Atrioventricular Valve, spread out

446.1 Aortic Valve, closed, ventricular aspect

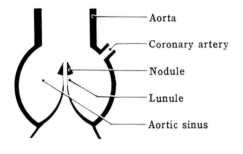

Aorta

Coronary artery

Nodule

Lunule

Aortic sinus

A. Closed, on longitudinal section.

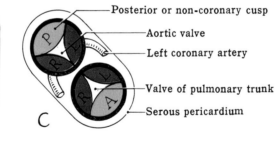

Lunule

Nodule

B. Spread out.

446.2 Diagram of the Aort Valve, closed and spread o

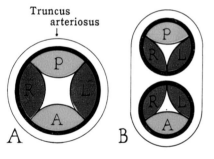

Truncus
arteriosus

A   B   C

Posterior or non-coronary cusp

Aortic valve

Left coronary artery

Valve of pulmonary trunk

Serous pericardium

446.3 Names applied to the V vules, or cusps, of the Aortic Val and Valve of the Pulmonary Tru explained on a development ba

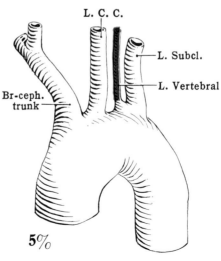

R. C. C.

R. Subcl.

Br-ceph.
trunk

L. C. C.

L. Subcl.

11%

L. C. C.

Br-ceph.
trunk

L. Subcl.

L. Vertebral

5%

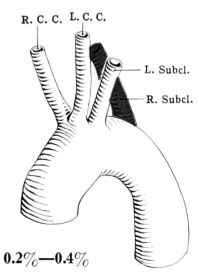

R. C. C. L. C. C.

L. Subcl.

R. Subcl.

0.2%—0.4%

446.4   Variations in the Origins of the Branches of the Aortic Arch

Approximate incidence: 11% of 1220 arches, 5% of 1000 arches, and 0.2% — 0.4% of 1500 arches. (Data on British and Japanese after Quain; Thomson; Adachi; and Loth.)

447 Scheme of Varieties of Aortic Arches

Note: The double aortic arch of the frog; the right aortic arch of the bird; the left aortic arch of the mammal, including man; and a variant.

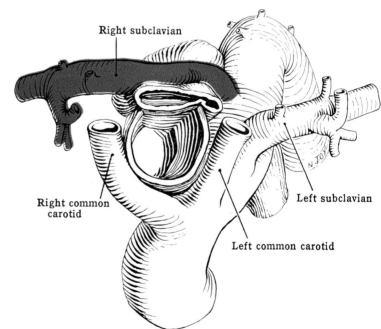

447.1 Specimen of a Double Aortic Arch, in an adult

Note: Both the right and the left aortic arch persist completely, as in the frog. The esophagus and trachea pass through the "aortic ring" so-formed. The condition is rare, and rarely do cases survive childhood.

447.2 Retro-esophageal Right Subclavian Artery

Note: The artery arises as the last branch of the aortic arch. It passes behind the esophagus and trachea. The right recurrent laryngeal nerve, having no vessel around which to recur, takes a direct course to the larynx, as in figure 532 drawn from the same subject. This condition was found in 14 or about 1% of 1,453 White, Negro, and Japanese cadavera (J. J. McDonald and Barry J. Anson).

VARIATIONS AND ANOMALIES

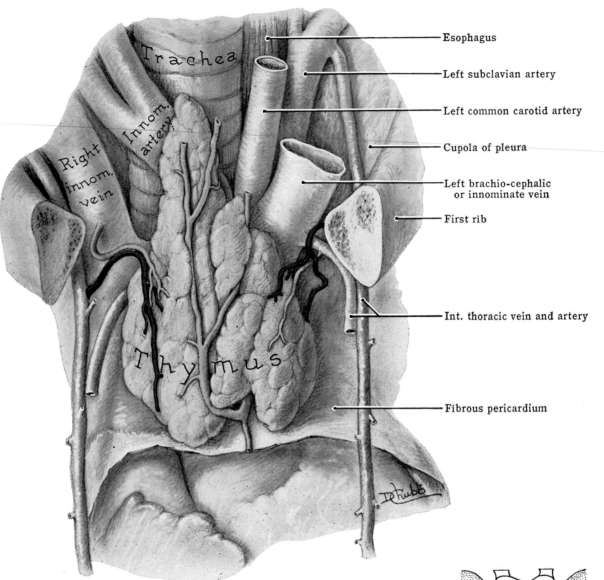

Esophagus

Left subclavian artery

Left common carotid artery

Cupola of pleura

Left brachio-cephalic
or innominate vein

First rib

Int. thoracic vein and artery

Fibrous pericardium

448   Thymus: Superior Mediastinum—I

The sternum and ribs have been excised and the pleurae removed.

Observe:

1. The thymus lying in the superior mediastinum; overlapping the upper
   limit of the pericardial sac below; and extending into the neck, here farther than usual, above.

2. The longitudinal fissure that divides the thymus into two asymmetrical
   lobes, a larger right and a smaller left. These two developmentally
   separate parts are easily separated from each other by blunt dissection.

3. The blood supply—arteries from the internal thoracic arteries; veins to
   the brachio-cephalic and internal thoracic veins and communicating
   above with the inferior thyroid veins.

4. The posterior relations, shown in figure 449.

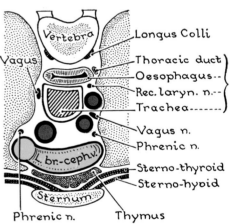

448.1

Diagram of the superior mediastinum, o
cross-section, above the level of the aorti
arch.

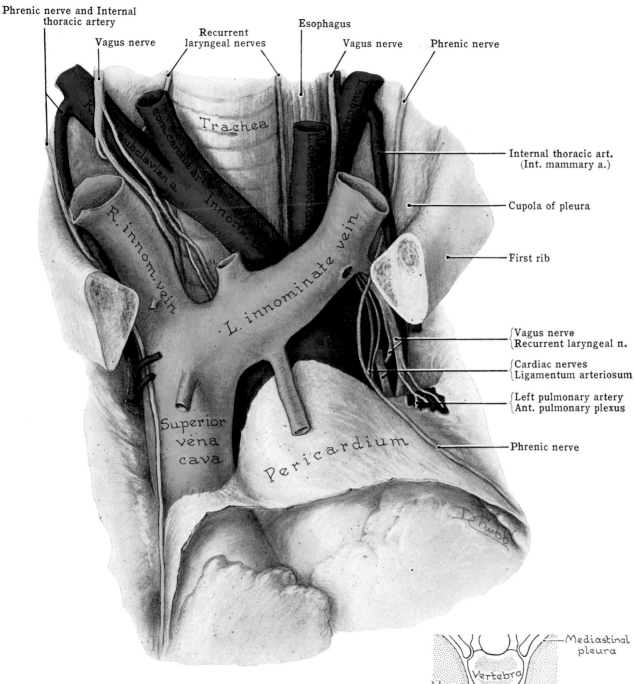

Phrenic nerve and Internal thoracic artery

Vagus nerve

Recurrent laryngeal nerves

Esophagus

Vagus nerve

Phrenic nerve

Trachea

R. innom. vein

L. innominate vein

Superior vena cava

Pericardium

Internal thoracic art. (Int. mammary a.)

Cupola of pleura

First rib

Vagus nerve
Recurrent laryngeal n.

Cardiac nerves
Ligamentum arteriosum

Left pulmonary artery
Ant. pulmonary plexus

Phrenic nerve

449 Root of the Neck: Superior Mediastinum—II

This is figure 448 with the thymus removed.

Observe:

The great veins, anterior to the great arteries.

The backward direction of the aortic arch and the nerves crossing its left side.

The lig. arteriosum, outside the pericardial sac and having the left recurrent nerve on its left side and the vagal and sympathetic branches to the superficial cardiac plexus on its right.

The right vagus, crossing the right subclavian a. (4th right primitive aortic arch), there giving off its recurrent branch, and passing medially to reach the trachea and esophagus.

The left vagus, crossing the aortic arch (4th left primitive aortic arch), there giving off its recurrent branch, and passing medially to reach the esophagus (fig. 450).

The left phrenic nerve, crossing the path of the vagus, but $\frac{1}{2}''$ anterior to it.

Mediastinal pleura

Vertebra

Vagus

Unit of 4 parallel structures

L. vagus n.

S.V.C.

Arch

Cardiac brs. of sympathetic & vagus nn.

Sternum

R. phrenic n.   L. phrenic n.

449.1

Diagram of the superior mediastinum, on cross-section, at the level of the aortic arch.

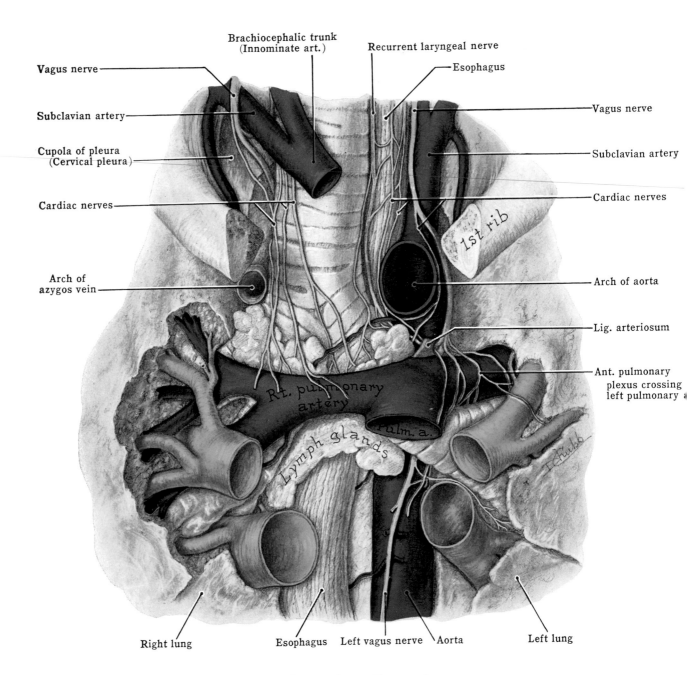

Vagus nerve

Brachiocephalic trunk
(Innominate art.)

Recurrent laryngeal nerve

Esophagus

Subclavian artery

Vagus nerve

Cupola of pleura
(Cervical pleura)

Subclavian artery

Cardiac nerves

Cardiac nerves

1st rib

Arch of
azygos vein

Arch of aorta

Lig. arteriosum

Ant. pulmonary
plexus crossing
left pulmonary a.

Rt. pulmonary
artery

Pulm. a.

Lymph glands

Right lung

Esophagus

Left vagus nerve

Aorta

Left lung

450 Pulmonary Arteries: Superior Mediastinum—III

Observe:

1. The pulmonary trunk, dividing below the aortic arch into the right and left pulmonary arteries. These arteries, running a straight, but oblique, course.—i.e. it is not horizontal. The right artery crossing just below the bifurcation of the trachea and separated from the esophagus by lymph nodes (glands).

2. The ligamentum arteriosum, passing from the beginning of the left pulmonary artery to the aorta beyond the point of origin of the left subclavian artery.

3. Cardiac branches of the vagus and sympathetic, streaming down the sides of the trachea and forming the cardiac plexuses.

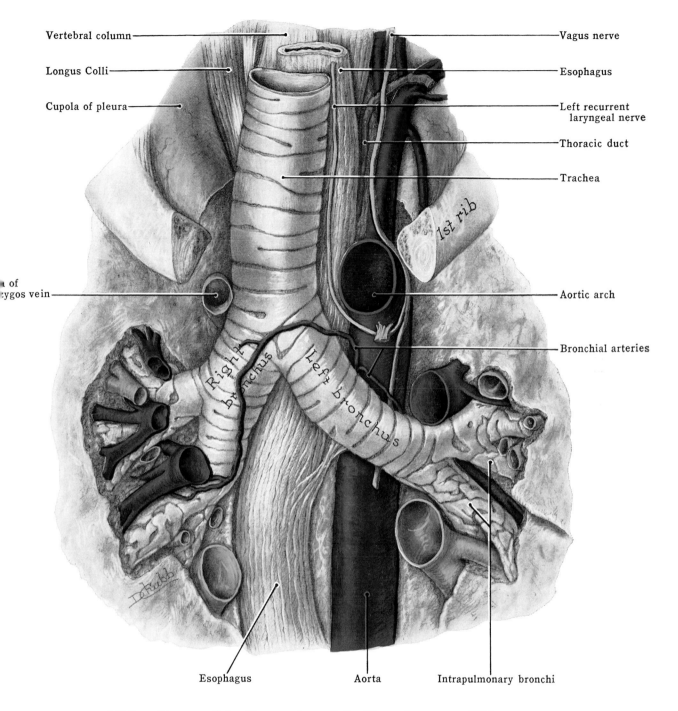

Vertebral column

Longus Colli

Cupola of pleura

...of ...ygos vein

Vagus nerve

Esophagus

Left recurrent laryngeal nerve

Thoracic duct

Trachea

1st rib

Aortic arch

Bronchial arteries

Right bronchus

Left bronchus

Esophagus

Aorta

Intrapulmonary bronchi

451 Bronchi: Superior Mediastinum—IV

Observe:

1. Four longitudinally running structures—trachea, esophagus, left recurrent laryngeal nerve, and thoracic duct. Of these, the esophagus bulges to the left of the median plane; the recurrent nerve lies in the angle between the trachea and esophagus; and the thoracic duct is at the side of the esophagus.

2. The arch of the aorta passing backwards on the side of these four structures, and the arch of the azygos vein passing forwards on the right.

3. The trachea inclining slightly to the right with the result that the right bronchus is more vertical that the left bronchus. The stem of the right bronchus is also shorter and wider, its first branch arising about 1″ from the bifurcation, whereas the first branch of the left stem arises about 2″ from the bifurcation.

4. The U-shaped rings of the trachea, commonly bifurcated; the ring at the bifurcation of the trachea being V-shaped; the intrapulmonary rings forming a mosaic around the bronchi.

5. The occasional muscular band, broncho-esophageal muscle, attaching the esophagus to the left bronchus.

Esophagus

Trachea

Vertebral artery

Thyro-cervical trunk

Costo-cervical trunk

Internal thoracic artery
(Int. mammary art.)

1st Rib

Right subclavian artery

Right common carotid artery

Brachiocephalic trunk

Arch of azygos vein

Lymph nodes

Right bronchus

Esophagus

Thoracic duct

Diaphragm

Left subclavian artery

Left common carotid artery

Aortic arch

Left bronchus

Aorta

Cisterna chyii

N.Joy

452 Esophagus, Trachea and Aorta, thoracic parts, anterior view

Observe:

1. The arch of the aorta, arching backwards on the left side of the trachea and esophagus, and the arch of the azygos vein arching forwards on their right sides. Each arches above the respective root of the lung (figs. 415 and 416).

2. The posterior relation of the trachea is the esophagus.

3. The anterior relations of the thoracic part of the esophagus from above downwards are: trachea (throughout its entire length), the right and left bronchi, the inferior tracheobronchial lymph nodes (in front of which lies the right pulmonary artery, fig. 450), the pericardium (removed, in front of which lies the oblique pericardial sinus and the left atrium of the heart, figs. 441 & 442), and finally, the diaphragm.

4. Above the level of the aortic arch, the esophagus bulges to the left beyond the trachea.

Broncho-mediastinal trunk

Jugular trunk

Right lymphatic duct

Subclavian trunk

Superior vena cava

Azygos vein

Collecting trunk

Thoracic duct

Collecting trunk

Inferior vena cava

L. Innominate Vein

Jugular trunk

Thoracic duct

Subclavian trunk

Left superior intercostal vein

Collecting trunk

Descending thoracic aorta

Esophagus

N. Joy

Diaphragm

453 Thoracic Duct

(A composite sketch made from photographs of two specimens dissected by Miss M. G. Gray.)

Observe

1. The thoracic duct (a) ascending on the vertebral column between the azygos vein and the descending aorta; and (b) at the junction of the posterior and superior mediastina, passing to the left and continuing its ascent to the neck where (c) it arches laterally to open near, or at, the angle of union of the internal jugular and subclavian veins.

2. The duct, here, as commonly, (a) plexiform in the posterior mediastinum and (b) splitting in the neck.

3. The duct receiving branches from the intercostal spaces of both sides via several collecting trunks and also branches from posterior mediastinal structures.

4. The duct finally receiving the jugular, subclavian, and broncho-mediastinal trunks.

5. The right lymph duct, very short and formed by the union of the right jugular, subclavian, and broncho-mediastinal trunks.

For origin of duct in cisterna chyli see figure 452; for termination of duct in the neck see figures 533 and 536.

Brachiocephalic trunk
(Innominate artery)

Thyroid
Gland

Right inferior
thyroid artery

Right supreme
intercostal artery

Right third posterior
intercostal artery

Arch of azygos vein

Thoracic duct

Azygos vein

454 Arterial Supply to the Trachea and Esophagus (right three-quarter view)

Observe:

1. The four unpaired median branches of the descending thoracic aorta (2 bronchial & 2 esophageal), which supply the trachea, bronchi, and esophagus. They are in series with the three unpaired median branches of the abdominal aorta (celiac, sup. mesenteric, and inf. mesenteric arteries), which supply the gastro-intestinal tract. (Continued on next page.

N. JOY

Branches of left gastric artery

Diaphragm

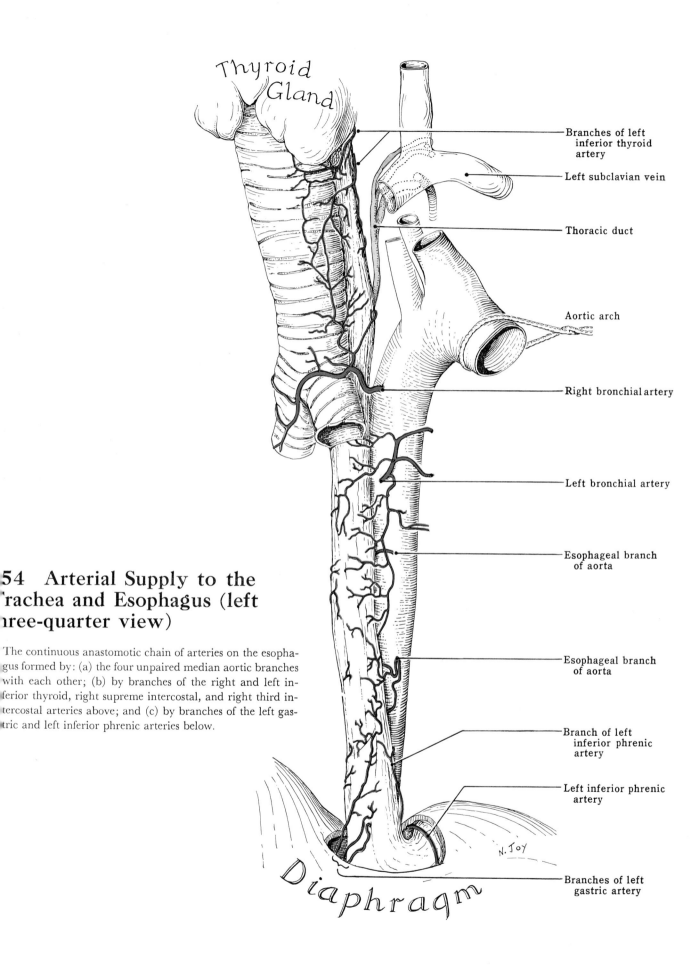

Thyroid Gland

Branches of left inferior thyroid artery

Left subclavian vein

Thoracic duct

Aortic arch

Right bronchial artery

Left bronchial artery

Esophageal branch of aorta

Esophageal branch of aorta

Branch of left inferior phrenic artery

Left inferior phrenic artery

Branches of left gastric artery

Diaphragm

N. Joy

54 Arterial Supply to the Trachea and Esophagus (left three-quarter view)

The continuous anastomotic chain of arteries on the esophagus formed by: (a) the four unpaired median aortic branches with each other; (b) by branches of the right and left inferior thyroid, right supreme intercostal, and right third intercostal arteries above; and (c) by branches of the left gastric and left inferior phrenic arteries below.

Right brachio-cephalic
or innominate vein

Left innom. vein

Left superior
intercostal vein

Aortic arch

Superior vena cava

Azygos vein

Accessory (Superior)
hemiazygos vein

Right posterior
intercostal veins

(Inferior)
Hemiazygos vein

Cut edge of pleura

Costo-diaphragmatic recess
(Phrenico-costal sinus)

Diaphragm

T12

Celiac artery

Sup. mesenteric artery

Left renal vein

Inf.
vena
cava

Aorta

455   Azygos System of Veins

Observe:

1. The left renal vein anterior to the aorta, and the left innominate or brachiocephalic vein anterior to the three branches of the aortic arch. These two cross-channels conduct blood from the left side of the body to the right side—and so to the right atrium.

2. The paired and approximately symmetrical, right and left, veins in front of the vertebral column. The right, or azygos, vein communicating below with the i. v. cava; the left vein communicating with the left renal vein; and each receiving the respective right and left posterior intercostal veins. The right vein ending above in the s. v. cava; the left in the left brachio-cephalic, or innominate, vein.

3. The left vein being a chain of veins—hemiazygos, accessory hemiazygos, and left superior intercostal—which here are continuous, but commonly are discontinuous. It is united to the right, or azygos, vein by several (here 4) cross-connecting channels. (Sieb.)

56 Persisting Left superior Vena Cava

The vessel connecting the left brachiocephalic innominate vein to the coronary sinus is the rimitive left superior vena cava. It has 3 component segments: (1) an upper, the stem of the ft superior intercostal vein; (2) a lower, the blique vein of the left atrium; and (3) a middle, e vein uniting the intercostal vein to the blique vein.

This channel to the right atrium functioned til the left superior vena cava established conction with the right by means of the left achiocephalic vein, after which the blood as re-routed, and the middle segment disap-ared, though it may persist as a vestigial thread ithin the fold of the left vena cava.

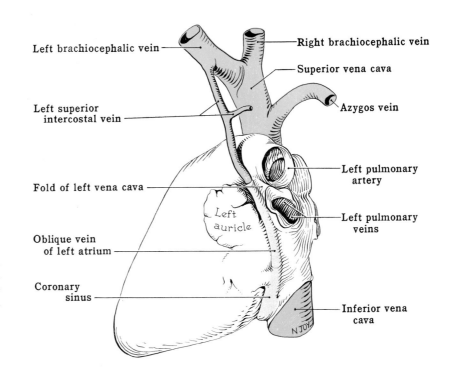

Left brachiocephalic vein
Right brachiocephalic vein
Superior vena cava
Left superior intercostal vein
Azygos vein
Left pulmonary artery
Fold of left vena cava
Left auricle
Left pulmonary veins
Oblique vein of left atrium
Coronary sinus
Inferior vena cava

457 Lobe of the Azygos Vein

This lobe, said to be constant in the porpoise, really part of a bifid apex. It results during mbryonic life when the apex of a developing ight lung encounters the arch of the azygos ein and is cleft by it, a portion of the apex com-g to lie on each side of the venous arch. The enous arch is suspended, so to speak, within pleural mesentery.

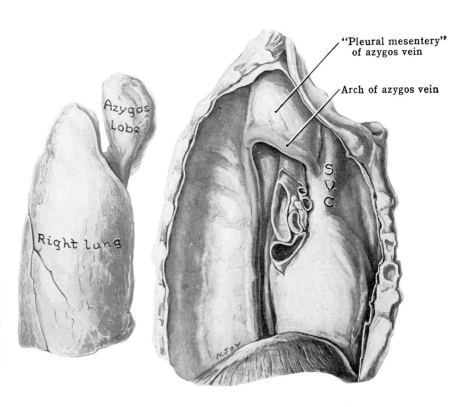

Azygos Lobe
Right lung
"Pleural mesentery" of azygos vein
Arch of azygos vein
S.V.C.

Variation and Anomaly

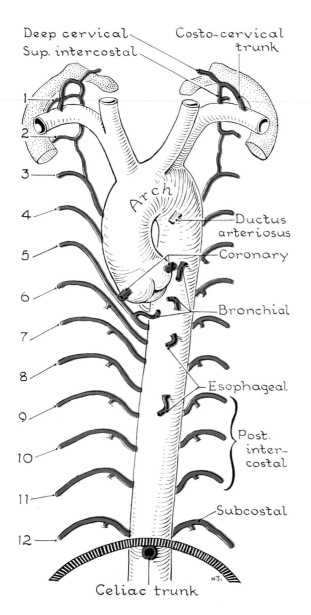

Deep cervical
Sup. intercostal

Costo-cervical trunk

1
2
3
4
5
6
7
8
9
10
11
12

Arch

Ductus arteriosus

Coronary

Bronchial

Esophageal

Post. inter-costal

Subcostal

Celiac trunk

N.J.

457.1 Thoracic Aorta and its Branches

The three parts of this artery give off branches as follows:

From the Ascending Aorta:
    Right coronary
    Left coronary

From the Arch of the Aorta:
    Brachiocephalic trunk
        Right subclavian
        Right common carotid
    Left common carotid
    Left subclavian
    (Occasional patent ductus arteriosus)

From the Descending Thoracic Aorta:
    Visceral branches:
        Esophageal
        Bronchial, left upper & lower
        Right bronchial
        Pericardial
        Mediastinal
    Parietal branches, paired:
        Posterior intercostal (Th. 3—11)
        Subcostal (Th. 12)
        Superior phrenic

Note:

When the ductus arteriosus remains patent, there is, of course, no ligamentum arteriosum. The right bronchial artery usually arises from either the upper left bronchial artery or the third right posterior intercostal artery (here the fifth) or the aorta direct. The small arteries to the pericardium, the tissues in the posterior mediastinum, and the upper surface of the diaphragm are not shown.

(For variations in the branching of the aortic arch, see figs. 446.4 & 447.)
(For abdominal aorta and its branches, see fig. 188.)

The Head and Neck

Superior sagittal sinus

Skin

Subcutaneous tissue

Occipito-frontalis

"Dangerous area"

Pericranium

Falx Cerebri

Corpus callosum

Tentorium cerebelli

Fornix
Septum pellucidum

Frontal sinus

Mid-brain

Pons

Cerebellum

Medulla

Lamina cribrosa

Palate

Septum nasi

Ext. occipital protuberanc

Int. occipital protuberanc

Falx cerebelli

Apical recess

Tongue

2

Atlas (post. arch)

Dens of axis

Geniohyoid

Epiglottis

Posterior wall of pharynx

Mylohyoid

Mandible

Retropharyngeal space

Thyroid cartilage

Plica vocalis
Larynx

6

Cricoid cartilage, lamina of

Cricoid cartilage, arch of

Trachea

Thyroid gland

Suprasternal space

Spinal cord or medulla

Thymus
Brachioceph. trunk
L. brachioceph. vein

2

Manubrium sterni

Esophagus

Sternal angle

Lig. flavum

Aorta

Pleural cavity

Pericardial cavity

Right bronchus

Observe:

1. The 3 adherent layers of the scalp—skin, subcutaneous tissue, and occipito-frontalis muscle—separated from the pericranium by loose areolar tissue (the dangerous area) in which, following injury, blood or pus may collect.

2. The tentorium cerebelli suspended by the falx cerebri, sloping to the internal occipital protuberance, and forming a floor for the cerebrum (removed) and a roof for the cerebellum. The external occipital protuberance, nearly level with the internal protuberance, marking the line between scalp and thick bone above and nuchal muscles and thin bone below.

3. Behind the tip or apex of the nose, a shelf above which is the apical recess of the nasal cavity.

4. The nasal septum extending from the apical recess in front to the nasopharynx behind, where it ends in a free posterior border, and from the sieve-like lamina cribrosa (cribriform plate) above to the palate below.

5. The palate, the anterior $\frac{2}{3}$ of which contains bone and is known as the hard palate, and the posterior $\frac{1}{3}$ which contains gland and muscle and is called soft palate. The Levator Palati (in contraction, as it is during the act of swallowing) pulling the soft palate upward and backward (it retracts as well as elevates) thereby closing the oral pharynx (not labelled), which lies below the soft palate, from the nasopharynx which lies above. A small mass, the pharyngeal tonsil, projecting from the roof of the nasopharynx.

6. The Orbicularis Oris in the upper and lower lips, with free margins curved forward. The incisor teeth in modern man, not biting edge to edge but edge to lingual surface.

7. The Geniohyoid passing from the mental spine (genial tubercle) of the mandible to the hyoid bone (not labelled), and above it the Genioglossus (not labelled) radiating into the tongue. The anterior $\frac{2}{3}$ of the tongue forming part of the floor of the mouth; the posterior $\frac{1}{3}$ forming the anterior wall of the oral pharynx. Behind the tongue, the epiglottis.

8. The larynx, guarded in front by the thyroid cartilage and extending from the tip of the epiglottis above to the lower border of the cricoid cartilage below, where it becomes the trachea. A horizontal slit that runs posteriorly from the thyroid cartilage separating an upper or false cord from a lower or true vocal cord, the plica vocalis.

9. The 4″ to $4\frac{1}{2}$″ long trachea, half in the neck and half in the thorax, bifurcating below into a right and a left bronchus, the mouth of the right bronchus being in view.

10. The cut ends of 19 tracheal rings (they may be counted) below the arch of the cricoid cartilage which always projects in front of the rings and is therefore palpable and readily identified. It is a valuable landmark. It is also a guide to the level of the 6th cervical vertebra which lies behind it. The isthmus of the thyroid gland crossing several tracheal rings, but leaving the upper one or two uncovered. The brachio-cephalic trunk (innominate artery), here as commonly, impressing the trachea.

11. The cricoid cartilage lying at the level of the body of the 6th cervical vertebra. At the lower border of this cartilage the larynx becoming the trachea and the pharynx becoming the esophagus. The diameter of the alimentary canal is here at its narrowest and least dilatable part. In the neck the esophagus projects to the left of the trachea, hence the right wall of the upper part of the esophagus is cut longitudinally and no lumen is seen.

12. The retropharyngeal space extending from the level of the atlas downward into the superior mediastinum.

13. The manubrium sterni is 2″ in length and is its own length of 2″ from the body of the 2nd thoracic vertebra.

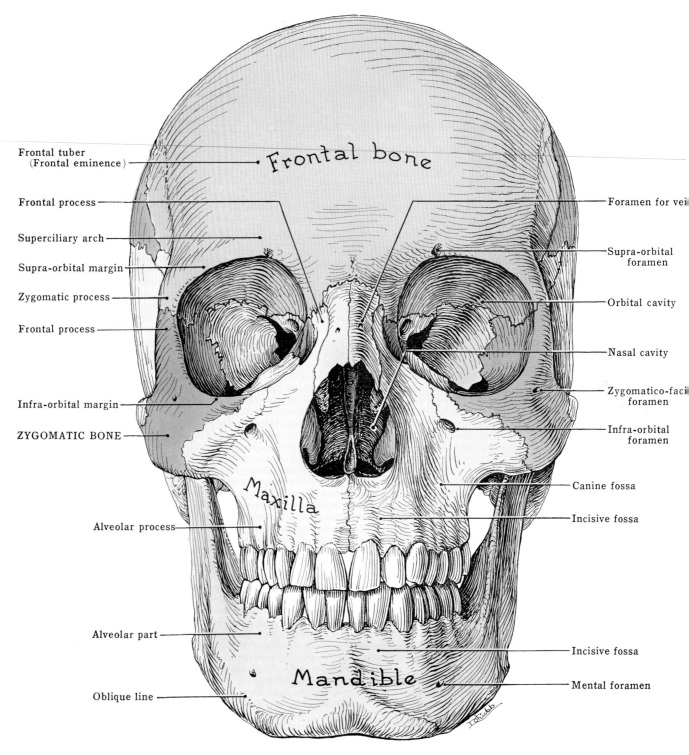

Frontal tuber
(Frontal eminence)

Frontal bone

Foramen for vei

Frontal process

Supra-orbital
foramen

Superciliary arch

Supra-orbital margin

Zygomatic process

Orbital cavity

Frontal process

Nasal cavity

Zygomatico-faci
foramen

Infra-orbital margin

Infra-orbital
foramen

ZYGOMATIC BONE

Maxilla

Canine fossa

Incisive fossa

Alveolar process

Alveolar part

Incisive fossa

Mandible

Mental foramen

Oblique line

459 Skull, front view (Norma Frontalis)

On the right side of the skull—surface features.

On the left side—foramina, fossae, and cavities.

Vertex

Temporal lines

Temporal fossa

Zygomatic arch

Post. border of ramus
of mandible

Angle of mandible

Base of mandible
(Inferior border)

Mental tubercle

Mental protuberance

(Interfrontal)
Metopic suture,
remains of

Glabella

Nasion

Internasal suture

Perpendicular plate
of ethmoid

Vomer

Anterior nasal spine

Intermaxillary suture

Symphysis menti

460 Skull, front view (Norma Frontalis)

On the right side of the skull—marginal or outline features.

On the left side—median line features.

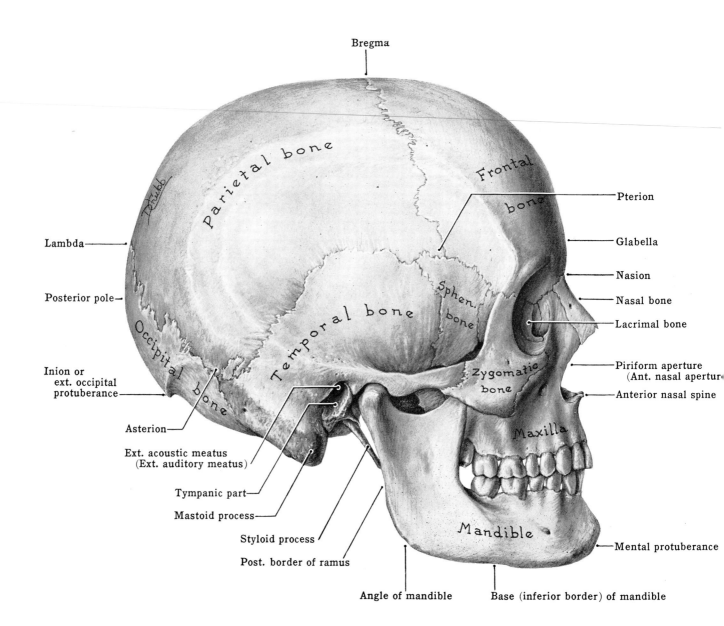

Bregma

Parietal bone

Frontal bone

Schubb

Pterion

Lambda

Glabella

Posterior pole

Nasion

Sphen. bone

Nasal bone

Temporal bone

Lacrimal bone

Inion or
ext. occipital
protuberance

Occipital bone

Zygomatic bone

Piriform aperture
(Ant. nasal aperture)

Anterior nasal spine

Asterion

Maxilla

Ext. acoustic meatus
(Ext. auditory meatus)

Tympanic part

Mastoid process

Mandible

Styloid process

Mental protuberance

Post. border of ramus

Angle of mandible

Base (inferior border) of mandible

461 Skull, from the side (Norma Lateralis)

Names of bones, outline features, and anthropological points.

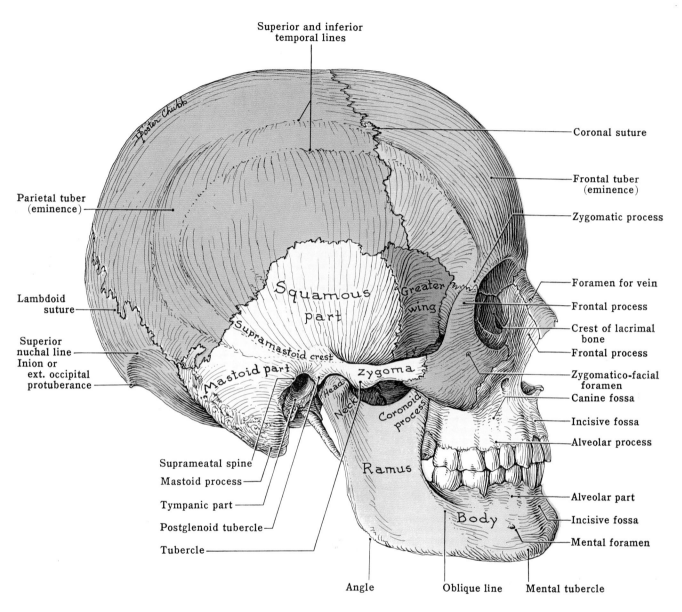

Superior and inferior
temporal lines

Coronal suture

Frontal tuber
(eminence)

Zygomatic process

Parietal tuber
(eminence)

Foramen for vein
Frontal process
Crest of lacrimal
bone
Frontal process
Zygomatico-facial
foramen
Canine fossa
Incisive fossa
Alveolar process

Greater wing

Squamous part

Supramastoid crest

zygoma

Head

Neck

Coronoid process

Mastoid part

Lambdoid
suture

Superior
nuchal line
Inion or
ext. occipital
protuberance

Alveolar part
Incisive fossa
Mental foramen

Ramus

Body

Suprameatal spine
Mastoid process
Tympanic part
Postglenoid tubercle
Tubercle

Angle

Oblique line

Mental tubercle

462 Skull, from the side (Norma Lateralis)

Names of parts of bones and surface features.
(Zygoma is short for zygomatic process of the temporal bone.)

SIDE VIEW

ABC

FRONT VIEW

463   The Buttresses of the Face

The mandible and the maxillae and the zygomatic bones are removed together with the smaller fragile bones of the face (nasal, lacrimal, inferior concha, vomer, and palatine).

Observe:

1. The three buttresses (yellow) on each side that prevent the bones of the face from being driven or displaced backward under the cranium are:
   (1) the zygomatic process of the temporal bone—horizontal,
   (2) the pterygoid process of the sphenoid bone—oblique,
   (3) the greater wing of the sphenoid bone—vertical.

2. The three buttresses (red) on each side that prevent the bones of the face from being driven or displaced upward are
   (A) the zygomatic process of the frontal bone,
   (B) the nasal part of the frontal bone,
   (C) the roof of the mandibular fossa for what it is worth—thin and translucent and easily fractured (see fig. 619.2.)

464 Buttresses of the Nose

A. The margin of the Piriform Aperture, or Bony Anterior Nasal Aperture, is sharp and is formed by the maxillae and the nasal bones.

B. On Removing the Nasal Bones the areas on the frontal processes of the maxillae (yellow) and on the frontal bone (blue) that articulate with and buttress the nasal bones are seen; so is the nasal septum (fig. 605).

B 1. Postero-superior view of the Nasal Bones in Articulation with each other shows the median crest which forms part of the nasal septum, the surfaces covered with mucous membrane (pink) and the grooves for the internal nasal nerves.

C. On Removing the Frontal Processes of the Maxillae and tilting the specimen, one sees:

. The areas of the frontal bone (yellow) against which the frontal processes of the maxillae abut,

. The areas of the labyrinths of the fragile ethmoid bone and the thin anterior borders of the lacrimal bones with which the maxillae articulate (red), and also

. The delicate and narrow lamina cribrosa (cribriform plate) of the ethmoid bone, which separates the roof of the nasal cavities from the floor of the anterior cranial fossa.

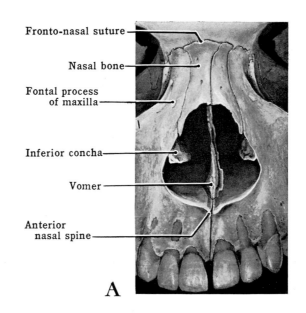

Fronto-nasal suture
Nasal bone
Fontal process of maxilla
Inferior concha
Vomer
Anterior nasal spine

A

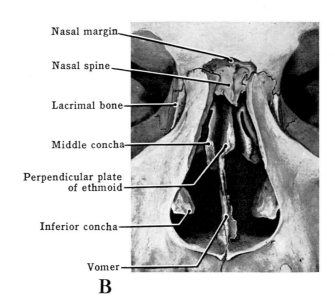

Nasal margin
Nasal spine
Lacrimal bone
Middle concha
Perpendicular plate of ethmoid
Inferior concha
Vomer

B

Frontal margin
Maxillary margin
Groove   Nasal surface

B 1

4 parts of the ethmoid bone:

a) Lamina cribrosa
b) Labyrinth
c) Perpendicular plate
d) Middle concha

for Frontal process of maxilla
Lacrimal bone
Naso-lacrimal canal

C

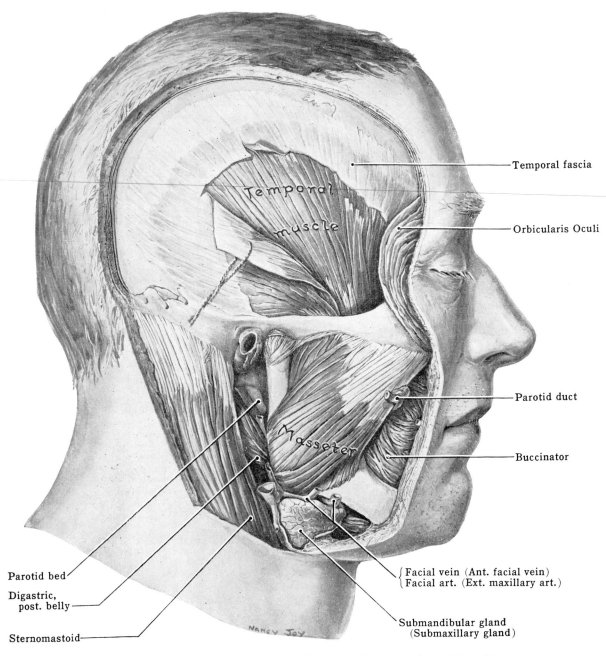

Temporal fascia

Orbicularis Oculi

Parotid duct

Buccinator

{ Facial vein (Ant. facial vein)
{ Facial art. (Ext. maxillary art.)

Submandibular gland
(Submaxillary gland)

Parotid bed

Digastric,
post. belly

Sternomastoid

NANCY JOY

465 Great Muscles on the Side of the Skull

Observe:

1. The temporal and masseteric muscles, both of which are supplied by the trigeminal nerve and both of which close the jaw. Temporalis, arising in part from the overlying temporal fascia, c.f. Gluteus Medius, (fig. 271), and Tibialis Anterior (fig. 305).

2. The Orbicularis Oculi and Buccinator, both of which are supplied by the facial nerve. One of these closes the eye; the other prevents food from collecting between the cheeks and the teeth.

3. Sternomastoid, which is the chief flexor of the head and neck, forming the posterior boundary of the parotid region; and the posterior belly of the Digastric which limits this region below.

4. The submandibular gland with the facial artery passing deep to it and the facial vein passing superficial.

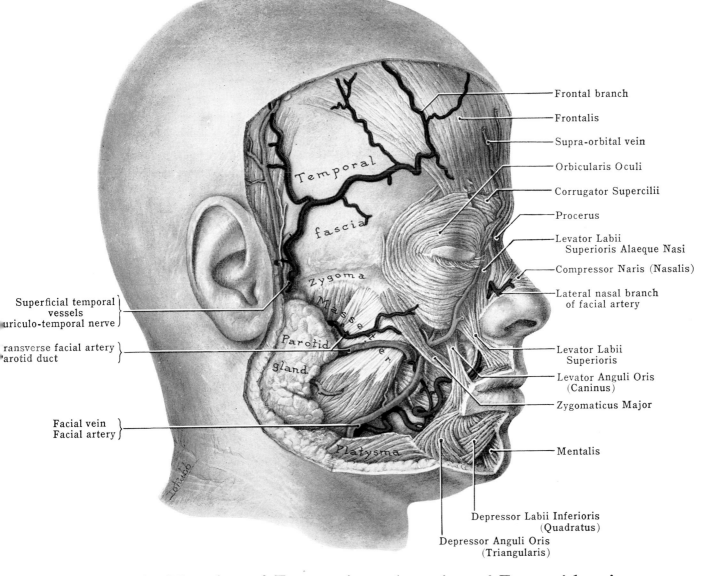

Frontal branch

Frontalis

Supra-orbital vein

Orbicularis Oculi

Corrugator Supercilii

Procerus

Levator Labii
Superioris Alaeque Nasi

Compressor Naris (Nasalis)

Lateral nasal branch
of facial artery

Levator Labii
Superioris

Levator Anguli Oris
(Caninus)

Zygomaticus Major

Mentalis

Superficial temporal
vessels
uriculo-temporal nerve

ransverse facial artery
·arotid duct

Facial vein
Facial artery

Depressor Labii Inferioris
(Quadratus)

Depressor Anguli Oris
(Triangularis)

466 Muscles of Expression; Arteries of Face, side view

Observe:

1. Around the eye—Orbicularis Oculi, Corrugator Supercilii, also Frontalis.

2. Around the nose—Compressor Naris, Procerus, and Levator Labii Superioris Alaeque Nasi.

3. Around the mouth—Orbicularis Oris (see fig. 470):

   In upper lip { Levator Labii Superioris Alaequae Nasi, Levator Labii Superioris, Zygomaticus Minor (= angular, infra-orbital and zygomatic heads of Quadratus Labii Superioris, fig. 470, A, B, C), Zygomaticus Major, Levator Anguli Oris.

   In cheek Buccinator (figs. 559, 574).

   In lower lip { Platysma (fig. 526), Risorius (not shown), Depressor Anguli Oris, and Depressor Labii Inferioris.

   In chin: Mentalis (fig. 470).

4. Around the Ear—Auriculares Anterior, Superior et Posterior (see fig. 467).
   All the above named muscles are supplied by the facial (VII) nerve.

5. The facial artery, usually sinuous but here tortuous, crossing the base of the mandible at the anterior border of Masseter, passing within half an inch of the angle of the mouth, and lying in front of the facial vein which takes a straight and more superficial course.

6. The transverse facial artery, crossing Masseter between the zygoma and the parotid duct.

Note: Assisting the facial and transverse facial arteries to supply the face are branches or twigs that accompany each branch of the trigeminal (V) nerve, shown in figure 470. Those accompanying V^1 are derived from the ophthalmic branch of the internal carotid artery; those accompanying V^2 and V^3, from the maxillary branch of the external carotid artery.

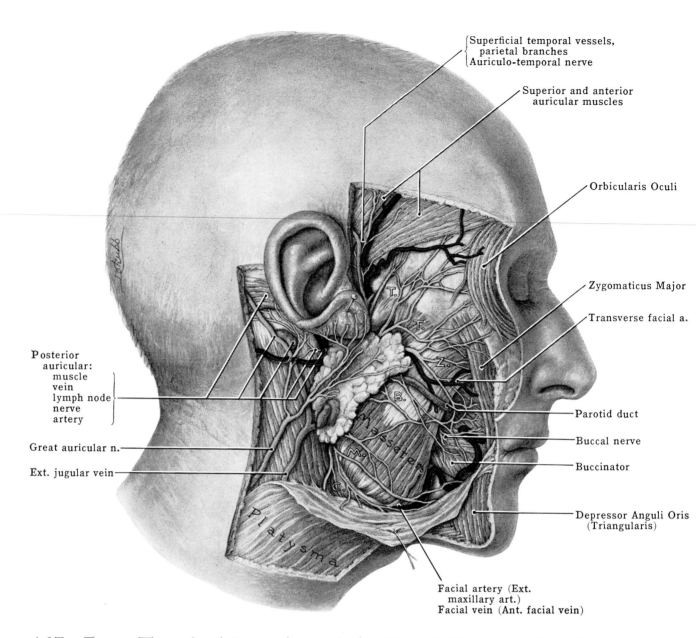

Superficial temporal vessels,
parietal branches
Auriculo-temporal nerve

Superior and anterior
auricular muscles

Orbicularis Oculi

Zygomaticus Major

Transverse facial a.

Parotid duct

Buccal nerve

Buccinator

Depressor Anguli Oris
(Triangularis)

Posterior
auricular:
muscle
vein
lymph node
nerve
artery

Great auricular n.

Ext. jugular vein

Facial artery (Ext.
maxillary art.)
Facial vein (Ant. facial vein)

467   Face: Terminal Branches of the Facial Nerve, side view

General: Deep fascia is absent from the face, but present over the Temporal and Masseter muscles.

The facial nerve supplies the muscles of expression and, though motor, is superficial. Masseter is a muscle of mastication and is supplied by the trigeminal nerve.

Observe:

1. The parotid gland, and the parotid duct crossing Masseter a finger's breadth below the zygomatic arch and turning medially to pierce Buccinator (fig. 574).
2. The branches of the facial nerve, radiating from under cover of the margin of the parotid gland like digits from an outstretched hand, anastomosing with each other and with the branches of the trigeminal nerve, and entering the muscles on their deep surfaces except where the muscles are two layers thick, when the deeper layer is entered on its superficial surface, e.g., Buccinator, Levator Anguli Oris (Caninus). These are divided somewhat arbitrarily into T = temporal, Z = zygomatic, B = Buccal, M = Mandibular, and C = cervical branches.
3. The cervical branch, running less than a finger's breadth

below the angle of the jaw and, after supplying branches to Platysma, crossing the base of the jaw at the anterior border of Masseter, crossing superficial to the facial vein and facial artery, anastomosing with the mandibular branch, and supplying the muscles of the lower lip and chin.

4. The buccal branch, which is motor to Buccinator, anastomosing with the buccal nerve (a branch of the trigeminal nerve) which is sensory.
5. The great auricular nerve (C. 2, 3), here lying ½″ behind the external jugular vein, but commonly in contact with it (fig. 472), and dividing into facial, auricular, and mastoid branches.
6. The posterior auricular nerve (a branch of the facial nerve), which is motor to Auricularis Posterior and Occipitalis, joined by a twig from the great auricular nerve.
7. The retro-auricular (posterior auricular) and superficial parotid lymph nodes.
8. The auriculo-temporal nerve, ascending with the superficial temporal vessels. Their relationships vary (fig. 466); when the nerve is deep, a layer of fascia commonly separates it from the vessels.

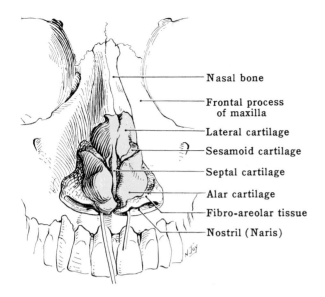

Nasal bone
Frontal process of maxilla
Lateral cartilage
Sesamoid cartilage
Septal cartilage
Alar cartilage
Fibro-areolar tissue
Nostril (Naris)

Alar cartilages pulled down in order to expose the sesamoid cartilages.

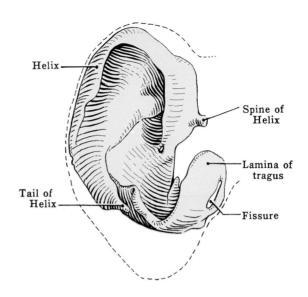

Helix
Spine of Helix
Lamina of tragus
Tail of Helix
Fissure

Cartilage of Right Auricle.

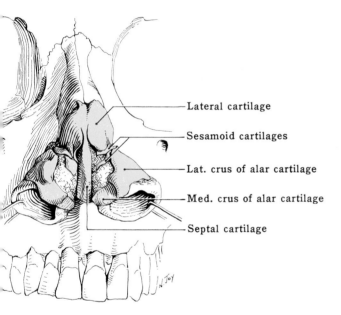

Lateral cartilage
Sesamoid cartilages
Lat. crus of alar cartilage
Med. crus of alar cartilage
Septal cartilage

Alar cartilages separated by dissection and retracted to right and left.

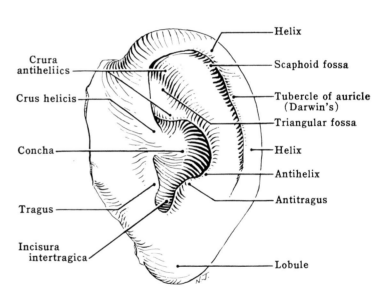

Crura antiheliics
Crus helicis
Concha
Tragus
Incisura intertragica
Helix
Scaphoid fossa
Tubercle of auricle (Darwin's)
Triangular fossa
Helix
Antihelix
Antitragus
Lobule

Auricle of Opposite Side.

468 Cartilages of the Nose

Observe:

1. The lateral nasal cartilages, fixed by suture to the nasal bones and continuous with the septal cartilage.
2. The alar nasal cartilages, free, movable, and U-shaped.
3. The medial crus of the right and of the left U, when in apposition, forming part of the septum of the nose.
4. The lower part of the ala of the nose, formed of fibro-areolar tissue, cf. the lobule of the auricle.

Note: The nasal cartilages are hyaline cartilage; the cartilage of the auricle is elastic cartilage.

469 The Auricle

Note:

The cartilage of the auricle is yellow or elastic cartilage. It is continuous with the cartilage of the external acoustic meatus. It does not extend into the lobule, the basis of which is fibro-areolar tissue.

There being very little subcutaneous tissue on the lateral surface of the auricle, the skin adheres to the cartilage and follows its irregularities. On the cranial surface, there being more subcutaneous tissue, the skin can be felt to be more movable.

The foramen at the root of the crus of the cartilage of the helix transmits an artery (fig. 551); the fissure in the cartilage of the external meatus is an unchondrified area, closed with fibrous tissue (fig. 577).

Infratrochlear nerve   Procerus

Supra-orbital nerve   Supratrochlear nerve   Corrugator Supercilii

Frontalis

Lacrimal nerve   Levator Palpebra

Lacrimal gland

Check ligament

Zygomatico-facial nerve

Zygomaticus Major

Infra-orbital nerve

Levator Anguli Oris (Caninus)

Buccal nerve   Buccal pad of fat

Platysma   Masseter

Depressor Anguli Oris (Triangularis)

Mental nerve   Inf. Incisive muscle

Depressores (Triangularis and Quadratus), reflected

Mentalis

470 Cutaneous Branches of Trigeminal Nerve: Dissection of Eyelid

Observe:

1. The 5 cutaneous branches of the ophthalmic nerve (V¹). Of these, the external nasal branch is shown but not labelled; and a sixth set of branches, for the supply of the cornea, is not shown, viz., the ciliary branches of the naso-ciliary nerve (fig. 520).

2. The 3 cutaneous branches of the maxillary nerve (V²):—(a) The infra-orbital branch, appearing through the infra-orbital foramen, 1 cm. below the orbital margin, between Levator Labii Superioris and Levator Anguli Oris; its branches radiating to the lower eyelid, to the dorsum of the nose, to the vestibule of the nose by branches that pierce the ala and by branches that enter from below, and to the upper lip. (b) The zygomatico-facial; and (c) the zygomatico-temporal (fig. 551).

3. The 3 cutaneous branches of the mandibular nerve (V³):— (a) The mental branch, appearing through the mental foramen, deep to Depressor Anguli Oris, and spreading out in the lower lip and chin. (b) The buccal branch, appearing at the anterior border of Masseter, below the level of the parotid duct, applied to Buccinator, and piercing it to supply the mucous membrane of the cheek; and (c) the auriculo-temporal branch (fig. 466).

4. A, B, C. A = Levator Labii Superioris Alaeque Nasi; B = Levator Labii Superioris; C = Zygomaticus Minor (angular, infra-orbital, and zygomatic heads of Quadratus Labii Superioris).

5. The buccal pad of lobulated fat, filling the space between Buccinator medially and the ramus of the jaw and Masseter laterally.

Continued on page facing

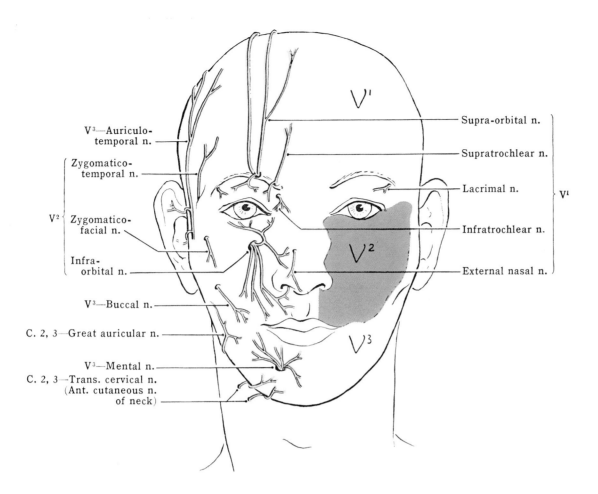

V¹

V³—Auriculo-
temporal n.

Zygomatico-
temporal n.

V² Zygomatico-
facial n.

Infra-
orbital n.

V³—Buccal n.

C. 2, 3—Great auricular n.

V³—Mental n.
C. 2, 3—Trans. cervical n.
(Ant. cutaneous n.
of neck)

Supra-orbital n.

Supratrochlear n.

Lacrimal n.

Infratrochlear n.   V¹

External nasal n.

V²

V³

470.1   Diagram of Sensory Nerves of Face, front view

The 3 divisions of the trigeminal nerve (N.V.) correspond in their distribution, nearly but not absolutely, to the 3 embryological regions of the face. Thus, the ophthalmic nerve (V¹) supplies the fronto-nasal process; the maxillary nerve (V²), the maxillary process (colored pink); and the mandibular nerve (V³), the mandibular process.

Cutaneous branches (supra-orbital and auriculo-temporal) have spread backwards in the scalp beyond a line that joins the auricles across the vertex, and there they meet the greater and lesser occipital nerves (fig. 500). Conversely, the great auricular nerve has spread across the masseteric region nearly to the angle of the mouth, and the anterior cutaneous nerve of the neck just reaches the face.

---

470   Cutaneous Branches of the Trigeminal Nerve: Dissection of the Eyelid

Continued from page facing

6. Levator Anguli Oris, continuous medially with the nasal muscles (Depressor Alae Nasi and Depressor Septi Nasi—not in view).

7. The orbital septum (palpebral fascia), attached to the orbital margin and, medially, passing behind the lacrimal sac to the crest of the lacrimal bone (post. lacrimal crest).

8. The medial palpebral ligament, crossing in front of the lacrimal sac, and attaching the elliptical upper and the rodlike lower tarsus to the frontal process of the maxilla.

9. The fan-shaped aponeurosis of Levator Palpebrae Superioris, attached to the front of the superior tarsus. Its medial edge, which is attached behind the lacrimal sac, and its lateral edge, which is attached to a tubercle within the orbital margin, are said to check the over-action of Levator Palpebrae.

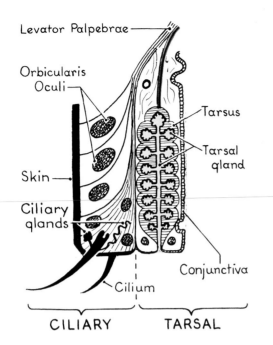

Levator Palpebrae

Orbicularis
Oculi

Skin

Ciliary
glands

Cilium

Tarsus

Tarsal
gland

Conjunctiva

CILIARY   TARSAL

471   Diagram of the Superior Palpebra or Eyelid, on sagittal section

(After Whitnall.)

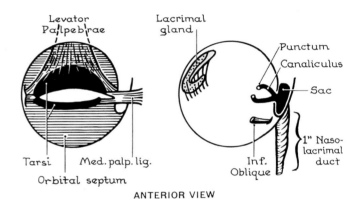

Levator
Palpebrae

Lacrimal
gland

Punctum

Canaliculus

Sac

1" Naso-
lacrimal
duct

Inf.
Oblique

Tarsi   Med. palp. lig.

Orbital septum

ANTERIOR VIEW

Zygomatic bone   Pars lacrimalis

EYE
BALL

Tarsus
&
Palpebral liqs.

Tear sac

HORIZONTAL SECTION

471.1   Diagram of the Lacrimal Apparatus

Note:

lacrimal gland and its ductules; conjunctival sac; lacrimal puncta, canaliculi and sac, and nasolacrimal duct. Also Pars lacrimalis of the Orbicularis Oculi. (*After Whitnall.*)

Levator Palpebrae

Superior Rectus

Space within cone
of muscles

Orbicularis
Oculi

Sup. tarsal
muscle

Tarsus (upper)

Bulbus
oculi

Optic nerve

Conjunctival sac

Orbital septum

Inf. tarsal
muscle

Subarachnoid
space

Inferior Rectus   Inferior Oblique

Fascia bulbi (Tenon's capsule)

471.2   Diagram of the Orbital Contents, on sagittal section

71.3   Diagram of the Superficial Veins of the Head and Neck

Labels (71.3): ccipital, Supra-orbital, Supra-trochlear, Superf. temp., Maxillary, t. aricular, (Post. facial) Retro-mandibular, (Ant.) Facial, C. facial, cessory n., ans-ervical, Ext. jugular, Communicating branch, Ant. jugular, prascapular, Omo-hyoid, SPLENIUS, LEV. SCAP., SC. MED. & POST.

Labels (471.4): P. aur., Superf. temporal, Occip., Maxillary, Facial, Lingual, Asc. phar., Int. carotid, M. Const., Car. sinus, Sup. thyroid, Com. carotid, Asc. cervical, Vertebral, Inf. thyroid, Costo-cerv. tr., Trans. cerv., Suprascap., Subclav., xillary V., Int. thor., Brachio-ceph. tr. (Innom. a.)

471.4   Diagram of the Subclavian and Carotid Arteries and their Branches

71.5   Branches of the Third Part of the Subclavian Artery

Almost as a rule some branch springs from the 3rd part of s artery, or else from its short 2nd part, and passes laterally rough the brachial plexus, usually behind nerve segments & 6 or 5, 6 & 7 (figs. 531, 536 both sides, & 537).
us:

(a) "The dorsal scapular art." (art. to Rhomboids, or de-nding branch of trans. cervical art.) so behaves in about % of cases;

(b) the transverse cervical art. in about 20% of cases, when may be said to spring from the dorsal scapular art. rather in vice versa; and

(c) the suprascapular art. in about 10% of cases. (*For details,* D. F. Hulke; and D. MacIntosh and G. G. Smith.)

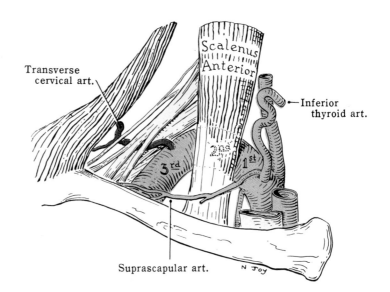

Labels: Transverse cervical art., Scalenus Anterior, Inferior thyroid art., 3rd, 2nd, 1st, Suprascapular art., N Joy

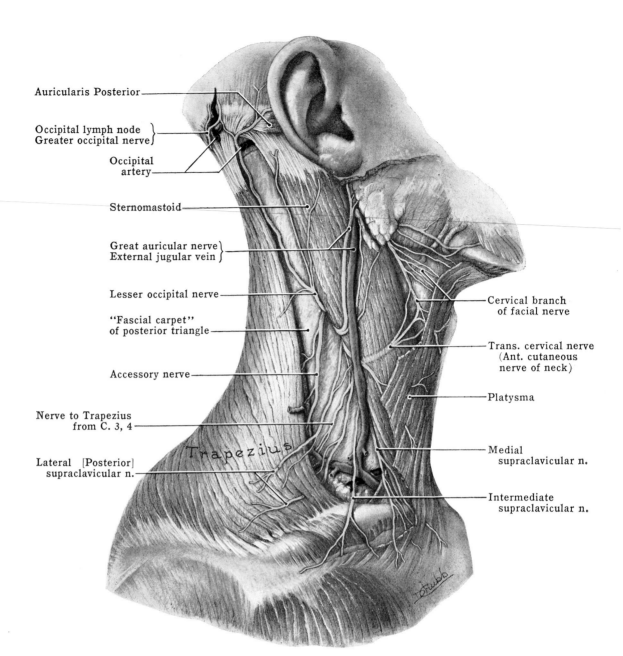

Auricularis Posterior

Occipital lymph node ⎱
Greater occipital nerve ⎰

Occipital
artery

Sternomastoid

Great auricular nerve ⎱
External jugular vein ⎰

Lesser occipital nerve

"Fascial carpet"
of posterior triangle

Accessory nerve

Nerve to Trapezius
from C. 3, 4

Lateral [Posterior]
supraclavicular n.

Trapezius

Cervical branch
of facial nerve

Trans. cervical nerve
(Ant. cutaneous
nerve of neck)

Platysma

Medial
supraclavicular n.

Intermediate
supraclavicular n.

472 Posterior Triangle of the Neck: Superficial Structures—I

Observe:

1. The 3 sides of the triangle—Trapezius, Sternomastoid, middle third of the clavicle—the apex being where the aponeuroses of the two muscles blend a little below the superior nuchal line.

2. Platysma (partly cut away), covering the lower part of the triangle.

3. The external jugular vein, descending vertically from behind the angle of the jaw, across Sternomastoid to its posterior border where, an inch above the clavicle, it pierces the investing deep fascia.

4. The "fascial carpet" that covers the muscular floor.

5. The accessory nerve—the only motor nerve superficial to the "fascial carpet"—descending within the deep fascia, and disappearing 2 fingers' breadth or more above the clavicle.

6. The cutaneous nerves (C. 2, 3, 4), radiating from the posterior border of Sternomastoid, below the accessory nerve.

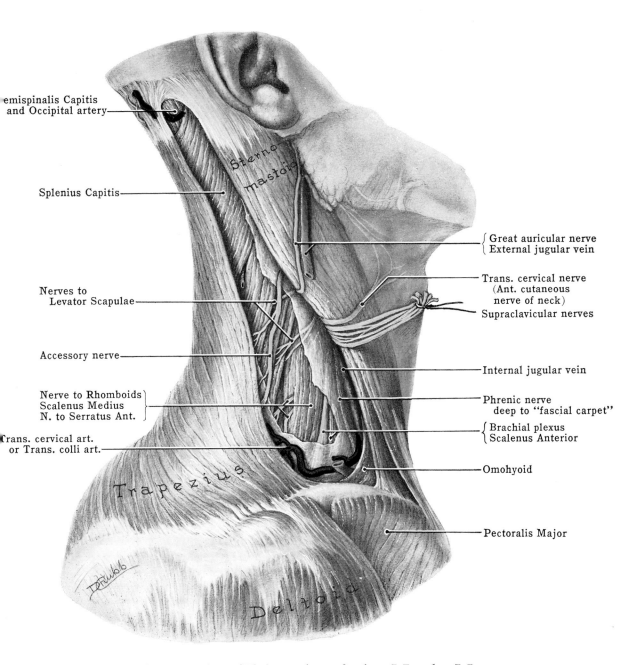

emispinalis Capitis
and Occipital artery

Splenius Capitis

Nerves to
Levator Scapulae

Accessory nerve

Nerve to Rhomboids
Scalenus Medius
N. to Serratus Ant.

Trans. cervical art.
or Trans. colli art.

Great auricular nerve
External jugular vein

Trans. cervical nerve
(Ant. cutaneous
nerve of neck)
Supraclavicular nerves

Internal jugular vein

Phrenic nerve
deep to "fascial carpet"

Brachial plexus
Scalenus Anterior

Omohyoid

Pectoralis Major

473   Posterior Triangle of the Neck: Motor Nerves deep to Fascial Carpet—II

Observe:

1. The muscles forming the floor of the upper part of the triangle (Semispinalis Capitis, Splenius, Levator Scapulae); those forming the lower part are shown in figure 474.

2. The accessory nerve (i.e., nerve to Sternomastoid and Trapezius), lying along Levator Scapulae but separated by the "fascial carpet".

3. Three motor nerves to upper limb muscles, lying (a) in the plane between the fascial carpet and the muscular floor, and (b) between the accessory nerve above and the brachial plexus below. They are the nerves to Levator Scapulae (C. 3, 4), to Rhomboids (C. 5), and to Serratus Anterior (C. 5, 6—the branch from C. 7 lies behind the plexus, fig. 23).

4. Two structures of surgical importance, situated just beyond the geometrical confines of the triangle: (a) a fourth motor nerve, viz. the phrenic nerve to the Diaphragm (C. 3, 4, 5), placed between carpet and floor; (b) the internal jugular vein, superficial to the carpet.

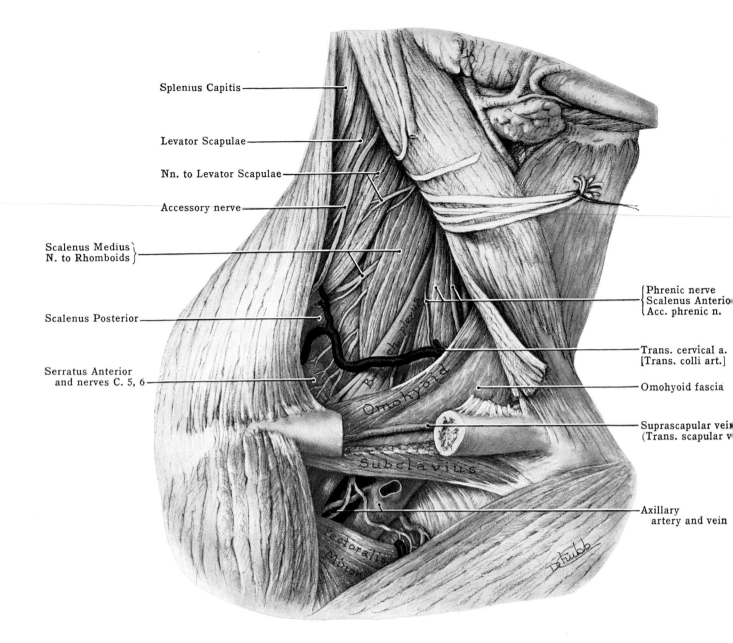

Splenius Capitis

Levator Scapulae

Nn. to Levator Scapulae

Accessory nerve

Scalenus Medius
N. to Rhomboids

Scalenus Posterior

Serratus Anterior
and nerves C. 5, 6

B...ch plexus

Omohyoid

Subclavius

Pectoralis Minor

Phrenic nerve
Scalenus Anterio
Acc. phrenic n.

Trans. cervical a.
[Trans. colli art.]

Omohyoid fascia

Suprascapular vei
(Trans. scapular v

Axillary
artery and vein

474 Posterior Triangle of the Neck: Omohyoid and its Fascia—III

The clavicular head of Pectoralis Major and part of the clavicle have been excised.

Observe:

1. The posterior belly of Omohyoid, held down by a sheet of fascia to the fascia ensheathing Subclavius; and the resulting pocket between this fascia posteriorly and the investing deep fascia and Sternomastoid anteriorly (fig. 542).

2. The brachial plexus, appearing between Scalenus Anterior and Scalenus Medius and here, as commonly, giving off an accessory phrenic nerve (see next figure) from C. 5.

3. The posterior border of Scalenus Anterior, nearly parallel to the posterior border of Sternomastoid, and slightly behind it; hence one is a guide to the other.

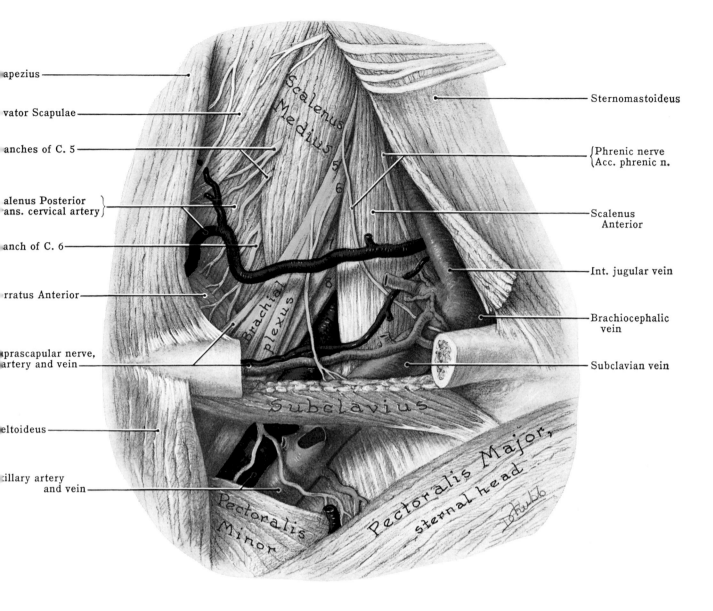

Trapezius ——

Levator Scapulae——

Branches of C. 5 ——

Scalenus Posterior
Trans. cervical artery

Branch of C. 6——

Serratus Anterior——

Suprascapular nerve,
artery and vein——

Deltoideus——

Axillary artery
and vein——

—— Sternomastoideus

{ Phrenic nerve
  Acc. phrenic n.

—— Scalenus Anterior

—— Int. jugular vein

—— Brachiocephalic vein

—— Subclavian vein

475 Posterior Triangle of the Neck: Brachial Plexus and Subclavian Vessels—IV

The 3rd part of the subclavian artery and the 1st part of the axillary artery are labelled.

Observe:

1. The muscles forming the floor of the lower part of the triangle (Scaleni Posterior, Medius et Anterior and Serratus Anterior).

2. The brachial plexus and subclavian artery, appearing between Scalenus Medius and Scalenus Anterior; the lowest root of the plexus (T. 1), concealed by the 3rd part of the artery.

3. The suprascapular nerve, found by following the lateral border of the plexus downwards.

4. The subclavian vein, hardly rising above the level of the clavicle, and separated from the 2nd part of the subclavian artery by Scalenus Anterior.

5. Subclavius, unimportant as a muscle, but valuable as a buffer between a fractured clavicle and the subclavian vessels.

Note how, by voluntarily forcing the upper limb backwards and downwards, the clavicle and Subclavius compress the subclavian vessels against the first rib and so arrest the pulse.

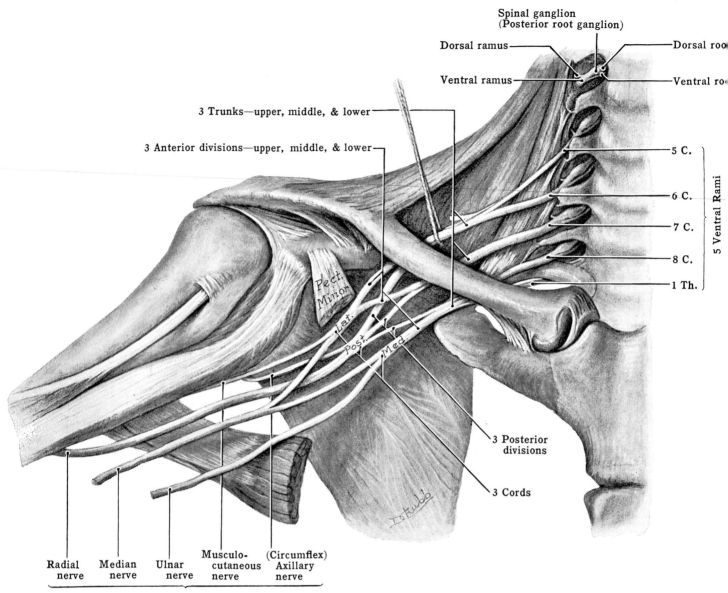

Spinal ganglion
(Posterior root ganglion)

Dorsal ramus — Dorsal roo

Ventral ramus — Ventral ro

3 Trunks—upper, middle, & lower

3 Anterior divisions—upper, middle, & lower

5 C.

6 C.

7 C.

8 C.

1 Th.

5 Ventral Rami

Pect. Minor

Lat.

Post.

Med.

3 Posterior
divisions

3 Cords

| Radial
nerve | Median
nerve | Ulnar
nerve | Musculo-
cutaneous
nerve | (Circumflex)
Axillary
nerve |

5 Terminal Branches

476 Brachial Plexus

Observe:

1. A dorsal (sensory) root of a spinal nerve larger than a ventral (motor) root.
2. The 2 roots uniting beyond the ganglion to form a very short mixed spinal nerve.
3. The mixed nerve at once dividing into a small dorsal ramus and a large ventral ramus.
4. The 5 ventral rami forming the brachial plexus (of these the middle ramus, C.7, is the largest).
5. The 5 rami uniting to form the 3 trunks of the plexus.
6. Each trunk dividing into 2 divisions, an anterior and a posterior.
7. From the divisions 3 cords resulting.
8. The 3 cords lying behind Pectoralis Minor.
9. The posterior cord and the radial nerve derived from segments C.5, 6, 7 and 8, and slightly from Th. 1.
10. The median nerve derived from segments C.6, 7, 8 and Th. 1, and slightly from C.5.

Occipitalis

Occipital artery
Occipital lymph
nodes

Levator Scapulae

Rhomboideus Minor

Rhomboideus Major

Deltoideus

Accessory nerve

Trapezius

Latissimus Dorsi

Obliquus Abdominis
Externus

Lumbar triangle

Fascia covering
Gluteus Medius

Gluteus Maximus

Greater occipital nerve
(dorsal ramus C. 2)

3rd occipital nerve
(dorsal ramus C. 3)

Lesser occipital nerve
(ventral ramus C. 2)

Cutaneous branches of
dorsal rami

Triangle of
auscultation

Cutaneous branches of
dorsal rami

Posterior branches of
lateral cutaneous nn.

Lateral cutaneous br. of ilio-
hypogastric n. (ventral
ramus of L. 1)

Cutaneous branches of
dorsal rami of
L. 1, 2, & 3

477 Superficial Muscles of the Back—I

On the left side, Trapezius is reflected.

Note: 1st layer—Trapezius and Latissimus Dorsi.
        2nd layer—Levator Scapulae and Rhomboidei Minor et Major.

These muscles help to attach the upper limb to the trunk.

Sternomastoideus

Splenius

Levator Scapulae

Scalenus Posterior

Trapezius, cut surface

Rhomboideus Minor

Rhomboideus Major

Semispinalis Capitis

Sternomastoideus

Splenius

Levator Scapulae

Serratus Posterior Superior, upper border

Serratus Anterior

Angle of rib

Serratus Posterior Inferior

Obliquus Externus

Obliquus Internus

Transversus aponeurosis

Iliac crest

Obliquus Externus

Lumbar triangle

Gluteus Medius

Gluteus Maximus

Trapezii

Serratus Post. Superior

Rhomb. Minor

Rhomboideus Major

Deltoid

Serratus Anterior

Lumbar (Lumbo-dorsal) fascia

Serratus Posterior Inferior

Latissimus Dorsi

Teres Major

478 Intermediate Muscles of the Back—II

Trapezius and Latissimus Dorsi are largely cut away on both sides.

Observe:

1. On the right side—Levator Scapulae and Rhomboidei, in situ. Serratus Superior, rising above Rhomboideus Minor. It is apt to be divided when Rhomboidei are severed.

2. On the left side—Rhomboidei, severed and allowing the vertebral border of the scapula to part from the thoracic wall. The 3 (usually 4) digitations of Levator Scapulae.

3. Serrati Posteriores Superior et Inferior, constituting the 3rd or intermediate layer of muscles, bridging the deep muscles, passing from spines to ribs, and sloping in opposite directions. These are muscles of inspiration.

4. The thoraco-lumbar (lumbo-dorsal) fascia, extending laterally to the angles of the ribs, becoming thin superiorly, passing deep to Serratus Superior, and reinforced inferiorly by Latissimus Dorsi and Serratus Inferior.

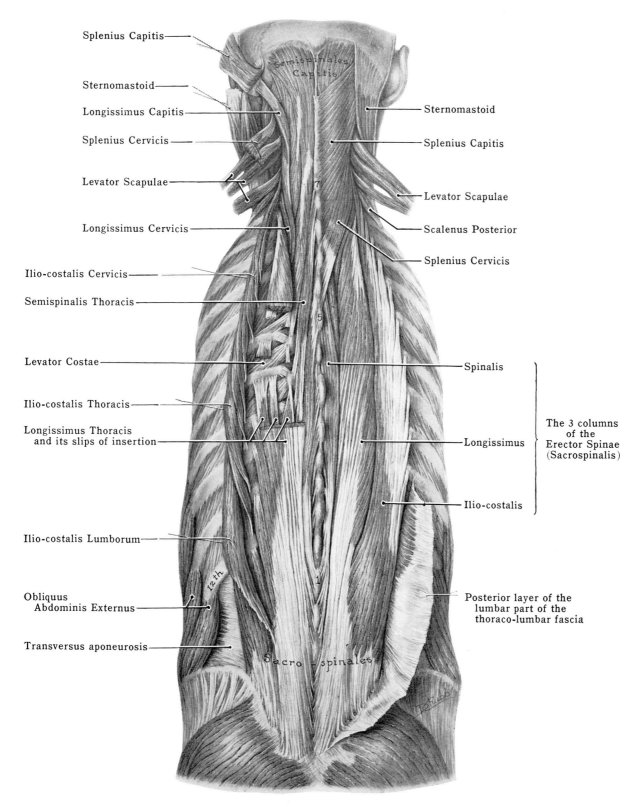

Splenius Capitis

Sternomastoid

Longissimus Capitis

Splenius Cervicis

Levator Scapulae

Longissimus Cervicis

Ilio-costalis Cervicis

Semispinalis Thoracis

Levator Costae

Ilio-costalis Thoracis

Longissimus Thoracis
and its slips of insertion

Ilio-costalis Lumborum

Obliquus
Abdominis Externus

Transversus aponeurosis

Semispinalis Capitis

Sternomastoid

Splenius Capitis

Levator Scapulae

Scalenus Posterior

Splenius Cervicis

Spinalis

The 3 columns
of the
Erector Spinae
(Sacrospinalis)

Longissimus

Ilio-costalis

Posterior layer of the
lumbar part of the
thoraco-lumbar fascia

Sacro-spinales

479 Deep Muscles of the Back—III

Observe:

1. Splenius Capitis et Cervicis, in situ on the right side and constituting the 4th layer of muscles; reflected on the left side and attached (Splenius Capitis) to the mastoid process deep to Sternomastoid and (Splenius Cervicis) to 1st, 2nd (and 3rd) transverse processes deep to Levator Scapulae.

2. Erector Spinae, which constitutes the 5th layer, in situ on the right side, lying between the spines medially and the angles of the ribs laterally, and splitting into 3 columns—lateral,

middle, and medial. On the left side, the lateral column is everted, a section is taken from the middle column, the medial column is in situ. Only the middle or Longissimus column extends to the skull, and is there inserted into the mastoid process deep to Splenius Capitis.

3. Semispinalis (thoracis, cervicis et capitis) in situ and belonging to the 6th, or oblique, or transverso-spinalis group of muscles.

4. For suboccipital muscles see figs. 490 & 491.

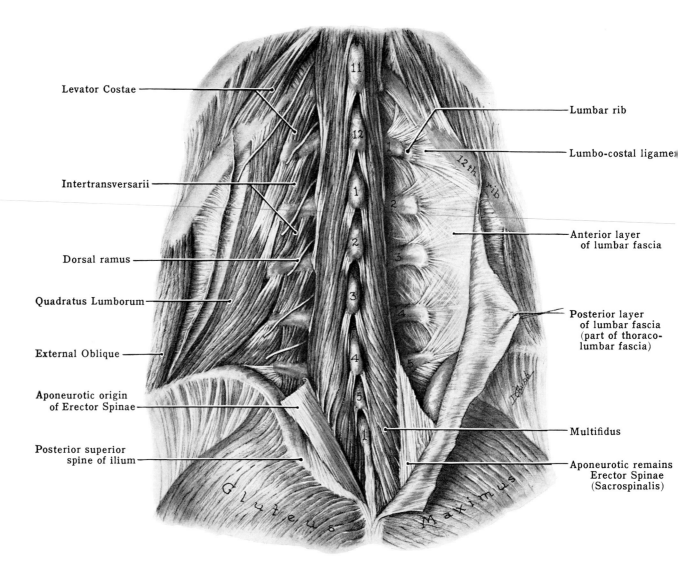

Levator Costae

Intertransversarii

Dorsal ramus

Quadratus Lumborum

External Oblique

Aponeurotic origin
of Erector Spinae

Posterior superior
spine of ilium

Lumbar rib

Lumbo-costal ligamen

Anterior layer
of lumbar fascia

Posterior layer
of lumbar fascia
(part of thoraco-
lumbar fascia)

Multifidus

Aponeurotic remains
Erector Spinae
(Sacrospinalis)

480 Multifidus: Quadratus Lumborum:
Lumbar Fascia—IV

Semispinalis, Multifidus, and Rotatores constitute the transverso-spinal, oblique,
or 6th layer (group) of muscles of the back. In general, their bundles pass obliquely
upwards from transverse processes to spines and occupy successively deeper layers.
The bundles of Semispinalis span about 5 interspaces, those of Multifidus about 3,
and those of Rotatores, 1 or 2.

(a) Semispinalis extends from the lower thoracic region to the skull (figs. 479,
490).

(b) Multifidus extends from the sacrum to the spine of the axis (fig. 493).

(c) Rotatores are well developed only in the thoracic region (fig. 411).

Observe:

1. Multifidus in the lumbo-sacral region, arising from the aponeurosis of Erector Spinae, from
mamillary processes and from the dorsum of the sacrum (not seen), and inserted into
spinous processes several segments higher up.

2. On the right side, after removal of Erector Spinae and Intertransversarii—the anterior
layer of lumbar fascia (ant. layer of lumbo-dorsal fascia), attached in fan-shaped manner
to the tips of transverse processes. Also, a short lumbar rib.

3. On the left side, after removal of the anterior layer of lumbar fascia—the oblique lateral
border of Quadratus Lumborum; the medial border in continuity with Intertransversarii;
and Intertransversarii in series with Levatores Costarum.

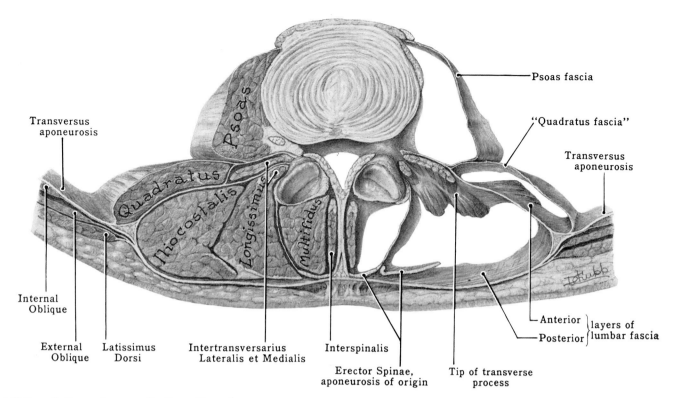

Transversus
aponeurosis

Psoas fascia

"Quadratus fascia"

Transversus
aponeurosis

Internal
Oblique

External
Oblique

Latissimus
Dorsi

Intertransversarius
Lateralis et Medialis

Interspinalis

Erector Spinae,
aponeurosis of origin

Tip of transverse
process

Anterior ⎱ layers of
Posterior ⎰ lumbar fascia

481   Muscles of the Back, on cross section—V

On the left side, the muscles are seen within their sheaths or compartments.
On the right side, the empty sheaths are seen.

Observe:

1. The posterior aponeurosis of Transversus Abdominis,
splitting into two strong sheets—the anterior and the posterior layer of the lumbar fascia (being part of the thoraco-
lumbar fascia) which enclose the deep muscles of the back.

2. The posterior layer, reinforced by Latissimus Dorsi and
at a higher level (fig. 478) by Serratus Posterior Inferior.

3. The weak areolar layer covering Quadratus Lumborum
and that covering Psoas.

4. Ends of Intertransversarius, Longissimus, and Quadratus
Lumborum, attached to a transverse process.

482   Spinal Cord within Its Membranes, from behind

Observe:

1. The denticulate lig., running like a band along each side
of the spinal cord and, by means of strong tooth-like
processes, anchoring the cord to the dura between
successive nerve roots.

2. The ventral nerve roots, lying in front of the denticulate lig. and the dorsal nerve roots lying behind it.

3. The ventral and the dorsal root of each nerve, leaving the
dura by a separate opening. The lowest right dorsal root
in this specimen leaves by three openings.

4. The fila of the various dorsal roots, having a linear attachment to the cord.

5. One filum of the lowest left dorsal root, deserting its own
root and joining the root above.

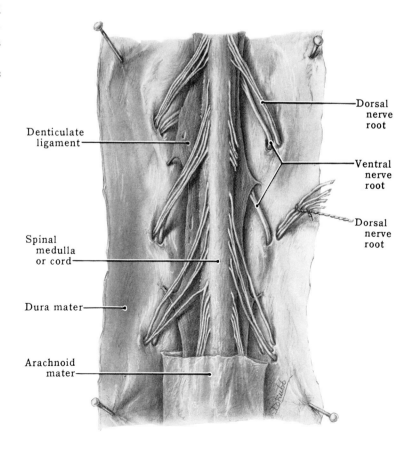

Dorsal
nerve
root

Ventral
nerve
root

Dorsal
nerve
root

Denticulate
ligament

Spinal
medulla
or cord

Dura mater

Arachnoid
mater

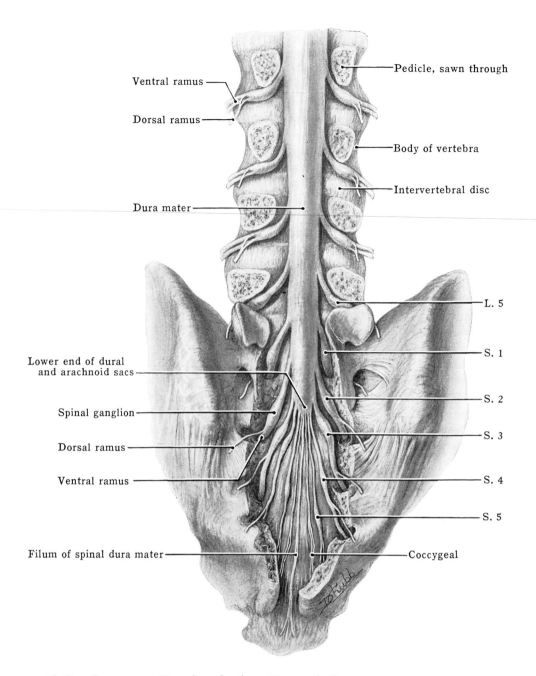

Ventral ramus

Dorsal ramus

Dura mater

Pedicle, sawn through

Body of vertebra

Intervertebral disc

L. 5

S. 1

S. 2

S. 3

S. 4

S. 5

Lower end of dural
and arachnoid sacs

Spinal ganglion

Dorsal ramus

Ventral ramus

Filum of spinal dura mater

Coccygeal

483 Lower End of the Dural Sac, from behind—I

The posterior parts of the lumbar and sacral vertebrae are sawn and nibbled away

Observe:

1. The lower limit of the dural (and the contained arachnoid) sac, at the level of the posterior superior iliac spine (= body of 2nd sacral vertebra), and the continuation of the dura as the filum of spinal dura mater.

2. The lumbar spinal ganglia in the intervertebral foramina; the sacral spinal ganglia, somewhat asymmetrical, within the sacral canal.

3. The dorsal nerve rami, smaller than ventral rami, and having both efferent and afferent components.

4. The superior articular processes of the sacrum, asymmetrical.

Spinal medulla
(Spinal cord)

Dura mater

Arachnoid mater

orsal nerve root

Lowest
denticulate ligaments

Th. XII

Conus medullaris

L. 1

Dorsal root fila

L. 2

Filum terminale

Dorsal Root

Ventral root

L. 3

Cauda equina

L. 4

Subarachnoid space

Pedicle of
vertebra L. 5

Superior
articular
process
of sacrum

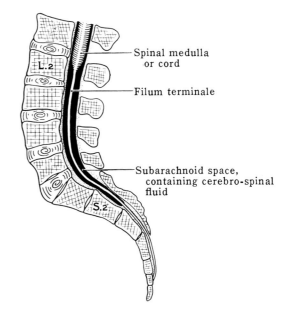

Spinal medulla
or cord

Filum terminale

Subarachnoid space,
containing cerebro-spinal
fluid

484.1

Diagram of the Spinal Cord or Medulla, in situ

Note:

1. The spinal cord ends at the level of the disc between the 1st and 2nd lumbar vertebrae.

2. The subarachnoid space ends at the level of the disc between the 1st and 2nd sacral vertebrae—but it may be lower (figs. 203 & 236).

3. Variations: 95% of 801 cords ended within the limits of the bodies of vertebrae L.1 and L.2; whereas 3% ended behind the lower half of vertebra T.12, and 2% behind vertebra L.3. (Observations and collected data after Reimann, A. F. and Anson, B. J.; also Jit, l. and Charnalia, V. M.).

84   Lower Ends of the Dural
nd Arachnoid Sacs, opened,
om behind—II

serve:

The lowest tooth or dens of the denticulate ligament, variable in level and asymmetrical (MacDonald, I. B. et al.).

A radicular branch of a spinal vein accompanying the dorsal root of nerve L. 1. There are only four or five radicular veins and arteries on each side of the cord to accompany the 31 pairs of spinal nerves. (Suh, T. H. and Alexander, L.)

The conus medullaris, or conical lower end of the spinal medulla, continued as a glistening thread, the filum terminale, which descends with the dorsal and ventral nerve roots. These constitute the cauda equina.

The hook retracting the elongated nerve roots, which surround a tubular space.

The subarachnoid space enclosed by arachnoid mater; the subdural space, which is the potential space between the dural and arachnoid maters.

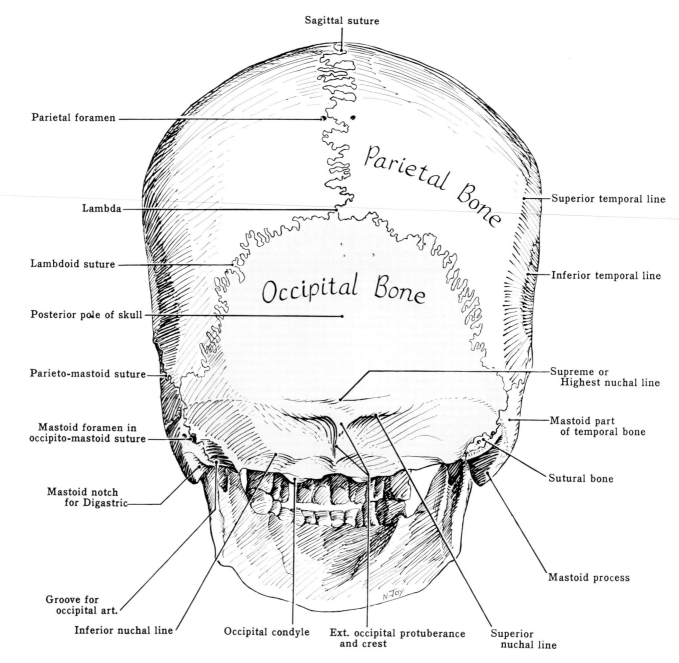

Sagittal suture

Parietal foramen

Parietal Bone

Superior temporal line

Lambda

Lambdoid suture

Occipital Bone

Inferior temporal line

Posterior pole of skull

Parieto-mastoid suture

Supreme or
Highest nuchal line

Mastoid foramen in
occipito-mastoid suture

Mastoid part
of temporal bone

Sutural bone

Mastoid notch
for Digastric

Mastoid process

Groove for
occipital art.

Inferior nuchal line   Occipital condyle   Ext. occipital protuberance
and crest

Superior
nuchal line

N Joy

485 Skull from behind—Norma Occipitalis

The outline is horseshoe-shaped from the tip of one mastoid process, over the vertex to the tip of the other. On each side, it crosses the parieto-mastoid suture and the temporal lines.

1. At the base of the skull, the outline is nearly straight (slightly convex) from one mastoid process to the other, except where the occipital condyles project downwards. On each side, it crosses two grooves (for the origin of the posterior belly of Digastric laterally, and for the occipital artery medially), the occipito-mastoid suture, the jugular process, and an occipital condyle. Between the condyles is the foramen magnum.

2. The surface is convex and includes parts of the parietal, occipital, and temporal bones. Near the centre is the lambda. From it a triradiate suture runs:

the sagittal (interparietal) upwards in the median plane, and the lambdoid (parieto-occipital) infero-laterally to the blunt postero-inferior angles of the parietal bones where it bifurcates on each side into the parieto-mastoid and occipito-mastoid sutures.

3. On each side are three inconstant foramina for emissary veins and meningeal arteries: parietal and mastoid foramina, and condylar canal (fig. 569).

Midway between the lambda and the foramen magnum is the external occipital protuberance. From it the superior nuchal line curves laterally and crosses the lateral aspect of the mastoid bone, dividing it into a smooth upper and a rough lower part.

The surface below the superior nuchal line is the nuchal area for the muscles of the neck or nucha.

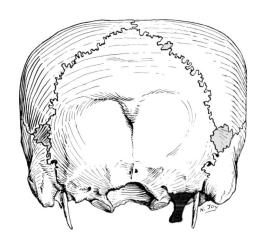

486   Occipital Bone at Birth

At birth, the bone is in 4 parts. The blue parts develop in cartilage; the red part develops in membrane. Note: (a) the double origin of the squamous part; (b) the early position of the hypoglossal canal—in the synchondrosis between the lateral and basilar parts.

487   Paramastoid Process

Rarely, a process descends from the jugular process of the occipital bone towards, or to, the transverse process of the atlas.

488   Interparietal Bone (Os Incae)

Occasionally, the several centres of ossification of the interparietal part of the occipital bone fail (A and B) in part or (C) in whole to coalesce with the supra-occipital part (fig. 486). The result is an independent interparietal bone.

Sutural bones (yellow) are commonly present, as in this specimen and in figure 487, notably at the inferior angles of the parietal bone.

489   Two Varieties of Synostosis of Occipital Bone and Atlas

OSSIFICATION and ANOMALIES

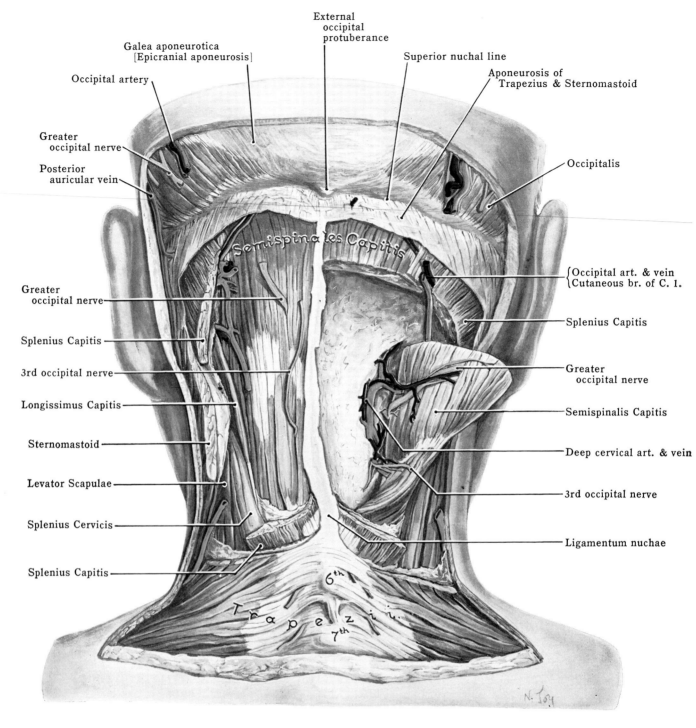

Occipital artery

Galea aponeurotica
[Epicranial aponeurosis]

External
occipital
protuberance

Superior nuchal line

Aponeurosis of
Trapezius & Sternomastoid

Greater
occipital nerve

Posterior
auricular vein

Occipitalis

Semispinales Capitis

Greater
occipital nerve

Occipital art. & vein
Cutaneous br. of C. I.

Splenius Capitis

Splenius Capitis

Greater
occipital nerve

3rd occipital nerve

Longissimus Capitis

Semispinalis Capitis

Sternomastoid

Deep cervical art. & vein

Levator Scapulae

3rd occipital nerve

Splenius Cervicis

Ligamentum nuchae

Splenius Capitis

6th

Trapezii.

7th

490   Suboccipital Region—I

Trapezius, Sternomastoid, and Splenius are largely excised.

Observe:

1. Semispinalis Capitis, forming the posterior wall of the sub-occipital region, pierced by the greater and third occipital nerves, and having a free medial border applied to the ligamentum nuchae. On the left side, Semispinalis Capitis is in situ; on the right side it is divided and turned laterally.

2. The remains of a thin sheet of fascia superficial to Semispinalis Capitis, and deep to it a tough, dense, areolar tissue in which run vessels and nerves.

3. The posterior border of the ligamentum nuchae, which, as the cervical part of the supraspinous ligament, extends upwards to the external occipital protuberance. Trapezius has been cut away from each side of it.

4. The aponeurosis of Trapezius and Sternomastoid arising from the superior nuchal line.

5. The right and left Occipitales united by the galea aponeurotica and arising from the highest nuchal lines.

Posterior auricular vein

C. 1, cutaneous br.

Mastoid emissary vein

Splenius Capitis

Occipital veins

Descending branch of occipital art.

Greater occipital nerve

Semispinales Capitis

Semispinalis Capitis

Minor Major

Occipital artery

Superior Oblique

C. 1, dorsal ramus

Inferior Oblique

C. 2, dorsal ramus [Gtr. occipital n.]

Longissimus Capitis

C. 3, dorsal ramus

Deep cervical art. & vein

C. 4, dorsal ramus (to Spinalis)

C. 5, dorsal ramus (cutaneous br.)

Semispinalis Cervicis

Semispinalis Cervicis

Semispinalis Capitis

Ligamentum nuchae

Splenius Capitis

Splenius Cervicis

Trapezius

Trapezius

491   Suboccipital Region—II

Semispinalis Capitis, which forms the posterior wall of the suboccipital region, is reflected on the left side and excised on the right side, and the underlying dense areolar tissue is mosly removed.

Observe:

1. The lig. nuchae forming a thin, median partition attached to the spines of the cervical vertebrae anteriorly and to the external crest of the occipital bone superiorly.

2. The greater occipital nerve (C. 2), when followed caudally, leading to the lower border of Obliquus Capitis Inferior around which it turns and to which it is the guide. This border, when followed medially, leading to the spine of the axis; when followed laterally, to the transverse process of the atlas.

3. The occipital artery appearing between Superior Oblique

and Longissimus Capitis. Longissimus is the only section of Erector Spinae to reach the skull.

4. The 1st cervical nerve, here delivering a cutaneous branch—which is unusual.

5. The descending branch of the occipital artery anastomosing with the deep cervical artery (a branch of the subclavian).

6. The posterior vertebral venous plexus. This plexus is largely imbedded in fascia, is usually empty and therefore inconspicuous, and hence is removed unnoticed with the fascia unless specially injected, as here, or engorged with blood.

Occipital veins

Mastoid emissary vein

Digastric, post. belly

Mastoid process

Communicating nerve

Transverse process of atlas

Joint cavities between articular processes:
C. 2 & C. 3

C. 3 & C. 4

Deep cervical art. & vein   Semispinalis Cervicis   Interspinales

Rectus Capitis Posterior Minor

Rectus Capitis Posterior Major

Cutaneous br. of C. (unusual)

Digastric

Superior Oblique

Suboccipital triangle and nerve C. 1 (dorsal ramus)

Greater occipital ner

Inferior Oblique

Bifid spine of axis

Semispinalis Cervici

Longissimus Capitis

Semispinalis Capitis

492   Suboccipital Region—III

On the left side, Rectus Capitis Posterior Major and Obliquus Capitis Inferior are removed.

Observe:

1. Rectus Capitis Posterior Major ascending from the spine of the axis to the occipital bone. Obliquus Capitis Superior ascending from the tip of the transverse process of the atlas to the occipital bone. Obliquus Capitis Inferior passing from spine to axis to tip of transverse process of atlas.

2. The foregoing 3 muscles, (viz. Inf. Oblique, Rectus Major, and Sup. Oblique), forming the sides of the suboccipital triangle which lies within the suboccipital region whose lower limit is the axis.

3. Rectus Capitis Posterior Minor arising from the posterior tubercle of the atlas and therefore lying on a deeper plane than the Posterior Major which arises from a spine.

4. The posterior arch of the atlas forming the floor of the suboccipital triangle. The posterior atlanto-occipital membrane (not labelled) passing from that arch to the margin of the foramen magnum above, and the posterior atlanto-axial membrane passing to the lamina of the axis below. The vertebral artery lying on the arch; the suboccipital nerve appearing between arch and artery and supplying the two straight muscles (minor and major) and the two oblique muscles (superior and inferior).

5. The gaps in these membranes through which pass nerve C. 1 (suboccipital n.), nerve C. 2 (greater occipital nerve) also the vertebral artery, the veins accompanying this artery, and veins passing independently.

6. A communicating branch passing from the dorsal ramus of nerve C. 1 to nerve C. 2 behind the posterior arch of the atlas. In figure 561 the ventral rami of these nerves are seen in communication.

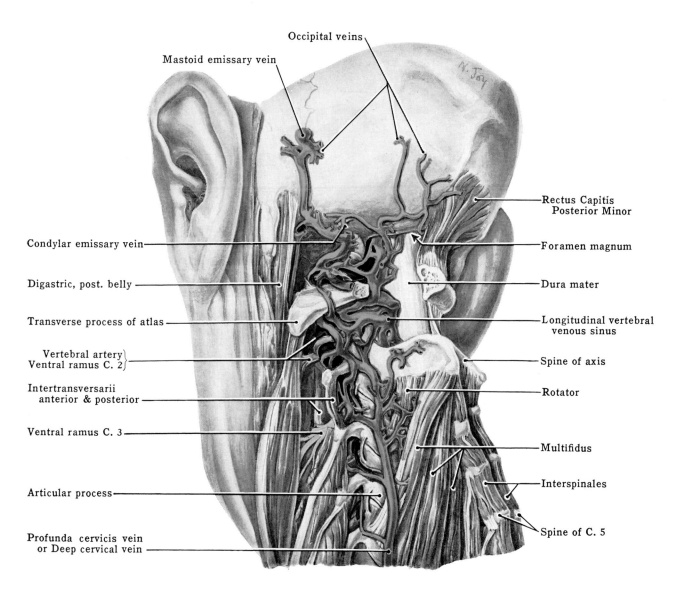

Occipital veins

Mastoid emissary vein

Condylar emissary vein

Digastric, post. belly

Transverse process of atlas

Vertebral artery
Ventral ramus C. 2

Intertransversarii
anterior & posterior

Ventral ramus C. 3

Articular process

Profunda cervicis vein
or Deep cervical vein

Rectus Capitis
Posterior Minor

Foramen magnum

Dura mater

Longitudinal vertebral
venous sinus

Spine of axis

Rotator

Multifidus

Interspinales

Spine of C. 5

493 Suboccipital Region—IV

(Postero-lateral view.)

Part of the posterior arch of the atlas is removed and with it the atlanto-occipital and the atlanto-axial membranes.

Observe:

1. The vertebral venous system of veins and its numerous intercommunications and connections, e.g., through the foramen magnum and the mastoid foramen and condylar canal with the intracranial venous sinuses; between the laminae and through the intervertebral foramina with the longitudinal vertebral venous sinuses (figs. 390 and 494); communicating with the veins of the scalp above, with the veins around the vertebral artery and, via the deep cervical vein, with brachio-cephalic vein below.

2. The Interspinales and the Multifidi extending up to, but not above, the spine of the axis.

Internal jugular vein

Vertebral artery

Accessory nerve

Vertebral venous plexus

Ventral ramus of C. 2

Intertransversarius
Scalenus Medius

Levator Scapulae
Splenius Cervicis

Axis

Lymph
nodes

Sternomastoid

Spinal
ganglion
of C. 2

Inferior
oblique

Longissimus
Capitis

Descending
branch of
occipital art.

Splenius Capitis

Dorsal ramus of C. 2
= greater occipital nerve

Trapezius

Semispinalis Capitis

Dorsal ramus of C. 3
= third occipital nerve

Rectus Capitis Posterior Major

Ligamentum nuchae

494   Cross Section of the Nuchal Region, at the level of the axis

The section, clearly, passes above the level of the spine and lamina of the axis, for Obliquus Inferior and Rectus Capitis Major are present, whereas Semispinalis Cervicis and Multifidus are not. Clearly, also, it passes below the posterior arch of the atlas, for Obliquus Superior and Rectus Capitis Minor do not appear.

Observe:

1. Trapezius, Splenius, and Semispinalis Capitis forming a covering or roof for the suboccipital region.

2. Two muscles that ascend from the spine of the axis divided, viz., Inferior Oblique and Rectus Capitis Posterior Major.

3. Many anastomosing veins: (a) those around the vertebral artery unite, before leaving the 6th cervical transverse foramen to form the vertebral vein (fig. 567); (b) the vertebral venous plexus, which followed cranially communicates through the foramen magnum with the basilar and occipital venous sinuses.

4. The ventral ramus of C. 2 passing forwards lateral to the vertebral artery; and the dorsal ramus ascending behind Inferior Oblique.

5. The spinal cord having plenty of room at this high level.

Trochlear nerve (IV)

Trigeminal nerve (V)

IV Ventricle

Facial n. (VII) and Vestibulocochlear n. (Acoustic n., VIII)

Glosso-pharyngeal nerve (IX)

Vagus nerve (X)

Accessory n. (XI): cranial } roots spinal }

Jugular process

Rectus Capitis Lateralis

Transverse process of atlas

Intertransversarius

Vertebral artery

Spinal (Post. root) ganglion of C. 2.

Lateral recess

Atlanto-occipital joint

Denticulate lig.

1st cervical nerve, dorsal ramus

Atlanto-axial joint

2nd cervical nerve: { ventral ramus { dorsal ramus

Capsule

Atlas

Dura

Axis

495 Cranial Nerves, exposed from behind

The posterior part of the skull and the cerebellum are removed.

Observe:

1. The trochlear (IV) nerves, arising from the dorsal aspect of midbrain just below the inferior colliculi; the trigeminal (V) nerves, ascending to enter the mouths of the trigeminal caves (Meckel's caves); the facial (VII) and vestibulo-cochlear (VIII) nerves ascending to enter the internal acoustic meatuses; the glossopharyngeal (IX) nerves, piercing the dura mater separately and passing with the vagus (X) and accessory (XI) nerves through the jugular foramina; the fila of the accessory nerves of opposite sides, leaving the medulla and spinal cord asymmetrically; and the gnarled appearance of the spinal roots.

2. The abducent (VI) nerves are not in view; the hypoglossal (XII) nerves are seen vaguely in front of the spinal roots of nerves XI and just above the vertebral arteries.

3. The transverse process of the atlas, joined to the jugular process (i.e., transverse process) of the occipital bone by Rectus Capitis Lateralis which morphologically is an Intertransverse muscle.

4. The vertebral arteries, raised from their beds on the posterior arch of the atlas.

5. The 1st cervical or suboccipital nerve, here having no sensory component. Its dorsal ramus, passing between the vertebral artery and the posterior arch of the atlas. Its ventral ramus (not labelled), curving around the atlanto-occipital joint.

6. The 2nd cervical nerve (largely sensory), having a large spinal ganglion, a large dorsal ramus, and a smaller ventral ramus. The fila of its dorsal root are seen just above the cut edge of the dura and behind the spinal root of nerve XI.

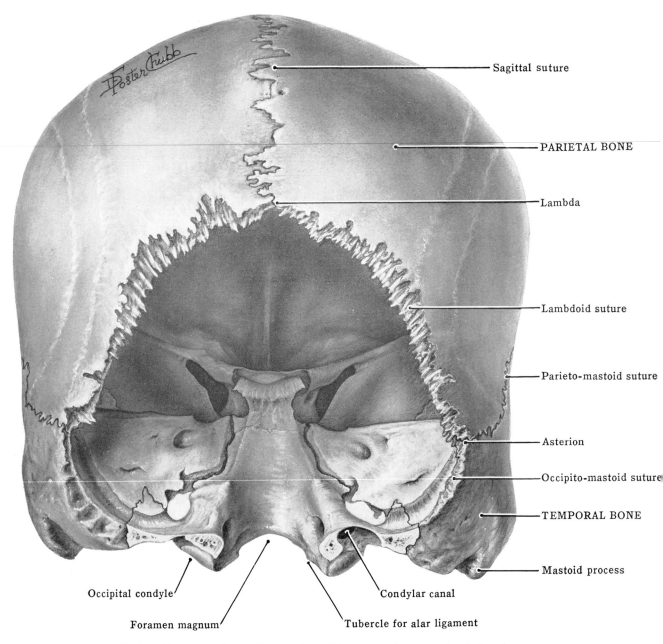

Sagittal suture

PARIETAL BONE

Lambda

Lambdoid suture

Parieto-mastoid suture

Asterion

Occipito-mastoid suture

TEMPORAL BONE

Mastoid process

Occipital condyle

Foramen magnum

Condylar canal

Tubercle for alar ligament

496 Posterior Cranial Fossa, from behind

The squamous part of the occipital bone was removed, after the right and left lateral parts had been sawn through. (Figure 497 is a key to this figure.)

Note:

1. The *dorsum sellae* is the squarish plate of bone rising from the body of the sphenoid. At its superior angles are the posterior clinoid processes.

2. The *clivus* is the sloping surface between the dorsum sellae and the foramen magnum. It is formed by the basilar part of the occipital bone (basi-occipital) with some assistance from the body of the sphenoid, as figure 511 makes clear.

3. The *sulci*, or grooves, for the sigmoid sinus and the inferior petrosal sinus both lead downwards to the jugular foramen.

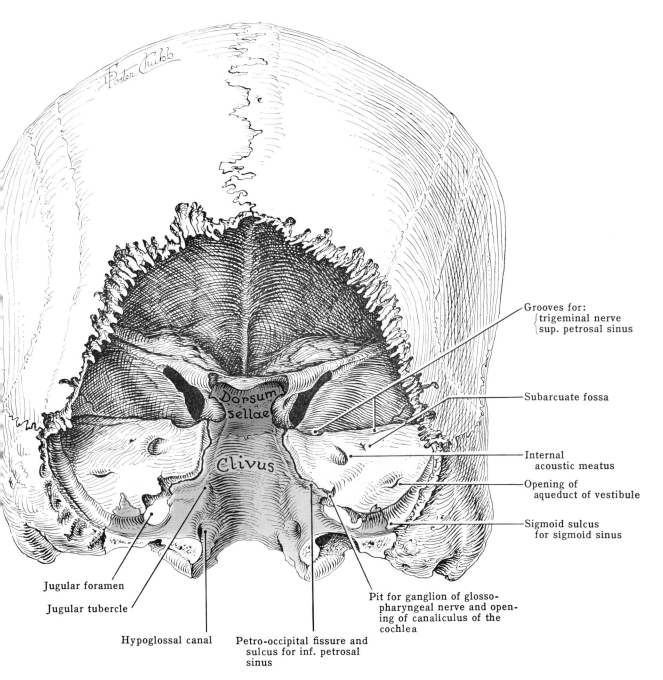

Grooves for:
{ trigeminal nerve
{ sup. petrosal sinus

Subarcuate fossa

Internal
acoustic meatus

Opening of
aqueduct of vestibule

Sigmoid sulcus
for sigmoid sinus

Dorsum
sellae

Clivus

Jugular foramen

Jugular tubercle

Hypoglossal canal

Petro-occipital fissure and
sulcus for inf. petrosal
sinus

Pit for ganglion of glossopharyngeal nerve and opening of canaliculus of the
cochlea

497 Posterior Cranial Fossa, from behind

Note: (1) That at birth the subarcuate fossa was large and extended laterally,
under the arc of the anterior semicircular canal (see fig. 645.1).

2. That the aqueduct of the vestibule opened under the arc of the posterior semicircular canal. This aqueduct transmits the endolymphatic duct (see figs. 644 and
650).

3. That the perilymphatic duct (within the canaliculus of the cochlea, figs. 633
& 644) opens at the bottom of the pyramidal pit for the glossopharyngeal ganglion.
This capillary aqueduct is said to allow the perilymph of the internal ear to mix with
the cerebrospinal fluid in the posterior cranial fossa; but there is evidence that it
ends as a closed sac. (*Wharton Young.*)

(*For posterior cranial fossa from above, see figs. 508 & 512.*)

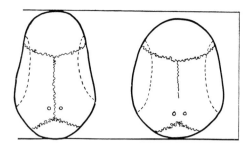

DOLICHOCEPHALIC SKULL.   BRACHYCEPHALIC SKULL.

498   Skulls, viewed from above

When the maximum width of a skull is less than 75 % of the maximum length, the skull is called dolichocephalic or long headed; when more than 80 %, it is brachycephalic or broad headed; and when between 75 % and 80 %, it is mesaticephalic.

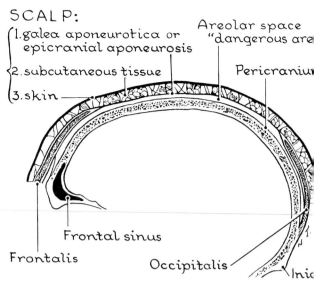

SCALP:
1. galea aponeurotica or epicranial aponeurosis
Areolar space "dangerous area
2. subcutaneous tissue
Pericranium
3. skin
Frontal sinus
Frontalis
Occipitalis
Inion

498.1   Diagram of the skull cap and its covering on median section, to show the 3 layers of the scalp and the subaponeurotic, areolar space.

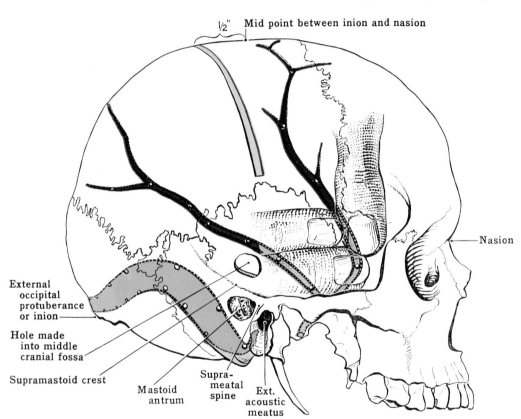

½"   Mid point between inion and nasion

Nasion

External occipital protuberance or inion

Hole made into middle cranial fossa

Supramastoid crest

Mastoid antrum

Supra-meatal spine

Ext. acoustic meatus

499   Surface Anatomy of the Cranium

The artery and the venous sinus were related to the outside of the skull by drilling holes along the grooves on the inside.

Note: The pterion, two fingers' breadth above the zygomatic arch and a thumb's breadth behind the frontal process of the zygomatic bone. The ant. branch of the middle meningeal a. crosses the pterion; the post. branch curves backwards less than a finger's breadth above the zygomatic arch and supramastoid crest; the stem of the artery traverses the foramen spinosum medial to the head of the mandible (fig. 508).

The lesser wing of the sphenoid extends almost to the pterion (fig. 508); hence, the pterion marks also the stem of the lateral cerebral fissure, the ant. perforated substance, etc. (fig. 506).

The central sulcus (yellow) has its upper end where indicated: its lower end lies 2″ above the external acoustic meatus.

The supramastoid crest approximately at the level of the floor of the middle cranial fossa; hence, a hole drilled below the crest and behind the suprameatal spine enters the mastoid antrum; whereas one drilled above the crest enters the middle cranial fossa.

The transverse and sigmoid sinuses (blue) curve from the inion, across the asterion, to a point less than ¾″ behind the ext. meatus, and thence forwards and downwards to a point in front of the mastoid process and below the ext. meatus where (on the post. transverse line, fig. 571) it becomes the int. jugular vein.

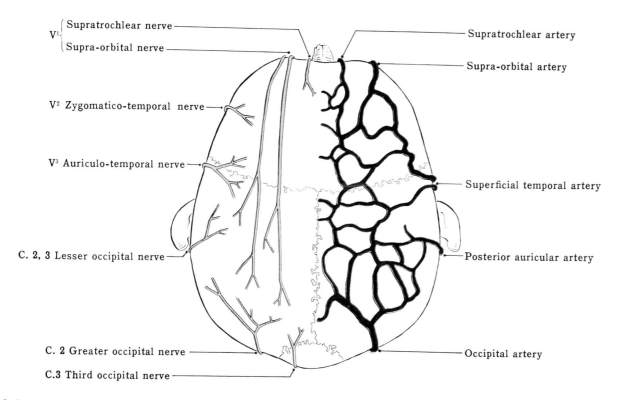

Supratrochlear nerve — V¹ {
Supra-orbital nerve —

V² Zygomatico-temporal nerve →

V³ Auriculo-temporal nerve →

C. 2, 3 Lesser occipital nerve —

C. 2 Greater occipital nerve —

C.3 Third occipital nerve —

Supratrochlear artery

Supra-orbital artery

Superficial temporal artery

Posterior auricular artery

Occipital artery

500 Diagram of the Arteries and Nerves of the Scalp

Observe:

1. The arteries, anastomosing freely with each other. The supra-orbital and supratrochlear are derived from the internal carotid artery via the ophthalmic artery; the three others are branches of the external carotid artery.

2. The nerves, appearing in sequence: V¹, V², V³, ventral rami of C. 2 & 3, and dorsal rami of C. 2 & 3. (C. 1 has no cutaneous branch.)

Anterior temporal diploic vein

Posterior temporal diploic vein —

Frontal diploic vein

Occipital diploic vein —

501 Diploic Veins

The outer table of the skull has been filed away and the channels for the diploic veins thereby opened.

Note:

Of the four (paired) diploic veins, the frontal opens into the supra-orbital vein at the supra-orbital notch; the anterior temporal opens into the spheno-parietal sinus; the posterior temporal and the occipital both open into the transverse sinus—but they may open into surface veins. There are no accompanying diploic arteries; the meningeal and pericranial arteries provide the arterial blood.

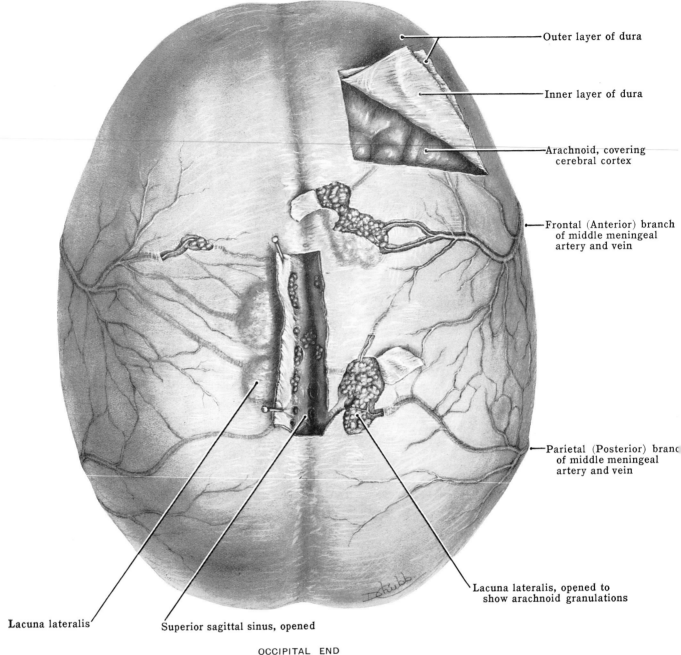

Outer layer of dura

Inner layer of dura

Arachnoid, covering
cerebral cortex

Frontal (Anterior) branch
of middle meningeal
artery and vein

Parietal (Posterior) branc
of middle meningeal
artery and vein

Lacuna lateralis, opened to
show arachnoid granulations

Lacuna lateralis

Superior sagittal sinus, opened

OCCIPITAL END

502   External Surface of the Dura Mater: Arachnoid Granulations

The skull cap is removed. In the median plane, the thick roof of the superior sagittal venous sinus is partly pinned aside and, laterally, the thin roofs of two lacunae laterales are reflected.

At the right front, an angular flap of both layers of dura is turned forwards; the subdural space is thereby opened; and the convolutions of the cerebral cortex are visible through the cobweb-like arachnoid mater.

Observe:

1. The frontal and parietal branches of the middle meningeal artery, arborising and anastomosing within the external or periosteal layer of the dura.

2. Each artery lying in a venous channel (middle meningeal vein) which enlarges above into a lake, lacuna lateralis.

3. Cauliflower-like masses, arachnoid granulations, dangling in the lakes, cf. chorionic villi of the placenta.

4. A channel or channels, draining the lake into the superior sagittal sinus which is triangular on cross section and has many discrete granulations protruding into it.

Labels on figure (clockwise/as positioned):
- Superior sagittal sinus
- Arachnoid granulations
- Cerebral veins
- Falx cerebri
- Frontal air sinus
- Crista galli
- Diaphragma sellae
- p.comm. a.cer.
- p.cer. m.cer. i.car.
- Straight sinus
- Falx cerebelli
- Tentorium cerebelli
- Vertebral aa.
- Basilar art.
- Superior cerebellar aa.

503 Folds of the Dura Mater

Observe:

1. The 4 reduplications of the inner layer of the dura mater, namely: the 2 sickle-shaped folds, (a) falx cerebri and (b) falx cerebelli, which lie vertically in the median plane; and the 2 roof-like folds, (c) tentorium cerebelli and (d) diaphragma sellae, which lie horizontally. The tentorium is perforated by the mid brain; the diaphragma, by the stalk of the hypophysis cerebri.
2. The 2 paired arteries that supply the brain—internal carotid and vertebral.

04 Diagram of Venous Sinuses of Dura Mater

bserve:

(a) The superior sagittal sinus at the upper or convex border of the falx cerebri; (b) the inferior sagittal sinus in the concave of free border; (c) the great cerebral vein joining the inf. sagittal sinus to form (d) the straight sinus which runs obliquely in the junction between falx cerebri and tentorium; (e) the occipital sinus in the attached border of the falx cerebelli.

The sup. sagittal sinus usually becomes—right transverse sinus—right sigmoid sinus—right int. jugular vein; the straight sinus behaves similarly on the left side.

The cavernous sinus communicating with the veins of the face via the ophthalmic veins and the pterygoid plexus, and emptying via the two petrosal sinuses (fig. 643).

The basilar sinus connecting the inf. petrosal sinuses of opposite sides and, like the occipital sinus, communicating below with the vertebral plexus (fig. 493).

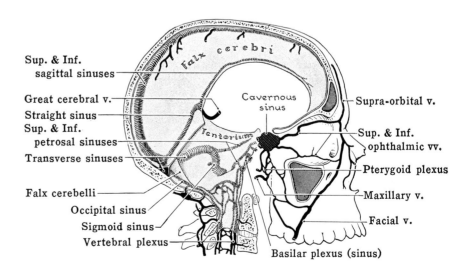

Labels on figure:
- Sup. & Inf. sagittal sinuses
- Great cerebral v.
- Straight sinus
- Sup. & Inf. petrosal sinuses
- Transverse sinuses
- Falx cerebelli
- Occipital sinus
- Sigmoid sinus
- Vertebral plexus
- Falx cerebri
- Cavernous sinus
- Tentorium
- Supra-orbital v.
- Sup. & Inf. ophthalmic vv.
- Pterygoid plexus
- Maxillary v.
- Facial v.
- Basilar plexus (sinus)

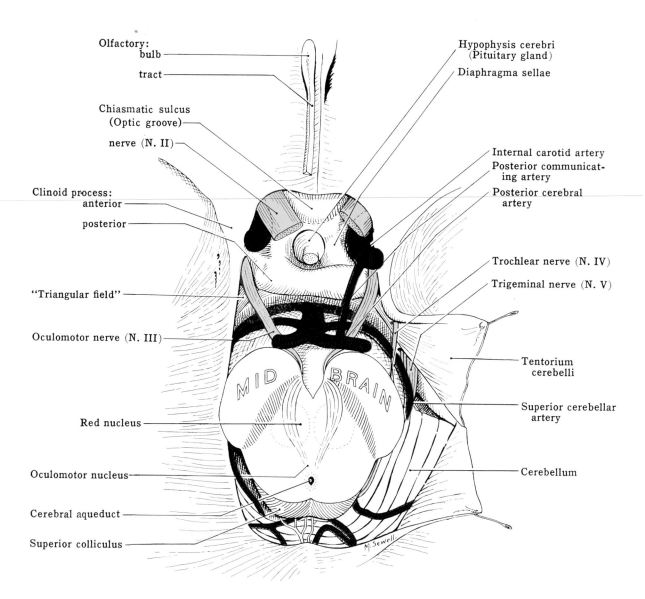

Olfactory:
bulb
tract

Chiasmatic sulcus
(Optic groove)
nerve (N. II)

Clinoid process:
anterior
posterior

"Triangular field"

Oculomotor nerve (N. III)

Red nucleus

Oculomotor nucleus

Cerebral aqueduct

Superior colliculus

Hypophysis cerebri
(Pituitary gland)
Diaphragma sellae

Internal carotid artery
Posterior communicat-
ing artery
Posterior cerebral
artery

Trochlear nerve (N. IV)

Trigeminal nerve (N. V)

Tentorium
cerebelli

Superior cerebellar
artery

Cerebellum

MID BRAIN

M. Sewell

505   A Stage in the Removal of the Brain

The forebrain is removed intact by carrying the knife postero-superiorly along the free curved border of the tentorium cerebelli and cutting through the midbrain (as in figs. 513 & 514). In so doing, the olfactory nerves (or else the olfactory tracts) and the optic nerves must be severed, but the remaining ten pairs of cranial nerves are not disturbed.   The internal carotid arteries, the posterior cerebral arteries and the stalk of the hypophysis cerebri must also be divided. On the right side, the tentorium is divided and reflected.

Observe:

1. The circular opening in the diaphragma sellae for the stalk of the hypophysis cerebri.
2. The free margin of the tentorium, extending forwards to the anterior clinoid process, and crossing the attached border which extends to the posterior clinoid process.
3. The triangular field or area between the free and attached borders and, within this, the oculomotor nerve bending round the posterior clinoid process. Followed backwards, this nerve passing between the posterior cerebral and superior cerebellar arteries.
4. On the right side, the long and slender trochlear nerve, curving round the midbrain under cover of the free edge of the tentorium, and piercing the triangular field at its posterior angle. Also, the trigeminal nerve entering the mouth of the trigeminal cave.

Olfactory bulb

Olfactory tract

mporal pole

teral
cerebral fissure

it. perforated
substance

fundibulum
amillary body

idbrain

iddle cerebellar
peduncle
rachium pontis)

la chorioidea
of IV ventricle

ateral recess
of IV ventricle

live

erebellum

Chiasma

Uncus

Pons

Pyramid

XII

II

Spinal
cord

Optic:
nerve—II
tract

Oculomotor nerve—III

Trochlear nerve—IV

Trigeminal nerve—V
sensory root
motor root

Abducent nerve—VI

Facial nerve—VII

Vestibulo-
cochlear nerve—VIII

Glossopharyngeal nerve—IX

Vagus nerve—X

Accessory nerve—XI:
cranial root
spinal root

506 Base of the Brain: The Superfical Origins of the Cranial Nerves

Note:

1. The olfactory bulb, in which the olfactory (1) nerves (not shown) end.

2. The superficial origin of the trochlear (IV) nerve is shown in figure 495.

3. The slender nervus intermedius, or so-called sensory root of the facial nerve (seen, but not labelled) between the facial (VII) and vestibulo-cochlear (acoustic, VIII) nerves.

4. The fila of the hypoglossal (XII) nerve, arising between the pyramid and the olive, and in line with the ventral root of the 1st cervical nerve.

FRONTAL BONE

ETHMOID BONE

SPHENOID BONE

MANDIBLE

Orbital part
(Orbital plate)

Lesser wing

Greater wing

Jugum

Body

Dorsum
sellæ

Head

Basilar part
(Basi-occipital)

Lateral part
(Condylar part)

Foramen
magnum

Squamous part
or squama

PARIETAL BONE

PARIETAL BONE

OCCIPITAL BONE

507   Interior of the Base of the Skull

The temporal bones are removed, but the heads of the mandible remain in situ.

Observe:

1. The head of the mandible, lying lateral to the spine of the sphenoid, at which there is a perforation, the foramen spinosum, for the transmission of the middle meningeal vessels.
2. The long axes of the right and left heads, when produced medially, meet near the anterior border of the foramen magnum.
3. The 3 bones contributing to the anterior cranial fossa.
4. The 4 parts of the occipital bone—basilar, right and left lateral, and squamous.

Jug   um

Body

Optic canal

507.1   Lesser Wings of Sphenoid before birth, posterior view

Note:

1. These wings, like sliding doors, close above the body of the sphenoid to form the jugum or yoke.
2. The posterior edge of the jugum becomes the anterior edge of the chiasmatic sulcus, which leads to the optic canals.
3. The left canal is not yet pinched off from the superior orbital fissure, but the right is.

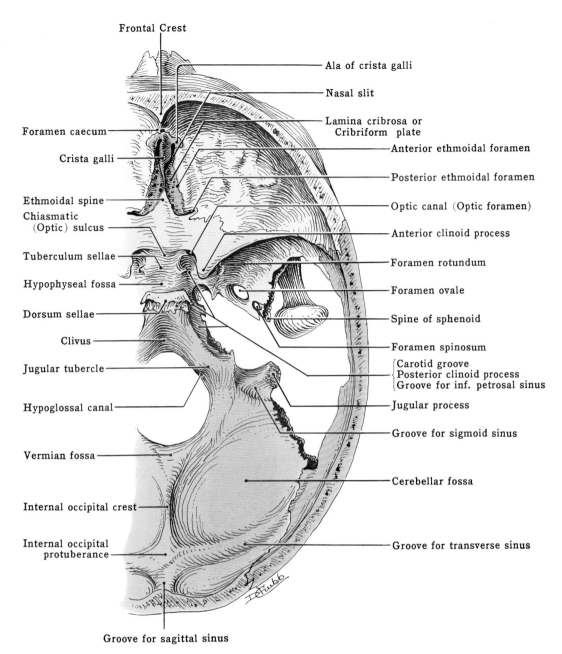

Frontal Crest

Ala of crista galli

Nasal slit

Lamina cribrosa or
Cribriform plate

Foramen caecum

Anterior ethmoidal foramen

Crista galli

Posterior ethmoidal foramen

Ethmoidal spine

Optic canal (Optic foramen)

Chiasmatic
(Optic) sulcus

Anterior clinoid process

Tuberculum sellae

Foramen rotundum

Hypophyseal fossa

Foramen ovale

Dorsum sellae

Spine of sphenoid

Clivus

Foramen spinosum

Jugular tubercle

Carotid groove
Posterior clinoid process
Groove for inf. petrosal sinus

Hypoglossal canal

Jugular process

Groove for sigmoid sinus

Vermian fossa

Cerebellar fossa

Internal occipital crest

Internal occipital
protuberance

Groove for transverse sinus

Groove for sagittal sinus

508 Interior of the Base of the Skull

(*Key to figure 407*).

Features in the median plane:

of the anterior cranial fossa—frontal crest and crista galli (for attachment of falx cerebri) with foramen caecum in between, and jugum whose free posterior edge limits this fossa posteriorly.

of the middle cranial fossa—chiasmatic sulcus (leading from one optic canal to the other, but not lodging the chiasma, see fig. 521), tuberculum sellae, hypophyseal fossa, and dorsum sellae which limits this fossa posteriorly.

of the posterior cranial fossa—dorsum sellae, clivus, foramen magnum, vermian fossa (below vermis of cerebellum), internal occipital crest (for falx cerebelli), and internal occipital protuberance from which the sulci for the transverse sinuses curve laterally, limiting this fossa postero-superiorly.

509 Crescent of Foramina in the Middle Cranial Fossa

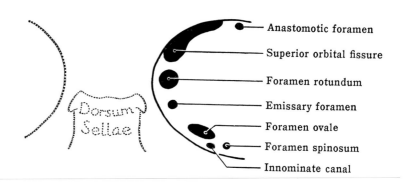

- Anastomotic foramen
- Superior orbital fissure
- Foramen rotundum
- Emissary foramen
- Foramen ovale
- Foramen spinosum
- Innominate canal

Note: Seven paired foramina, of which 4 (black) are constant and 3 (red) are inconstant, open from the sphenoid bone into the middle cranial fossa. Because of the crescentic design made by these foramina, it is simple to relate one foramen to another.

Anastomotic foramen transmits a branch from middle meningeal art. to lacrimal art. (fig. 524). *Emissary foramen* transmits a vein from cavernous sinus to pterygoid plexus. *Innominate canal*, in lieu of foramen ovale, transmits lesser petrosal nerve to otic ganglion.

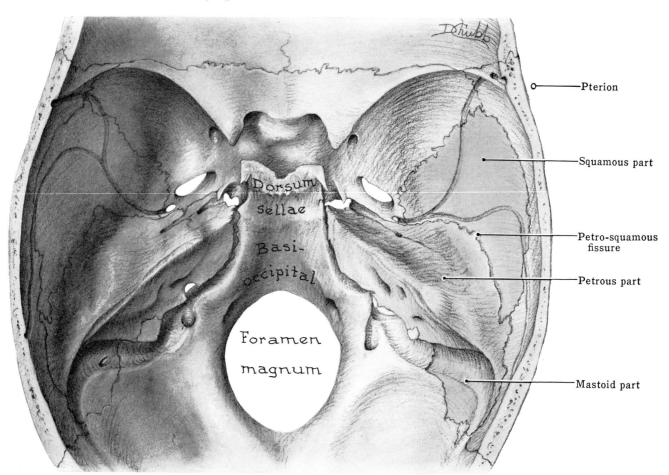

- Pterion
- Squamous part
- Petro-squamous fissure
- Petrous part
- Mastoid part

Dorsum sellae

Basi-occipital

Foramen magnum

510 Temporal Bone, in its setting, at the interior of the base of the skull

(Figures 509 and 512 are keys to figure 510.)

511 Spheno-occipital Synchondrosis (Basilar Suture), in paramedian section, aged about ten years

This synchondrosis is usually obliterated (becomes a synostosis) by the 17th or 18th year, and always by the 21st year (McKern & Stewart).

Note the right sphenoidal sinus, like an inflated rubber balloon, invading the cancellous bone.

Sella Turcica
Dorsum sellae
Body of sphenoid bone
Basi-occipital
sinus
Spheno-occipital synchondrosis

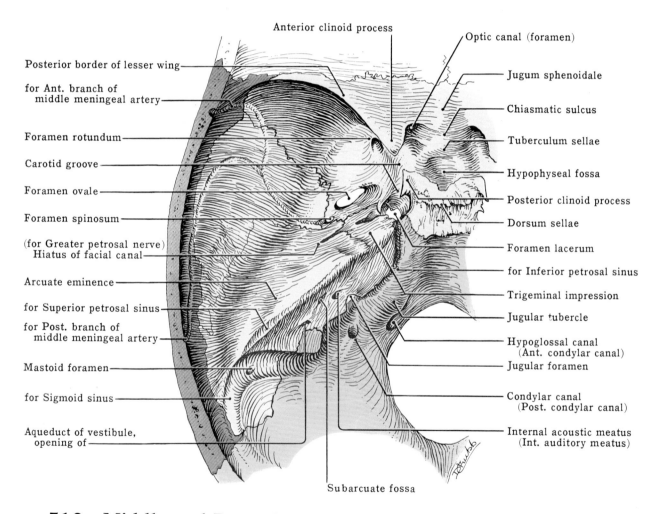

Anterior clinoid process
Posterior border of lesser wing
for Ant. branch of middle meningeal artery
Foramen rotundum
Carotid groove
Foramen ovale
Foramen spinosum
(for Greater petrosal nerve) Hiatus of facial canal
Arcuate eminence
for Superior petrosal sinus
for Post. branch of middle meningeal artery
Mastoid foramen
for Sigmoid sinus
Aqueduct of vestibule, opening of

Optic canal (foramen)
Jugum sphenoidale
Chiasmatic sulcus
Tuberculum sellae
Hypophyseal fossa
Posterior clinoid process
Dorsum sellae
Foramen lacerum
for Inferior petrosal sinus
Trigeminal impression
Jugular tubercle
Hypoglossal canal (Ant. condylar canal)
Jugular foramen
Condylar canal (Post. condylar canal)
Internal acoustic meatus (Int. auditory meatus)

Subarcuate fossa

512 Middle and Posterior Cranial Fossae, from above

Note:

1. Three features—tuberculum sellae, hypophyseal fossa, and dorsum sellae—constitute the sella turcica or Turkish saddle.

2. Of the two, paired clinoid processes (for the attachment of the tentorium, fig. 514) the anterior, on the lesser wing of the sphenoid, is conical; the posterior, on the angle of the dorsum sellae, is beak-like.

3. The foramen lacerum is situated between the hypophyseal fossa and the apex of the petrous bone. There the carotid canal discharges the internal carotid art. into the upper half of the foramen lacerum.

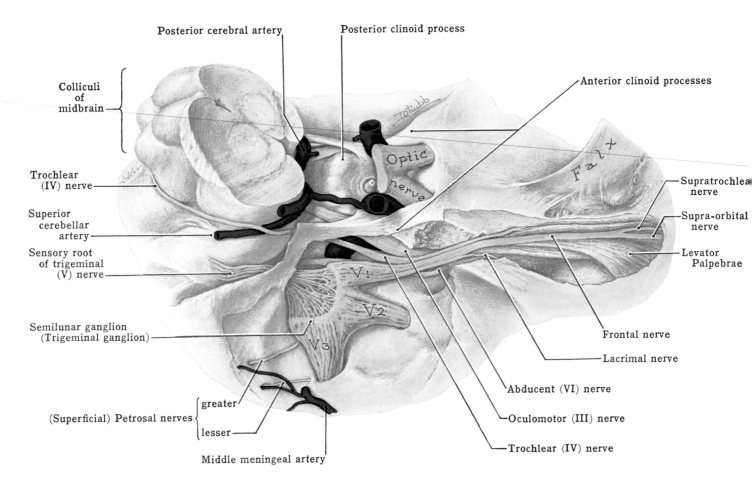

Posterior cerebral artery

Posterior clinoid process

Anterior clinoid processes

Colliculi of midbrain

Tubub

Optic nerve

Falx

Trochlear (IV) nerve

Supratrochlear nerve

Superior cerebellar artery

Supra-orbital nerve

Sensory root of trigeminal (V) nerve

V1

Levator Palpebrae

V2

Semilunar ganglion (Trigeminal ganglion)

V3

Frontal nerve

Lacrimal nerve

(Superficial) Petrosal nerves { greater / lesser

Abducent (VI) nerve

Oculomotor (III) nerve

Trochlear (IV) nerve

Middle meningeal artery

513 Nerves in the Middle Cranial Fossa—I

(Nerves II–VI and the superficial petrosal nerves.)

The tentorium cerebelli is cut away in order to reveal the courses of the trochlear (IV) and trigeminal (V) nerves in the posterior cranial fossa, i.e., below the level of the tentorium. The dura mater is largely removed from the middle fossa; the roof of the orbital cavity is partly removed.

Observe:

1. The semilunar ganglion and its 3 divisions.
2. The mandibular nerve (V³), dropping down through the foramen ovale (into the infratemporal fossa).
3. The maxillary nerve (V²), passing forwards through the

foramen rotundum (into the pterygo-palatine fossa).

4. The ophthalmic nerve (V¹), ascending slightly, closely applied to the trochlear (IV) nerve, and dividing into frontal and lacrimal branches. These 3 (trochlear, frontal, lacrimal) nerves, running forwards through the superior orbital fissure and applied to the roof of the orbital cavity (removed).

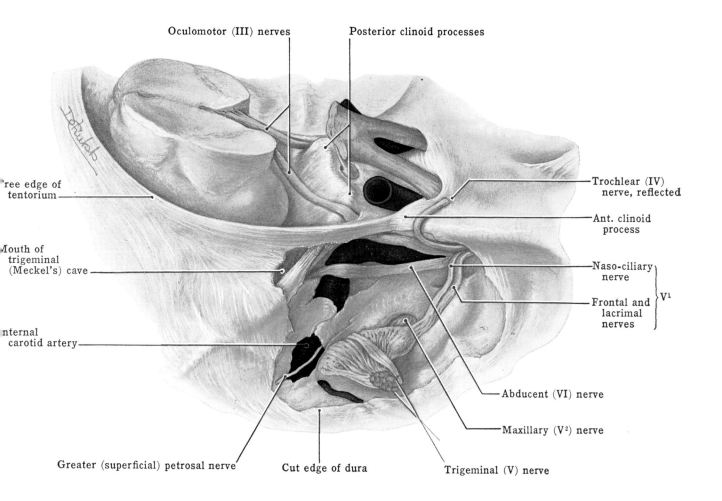

Oculomotor (III) nerves

Posterior clinoid processes

Free edge of tentorium

Mouth of trigeminal (Meckel's) cave

Internal carotid artery

Greater (superficial) petrosal nerve

Cut edge of dura

Trigeminal (V) nerve

Trochlear (IV) nerve, reflected

Ant. clinoid process

Naso-ciliary nerve

Frontal and lacrimal nerves

V^1

Abducent (VI) nerve

Maxillary (V^2) nerve

514 Nerves in the Middle Cranial Fossa—II

The trigeminal nerve is divided, withdrawn from the mouth of the trigeminal cave, and turned forwards. The trochlear nerve also is turned forwards.

Observe:

1. The bed of the semilunar ganglion partly formed by the greater petrosal nerve and the internal carotid artery, dura intervening.

2. The motor root of nerve V (the nerve to the muscles of mastication), crossing the ganglion diagonally, from medial to lateral side, to join V^3.

3. V^1, giving off the naso-ciliary nerve, and crowding with nerves III, IV, and VI through the superior orbital fissure.

4. The anterior clinoid process, "pulled backwards" by the free edge of the tentorium between the optic nerve and internal carotid artery medially, and the oculo-motor nerve below.

5. The abducent (VI) nerve, making a right-angled turn at the apex of the petrous bone and then, as it runs horizontally forwards, hugging the internal carotid artery which flattens it.

6. The sinuous course of the internal carotid artery.

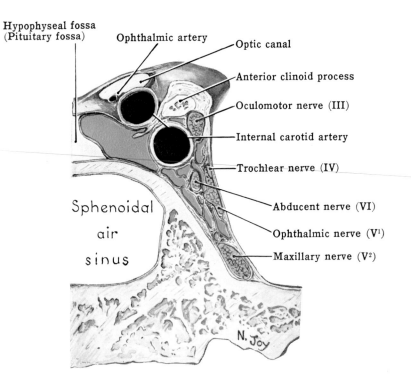

Hypophyseal fossa (Pituitary fossa)

Ophthalmic artery

Optic canal

Anterior clinoid process

Oculomotor nerve (III)

Internal carotid artery

Trochlear nerve (IV)

Abducent nerve (VI)

Ophthalmic nerve (V¹)

Maxillary nerve (V²)

Sphenoidal air sinus

N. Joy

515 Cavernous Sinus, on coronal section

Observe:

1. This venous sinus, situated at the side of the sphenoidal air sinus and of the hypophyseal fossa.

2. The internal carotid artery, surrounded by the internal carotid plexus (not drawn), and the abducent nerve (fig. 643), passing through the sinus.

3. The internal carotid artery, having made an acute bend, is cut twice. This artery and the oculomotor nerve grooving the anterior clinoid process.

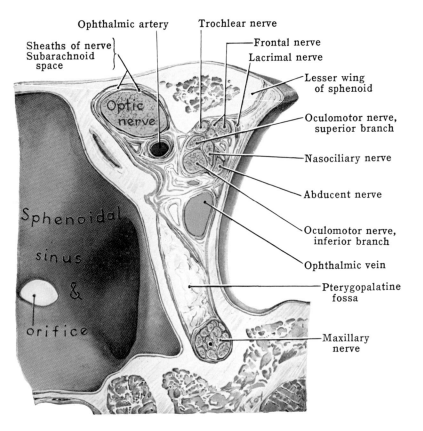

Ophthalmic artery

Trochlear nerve

Sheaths of nerve Subarachnoid space

Frontal nerve

Lacrimal nerve

Lesser wing of sphenoid

Optic nerve

Oculomotor nerve, superior branch

Nasociliary nerve

Abducent nerve

Sphenoidal sinus & orifice

Oculomotor nerve, inferior branch

Ophthalmic vein

Pterygopalatine fossa

Maxillary nerve

516 Nerves and Vessels at the Apex of the Orbital Cavity on coronal section

Observe:

1. The optic nerve within its pial, arachnoid, and dural sheaths and the subarachnoid space. The ophthalmic artery emerging from the optic canal.

2. Other nerves crowded together, tightly packed passing through the medial end of the superior orbital fissure. They are: the upper and the lower branch of the oculomotor nerve (III), the trochlear nerve (IV); the frontal, lacrimal and naso-ciliary branches of the ophthalmic nerve (V¹); and the abducent nerve (VI).

3. The ophthalmic vein, about to open into the cavernous sinus, in turn to be drained by the superior and inferior petrosal sinuses (fig. 643).

(For posterior half of orbital cavity on coronal section, see figures 591 & 592.)

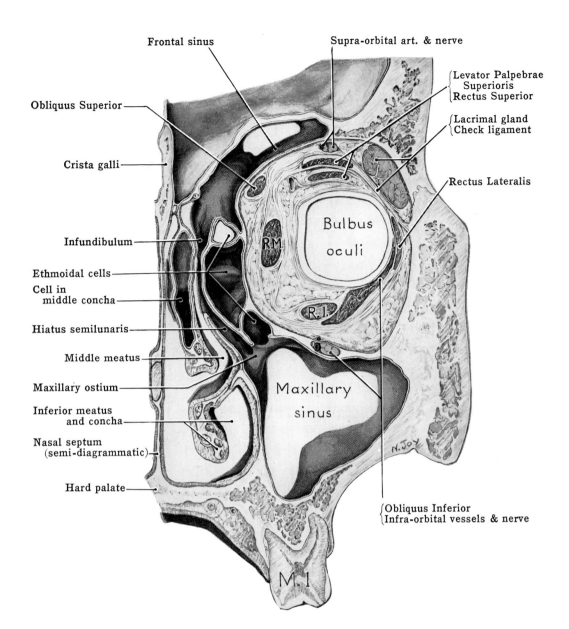

Frontal sinus

Supra-orbital art. & nerve

Levator Palpebrae
Superioris
Rectus Superior

Obliquus Superior

Lacrimal gland
Check ligament

Crista galli

Rectus Lateralis

Bulbus
oculi

Infundibulum

R M

Ethmoidal cells
Cell in
middle concha

R. I.

Hiatus semilunaris

Middle meatus

Maxillary ostium

Maxillary
sinus

Inferior meatus
and concha

Nasal septum
(semi-diagrammatic)

N. Joy

Hard palate

Obliquus Inferior
Infra-orbital vessels & nerve

M. I

517 Right Side of the Head, on coronal section, viewed from behind

Observe:

1. The bulbus oculi (eyeball) within the somewhat circular orbital cavity. The stout, thick lateral bony wall; the thin, papery roof, medial wall, and floor surrounded with air sinuses—frontal, ethmoidal, and maxillary.

2. The 4 Recti Oculi and 2 Obliqui Oculi arranged around the bulb, Obliquus Inferior inserted by tendon. Levator Palpebrae Superioris above Rectus Superior, and the check ligament passing from it.

3. The lacrimal gland lying between the check ligament and the frontal bone.

4. The 4 Recti and the fascia uniting them forming a circle around the bulb—it is a section of the cone of muscles.

5. The nasal septum (semidiagrammatic). The middle concha, here, containing an air cell. The entrance to the frontal sinus through the infundibulum, which is at the lowest point of the sinus.

6. The entrance to the maxillary sinus through the hiatus semilunaris, which is at the level of the roof of the sinus. The lowest point of the sinus, here as commonly, below the level of the floor of the nasal cavity. The nasal wall of the sinus is very thin in the inferior meatus, well above the floor of the nose.

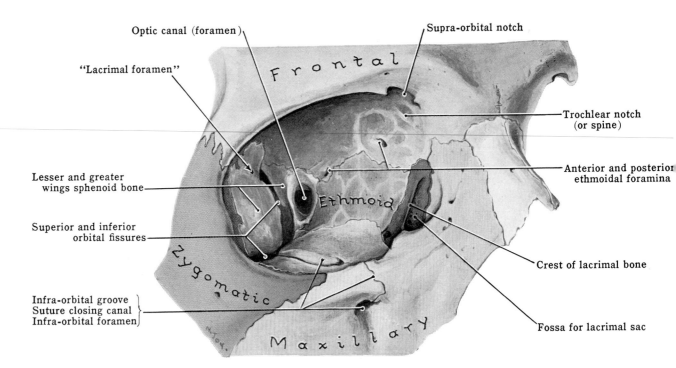

Optic canal (foramen)

"Lacrimal foramen"

Supra-orbital notch

Frontal

Trochlear notch
(or spine)

Anterior and posterior
ethmoidal foramina

Lesser and greater
wings sphenoid bone

Ethmoid

Superior and inferior
orbital fissures

Crest of lacrimal bone

Zygomatic

Infra-orbital groove
Suture closing canal
Infra-orbital foramen

Fossa for lacrimal sac

Maxillary

518 Orbital Cavity

Observe:

1. The quadrangular orbital margin, at the base of the cavity, to which the frontal, maxillary, and zygomatic bones contribute.

2. The spiral form of the medial part of this margin. It is spiral since the supra-orbital margin leads to the crest of the lacrimal bone (post. lacrimal crest); whereas the infra-orbital margin is continuous with the crest on the frontal process of the maxilla (ant. lacrimal crest).

3. The fossa for the lacrimal sac, between these two crests.

4. The optic canal, situated at the apex of the pear-shaped orbital cavity, and placed between the body of the sphenoid and the two roots of the lesser wing. A straight probe must pass along the lateral wall of the cavity, if it is to traverse the canal.

5. The superior wall or roof, formed by the orbital plate of the frontal bone.

6. The inferior wall or floor, formed by the orbital plate of the maxilla and slightly by the zygomatic bone, and crossed by the infra-orbital groove, the anterior end of which is converted into the infra-orbital canal which ends at the infra-orbital foramen.

7. The stout lateral wall, formed by the frontal process of the zygomatic bone and by the greater wing of the sphenoid. The superior and inferior orbital fissures, together forming a V-shaped fissure which limits the greater wing of the sphenoid.

8. The fragile medial wall, formed by the papery lacrimal bone and the papery orbital plate (lamina papyracea) of the ethmoid bone. The anterior and posterior ethmoidal foramina, which developed in the suture between the frontal and ethmoidal bones, but are now, in this specimen, enveloped by the frontal bone.

9. The "lacrimal foramen", just beyond the supero-lateral end of the superior orbital fissure, for the anastomosis between the middle meningeal and lacrimal arteries. The zygomatic foramen on the orbital surface of the zygomatic bone is not in view.

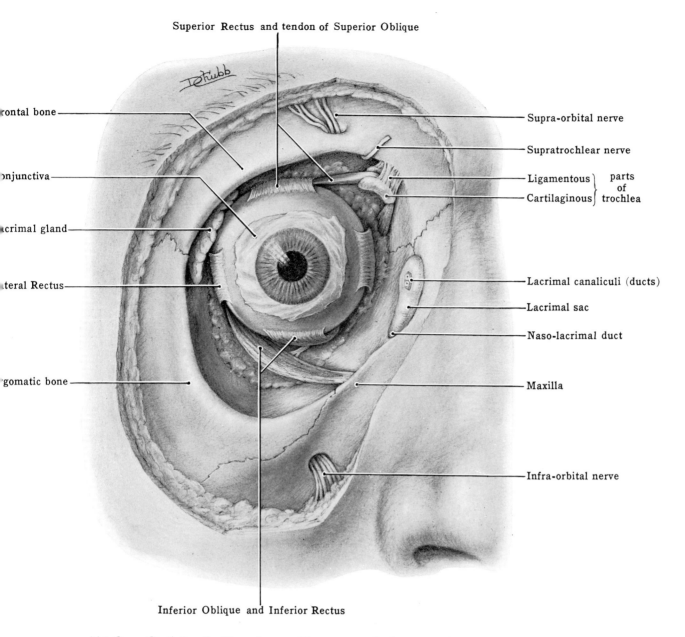

Superior Rectus and tendon of Superior Oblique

rontal bone

onjunctiva

crimal gland

teral Rectus

gomatic bone

Supra-orbital nerve

Supratrochlear nerve

Ligamentous } parts
Cartilaginous } of trochlea

Lacrimal canaliculi (ducts)

Lacrimal sac

Naso-lacrimal duct

Maxilla

Infra-orbital nerve

Inferior Oblique and Inferior Rectus

519 Orbital Cavity, dissected from the front

The eyelids, orbital septum, Levator Palpebrae Superioris, and some fat are removed.

Observe:

1. The ocular conjunctiva, loose and wrinkled over the sclera, but adherent to the cornea.

2. The aponeurotic insertions of the four Recti, inserted 6 to 8 mm. behind the sclero-corneal junction.

3. The superior and inferior oblique muscles, crossing below the corresponding superior and inferior straight muscles.

4. The tendon of Obliquus Superior, playing in a cartilaginous pulley or trochlea, which is fixed by ligamentous fibres just behind the supero-medial angle of the orbital margin.

5. The nerve to Obliquus Inferior entering its posterior border.

6. The lacrimal gland, placed between the bony orbital wall laterally and the eyeball and Rectus Lateralis medially.

7. The lacrimal sac, receiving the superior and inferior lacrimal canaliculi (ducts) and becoming the naso-lacrimal duct which traverses the (bony) naso-lacrimal canal to open into the nose (fig. 610).

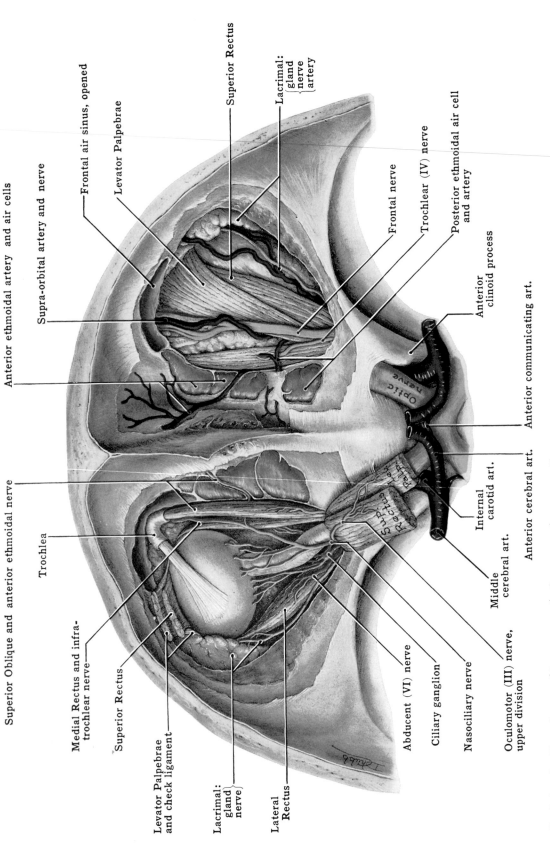

Anterior ethmoidal artery and air cells

Supra-orbital artery and nerve

Frontal air sinus, opened

Levator Palpebrae

Superior Rectus

Lacrimal: { gland nerve artery }

Frontal nerve

Trochlear (IV) nerve

Posterior ethmoidal air cell and artery

Anterior clinoid process

Optic nerve

Anterior communicating art.

Internal carotid art.

Superior Rectus

Middle cerebral art.

Anterior cerebral art.

Superior Oblique and anterior ethmoidal nerve

Medial Rectus and infra-trochlear nerve

Trochlea

Superior Rectus

Levator Palpebrae and check ligament

Lacrimal: { gland nerve }

Lateral Rectus

Abducent (VI) nerve

Ciliary ganglion

Nasociliary nerve

Oculomotor (III) nerve, upper division

520 Orbital Cavity, dissected from above—I

On the right side—The orbital plate of the frontal bone is removed.
On the left side—Levator Palpebrae and Rectus Superior are reflected.

Observe, on the right side:

1. Levator Palpebrae Superioris, overlying Rectus Superior.
2. The 3 nerves applied to the roof of the orbital cavity—trochlear, frontal, lacrimal.
3. Four of the branches of the ophthalmic artery.

Observe, on the left side:

4. The superior division nerve III, supplying Rectus Superior and Levator Palpebrae.
5. The entire course of Obliquus Superior, and the trochlear (IV) nerve supplying it.
6. Rectus Lateralis and the abducent (VI) nerve supplying it.
7. Rectus Medialis and a branch of the oculomotor (III) nerve supplying it.
8. The lacrimal nerve, running above Rectus Lateralis to the lacrimal gland.
9. The ciliary ganglion, placed between Rectus Lateralis and the optic nerve and giving

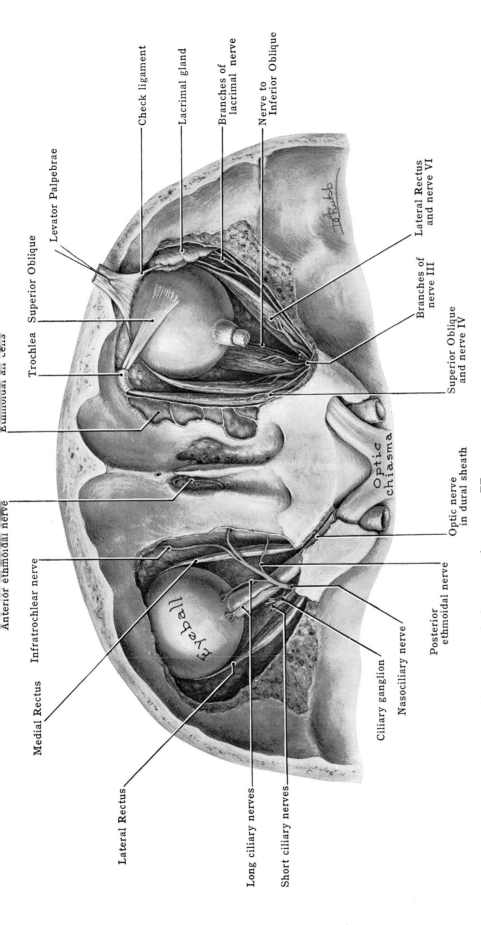

Ethmoidal air cells

Trochlea Superior Oblique

Levator Palpebrae

Check ligament

Lacrimal gland

Branches of
lacrimal nerve

Nerve to
Inferior Oblique

Branches of
nerve III

Lateral Rectus
and nerve VI

Superior Oblique
and nerve IV

Optic nerve
in dural sheath

Optic chiasma

Anterior ethmoidal nerve

Infratrochlear nerve

Medial Rectus

Lateral Rectus

Long ciliary nerves

Short ciliary nerves

Ciliary ganglion

Nasociliary nerve

Posterior
ethmoidal nerve

521   Orbital Cavity, dissected from above—II

Observe, on the right side:

1. The nerves to the six ocular muscles—4 Recti and 2 Obliqui—the trochlear to Obliquus Superior, the abducent to Rectus Lateralis, and the oculomotor to the remaining four and also to Levator Palpebrae Superioris.

2. The four Recti (Superior, Medialis, Inferior, Lateralis), supplied on their ocular surfaces; the two Obliqui (Superior, Inferior) near their borders. Rectus Superior and Obliquus Inferior are not in view.

Observe, on the left side:

3. The eyeball, occupying the anterior half of the 2″ long orbital cavity.

4. The ciliary ganglion, faintly brownish in colour, lying far back between Rectus Lateralis and the sheath of the optic nerve, receiving a twig (sensory and sympathetic) from the nasociliary nerve and a twig (motor to Sphincter Pupillae and Ciliary muscle) from the nerve to Obliquus Inferior, and giving off short ciliary nerves (cut short).

5. The nasociliary nerve, sending a twig to the ciliary ganglion, crossing the optic nerve, giving off two long ciliary nerves (sensory to the eyeball and cornea), and the posterior ethmoidal nerve (to the sphenoidal sinus and posterior ethmoidal cells), and dividing into the anterior ethmoidal and infratrochlear nerves.

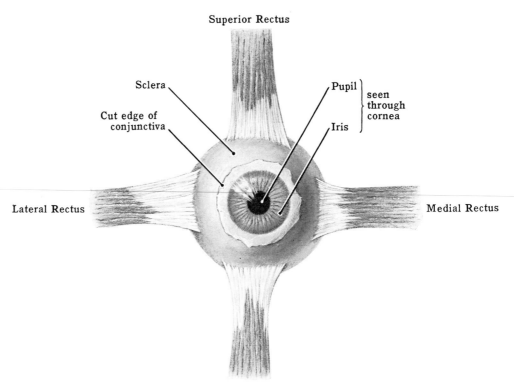

522   Eyeball and the Attachments of the Four Recti Oculi, front view

The 4 Recti are spread out to show the insertions of their aponeuroses into the anterior half of the bulb or eyeball, 6 to 8 mm. behind the sclero-corneal junction.

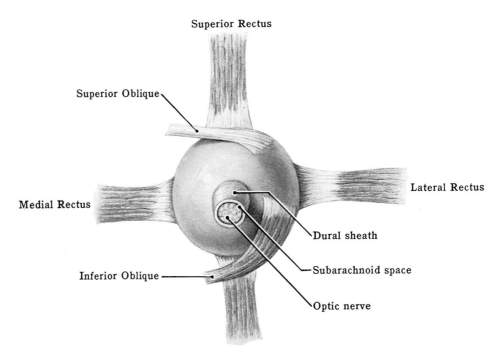

522.1   Eyeball and the Attachments of the Two Obliqui Oculi, posterior view

The 2 Obliques are inserted by aponeuroses into the postero-lateral quadrant of the eyeball.

   When in situ, Inferior Rectus passes above Inferior Oblique, as in figure 519.

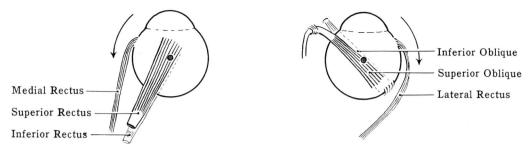

Medial Rectus ——

Superior Rectus ——

Inferior Rectus ——

Inferior Oblique

Superior Oblique

Lateral Rectus

ADDUCTORS   **VERTICAL AXIS**   ABDUCTORS

Inferior Oblique ——

Superior Rectus ——

Superior Oblique

Inferior Rectus

ELEVATORS   **HORIZONTAL AXIS**   DEPRESSORS

Sup. (Inf.) Oblique ——

Sup. (Inf.) Rectus ——

Superior Rectus

Superior Oblique

MEDIAL ROTATORS

Inferior Rectus

Inferior Oblique

MED. (LAT.) ROTATORS   LATERAL ROTATORS

SAGITTAL AXIS

523   Actions of the Six Ocular Muscles

In each instance it is the right eyeball that is represented

Note: Of the 6 ocular muscles, the Medial Rectus and the Lateral Rectus move the eyeball on one axis only; each of the four other muscles moves it on all three axes.

Rectus Superior   elevates,   adducts,   and rotates medially.
Rectus Inferior   depresses,   adducts,   and rotates laterally.
Obliquus Superior   depresses,   abducts,   and rotates medially.
Obliquus Inferior   elevates,   abducts,   and rotates laterally.

The 2 Obliqui also protract (protrude) the eyeball, whereas the 4 Recti retract it.

Clinical tests: It is true that Superior Rectus turns the eye up and, along with Inferior Rectus, assists Medial Rectus to turn the eye in. Clinical evidence, however, proves that the greatest upward action of Superior Rectus is when the eye is turned out—it is then working directly over the centre of rotation. Therefore, the test for the efficiency of Superior Rectus is to look up and out; whereas for Inferior Rectus it is to look down and out.

Similarly, the greatest upward action of Inferior Oblique is when the eye is turned up and in; whereas the greatest downwards action of Superior Oblique is when the eye is turned down and in. Hence, the test for the efficiency of these two muscles is to look in these directions.

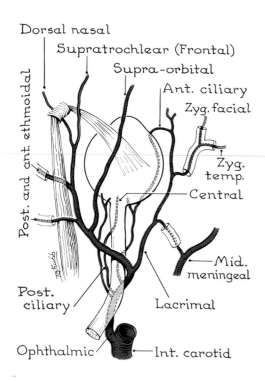

Dorsal nasal

Supratrochlear (Frontal)

Supra-orbital

Ant. ciliary

Zyg. facial

Zyg. temp.

Post. and ant. ethmoidal

Central

Mid. meningeal

Post. ciliary

Lacrimal

Ophthalmic

Int. carotid

524 Diagram of the Ophthalmic Artery

Note:

1. This branch of the internal carotid artery enters the orbit via the optic canal within the dural sheath of the optic nerve shown in figure 525. It supplies the contents of the orbit.

2. Of its branches: the central a. to the retina is an end artery. Of the 8 or so posterior ciliary arteries, 6 supply the choroid which in turn nourishes the outer non-vascular layer of the retina; whereas 2 long posterior ciliary arteries, one on each side of the eyeball, run between sclera and choroid to anastomose with anterior ciliary arteries which are derived from muscular branches.

3. Six branches pass beyond the orbit (a) supratrochlear a. and (b) supra-orbital a. to the forehead, (c) dorsal nasal a. to the face, (d) lacrimal a. to the eyelid and, via its zygomatic branches, to the cheek and the temporal region, and (e and f) anterior and posterior ethmoidal aa. to the nasal cavity. These 6 arteries which extend beyond the orbit anastomose freely with branches of the external carotid artery.

4. The lacrimal artery commonly anastomoses with the middle meningeal artery, via the foramen lacrimale (fig. 509), and may be derived from it.

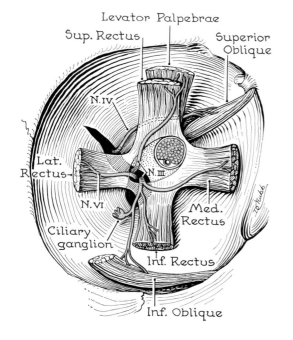

Levator Palpebrae

Sup. Rectus

Superior Oblique

N.IV

Lat. Rectus

N.III

N.VI

Med. Rectus

Ciliary ganglion

Inf. Rectus

Inf. Oblique

525 Diagram of the Motor Nerves the Orbit

Observe:

1. The optic nerve within its pial, arachnoid, and dural sheaths.

2. The 4 Recti arising from a fibrous cuff, called the anulus tendineus, that encircles:—the dural sheath of the optic nerve, nerve VI (abducent n.), and the upper and lower divisions of nerve III (oculomotor n.). The naso-ciliary nerve (not shown) also passes through this cuff, but nerve IV (trochlear n.) clings to the bony roof of the cavity.

3. Nerves IV and VI supplying one muscle each, and nerve III supplying the remaining five orbital muscles—2 via its upper division; 3 via its lower division and, via the ciliary ganglion, it supplies parasympathetic fibres to the ciliary muscle and sphincter iridis.

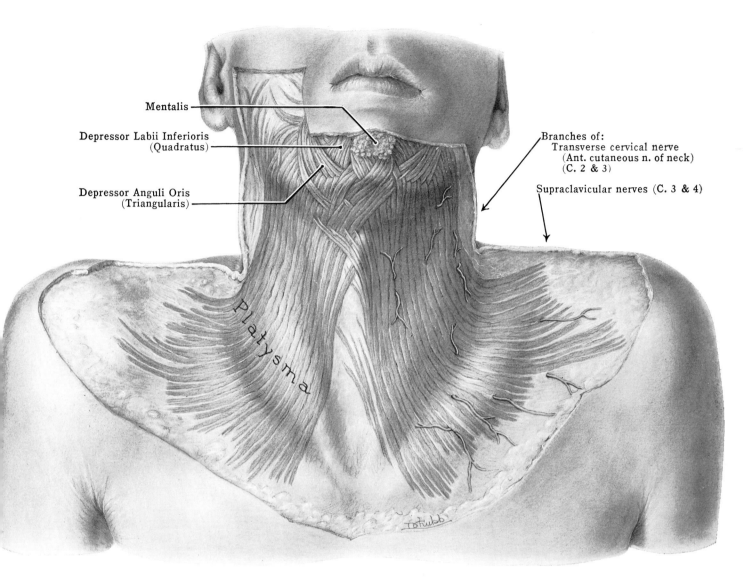

Mentalis

Depressor Labii Inferioris
(Quadratus)

Depressor Anguli Oris
(Triangularis)

Branches of:
Transverse cervical nerve
(Ant. cutaneous n. of neck)
(C. 2 & 3)

Supraclavicular nerves (C. 3 & 4)

Platysma

526 Platysma, front view

Observe:

1. The platysma, spreading subcutaneously like a sheet, pierced by cutaneous nerves, crossing the whole length of the lower border of the mandible above, crossing the whole length of the clavicle below, and extending downwards to the level of the 1st or 2nd rib and to (or towards) the acromion.

2. The anterior borders of the two Platysmas, decussating behind the chin (in the submental region) and, below that, free and diverging, and so leaving the median part of the neck uncovered.

3. Its posterior border, free, covering the antero-inferior part of the posterior triangle, and continuing upwards across the lower border of the jaw to the angle of the mouth.

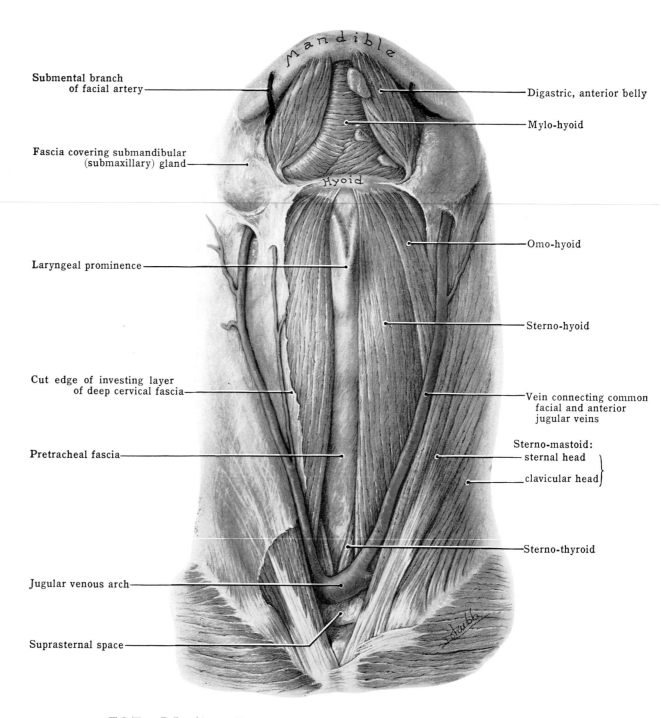

Submental branch of facial artery

Fascia covering submandibular (submaxillary) gland

Laryngeal prominence

Cut edge of investing layer of deep cervical fascia

Pretracheal fascia

Jugular venous arch

Suprasternal space

Mandible

Hyoid

Digastric, anterior belly

Mylo-hyoid

Omo-hyoid

Sterno-hyoid

Vein connecting common facial and anterior jugular veins

Sterno-mastoid:
sternal head
clavicular head

Sterno-thyroid

527 Median Part of the Front of the Neck—I

Observe:

1. This region, extending from the mandible above to the sternum below; and divided by the hyoid bone into a suprahyoid and an infrahyoid part.

2. The suprahyoid part or submental triangle, having the Digastrics (anterior bellies) for its sides, the hyoid bone for its base, the Mylohyoid for its floor, and some submental lymph nodes for contents. Actually, the submental triangle is part of the floor of the mouth. (Fig. 595).

3. The infrahyoid part, shaped like an elongated diamond, and bounded on each side by Sterno-hyoid above and Sterno-thyroid below.

4. The suprasternal (fascial) space, containing a cross-connecting vein called the jugular venous arch. In this specimen the anterior jugular veins were absent, as such, in the median part of the neck, but were present above the clavicles.

5. The connecting vein along the anterior border of Sternomastoid.

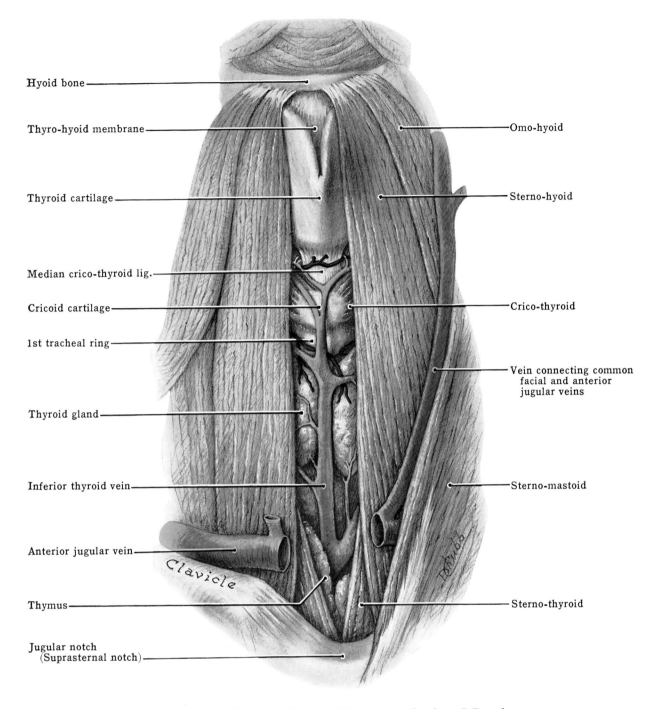

Hyoid bone

Thyro-hyoid membrane

Thyroid cartilage

Median crico-thyroid lig.

Cricoid cartilage

1st tracheal ring

Thyroid gland

Inferior thyroid vein

Anterior jugular vein

Clavicle

Thymus

Jugular notch
(Suprasternal notch)

Omo-hyoid

Sterno-hyoid

Crico-thyroid

Vein connecting common
facial and anterior
jugular veins

Sterno-mastoid

Sterno-thyroid

528 Median Part of the Front of the Neck: Depressors of the Larynx—II

On the left side of the picture, Sternomastoid is removed.

Observe:

1. The structures in the median plane, labelled on the left side of the picture; also the un-labelled anastomoses between the crico-thyroid arteries, between the superior thyroid arteries, and between the anterior jugular veins (excised). Also, the thymus (enlarged) projecting upwards from the thorax. On looking behind it, you might see, peeping above the jugular notch, the left brachiocephalic (innominate) vein and the trunk. (Figs. 449 & 529).

2. The two superficial Depressors of the larynx or "strap muscles"—Omo-hyoid (superior belly) and Sterno-hyoid.

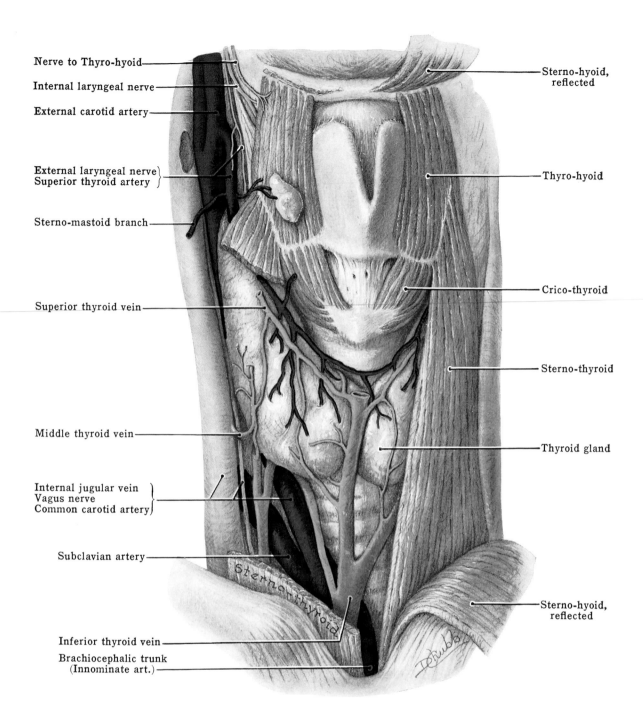

Nerve to Thyro-hyoid

Internal laryngeal nerve

External carotid artery

External laryngeal nerve
Superior thyroid artery

Sterno-mastoid branch

Superior thyroid vein

Middle thyroid vein

Internal jugular vein
Vagus nerve
Common carotid artery

Subclavian artery

Inferior thyroid vein

Brachiocephalic trunk
(Innominate art.)

Sterno-hyoid,
reflected

Thyro-hyoid

Crico-thyroid

Sterno-thyroid

Thyroid gland

Sterno-hyoid,
reflected

529 Front of the Neck: Depressors of the Larynx: Thyroid Gland—III

On the left side of the specimen, the two superficial Depressors (Sterno-hyoid and Omo-hyoid) are reflected and the two deep Depressors (Sterno-thyroid and Thyro-hyoid) are thereby uncovered. On the right side, Sterno-thyroid is largely excised.

Observe:

1. The two lobes of the thyroid gland, united across the median plane by an isthmus.

2. The surface network of veins on the gland, drained by the superior, middle, and inferior thyroid veins.

3. The right lobe of the gland, overlying the common carotid artery.

4. The upper pole of the right lobe, pushing the superior thyroid artery into the angle between the attachments of Sterno-thyroid and Inferior Constrictor to the thyroid cartilage, and, therefore, against the external laryngeal nerve (see also figs. 530 & 534).

5. An accessory thyroid gland, or detached lobule, occasionally present and situated in front of Thyro-hyoid.

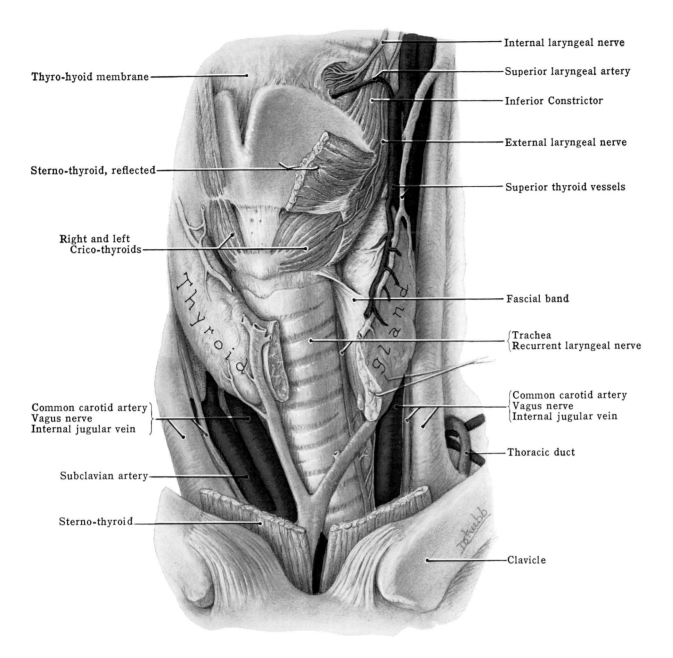

Thyro-hyoid membrane

Sterno-thyroid, reflected

Right and left
Crico-thyroids

Thyroid gland

Common carotid artery
Vagus nerve
Internal jugular vein

Subclavian artery

Sterno-thyroid

Internal laryngeal nerve

Superior laryngeal artery

Inferior Constrictor

External laryngeal nerve

Superior thyroid vessels

Fascial band

Trachea
Recurrent laryngeal nerve

Common carotid artery
Vagus nerve
Internal jugular vein

Thoracic duct

Clavicle

530   Front of the Neck: Thyroid Gland—IV

The left Sterno-thyroid is reflected; the isthmus of the thyroid gland is divided; and
the left lobe is retracted.

Observe:

1. The retaining fascial band, attaching the capsule of the thyroid gland to the crico-tracheal
   ligament and cricoid cartilage.
2. The left recurrent laryngeal nerve, on the side of the trachea, just in front of the angle between the trachea and esophagus, and behind the retaining band.
3. The internal laryngeal nerve, running along the upper border of Inferior Constrictor, and
   piercing the thyro-hyoid membrane as several branches.
4. The external laryngeal nerve, applied to Inferior Constrictor, running along the anterior
   border of the superior thyroid artery, passing deep to the insertion of Sterno-thyroid, and
   giving twigs to Inferior Constrictor and piercing it before ending in Crico-thyroid.
5. The fibrous arch, bridging Crico-thyroid and giving origin to Inferior Constrictor.

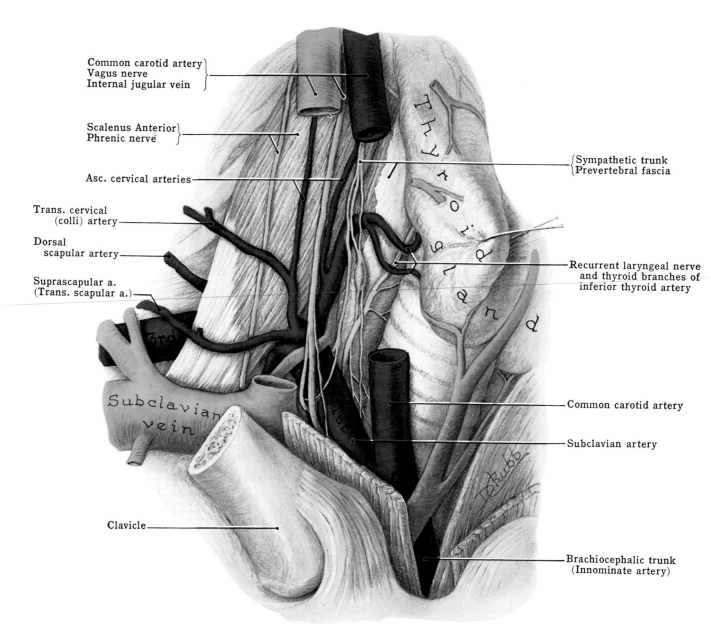

Common carotid artery
Vagus nerve
Internal jugular vein

Scalenus Anterior
Phrenic nerve

Asc. cervical arteries

Trans. cervical
(colli) artery

Dorsal
scapular artery

Suprascapular a.
(Trans. scapular a.)

Subclavian vein

Clavicle

Thyroid gland

Sympathetic trunk
Prevertebral fascia

Recurrent laryngeal nerve
and thyroid branches of
inferior thyroid artery

Common carotid artery

Subclavian artery

Brachiocephalic trunk
(Innominate artery)

531 Root of the Neck, right side

The clavicle is partly removed; sections are taken from the common cartoid art. and int. jugular vein; the right lobe of the thyroid gland and the trachea are retracted.

Observe:

1. The brachiocephalic trunk dividing behind the sterno-clavicular joint into the right common carotid and right subclavian arteries.

2. Scalenus Anterior, dividing the subclavian artery into three parts—1st, 2nd, and 3rd—and separating the 2nd part from the subclavian vein. This vein, lying antero-inferior to the artery, and joining the internal jugular vein at the medial border of Scalenus Anterior to form the brachiocephalic vein.

3. Running vertically on the obliquely placed Scalenus Anterior: (a) the common carotid artery, internal jugular vein, and vagus nerve (inside the carotid sheath); (b) the sympathetic trunk behind the common carotid artery (outside the sheath); (c) the ascending cervical artery (here represented by two vessels); and (d) most lateral of all, the phrenic nerve which is clamped down by two arteries and, therefore cannot be mistaken for the vagus nerve.

4. The vagus, crossing the 1st part of the subclavian artery, and giving off an (inferior) cardiac branch and the recurrent laryngeal nerve. The latter (a) recurring below the artery, (b) crossing behind the common carotid artery on its way to the side of the trachea, and (c) giving twigs to the trachea and esophagus, and receiving twigs from the sympathetic.

5. The sympathetic trunk, throwing a fine loop, the ansa subclavia, around the 1st part of the artery. The middle cervical ganglion is not labelled.

6. The thyro-cervical trunk (not labelled), dividing into the inferior thyroid artery which takes an S-shaped course, and the transverse cervical and suprascapular arteries which cross Scalenus Anterior.

7. The deep or dorsal scapular branch of the trans. cervical artery, here and commonly, springing from the 2nd or 3rd part of the subclavian artery. The vertebral vein (not labelled) crossing the 1st part of the artery.

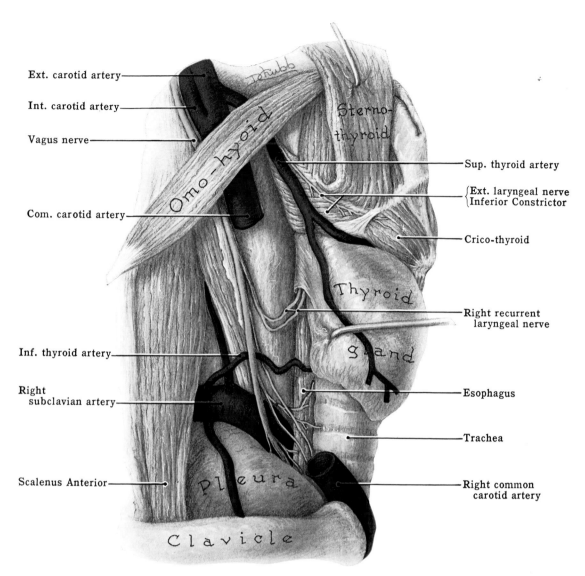

Ext. carotid artery

Int. carotid artery

Vagus nerve

Com. carotid artery

Inf. thyroid artery

Right subclavian artery

Scalenus Anterior

Sup. thyroid artery

Ext. laryngeal nerve
Inferior Constrictor

Crico-thyroid

Right recurrent laryngeal nerve

Esophagus

Trachea

Right common carotid artery

532 Anomalous Right Recurrent Laryngeal Nerve

From the same subject as figure 447.2

Occasionally the right subclavian artery springs directly from the aortic arch, as its fourth branch, and passes behind the trachea and esophagus. For embryological reasons, shown in figure 447, the right recurrent nerve, having then no artery around which to recur, takes an almost direct course to the larynx. As would be expected, many of its esophageal and tracheal branches then spring directly from the parent vagus nerve.

Note: The inferior thyroid artery here springs directly from the subclavian artery. The vertebral and internal thoracic arteries are not labelled.

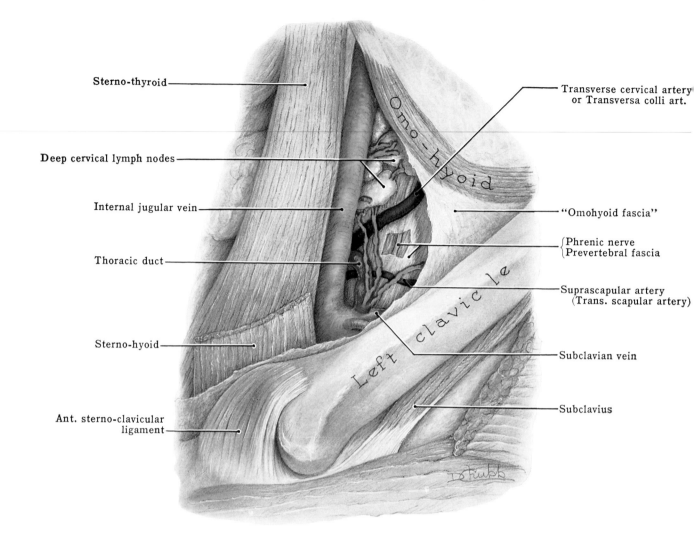

Sterno-thyroid

Deep cervical lymph nodes

Internal jugular vein

Thoracic duct

Sterno-hyoid

Ant. sterno-clavicular ligament

Omo-hyoid

Transverse cervical artery or Transversa colli art.

"Omohyoid fascia"

{ Phrenic nerve
Prevertebral fascia }

Suprascapular artery (Trans. scapular artery)

Left clavicle

Subclavian vein

Subclavius

533 Termination of the Thoracic Duct

Sternomastoid and the enveloping fascia of the neck are removed. The deeper layer of fascia, "the Omohyoid fascia", that binds Omohyoid to the fascia enclosing Subclavius, is partly snipped away.

Observe:

1. "The Omohyoid fascia", continuous in front of Sternohyoid and across the suprasternal space with the fascia of the opposite side.

2. The thoracic duct, receiving a tributary from the nodes of the neck (jugular trunk), another from the nodes of upper limb (subclavian trunk), and ending in the angle between the internal jugular and subclavian veins.

3. The phrenic nerve, descending in naked contact with Scalenus Anterior, i.e., deep to Scalenus Anterior fascia, which is a lateral prolongation of the prevertebral fascia, and clamped down by the 2 arteries labelled.

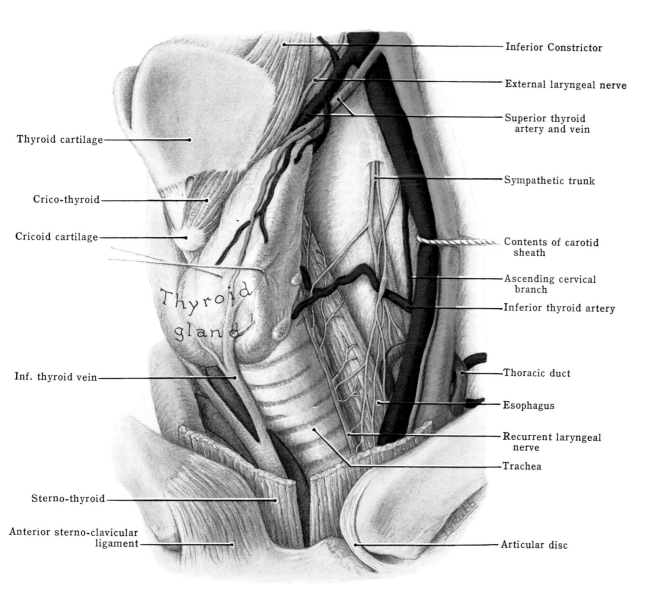

Thyroid cartilage

Crico-thyroid

Cricoid cartilage

Thyroid gland

Inf. thyroid vein

Sterno-thyroid

Anterior sterno-clavicular ligament

Inferior Constrictor

External laryngeal nerve

Superior thyroid artery and vein

Sympathetic trunk

Contents of carotid sheath

Ascending cervical branch

Inferior thyroid artery

Thoracic duct

Esophagus

Recurrent laryngeal nerve

Trachea

Articular disc

534   Root of the Neck, left side

(Esophagus, Trachea, Left Recurrent Laryngeal Nerve, Thoracic Duct.)

Observe:

1. The three structures contained in the carotid sheath (internal jugular vein, common carotid artery, and vagus nerve), retracted.

2. The esophagus, bulging to the left of the trachea. It does not bulge to the right.

3. The left recurrent nerve, ascending on the side of the trachea just in front of the angle between the trachea and esophagus, giving twigs to the esophagus and trachea (not in view), and receiving twigs from the sympathetic.

4. The thoracic duct, passing from the side of the esophagus to its termination (figs. 533 & 453) and, in so doing, arching immediately behind the 3 structures contained in the carotid sheath.

5. The middle cervical (sympathetic) ganglion, here in 2 parts: one in front of the inferior thyroid artery; the other, just above the thoracic duct, is called the vertebral ganglion.

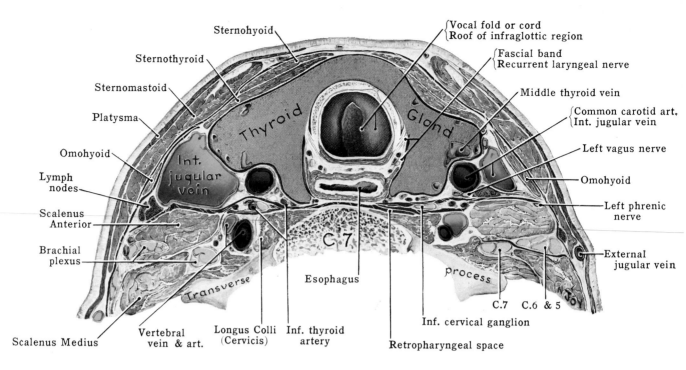

Sternohyoid

Sternothyroid

Sternomastoid

Platysma

Omohyoid

Lymph nodes

Scalenus Anterior

Brachial plexus

Scalenus Medius

Vertebral vein & art.

Longus Colli (Cervicis)

Inf. thyroid artery

Esophagus

Retropharyngeal space

Inf. cervical ganglion

Vocal fold or cord
Roof of infraglottic region

Fascial band
Recurrent laryngeal nerve

Middle thyroid vein

Common carotid art.
Int. jugular vein

Left vagus nerve

Omohyoid

Left phrenic nerve

External jugular vein

C.7 C.6 & 5

Int. jugular vein

Thyroid Gland

Transverse

C.7

Process

535 Neck on cross section at the level of the Thyroid Gland, seen from below

Observe:

1. The thyroid gland, within its sheath, asymmetrically enlarged and overflowing the carotid sheath and its contents (common carotid artery, internal jugular vein and vagus nerve) on one side and thrusting it laterally on the other.

2. The internal jugular veins, of unequal size, as sometimes happens; and also the vertebral arteries.

3. The retropharyngeal space of loose areolar tissue, extending far laterally behind the carotid sheath. The approach to the space is from the posterior border of Sternomastoid.

4. Scalenus Anterior deep to the posterior border of Sternomastoid.

5. The vertebral artery and vein near the apex of the "Triangle of the Vertebral Artery" (fig. 536A) between Longus Colli and Scalenus Anterior.

6. The brachial plexus passing infero-laterally between Scalenus Anterior and Scalenus Medius (see fig. 475).

7. The inferior thyroid artery (divided twice) and the middle cervical ganglion on a plane between the carotid sheath and the vertebral artery.

8. The fascial band that retains the thyroid gland and behind it the recurrent laryngeal nerve and the inferior laryngeal artery (see fig. 530).

9. The vocal folds and the conus elasticus (crico-vocal membranes), covered with mucous membrane and having the same shape as the tentorium cerebelli (fig. 572), hence, air expelled forcibly from the lungs would blow the vocal folds apart.

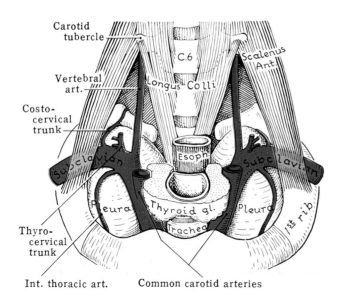

Carotid tubercle

Vertebral art.

Costo-cervical trunk

Thyro-cervical trunk

Int. thoracic art.

Common carotid arteries

C.6

Longus Colli

Scalenus Ant.

Subclavian

Subclavian

Pleura

Esoph.

Thyroid gl.

Trachea

Pleura

1st rib

536A Triangle of the Vertebral Artery

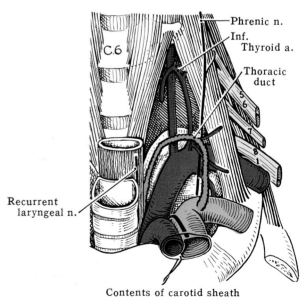

C.6

Recurrent laryngeal n.

Contents of carotid sheath

Phrenic n.

Inf. Thyroid a.

Thoracic duct

536B Course of the Thoracic Duct

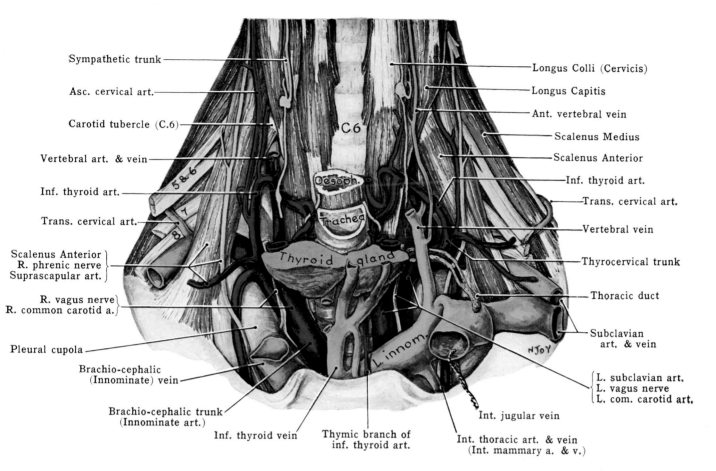

Sympathetic trunk

Asc. cervical art.

Carotid tubercle (C.6)

Vertebral art. & vein

Inf. thyroid art.

Trans. cervical art.

Scalenus Anterior
R. phrenic nerve
Suprascapular art.

R. vagus nerve
R. common carotid a.

Pleural cupola

Brachio-cephalic
(Innominate) vein

Brachio-cephalic trunk
(Innominate art.)

Inf. thyroid vein

Thymic branch of
inf. thyroid art.

Int. thoracic art. & vein
(Int. mammary a. & v.)

Int. jugular vein

L. subclavian art.
L. vagus nerve
L. com. carotid art.

Subclavian
art. & vein

Thoracic duct

Thyrocervical trunk

Vertebral vein

Trans. cervical art.

Inf. thyroid art.

Scalenus Anterior

Scalenus Medius

Ant. vertebral vein

Longus Capitis

Longus Colli (Cervicis)

C.6

Oesoph.

Trachea

Thyroid gland

L. innom.

5 & 6

7

8

NJoY

536 Root of the Neck, viewed obliquely from above

Observe:

1. *Laterally:* The pleural cupola, rising $1\frac{1}{2}$ inches above the sternal end of the 1st rib. The subclavian artery, which arches over the pleura, divided into 3 unequal parts by Scalenus Anterior. The 3rd part of the artery and the brachial plexus appearing between Scalenus Anterior and Scalenus Medius, the lowest trunk of the plexus (C.8 & T.1) being behind the artery.

2. The phrenic nerve, descending almost vertically and crossing the obliquely running Scalenus Anterior to which it is clamped by the suprascapular artery and, on leaving Scalenus Anterior, lying on the pleura and crossing the internal thoracic artery before meeting the right brachio-cephalic vein.

3. *In the Median Plane:* The esophagus applied to the vertebral column, the trachea applied to the esophagus, the thyroid gland applied to the trachea and overlapping the common carotid arteries. The inferior thyroid veins descending to the left brachio-cephalic (innominate) vein, and an occasional branch of the inferior thyroid artery descending to the thymus).

4. *Lateral to these Median Structures:* "The Triangle of the Vertebral Artery" (see above, A & B) bounded laterally by Scalenus Anterior, and medially by Longus Colli. The apex where these 2 muscles meet at the carotid tubercle (ant. tubercle of trans. process of C.6); the base being the 1st part

of the subclavian artery. The vertebral artery, which ascends from base to apex, dividing the triangle into 2 nearly equal parts.

Anterior to the triangle, the carotid sheath and its 3 contents (artery, vein and nerve). On the left side, between sheath and vertebral artery, and therefore below the level of the carotid tubercle, 2 vessels arching in opposite directions—the inferior thyroid artery and the thoracic duct. The artery of both sides arching medially, and on the left side the duct arching laterally. The artery reaching the thyroid gland as 2 branches, an upper and a lower. The recurrent laryngeal nerve bears a varying relationship to these 2 terminal arteries (being either anterior to, or posterior to, or between, them), here, between them.

The duct pulled down by the reflected internal jugular vein in which it ends. The arching duct lying immediately behind the carotid sheath and its 3 contents and sometimes, as here, a 4th structure, namely, the vertebral vein.

5. The right and left vagus nerves descending on the lateral side of the corresponding common carotid artery; the right vagus being conducted to the subclavian artery which it crosses, giving off its recurrent nerve (not labelled) as it does so; the left vagus being conducted to the aortic arch (not in view) where it behaves similarly. The vagus nerves, free, and not clamped down as are the phrenic nerves.

Scalenus Anterior intervening between the subclavian artery and vein.

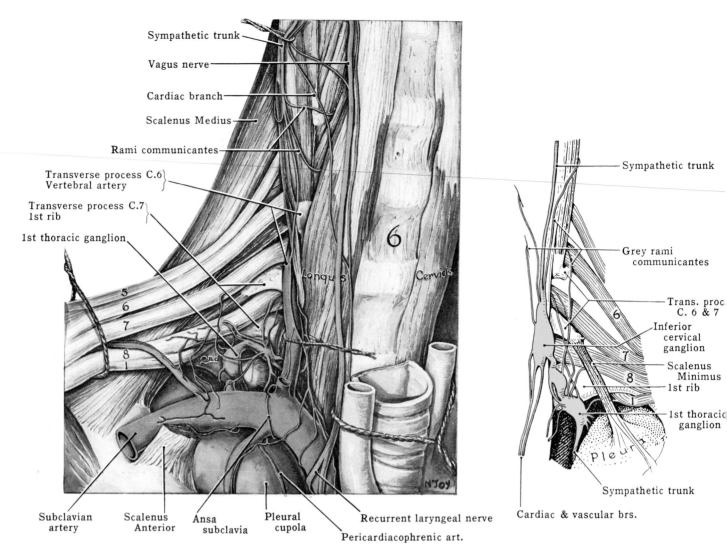

Sympathetic trunk

Vagus nerve

Cardiac branch

Scalenus Medius

Rami communicantes

Transverse process C.6
Vertebral artery

Transverse process C.7
1st rib

1st thoracic ganglion

Sympathetic trunk

Grey rami
communicantes

Trans. proc
C. 6 & 7

Inferior
cervical
ganglion

Scalenus
Minimus
1st rib

1st thoracic
ganglion

Sympathetic trunk

Subclavian
artery

Scalenus
Anterior

Ansa
subclavia

Pleural
cupola

Recurrent laryngeal nerve

Pericardiacophrenic art.

Cardiac & vascular brs.

537   Stellate Ganglion [Cervico-thoracic Ganglion]

The pleura has been depressed and the vertebral artery retracted. (Dissection by G. F. Lewis.)

Observe:

1. The lowest trunk of the brachial plexus (C. 8 & T. 1) raised from the groove it occupies on the 1st rib behind the sub-clavian artery; the transverse cervical artery (not labelled) here arising from the 3rd part of the artery and passing through the plexus (fig. 471.4).

2. The sympathetic trunk (retracted laterally) sending a communicating branch to the vagus, and gray rami communicantes (postganglionic fibres) to the roots of the cervical nerves, and cardiac branches.

3. The vertebral artery, retracted medially in order to uncover the stellate ganglion (i.e., the combined inferior cervical and 1st thoracic ganglia) which rests behind it on the 1st and 2nd ribs.

4. Fine branches passing from the ganglion to nerves C. 7, 8,

and T. 1, and to adjacent arteries.

5. The vertebral ganglion, quite small, just below the thread that retracts the vertebral artery. From this ganglion the sympathetic trunk passing behind the vertebral artery to join the stellate ganglion, but before so doing sending a slender branch around the subclavian artery as the ansa subclavia.

6. On the left side a pen and ink tracing of a photograph of a dissection of the left side of the same specimen, revealing a very different pattern. Thus, the inferior cervical ganglion occupies its more usual position between the transverse process of C. 7 and the 1st rib, ganglion T. 1 being on and below the 1st rib. Scalenus Minimus (Scalenus Pleuralis) here present (fig. 567).

Superior articular process

Capsular lig.

Transverse process

Anterior & Posterior Intertransversarii

Dorsal ramus

Ventral rami

Trans. process C. 5.

Dorsal ramus

Spinal nerve

Ventral ramus

Trans. process C. 6.

Vertebral artery

Dorsal nerve root

Ventral nerve root

Spinous process

Lamina

Right & Left Interspinales

Spinous process

Lig. flava

Dura mater

Arachnoid mater

rior articular process C. 6.

ynovial fold

Spinal ganglion

Dorsal ramus

Ventral ramus

Ventral root

Spinal nerve

Spinal cord

C 6

N JOY

C 3

C 4

538 A Cervical Nerve, in situ

Observe:

1. Two paired Interspinales uniting the bifid ends of 3 spinous processes.

2. Capsular ligaments uniting articular processes.

3. Anterior and Posterior Intertransversarii uniting anterior and posterior tubercles of transverse processes.

4. The ligamentum flavum attached to the upper border of one lamina and to the ventral surface of the lamina next above, and extending transversely from one articular capsule to the other.

5. Dura mater applied to ligamentum flavum; arachnoid mater applied to dura and separated from pia mater, which clothes the medulla or cord, by cerebrospinal fluid, which has escaped.

6. The fila of the dorsal nerve roots (7th & 8th) leaving the spinal medulla in single file. One filum of C. 8 joining C. 7.

7. Dura (and arachnoid) carried distally as a covering for the roots, nerve, and rami and gradually fading away.

8. A dorsal nerve root (here 6th and 7th) larger than a ventral

root; its swelling, the spinal ganglion. The 2 roots, each in a separate dural sheath, uniting beyond the ganglion to form a spinal nerve. The nerve, about 1 cm. long, dividing into a small dorsal and a large ventral ramus.

9. The roots and the nerve crossing behind the vertebral artery. The dorsal ramus of the spinal nerve curving dorsally, applied to the root of a superior articular process, and passing medial to a Posterior Intertransverse muscle. The ventral ramus resting on the transverse process, which is grooved to support it, and emerging between an anterior and a posterior intertransverse muscle. C. 5 raised from its grooved bed.

10. Inset: On vertebra C. 3, in contrast with C. 4, bony overgrowths at the intervertebral foramen (on sup. articular process and body) may constrict the roots of the nerve. This condition is not uncommon in the cervical vertebrae of dissecting-room subjects.

11. Synovial folds projecting between articular surfaces, as they do elsewhere.

A **A Normal Thyroid Gland** has a right and a left lobe and a connecting isthmus.

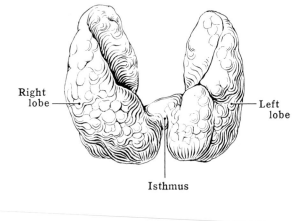

Right lobe — — Left lobe

Isthmus

B **An Accessory Thyroid Gland** may occur between the levels of the suprahyoid region and the aortic arch. (See fig. 529.)

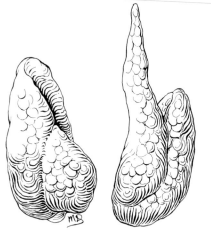

C **Pyramidal Lobe. Absence of Isthmus.** About 50% of glands have a pyramidal lobe which extends from near the isthmus to, or towards, the hyoid bone. The isthmus is occasionally absent, the gland being then in two parts.

D **Accessory Thyroid Tissue** may occur along the course of the thyroglossal duct.

E **Levator Glandulae Thyroideae** is a detached slip of a depressor muscle of the larynx which becomes attached to the thyroid gland.

539 Thyroid Gland

VARIATIONS AND ANOMALIES

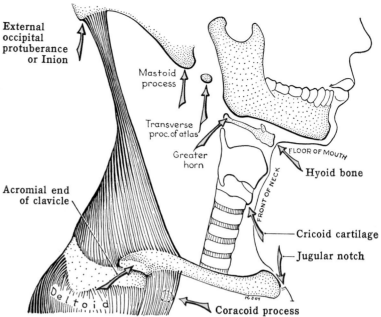

540 Triangles of the Neck

Note:

The obliquely set Sternomastoid divides the side of the neck into an anterior and a posterior triangle.

The anterior triangle is bounded by Sternomastoid, the median line of the neck, and the lower border of the mandible. It is subdivided into 3 smaller triangles—submandibular, carotid, and muscular. The posterior belly of Digastric (and Stylohyoid) separates the carotid triangle from the submandibular triangle; the superior belly of Omohyoid separates the carotid triangle from the muscular triangle. The region between the anterior bellies of the Digastrics and the body of the hyoid bone is the (unpaired) submental triangle.

The posterior triangle is bounded by Trapezius, Sternomastoid, and the middle third of the clavicle (figs. 472–475). It is divisible into a subclavian (supraclavicular) and an occipital triangle by the inferior belly of Omohyoid, but of much greater significance is the fact that it is divided by the accessory nerve (nerve XI) into nearly equal upper and lower parts. Of these, the upper contains little of importance, but the lower contains numerous structures of great importance. Hence, above the nerve your dissection may be carefree, whereas below it you must proceed very carefully.

540.1 Bony Landmarks of the Neck

Note:

The inion and the mastoid process (and the superior nuchal line uniting them) are created by the downward pull of Trapezius and Sternomastoid.

The transverse process of the atlas, being the most prominent of the cervical transverse processes, is felt with the finger-tip on pressing upwards between the angle of the jaw and the mastoid process.

The body of the hyoid bone lies at the angle between the floor of the mouth and the front of the neck.

The greater horn of one side of the hyoid bone is palpable only when the greater horn of the opposite side is steadied.

The arch of the cricoid cartilage projects beyond the rings of the trachea (figs. 458, 623), and is thereby readily identified in life, on running the finger-tip upwards. It is the guide to the level of C.6, where so many things happen.

The jugular (suprasternal) notch is visible and palpable between the medial ends of the clavicles.

The lateral end of the clavicle, being thicker than the acromion, is palpable on pressing medially, above the acromion.

The coracoid process, located 1″ below the clavicle under the edge of the Deltoid, is palpable on pressing laterally with the finger in the deltopectoral triangle.

540.2

Diagram of the posterior belly of the digastric muscle to demonstrate its superficial and key position.

Note:

1. Except for (a) cervical brs. of the facial nerve, (b) facial brs. of the great auricular nerve, and (c) the ext. jugular vein and its connections (figs. 467 & 471.3), all vessels and nerves crossing this belly cross deep to it—the great vein, all arteries great and small, the last three cranial nerves, and the sympathetic trunk (fig. 551).

2. This belly runs from mastoid process to hyoid bone, and crosses deep to the angle of the jaw.

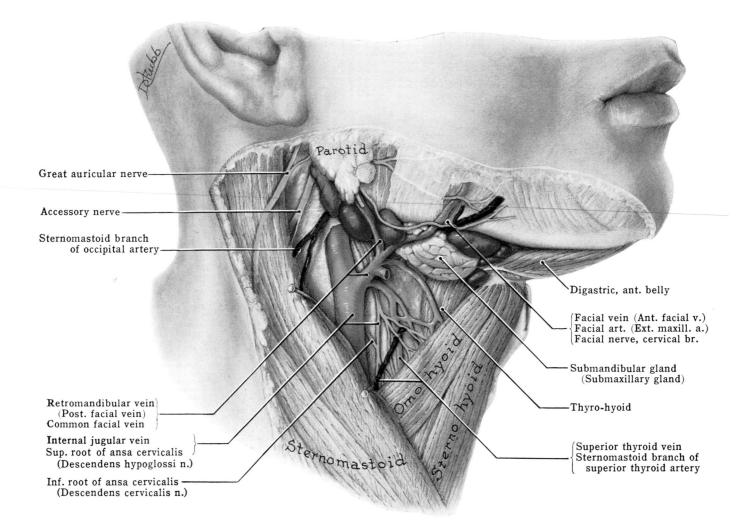

Great auricular nerve

Accessory nerve

Sternomastoid branch
of occipital artery

Parotid

Digastric, ant. belly

Facial vein (Ant. facial v.)
Facial art. (Ext. maxill. a.)
Facial nerve, cervical br.

Submandibular gland
(Submaxillary gland)

Thyro-hyoid

Retromandibular vein
(Post. facial vein)
Common facial vein

Internal jugular vein
Sup. root of ansa cervicalis
(Descendens hypoglossi n.)

Inf. root of ansa cervicalis
(Descendens cervicalis n.)

Omo-hyoid

Sterno-hyoid

Sternomastoid

Superior thyroid vein
Sternomastoid branch of
superior thyroid artery

541   Anterior Triangle of the Neck, superficial dissection—I

Observe:

1. The accessory nerve entering the deep surface of Sternomastoid between $1\frac{1}{2}$ and $2\frac{1}{2}$ inches below the tip of the mastoid process, and joined along its lower border by the sternomastoid branch of the occipital artery.

2. The internal jugular vein joined in front by several veins, notably, the common facial vein, about the level of the hyoid bone.

3. Branches of the ansa cervicalis (ansa hypoglossi) passing deep to Omohyoid.

4. The sternomastoid branch of the superior thyroid artery descending near the upper border of Omohyoid.

5. The submandibular gland and lymph nodes filling—and indeed overflowing—the submandibular triangle (digastric triangle). The retromandibular and facial veins running superficial to the gland.

Continued from page facing

6. Of these branches, note (a) the superior root of the ansa cervicalis arising from the hypoglossal nerve where the sternomastoid artery arises from the occipital artery, descending superficial to the internal and common carotid arteries outside their fascial sheath, and joining the inferior root (C.2 and 3) which appears on the medial side of the internal jugular vein (commonly on the lateral side) to form the ansa cervicalis near the upper border of Omohyoid; (b) the nerve to Thyrohyoid crossing the greater horn of the hyoid bone to enter the superficial surface of this muscle.

7. The internal and external laryngeal nerves appearing deep to the external carotid artery; the former following the upper border of Inferior Constrictor and piercing the thyrohyoid membrane; the latter applied to Inferior Constrictor and lying close to the superior thyroid artery and giving it twigs.

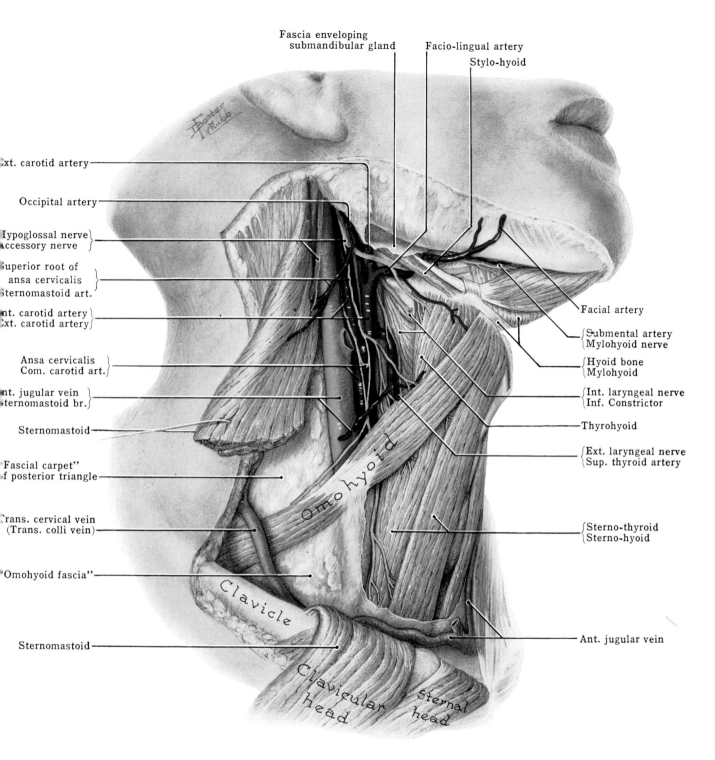

Fascia enveloping
submandibular gland

Facio-lingual artery

Stylo-hyoid

Ext. carotid artery

Occipital artery

Hypoglossal nerve
Accessory nerve

Superior root of
ansa cervicalis
Sternomastoid art.

Int. carotid artery
Ext. carotid artery

Ansa cervicalis
Com. carotid art.

Int. jugular vein
Sternomastoid br.

Sternomastoid

"Fascial carpet"
of posterior triangle

Trans. cervical vein
(Trans. colli vein)

"Omohyoid fascia"

Sternomastoid

Facial artery

Submental artery
Mylohyoid nerve

Hyoid bone
Mylohyoid

Int. laryngeal nerve
Inf. Constrictor

Thyrohyoid

Ext. laryngeal nerve
Sup. thyroid artery

Sterno-thyroid
Sterno-hyoid

Ant. jugular vein

Omohyoid

Clavicle

Clavicular head

Sternal head

542   Anterior Triangle of the Neck, deeper dissection—II

Sternomastoid is divided and reflected; the more superficial veins are removed, so
are the submandibular gland and lymph nodes.

Observe:

1. The intermediate tendon of Digastric held down to the
hyoid bone by a fascial sling; the intermediate tendon of
Omohyoid similarly held down to the clavicle.

2. The remains of the fascial sheath of the submandibular
gland which posteriorly, as the stylo-mandibular ligament,
separates this gland from the parotid gland.

3. The facial and lingual arteries, here arising by a common
stem, passing deep to Stylohyoid and Digastric to enter the

submandibular triangle The facial artery here giving off its
submental branch, which accompanies the mylohyoid nerve.

4. Thyrohyoid and Inferior Constrictor forming the floor (more
literally, the medial wall) of the carotid triangle.

5. The hypoglossal nerve curving into the carotid triangle and
curving out again; passing deep to Digastric twice; crossing
the internal and external carotid arteries and giving off two
branches from its convex side.

Continued on page opposite

543   Diagram of the Superficial Veins of the Neck

Occipital

Supra-orbital

Supra trochlear

Superf. temp.

Maxillary

Post. auricular

(Post. facial) Retro-mandibular

(Ant.) Facial

C. facial

SPLENIUS

LEV. SCAP.

SC. MED. & POST.

Accessory n.

Trans-cervical

Ext. jugular

Communicating branch

Ant. jugular

Suprascapular

Omo-hyoid

543.1   Diagram of the Laryngea Branches of Right Vagus Nerve

Lower ganglion

Pharyngeal br.

Sup. laryngeal nerve

Int. laryngeal nerve

Thyro-hyoid

Ext. laryngeal n.

Vagus nerve

Crico-thyroid

Recurrent laryngeal n.

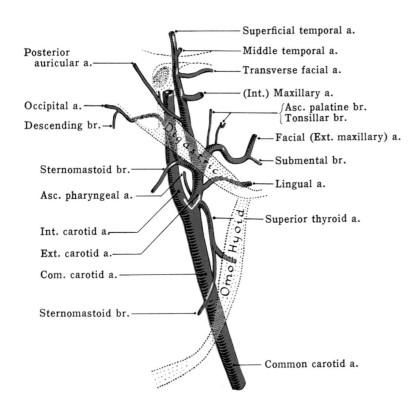

543.2   Diagram of the Carotid Arteries and their Branches in the Neck

Superficial temporal a.

Middle temporal a.

Transverse facial a.

Posterior auricular a.

(Int.) Maxillary a.

Asc. palatine br.
Tonsillar br.

Occipital a.

Descending br.

Facial (Ext. maxillary) a.

Submental br.

Sternomastoid br.

Lingual a.

Asc. pharyngeal a.

Omo-Hyoid

Superior thyroid a.

Int. carotid a.

Ext. carotid a.

Com. carotid a.

Sternomastoid br.

Common carotid a.

Note: The common carotid divides into 2 terminal branches, the internal and the external, and neither the common carotid nor the internal carotid gives off collateral branches in the neck.

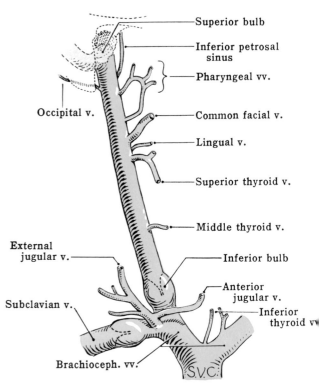

543.3   Diagram of the Internal Jugular Vein and its Tributaries

Superior bulb

Inferior petrosal sinus

Pharyngeal vv.

Occipital v.

Common facial v.

Lingual v.

Superior thyroid v.

Middle thyroid v.

External jugular v.

Inferior bulb

Anterior jugular v.

Subclavian v.

Inferior thyroid v

Brachioceph. vv.

S.V.C.

Note: The dilatation or bulb at each end of the internal jug lar vein. The superior jugular bulb is separated from the flo of the middle ear by a delicate bony plate. The inferior jugul bulb, like the corresponding bulb at the end of the subclavi vein, contains a bicuspid valve which permits the flow of blo towards the heart. There are no valves in the brachio-cephal veins or in the superior vena cava.

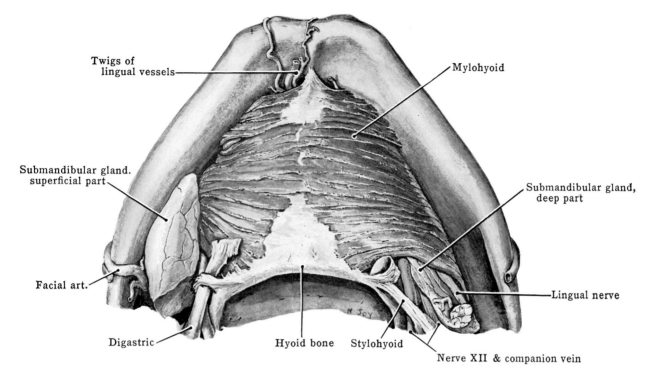

Twigs of
lingual vessels

Mylohyoid

Submandibular gland.
superficial part

Submandibular gland,
deep part

Facial art.

Lingual nerve

Digastric

Hyoid bone   Stylohyoid

Nerve XII & companion vein

544   Floor of the Mouth, from below—Mylohyoids 1

(The anterior bellies of the Digastrics are removed, fig. 527.)

Observe:

1. The right and left Mylohyoids, which together form the "oral diaphragm", arising from the mylohyoid line of the jaw (fig. 553.1), and inserted into an indefinite median raphe and into the hyoid bone (fig. 596).

2. The submandibular gland turning round the posterior border of the Mylohyoid.

3. The hypoglossal nerve and its companion vein passing deep to the same posterior border; and high up the lingual nerve applied to the jaw.

545   Floor of the Mouth, from below—Geniohyoids II

(The left Mylohyoid and part of the right are reflected.)

Observe:

1. The Geniohyoid, triangular, in contact with its fellow, and extending from the mental spine of the jaw to the front of the body of the hyoid bone.

2. The structures seen in figure 544 followed forwards: companion vein (distended), hypoglossal nerve, deep part of gland, and lingual nerve (appearing at anterior border of Medial Pterygoid).

3. The areolar covered sublingual gland, and lateral to it the mucous membrane of the mouth with twigs of the sublingual artery.
(For mouth from medial side and from above, see figs. 597, 598, & 599.)

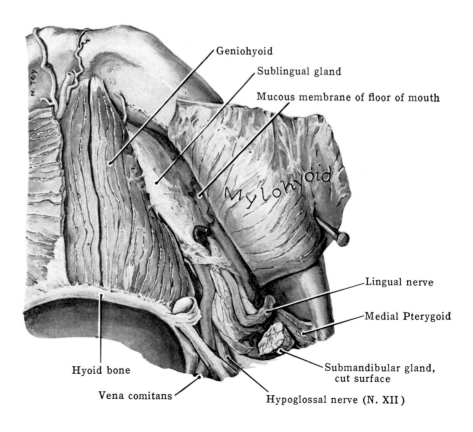

Geniohyoid

Sublingual gland

Mucous membrane of floor of mouth

Lingual nerve

Medial Pterygoid

Hyoid bone

Submandibular gland,
cut surface

Vena comitans

Hypoglossal nerve (N. XII)

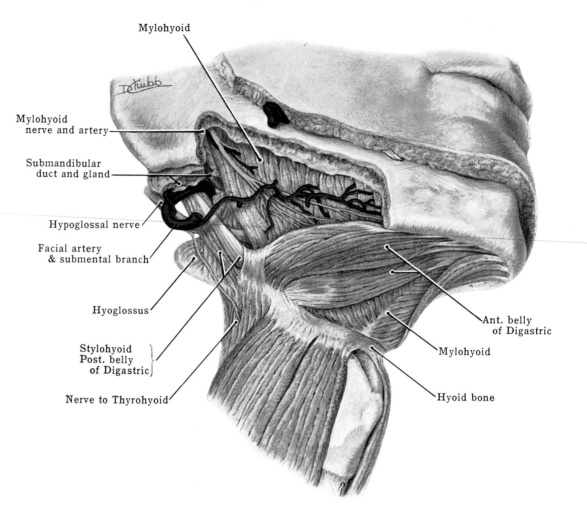

Mylohyoid

Mylohyoid
nerve and artery

Submandibular
duct and gland

Hypoglossal nerve

Facial artery
& submental branch

Hyoglossus

Stylohyoid
Post. belly
of Digastric

Nerve to Thyrohyoid

Ant. belly
of Digastric

Mylohyoid

Hyoid bone

546 Suprahyoid Region—I

The medial wall of the submandibular (digastric) triangle

Observe:

1. Stylohyoid and the posterior belly of Digastric forming the posterior side of the triangle; the facial artery arching over these. The anterior belly of the Digastric forming the anterior side. Here this belly has an extra origin from the hyoid bone.

2. Mylohyoid forming the medial wall of the triangle and having a free posterior border.

3. The mylohyoid nerve, which supplies Mylohyoid and anterior belly of Digastric, accompanied by the mylohyoid branch of the inferior alveolar artery (inf. dental art.) posteriorly and by the submental branch of the facial artery anteriorly.

4. The hypoglossal nerve, the submandibular gland, and the submandibular duct passing forwards deep to the posterior border of Mylohyoid.

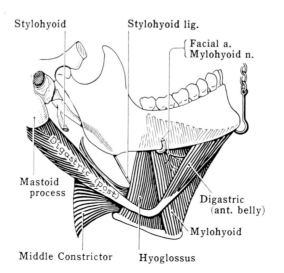

Stylohyoid

Stylohyoid lig.

{ Facial a.
  Mylohyoid n.

Mastoid
process

Digastric (post.)

Middle Constrictor

Digastric
(ant. belly)

Mylohyoid

Hyoglossus

546.1

Diagram of 4 layers of suprahyoid muscles:—Digastric, Mylohyoid, Hyoglossus, and Middle Constrictor.

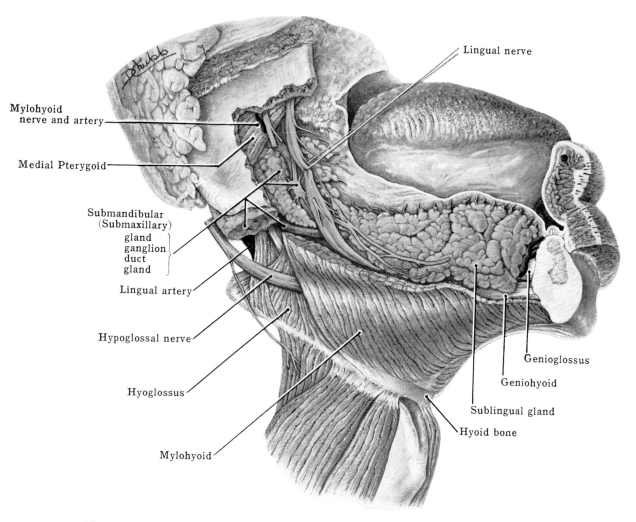

Mylohyoid nerve and artery

Medial Pterygoid

Submandibular (Submaxillary)
gland
ganglion
duct
gland

Lingual artery

Hypoglossal nerve

Hyoglossus

Mylohyoid

Lingual nerve

Genioglossus

Geniohyoid

Sublingual gland

Hyoid bone

547 Suprahyoid Region–II

The salivary glands, on lateral view.

Observe:

1. The sublingual salivary gland, almond-shaped, almost touching its fellow of the opposite side behind the symphysis menti and almost touching the deep part of the submandibular gland posteriorly.

2. The dozen or more fine ducts passing from the upper border of the sublingual gland to open on the plica sublingualis.

3. Several individual or detached lobules of the sublingual gland, each having a fine duct, behind the main mass of the gland, and labial glands in the lip (unlabelled).

4. The mylohyoid nerve and artery (cut short) and the lingual nerve clamped between Medial Pterygoid and the ramus of the jaw. The lingual nerve lying between the sublingual gland and the deep or oral part of the submandibular gland; the submandibular ganglion suspended from this nerve, and various sensory and secretory fibres leaving it.

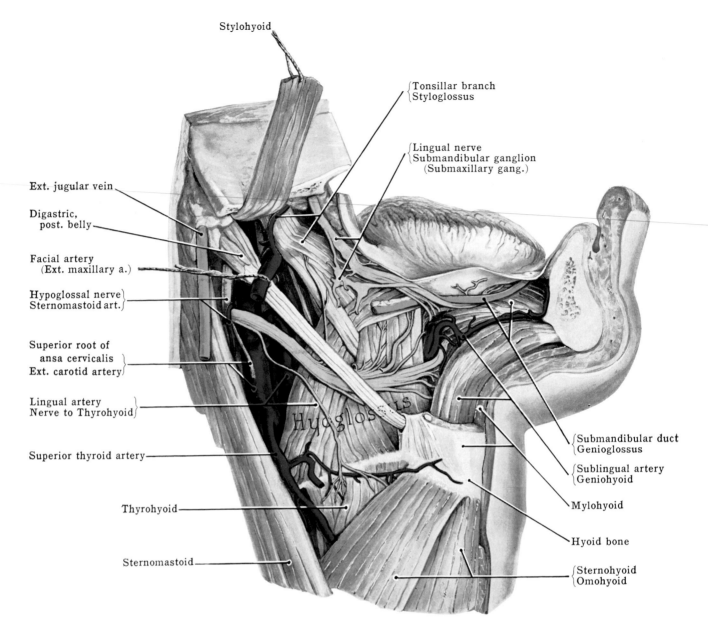

Stylohyoid

Tonsillar branch
Styloglossus

Lingual nerve
Submandibular ganglion
(Submaxillary gang.)

Ext. jugular vein

Digastric,
post. belly

Facial artery
(Ext. maxillary a.)

Hypoglossal nerve
Sternomastoid art.

Superior root of
ansa cervicalis
Ext. carotid artery

Lingual artery
Nerve to Thyrohyoid

Superior thyroid artery

Thyrohyoid

Sternomastoid

Hyoglossus

Submandibular duct
Genioglossus

Sublingual artery
Geniohyoid

Mylohyoid

Hyoid bone

Sternohyoid
Omohyoid

548 Suprahyoid Region—III

The relationships of Hyoglossus and of the side of the tongue.

Observe:

1. Stylohyoid, thrown up. Posterior belly of Digastric left in situ as a landmark.

2. Hyoglossus ascending from the greater horn and body of the hyoid bone to the side of the tongue; Styloglossus, postero-superiorly, crossed by the tonsillar branch of the facial artery and interdigitating with bundles of Hyoglossus; and Genioglossus, anteriorly, fanning out into the tongue.

3. The hypoglossal nerve, crossed twice by Digastric, crossing twice the lingual artery, and supplying all the muscles of the tongue, both extrinsic and intrinsic, Palatoglossus excepted. The branches of the hypoglossal nerve before the 2nd crossing of Digastric leaving its lower border; hence, the wise dissector works along the upper border.

4. The submandibular duct running forwards, across Hyoglossus and Genioglossus, to its orifice.

5. The lingual nerve in contact with the jaw posteriorly, making a partial spiral around the submandibular duct, and ending in the tongue. The submandibular ganglion suspended from the nerve, and twigs leaving the nerve to supply mucous membrane.

6. The 1st part of the lingual artery behind Hyoglossus, and the 3rd part in front.

Stylohyoid and Digastric

Medial Pterygoid

{ Styloglossus
{ Glossopharyngeal nerve

Hyoglossus, divided

{ Sublingual artery
{ Genioglossus

Facial artery

Ext. carotid art.

Hypoglossal nerve

Int. carotid art.

Stylopharyngeus }
Stylohyoid lig. }

Middle Constrictor }
Lingual artery }

Greater horn
of hyoid bone

Sternomastoid br. }
Cricothyroid br. }

Hypoglossal nerve

Dorsales linguae aa.
on Genioglossus

Body of hyoid bone

Fascial sling for
Digastric, pulled down

549   Suprahyoid Region—IV

The lingual artery displayed.

Stylohyoid and posterior belly of Digastric are thrown up; the hypoglossal nerve
is divided and thrown backwards and forwards; and the greater part of Hyoglossus
is removed, in order to uncover the 2nd part of the lingual artery.

Observe:

1. The 1st part of the lingual artery, as in figure 548.

2. The 2nd part, deep to Hyoglossus, parallel to the greater horn of the hyoid bone, and lying
   on Middle Constrictor, stylohyoid ligament, and Genioglossus.

3. The 3rd part, ascending at the anterior border of Hyoglossus, which partly overlaps it,
   and turning into the tongue as the profunda linguae artery (see fig. 592).

4. The branches of the lingual artery (a) muscular, (b) dorsales linguae from the 2nd part
   which reach the tonsil bed, and (c) the sublingual artery which supplies the sublingual
   gland and the front of the floor of the mouth.

5. Stylopharyngeus deep to Styloglossus, which in turn is deep to Stylohyoid. Stylopharyngeus
   passing deep to Middle Constrictor.

6. The glossopharyngeal nerve, not making the usual spiral descent lateral to Stylopharyngeus
   as in figure 574 but descending medial to it.

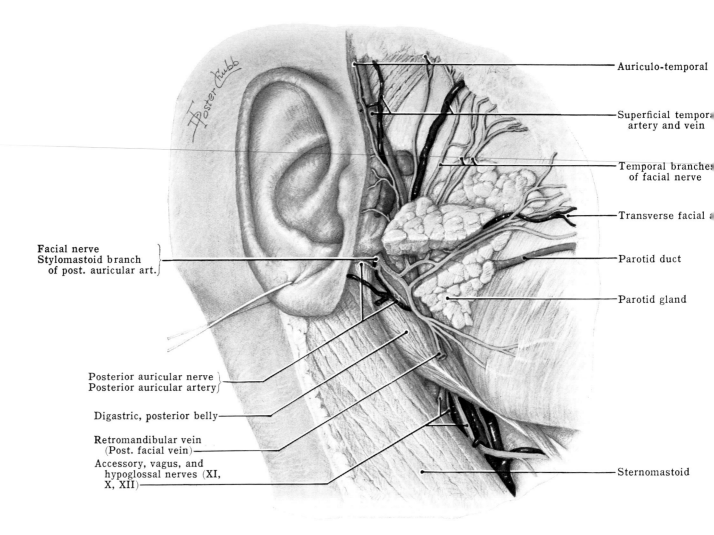

Auriculo-temporal

Superficial tempora[l]
artery and vein

Temporal branche[s]
of facial nerve

Transverse facial [a]

Parotid duct

Parotid gland

Facial nerve
Stylomastoid branch
of post. auricular art.

Sternomastoid

Posterior auricular nerve
Posterior auricular artery

Digastric, posterior belly

Retromandibular vein
(Post. facial vein)

Accessory, vagus, and
hypoglossal nerves (XI,
X, XII)

550   Parotid Region—II

(Stage I is represented in figure 467.) The parotid gland is partly cut away.

Observe:

1. The stem of the facial nerve descending from the stylomastoid foramen for $\frac{1}{4}''$ to $\frac{1}{2}''$ before curving forwards to penetrate the deeper part of the parotid gland.

2. The nerve to the posterior belly of Digastric arising from the stem of the facial nerve.

3. The posterior auricular artery giving off a branch, the stylomastoid art., which accompanies the facial nerve through the stylomastoid foramen into the facial canal.

4. The relatively superficial position of the great landmark in the upper part of the neck, namely: the posterior belly of Digastric. Only three structures cross superficial to it: (a) the cervical branch of the facial nerve, (b) branches of the retromandibular vein, and (c) branches of the great auricular nerve shown in figure 467. All other crossing structures cross deep to it.

5. Preauricular lymph nodes.

6. Auricular and temporal branches of the auriculo-temporal nerve.

Branch of superficial temporal artery

Branches of:
  post. auricular a.
  great auricular n.

Auricular branches of vagus nerve

Mastoid process

Temporo-mandibular lig.

Stylohyoid and
Digastric, post. belly

Accessory nerve
Int. jugular vein

Sternomastoid branch of occipital artery

Vagus nerve

Superior root of ansa cervicalis on int. carotid artery

Ext. carotid artery

Temporal muscle

Masseter

Zygomatico-temporal nerve

Zygomatic bone, cut surface

Nerve and artery to Masseter

Parotid duct

Mylohyoid

Hypoglossal nerve
Lingual artery

551   Parotid Bed: The Temporal Muscle: Auricular Vessels and Nerves—III

Observe:

1. The mastoid process, rough where Sternomastoid (and also Splenius Capitis and Longissimus Capitis) has been removed from it.

2. The posterior belly of Digastric, arising deep to the mastoid process and passing deep to the angle of the jaw.

3. The vessels and nerves passing deep to Digastric—notably: the internal jugular vein, internal carotid artery, external carotid artery and its lingual, facial, and occipital branches, and the last three cranial nerves.

4. The Temporal muscle, inserted into the beak-shaped coronoid process.

5. The nerve and artery to Masseter, crossing the mandibular notch behind the Temporal muscle—the nerve appearing from above Lateral Pterygoid and the artery from below it.

6. Vessels and nerves of the auricle, mostly turning round the free borders of the cartilage, but some piercing the cartilage.

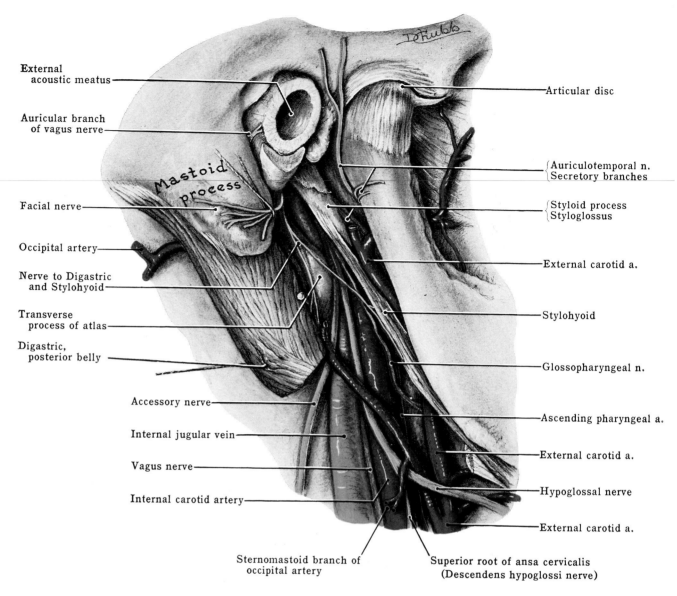

External acoustic meatus

Auricular branch of vagus nerve

Facial nerve

Occipital artery

Nerve to Digastric and Stylohyoid

Transverse process of atlas

Digastric, posterior belly

Accessory nerve

Internal jugular vein

Vagus nerve

Internal carotid artery

Articular disc

Auriculotemporal n.
Secretory branches

Styloid process
Styloglossus

External carotid a.

Stylohyoid

Glossopharyngeal n.

Ascending pharyngeal a.

External carotid a.

Hypoglossal nerve

External carotid a.

Mastoid process

Sternomastoid branch of occipital artery

Superior root of ansa cervicalis
(Descendens hypoglossi nerve)

552 Structures Deep to the Parotid Bed—IV

The facial nerve, the posterior belly of Digastric and the nerve to this belly are retracted, whereas the external carotid artery, Stylohyoid and the nerve to Stylohyoid remain in situ.

Observe:

1. The tip of the transverse process of the atlas, about midway between the tip of the mastoid process and the angle of the jaw.

2. The internal jugular vein, the internal carotid artery, and the last four cranial nerves crossing in front of the transverse process and deep to the styloid process.

3. The strange impression made on the internal jugular vein by the transverse process.

4. The internal and external carotids separated from each other by the styloid process.

5. The last four cranial nerves (XII concealing X) starting to diverge from each other as they cross the transverse process.

6. The two nerves that pass forwards to the tongue: (a) IX or glossopharyngeal being above the level of the angle of the jaw and passing between the two carotid arteries, and (b) XII or hypoglossal being below the angle of the jaw and passing superficial to both carotids, and indeed, to all the arteries it meets, except the occipital artery and its sternomastoid branch.

7. The thickness of the skin lining the cartilage of the meatus and the stems of the two nerves—auricular branch of the vagus and auriculo-temporal—that supply the meatus and the outer surface of the tympanic membrane.

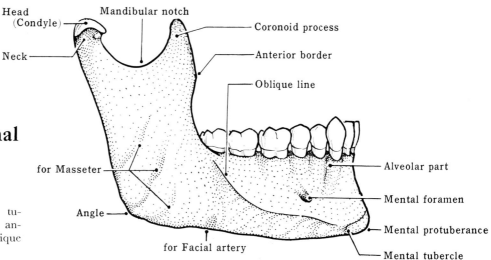

Head (Condyle) — Mandibular notch — Coronoid process

Neck — Anterior border

Oblique line

553 Mandible, external surface

Observe:

The coronoid process and the mental tubercle imperfectly connected by (a) the anterior border of the ramus, and (b) the oblique line that crosses the body diagonally.

for Masseter — Alveolar part

Mental foramen

Angle — Mental protuberance

for Facial artery — Mental tubercle

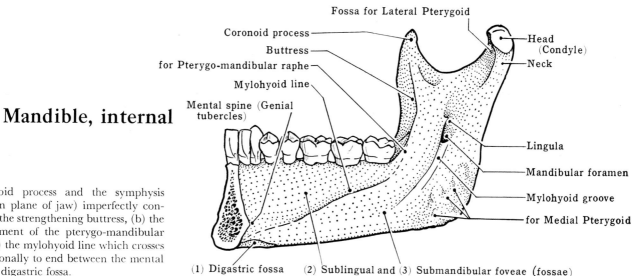

Fossa for Lateral Pterygoid

Coronoid process — Head (Condyle)

Buttress — Neck

for Pterygo-mandibular raphe

Mylohyoid line

Mental spine (Genial tubercles)

553.1 Mandible, internal surface

Observe:

The coronoid process and the symphysis menti (median plane of jaw) imperfectly connected by (a) the strengthening buttress, (b) the site of attachment of the pterygo-mandibular raphe, and (c) the mylohyoid line which crosses the body diagonally to end between the mental spine and the digastric fossa.

Lingula

Mandibular foramen

Mylohyoid groove

for Medial Pterygoid

(1) Digastric fossa   (2) Sublingual and (3) Submandibular foveae (fossae)

553.2 Mental Foramen, in edentulous jaws

Observe:

The position of the mental foramen in edentulous jaws varying with the extent of the absorption of the alveolus.

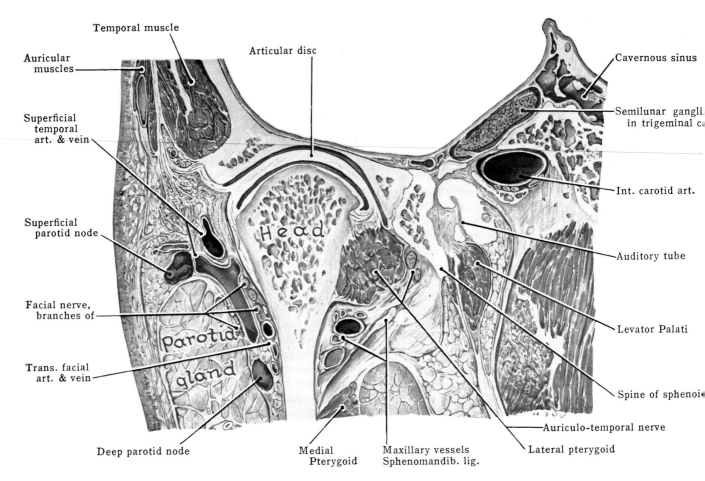

Temporal muscle

Auricular muscles

Articular disc

Cavernous sinus

Semilunar gangli in trigeminal c.

Superficial temporal art. & vein

Head

Int. carotid art.

Superficial parotid node

Auditory tube

Facial nerve, branches of

Parotid gland

Levator Palati

Trans. facial art. & vein

Spine of sphenoi

Auriculo-temporal nerve

Deep parotid node

Medial Pterygoid

Maxillary vessels Sphenomandib. lig.

Lateral pterygoid

554 Temporo-mandibular Joint, on coronal section

Observe:

1. The articular disc attached to the neck of the jaw medially and laterally, partly in conjunction with the Lateral Pterygoid.
2. The roof of the mandibular fossa, which separates head and disc from the middle cranial fossa, to be thin centrally (fig. 619.2) but thick elsewhere, cf., the acetabulum.
3. The spine of the sphenoid (figs. 569 & 571.1) at the medial end of the fossa, and the two roots of the auriculo-temporal nerve crossing lateral to it (fig. 560).
4. The auditory tube with closed slit-like lumen, and the Levator Palati lying below it.
5. The semilunar ganglion in its trigeminal cave, the mouth of which opens below the tentorium (fig. 565); and separated from the int. carotid artery by membrane (bone being deficient) and, therefore, subjected to the pulsations of that artery (figs. 513 & 514).
6. The maxillary vessels crossing the neck of the jaw on its medial side.
7. Superficial and deep parotid lymph nodes.
8. The "aponeurotic" tendon of Temporalis, buried in the muscle for it receives fleshy fibres from the temporal fossa on one side and from the temporal fascia on the other (figs. 465 & 591).

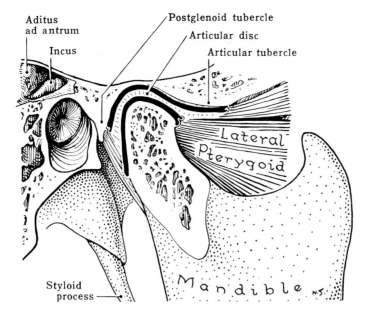

555 Temporo-mandibular Joint, on sagittal section

Note the articular disc dividing the articular cavity into an upper and a lower compartment, and the Lateral Pterygoid inserted in part into the disc.

(For orientation of head of jaw, see figure 507; for articular part of mandibular fossa and articular tubercle, see figures 558 & 619.2; for lateral, or temporo-mandibular, lig., see figure 551.)

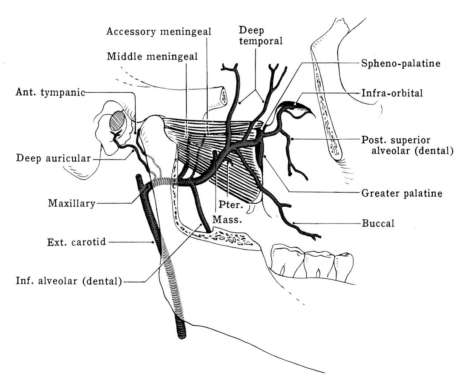

556 Diagram of the Maxillary Artery

Observe:

1. This, the larger of the two terminal branches of the external carotid art., arising at the neck of the jaw and divided into three parts by the Lateral Pterygoid.
2. The branches of the first part pass through foramina or canals: (a) deep auricular a. to the ext. acoustic meatus, (b) anterior tympanic a. to the tympanum (c, d) middle and accessory meningeal aa. to the cranial cavity, and (e) inf. alveolar a. to the jaw and teeth.
3. The branches of the second part supply muscles—by

Masseteric, deep temporal, pterygoid, and buccal branches.

4. The branches of the third part arise from the end of the artery within the pterygo-palatine fossa: (a) post superior alveolar a., (b) infra-orbital a., (c) greater palatine a., (d) artery of the pterygoid canal, (e) pharyngeal a., and (f) sphenopalatine a. These, accompanied by branches of the maxillary nerve, pass through bony canals or foramina.

The greater palatine a. gives rise to the lesser palatine aa. (fig. 583). The sphenopalatine a. ends as the post. lateral nasal and post. nasal septal aa. (fig. 607).

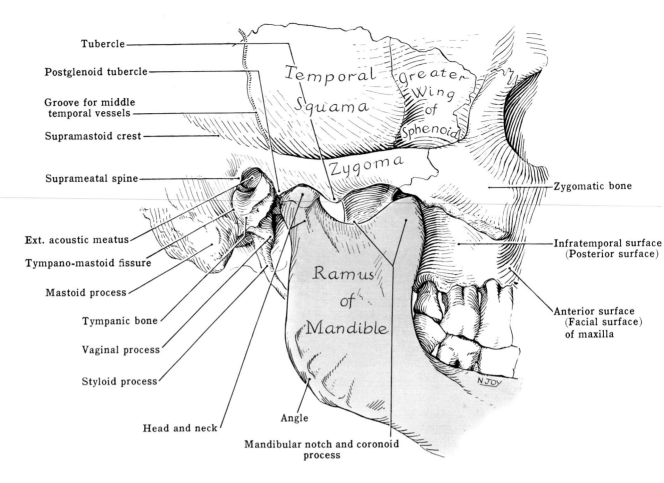

Tubercle

Postglenoid tubercle

Groove for middle temporal vessels

Supramastoid crest

Suprameatal spine

Ext. acoustic meatus

Tympano-mastoid fissure

Mastoid process

Tympanic bone

Vaginal process

Styloid process

Head and neck

Angle

Mandibular notch and coronoid process

Temporal Squama

Greater Wing of Sphenoid

Zygoma

Zygomatic bone

Ramus of Mandible

Infratemporal surface (Posterior surface)

Anterior surface (Facial surface) of maxilla

557   Lateral Wall of the Infratemporal Fossa—I

This wall is formed by the ramus of the mandible.

Note:

1. The zygoma [zygomatic process of the squamous part of the temporal bone] plus the zygomatic bone constitute the zygomatic arch. This arch is continued as a buttress downwards and forwards to the first or second molar tooth. The buttress forms the anterior limit of the infratemporal fossa and separates it from the facial aspect of the skull.

2. The zygoma lies at the boundary line between the temporal fossa above and the infratemporal fossa below.

3. Below the tubercle of the zygoma and in front of the neck of the jaw there is a clear passage across the base of the skull through which a pencil can be passed—see figure 571.

4. When in occlusion a tooth bites on two other teeth.

557.1   Bipartite Zygomatic Bone (Os Japonicum)

Rarely the zygomatic bone is divided either horizontally or vertically into two parts. In this instance the condition was bilateral. (Courtesy of Dr. J. E. Anderson.)

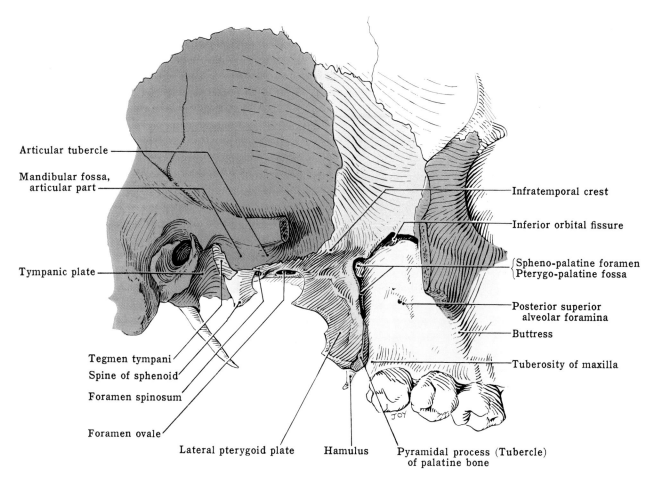

Articular tubercle

Mandibular fossa,
articular part

Tympanic plate

Tegmen tympani
Spine of sphenoid
Foramen spinosum

Foramen ovale

Lateral pterygoid plate

Hamulus

Pyramidal process (Tubercle)
of palatine bone

Infratemporal crest

Inferior orbital fissure

Spheno-palatine foramen
Pterygo-palatine fossa

Posterior superior
alveolar foramina

Buttress

Tuberosity of maxilla

558 Roof and the Medial and Anterior Walls of the Infratemporal Fossa, infero-lateral view—II

The jaw is removed and the zygomatic arch is cut away.

Note:

1. The medial wall of the fossa is formed by the lateral pterygoid plate.

2. The posterior free border of this plate, when followed upwards, leads to the foramen ovale in the roof of the fossa. Behind the foramen ovale, at the root of the spine of the sphenoid, is the foramen spinosum (Figs. 508 & 569). The roof is separated from the temporal fossa by the infratemporal crest.

3. Below, the anterior border of the lateral plate is separated from the maxilla by the pyramidal process of the palatine bone which is insinuated as a buffer between the two (figs. 569 & 570). Above, the border is free and forms the posterior limit of the pterygo-maxillary fissure, which is the entrance to the pterygo-palatine fossa on the medial wall of which can be seen the sphenopalatine foramen which leads to the nasal cavity.

4. The rounded anterior wall of the fossa is the infratemporal surface of the maxilla, which is of egg-shell thickness, is limited above by the inferior orbital fissure, and is pierced by two (or more) posterior superior alveolar (dental) foramina for the vessels and nerves of the same name.

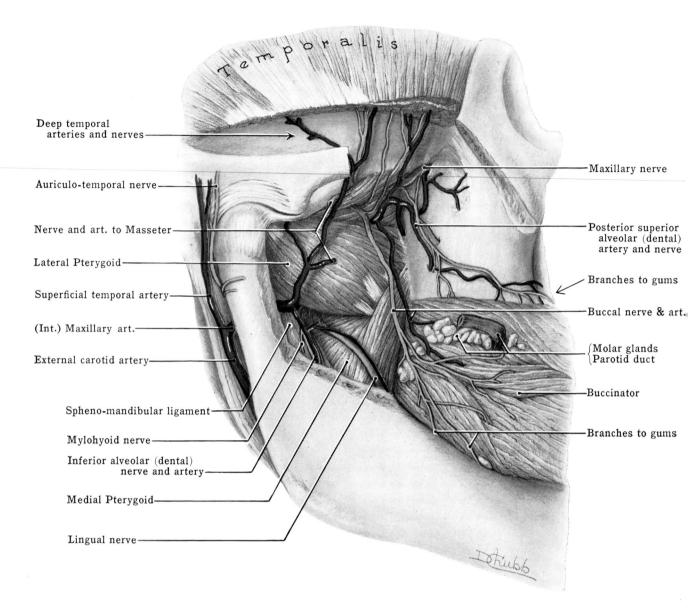

Deep temporal arteries and nerves

Auriculo-temporal nerve

Nerve and art. to Masseter

Lateral Pterygoid

Superficial temporal artery

(Int.) Maxillary art.

External carotid artery

Spheno-mandibular ligament

Mylohyoid nerve

Inferior alveolar (dental) nerve and artery

Medial Pterygoid

Lingual nerve

Temporalis

Maxillary nerve

Posterior superior alveolar (dental) artery and nerve

Branches to gums

Buccal nerve & art.

Molar glands
Parotid duct

Buccinator

Branches to gums

559 Infratemporal Fossa, superficial dissection—III

Observe:

1. Lateral Pterygoid, triangular in shape, arising from the medial wall and roof of the infratemporal fossa (fig. 558), the two heads being at a right angle to each other, and inserted into the articular disc of the temporo-mandibular joint and into the front of the neck of the jaw.

2. Below this, Medial Pterygoid is seen; in front of Medial Pterygoid, Buccinator is seen.

3. Appearing (a) between Lateral Pterygoid and the roof—the nerves to Masseter and Temporalis; (b) between the heads of Lateral Pterygoid—the buccal nerve and the maxillary artery (the nerve here pierces Lateral Pterygoid); and (c) between Lateral and Medial Pterygoids—the inferior alveolar and lingual nerves.

4. The maxillary nerve (V^2) becoming the infra-orbital nerve and passing through the inferior orbital fissure, after giving off the posterior superior alveolar nerve which sends two (or more) branches into the foramina of the same name.

5. The maxillary artery, which is the larger of the two end branches of the external carotid, running forwards deep to the neck of the jaw, disappearing deep to Lateral Pterygoid, and reappearing between its two heads before plunging into the pterygo-palatine fossa. It is seen sending branches to accompany each nerve mentioned above.

6. Buccinator, pierced by (a) the parotid duct, (b) the ducts of the molar glands, and (c) branches (sensory) of the buccal nerve.

7. At the upper and lower borders of Buccinator, branches of the posterior superior alveolar and buccal nerves sending branches to the upper and lower gums respectively.

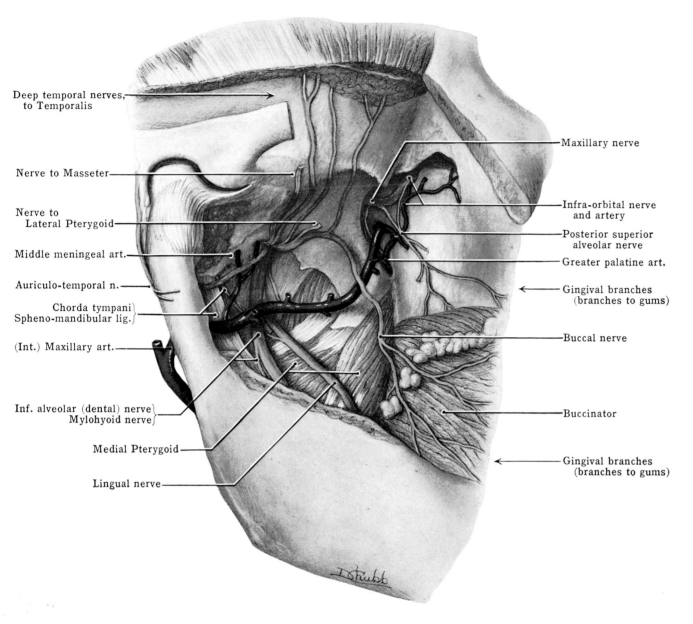

Deep temporal nerves,
to Temporalis

Nerve to Masseter

Nerve to
Lateral Pterygoid

Middle meningeal art.

Auriculo-temporal n.

Chorda tympani
Spheno-mandibular lig.

(Int.) Maxillary art.

Inf. alveolar (dental) nerve
Mylohyoid nerve

Medial Pterygoid

Lingual nerve

Maxillary nerve

Infra-orbital nerve
and artery

Posterior superior
alveolar nerve

Greater palatine art.

Gingival branches
(branches to gums)

Buccal nerve

Buccinator

Gingival branches
(branches to gums)

560   Infratemporal Fossa, deeper dissection—IV

Lateral Pterygoid is removed and so are most branches of the artery.

Observe:

1. Medial Pterygoid arising from the medial surface of the lateral pterygoid plate and having a small superficial head which arises from the pyramidal process of the palatine bone (fig. 558).

2. The spheno-mandibular ligament, which, as a fascial band, descends from the spine of the sphenoid to the lingula of the mandible (fig. 553).

3. The maxillary artery and the auriculo-temporal nerve passing between the ligament and the neck of the jaw.

4. The mandibular nerve (V³) entering the infratemporal fossa through the roof, via the foramen ovale which also transmits the accessory meningeal artery (not labelled).

5. The middle meningeal artery passing through the roof via the foramen spinosum.

6. The inferior alveolar and lingual nerves descending on Medial Pterygoid. The former giving off the mylohyoid nerve (to Mylohyoid and anterior belly of Digastric); the latter receiving the chorda tympani (which carries secretory fibres and fibres of taste).

7. The nerves to the 4 muscles of mastication: Masseter, Temporal, and Lateral Pterygoid, which are labelled, and the nerve to Medial Pterygoid which is not labelled. Note the buccal branch of the mandibular nerve is sensory; it is the buccal branch of the facial nerve that supplies Buccinator.

8. The maxillary nerve (V²) becoming the infra-orbital nerve which enters the infra-orbital groove at the inferior orbital fissure. Deep in the pterygo-palatine fossa the pterygo-palatine ganglion is seen suspended from the nerve.

Anterior tubercle of atlas   Nerves: XII, XI & X, IX

Jugular process
Rectus Capitis
Lateralis

Nerve C. 1

Occipital artery

Digastric (post. belly)

Sup. cervical ganglion

Nerve C. 2

Nerve C. 3

Sympathetic trunk

Nerve C. 4

Phrenic nerve

Nerve C. 5

Inf. cervical
ganglion

Ansa subclavia
Vertebral
ganglion

Brachiocephalic trunk

Internal jugular vein

Facial nerve

Mastoid process

{Rectus Capitis Anterior
{Rectus Capitis Lateralis

Trans. process of atlas

{Intertransversarius Anterior
{Intertransversarius Posterior

Levator Scapulae

Trans. process C. 3

Longus Capitis

Longus Colli (Cervicis)

Scalenus Medius

Carotid tubercle, on
trans. process C. 6

Vertebral artery

{Inferior thyroid art.
{Ascending cervical art.

Transverse cervical art.

Costo-cervical trunk

Suprascapular artery

Thyro-cervical trunk

Internal thoracic art.

Subclavian artery

Common carotid artery

561   Prevertebral Region: Root of the Neck

On the left side of the specimen, Longus Capitis is removed.

Observe:

1. The prevertebral and deep lateral muscles of the neck. Of these muscles, 3—Scalenus Anterior, Longus Capitis, and Longus Colli—are attached to the anterior tubercles of the transverse processes of vertebrae C. 3, 4, 5 and 6; hence, the prominence of these tubercles, as seen in figures 367 & 368.

2. The transverse process of the atlas joined to the transverse process of the axis by Intertransverse muscles; and joined similarly to the transverse process of the occipital bone (i.e.,

jugular process) by Rectus Capitis Lateralis which morphologically is an Intertransverse muscle. Note: the internal jugular vein crossing these structures.

3. The cervical plexus arising from ventral rami, C. 1, 2, 3 and 4; and the brachial plexus from C. 5, 6, 7, 8 and T. 1.

4. The sympathetic trunk and ganglia and its gray rami communicantes.

5. The subclavian artery and its branches.

462 Ligaments of the Atlanto-axial and Atlanto-occipital Joints, in median section

Observe:

The layers of tissue encountered in the median plane. From behind forwards they are: (a) dura mater, (b) posterior longitudinal lig., continued upwards as the membrana tectoria, stretching from axis to occipital bone, (c) transverse ligament of the atlas and the upper and lower longitudinal bands, which, like the membrana, stretch from axis to occipital bone and (d) the lig. apicis dentis (not labelled), which is a vestigial filament stretching from the apex of the dens to the occipital bone.

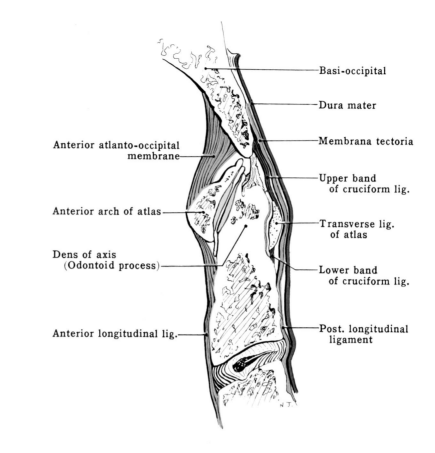

- Basi-occipital
- Dura mater
- Membrana tectoria
- Upper band of cruciform lig.
- Transverse lig. of atlas
- Lower band of cruciform lig.
- Post. longitudinal ligament

Anterior atlanto-occipital membrane

Anterior arch of atlas

Dens of axis (Odontoid process)

Anterior longitudinal lig.

463 Atlas and its Transverse Ligament and the Axis, from above

Observe:

The large vertebral foramen of the atlas which is divided into two foramina by the transverse ligament of the atlas. In the larger, posterior foramen the spinal cord lies loosely. In the smaller, anterior foramen the dens of the axis fits tightly. It articulates in front with the anterior arch of the atlas and behind with the transverse ligament which, like the annular ligament of the radius, forms an arc of a circle.

Anterior arch

Foramen for dens

Lateral mass

Foramen for spinal cord

Posterior arch

- Anterior tubercle
- Facet for dens
- Sup. articular facet
- Transverse ligament
- Transverse process
- Transverse foramen
- Groove for vertebral a.
- Posterior tubercle

Body

Dens of axis

Vertebral foramen for spinal cord

- Facet for atlas
- Superior articular facet
- Transverse process
- Transverse foramen
- Inf. articular process
- Lamina
- Spinous process or spine

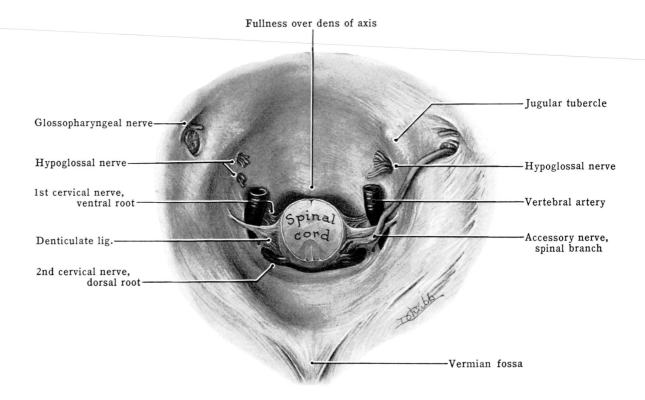

Fullness over dens of axis

Glossopharyngeal nerve

Hypoglossal nerve

1st cervical nerve, ventral root

Denticulate lig.

2nd cervical nerve, dorsal root

Spinal cord

Jugular tubercle

Hypoglossal nerve

Vertebral artery

Accessory nerve, spinal branch

Vermian fossa

564 Structures seen through the Foramen Magnum, from above

Observe:

1. In front, the fullness over the transverse ligament of the atlas (fig. 563), which curves tightly behind the dens of the axis.
2. Passing through the foramen magnum within the meninges: (a) the spinal cord or medulla, (b) the vertebral arteries, (c) the spinal roots of the accessory nerves (XI), and (d) the highest tooth of the ligamentum denticulatum of each side.
3. The hypoglossal nerves (XII) leaving the dura mater through two openings which are close together on the right side and separated on the left side.
4. In this specimen the first cervical nerve has no posterior (sensory) root.

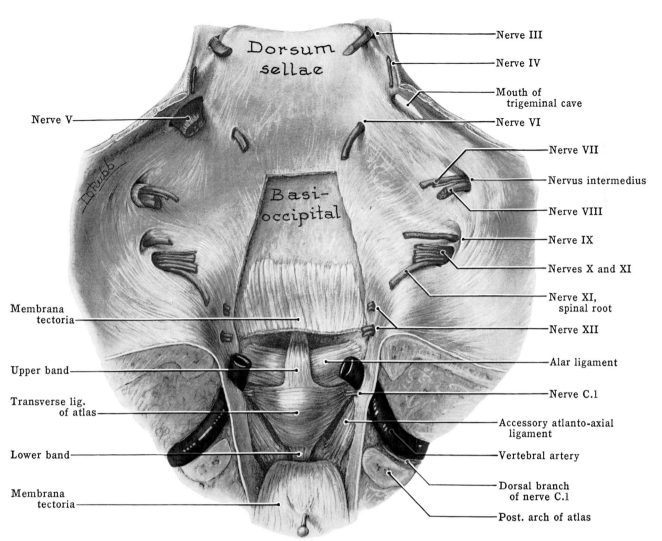

Dorsum sellae

Basi-occipital

Nerve V

Membrana tectoria

Upper band

Transverse lig. of atlas

Lower band

Membrana tectoria

Nerve III

Nerve IV

Mouth of trigeminal cave

Nerve VI

Nerve VII

Nervus intermedius

Nerve VIII

Nerve IX

Nerves X and XI

Nerve XI, spinal root

Nerve XII

Alar ligament

Nerve C.1

Accessory atlanto-axial ligament

Vertebral artery

Dorsal branch of nerve C.1

Post. arch of atlas

565 Ligaments of the Atlanto-axial and Atlanto-occipital joints, from behind

Observe:

1. The bow-shaped transverse ligament of the atlas, which, by the addition of an upper and a lower longitudinal band, becomes a cruciform ligament.

2. The alar or check ligaments passing from the sides of the apex of the dens postero-laterally, above the transverse ligament, to the medial sides of the occipital condyles.

3. The sites where the last ten pairs of cranial nerves and the first pair of cervical nerves pass through the dura, noting (a) that they are in numerical sequence, cranio-caudally, and (b) that nerves III, IV and VI, which supply the muscles of the eye, and XII, which supplies the muscles of the tongue, are nearly in vertical line with each other and with the ventral or motor root of C. 1.

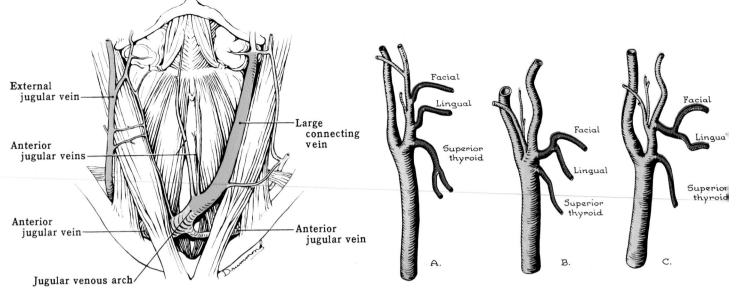

566 Large Connecting Vein

A small vein that lies along the anterior border of Sternomastoid and connects the common facial vein to the anterior jugular vein may attain great size. It may, indeed, be greater than even the internal jugular vein and it is at times mistaken for it.

566.1 Variations in the Origin of the Lingual Artery

A. The superior thyroid, lingual, and facial arteries arose separately in 80% of 211 specimens. B, C. In 20% the lingual and facial arteries arose from a common stem, either high or low. In one instance the superior thyroid and lingual arteries arose from a common stem. (*G. F. Lewis.*)

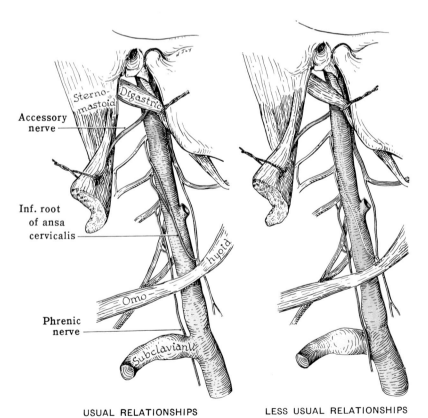

USUAL RELATIONSHIPS   LESS USUAL RELATIONSHIPS

566.2 Variable Relationships of the Accessory, Ansa Cervicalis, and Phrenic Nerves to the Great Veins

The accessory nerve crossed anterior to the internal jugular vein in 70% of 188 instances, and posterior to it in 30%. (J. C. B. G.)

The inferior root of the ansa cervicalis, while on its way to join the superior root, passed round the medial side of the internal jugular vein in 43% of 118 instances, and round the lateral side in 57%. (D. L. MacIntosh and G. G. Smith.)

The phrenic nerve (C.3, 4, and 5) passes behind the site of union of the subclavian, internal, jugular, and brachiocephalic veins, but occasionally the branch from C.5, or less commonly the entire phrenic nerve, passes anterior to the subclavian vein.

VARIATIONS AND ANOMALIES

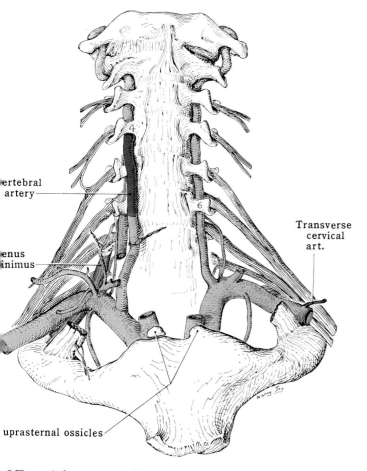

ertebral
artery

enus
inimus

Transverse
cervical
art.

uprasternal ossicles

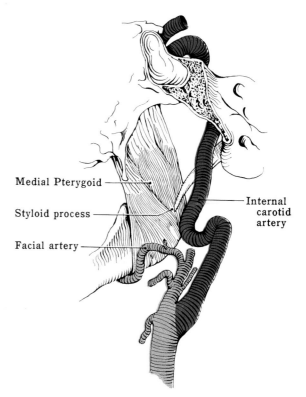

Medial Pterygoid

Styloid process

Facial artery

Internal
carotid
artery

567.1 Tortuous Internal Carotid Artery

This artery is always tortuous inside the skull. It may be tortuous outside also and come to lie close behind the tonsil.

67 Abnormal Vertebral Artery: uprasternal Ossicles: Scalenus Minimus

The Vertebral Artery, in 6.4% of 1,000 half heads (Japanese), enters not the foramen of the 6th cervical transverse process but another—the 5th in 4.5%, the 7th in 1.2%, and the 4th as here in 0.7% (Adachi).

Suprasternal Ossicles, which range in size between that of a small shot and an average female lunate bone, were found either paired or singly, and either separate from the manubrium or fused to it, in 6.8% of 544 white adult sterna examined by X-rays. (W. Montague Cobb.)

Scalenus Minimus, passing between subclavian artery and brachial plexus, is commonly present. (Also fig. 537.)

Aberrant Transverse Cervical Artery, see figure 471.5.

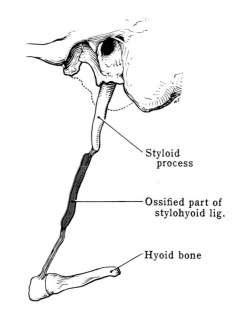

Styloid
process

Ossified part of
stylohyoid lig.

Hyoid bone

lo-hyoid lig.

oid bone

568 An Ossified Stylohyoid Ligament

here unites the styloid process (in 2 pieces) to the lesser horn. Thus, a chain of 4 bones with 4 joints attaches the body and greater horn of the hyoid to the skull.

568.1 Partial Ossification of Stylohyoid Ligament, left side

VARIATIONS AND ANOMALIES

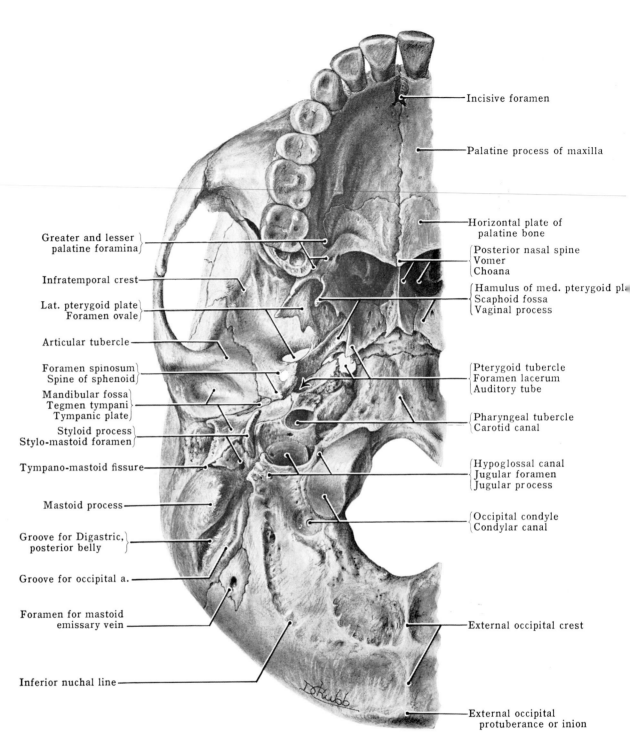

Incisive foramen

Palatine process of maxilla

Horizontal plate of palatine bone

Posterior nasal spine
Vomer
Choana

Hamulus of med. pterygoid pl.
Scaphoid fossa
Vaginal process

Greater and lesser palatine foramina

Infratemporal crest

Lat. pterygoid plate
Foramen ovale

Articular tubercle

Foramen spinosum
Spine of sphenoid

Mandibular fossa
Tegmen tympani
Tympanic plate

Styloid process
Stylo-mastoid foramen

Tympano-mastoid fissure

Mastoid process

Groove for Digastric, posterior belly

Groove for occipital a.

Foramen for mastoid emissary vein

Inferior nuchal line

Pterygoid tubercle
Foramen lacerum
Auditory tube

Pharyngeal tubercle
Carotid canal

Hypoglossal canal
Jugular foramen
Jugular process

Occipital condyle
Condylar canal

External occipital crest

External occipital protuberance or inion

569   Exterior of the Base of the Skull

Note:

(1) The unlabelled foramen between the carotid canal and the jugular foramen which transmits the tympanic branch of the glosso-pharyngeal nerve, shown in figure 659.

(2) The unlabelled foramen on the lateral wall of the jugular foramen which transmits the auricular branch of the vagus nerve, shown in figure 552. The auricular branch enters this foramen, crosses the stylomastoid foramen, and leaves through the tympano-mastoid fissure.

(3) The foramen for the mastoid emissary vein, in this specimen, lies in a sutural bone.

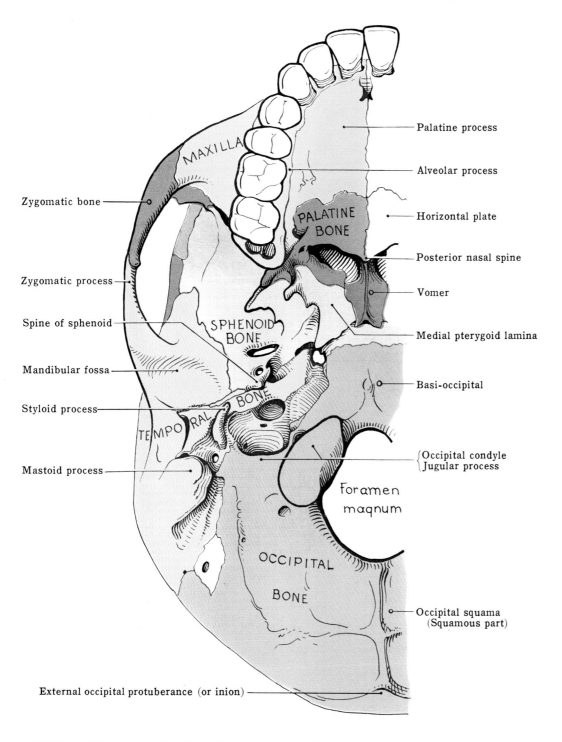

Zygomatic bone

Zygomatic process

Spine of sphenoid

Mandibular fossa

Styloid process

Mastoid process

MAXILLA

PALATINE BONE

SPHENOID BONE

TEMPORAL BONE

OCCIPITAL BONE

Foramen magnum

Palatine process

Alveolar process

Horizontal plate

Posterior nasal spine

Vomer

Medial pterygoid lamina

Basi-occipital

Occipital condyle
Jugular process

Occipital squama
(Squamous part)

External occipital protuberance (or inion)

570   Bones of the Exterior of the Base of the Skull

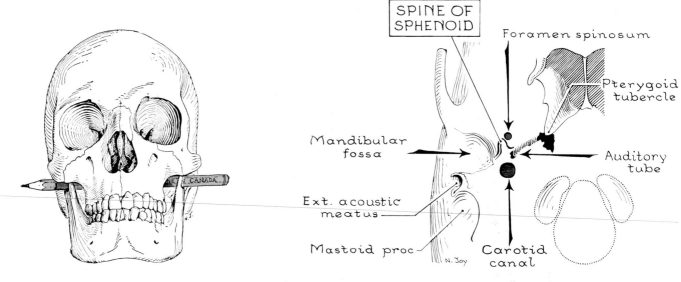

571 A Pencil Passed Across the Base of the Skull

Note:

There being nothing to stop it, a pencil can be passed through the mandibular notches and across the base of the skull; i.e., the pencil lies behind the pterygoid plates and occupies the anterior transverse line (see fig. 571.2, below).

571.1 Spine of the Sphenoid

Note: A blow delivered to the side of the jaw does not drive the jaw under the cranium, because the head of the jaw would require to descend the steep medial wall of the mandibular fossa and the spine of the sphenoid in which that wall ends. Like a sentinel, the spine "keeps guard over" 4 strategic points: (1) anteriorly, the foramen spinosum for the middle meningeal art.; (2) posteriorly, the entrance to the carotid canal; (3) medially, the entrance to the bony auditory tube; and (4) laterally, the mandibular fossa which lodges the head of the mandible, which therefore is the surface landmark to the spine.

571.2 Anterior and Posterior Transverse Lines at the Base of the Skull

Note: (1) The foramen ovale at the root of the lateral pterygoid plate; the foramen lacerum at the root of the medial pterygoid plate; and the synchondrosis between the basilar part of the occipital bone (basioccipital) and the body of the sphenoid.
(2) The posterior transverse line stretches across the base of the skull between the mastoid and the styloid processes of the two sides. The features it crosses are labelled.

THE 3 KEYS TO THE BASE OF THE SKULL

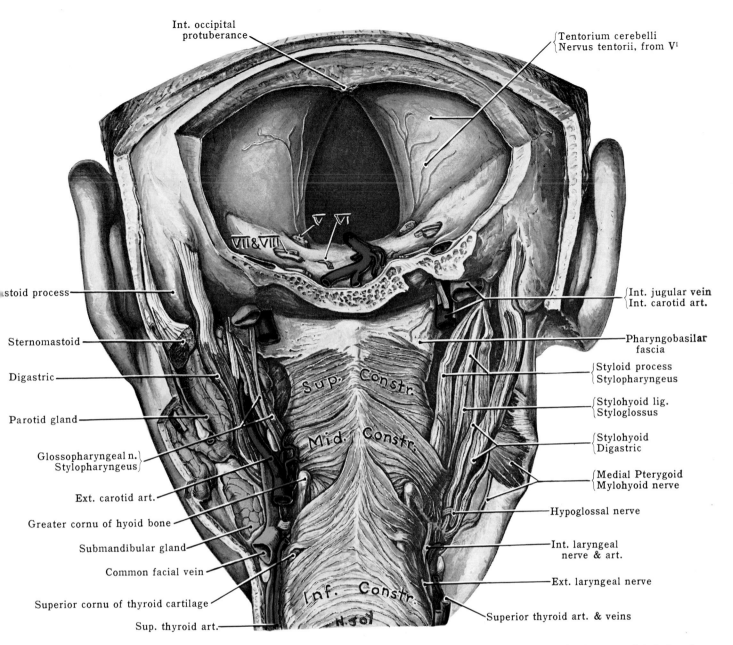

Int. occipital protuberance

Tentorium cerebelli
Nervus tentorii, from Vⁱ

V VI
VII & VIII

stoid process

Int. jugular **vein**
Int. carotid art.

Sternomastoid

Pharyngobasilar fascia

Digastric

Styloid process
Stylopharyngeus

Parotid gland

Stylohyoid lig.
Styloglossus

Stylohyoid
Digastric

Glossopharyngeal n.
Stylopharyngeus

Medial Pterygoid
Mylohyoid nerve

Ext. carotid art.

Hypoglossal nerve

Greater cornu of hyoid bone

Int. laryngeal nerve & art.

Submandibular gland

Common facial vein

Ext. laryngeal nerve

Superior cornu of thyroid cartilage

Sup. thyroid art.

Superior thyroid art. & veins

Sup. Constr.
Mid. Constr.
Inf. Constr.
N.Joy

572   Tentorium from below: Pharynx and Parotid Gland, from behind

Observe:

1. The tentorium cerebelli, forming the roof of the posterior cranial fossa, and its nerve. The basi-occipital, sawn across, and the basilar artery, formed by the union of the 2 unequal vertebral arteries, ascending on the dorsum sellae. (For bones, see fig. 497.)

2. The pharyngo-basilar fascia (i.e., the tough submucous coat) suspending the pharynx from the basi-occipital. Of the 3 Constrictors, Inferior overlapping Middle, and Middle overlapping Superior. This posterior aspect is flat or even slightly concave—not round—from side to side, being applied to the prevertebral region (fig. 561).

3. The tip of the greater horn of the hyoid bone and descending from it the thyrohyoid ligament which is the posterior border of the thyrohyoid membrane, not labelled.

4. *On the Right Side:* the styloid process of the temporal bone, slightly grooved on its medial side from contact with the internal jugular vein, and united to the lesser horn of the hyoid bone (not in view) by the stylohyoid ligament. Stylopharyngeus passing from the medial side of the styloid process for-

wards and medially to the interval between Superior and Middle Constrictors. Stylohyoid passing from the lateral side forwards and laterally to be split on its way to the hyoid bone by the Digastric. Styloglossus passing from the anterior aspect of the process and the ligament medially and forwards to the tongue.

5. *On the Left Side:* the glossopharyngeal nerve making a spiral round Stylopharyngeus and both entering the pharyngeal wall.

6. The posterior surface of the parotid gland grooved: by the mastoid process and below this by Sternomastoid, and more medially by Digastric and by the styloid process and the 3 muscles that arise from it (see cross-sections figs. 579 and 584). The external carotid artery approaching the gland from below. The parotid gland extending from the skin almost to the pharyngeal wall and separated from the submandibular gland merely by a strong layer of fascia. From the deep fascia processes extending between the lobules of the parotid gland but the submaxillary gland free within its fascial sheath.

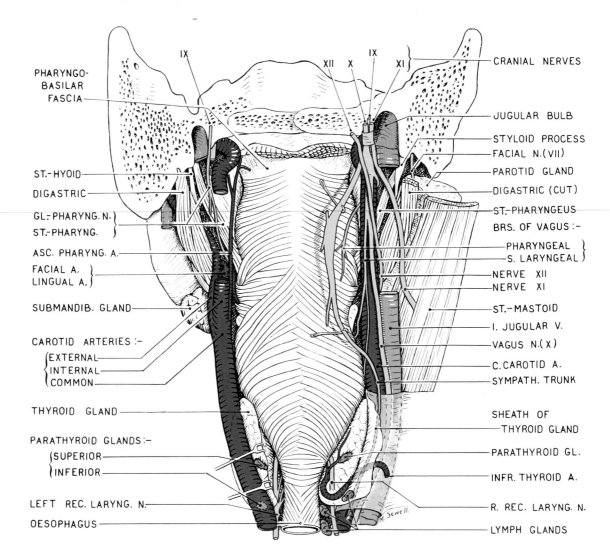

PHARYNGO-
BASILAR
FASCIA

IX

XII   X   IX   XI }   CRANIAL NERVES

ST.-HYOID

DIGASTRIC

GL.-PHARYNG. N. }
ST.-PHARYNG. }

ASC. PHARYNG. A.

FACIAL A. }
LINGUAL A. }

SUBMANDIB. GLAND

CAROTID ARTERIES :-
{EXTERNAL
{INTERNAL
{COMMON

THYROID GLAND

PARATHYROID GLANDS:-
{SUPERIOR
{INFERIOR

LEFT REC. LARYNG. N.

OESOPHAGUS

JUGULAR BULB

STYLOID PROCESS

FACIAL N.(VII)

PAROTID GLAND

DIGASTRIC (CUT)

ST.-PHARYNGEUS

BRS. OF VAGUS :-

PHARYNGEAL }
S. LARYNGEAL }

NERVE XII

NERVE XI

ST.-MASTOID

I. JUGULAR V.

VAGUS N.(X)

C. CAROTID A.

SYMPATH. TRUNK

SHEATH OF
THYROID GLAND

PARATHYROID GL.

INFR. THYROID A.

R. REC. LARYNG. N.

LYMPH GLANDS

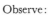

M. Sewell.

573   Pharynx and the Last Four Cranial Nerves, from behind

Observe:

1. The narrowest and least distensible part of the alimentary canal, where the pharynx becomes the esophagus.

2. Inferior Constrictor of the pharynx overlapping Middle Constrictor, and Middle overlapping Superior.

3. Between the Superior Constrictor and the base of the skull, the semilunar area on each side where the pharyngo-basilar fascia can be seen attaching the pharynx to the basi occipital bone.

4. The nerves and vessels that emerge from the foramina on "the posterior transverse line of the skull" (fig. 571 . 2) and which give this line its importance. They are: (a) the facial nerve, (b) the internal jugular vein, and (c) the last four cranial nerves. Of the 4 nerves: IX lies anterior to X and XI; and XII, which is the most medial, makes half spiral around X as it descends.

5. The internal carotid artery lies just behind the midpoint of the oblique line (fig. 571.1 and therefore anterior to the structures on the posterior line. Lying posterior to the artery and accompanying it into the carotid canal is the sympathetic trunk.

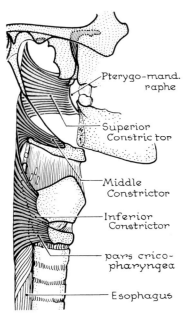

Pterygo-mand.
raphe

Superior
Constrictor

Middle
Constrictor

Inferior
Constrictor

pars crico-
pharynqea

Esophagus

573.1   Diagram of the 3 constrictors of the pharynx, showing their attachments and borders.

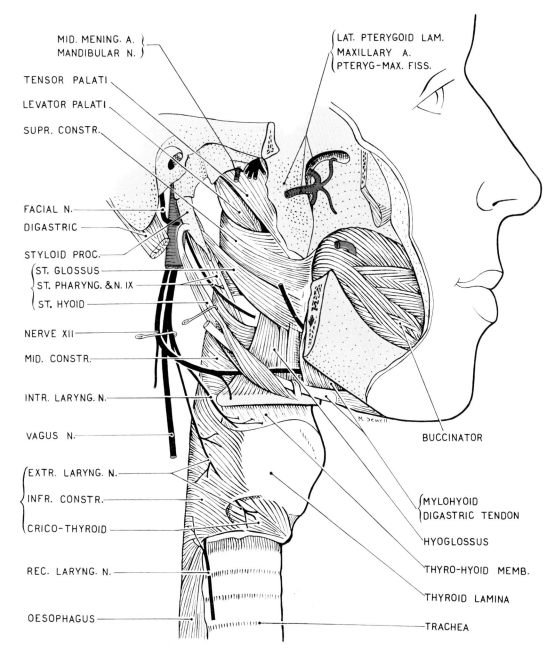

MID. MENING. A.
MANDIBULAR N.

LAT. PTERYGOID LAM.
MAXILLARY A.
PTERYG-MAX. FISS.

TENSOR PALATI

LEVATOR PALATI

SUPR. CONSTR.

FACIAL N.

DIGASTRIC

STYLOID PROC.

ST. GLOSSUS
ST. PHARYNG. & N. IX
ST. HYOID

NERVE XII

MID. CONSTR.

INTR. LARYNG. N.

VAGUS N.

EXTR. LARYNG. N.

INFR. CONSTR.

CRICO-THYROID

REC. LARYNG. N.

OESOPHAGUS

BUCCINATOR

MYLOHYOID
DIGASTRIC TENDON

HYOGLOSSUS

THYRO-HYOID MEMB.

THYROID LAMINA

TRACHEA

M. Sewell

574 Pharyngeal Muscles and the Buccinator, side view

Observe:

1. Superior Constrictor and Buccinator arising from opposite sides of the pterygo-mandibular raphe.

2. Middle Constrictor overlapped by Hyoglossus, and Hyoglossus in turn overlapped by Mylohyoid.

3. Inferior Constrictor arising from the oblique line of the lamina of the thyroid cartilage (fig. 623) and from the fibrous arch that joins the tubercle on the lower border of this lamina to the tubercle on the lower border of the cricoid cartilage.

4. Tensor and Levator Palati, behind the lateral pterygoid lamina or plate, helping to form the medial wall of the infratemporal fossa.

5. Levator Palati crossing the concave upper border of Superior Constrictor; and Tensor Palati passing between the fibres of origin of Superior Constrictor at the level of the hamulus (fig. 575).

6. The styloid process and the 3 muscles that arise from it—Stylo-glossus, Stylo-pharyngeus, Stylo-hyoid.

7. Styloglossus interdigitating with Hyoglossus on the side of the tongue; Stylopharyngeus and the glossopharyngeal nerve (IX) passing between Superior and Middle Constrictors; Stylohyoid split by the tendon of Digastric and attached to the hyoid bone.

8. The internal laryngeal nerve passing through the thyrohyoid membrane between Middle and Inferior Constrictors.

9. The recurrent laryngeal nerve passing deep to the lower border of Inferior Constrictor.

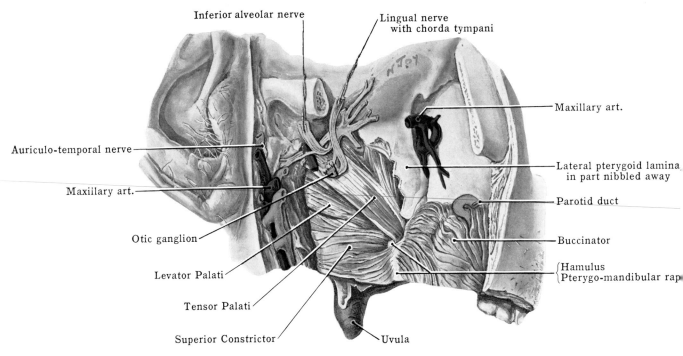

Inferior alveolar nerve

Lingual nerve
with chorda tympani

Maxillary art.

Auriculo-temporal nerve

Lateral pterygoid lamina
in part nibbled away

Maxillary art.

Parotid duct

Otic ganglion

Buccinator

Levator Palati

Hamulus
Pterygo-mandibular rap

Tensor Palati

Superior Constrictor

Uvula

575 Otic Ganglion, on lateral view

Note:

1. Levator Palati crossing the upper border of Sup. Constrictor.
2. Tensor Palati hooking round the hamulus.
3. The otic ganglion (fig. 659) lateral to Tensor Palati.

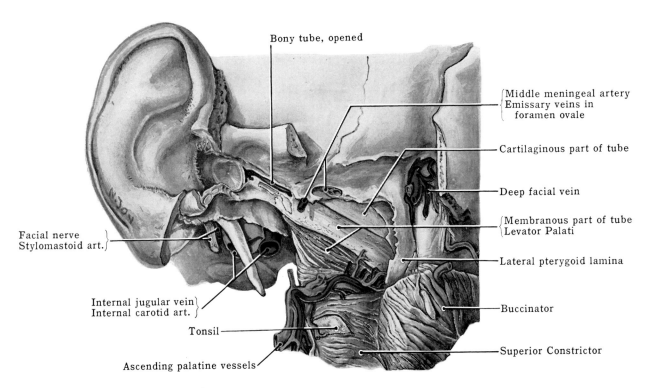

Bony tube, opened

Middle meningeal artery
Emissary veins in
foramen ovale

Cartilaginous part of tube

Deep facial vein

Membranous part of tube
Levator Palati

Facial nerve
Stylomastoid art.

Lateral pterygoid lamina

Internal jugular vein
Internal carotid art.

Buccinator

Tonsil

Superior Constrictor

Ascending palatine vessels

576 Auditory Tube (Pharyngo-tympanic Tube), lateral view
(Tensor Palati is removed.)

Note:

1. The tonsil, here bulging through Sup. Constrictor.
2. The cartilaginous part of the tube resting on a spine on the medial pterygoid lamina; the membranous part "resting on" Levator Palati.
3. Tube, Levator, and vessels crossing the upper border of Sup. Constrictor.
4. Emissary veins in the foramen ovale; and a vein connecting the maxillary and facial veins.

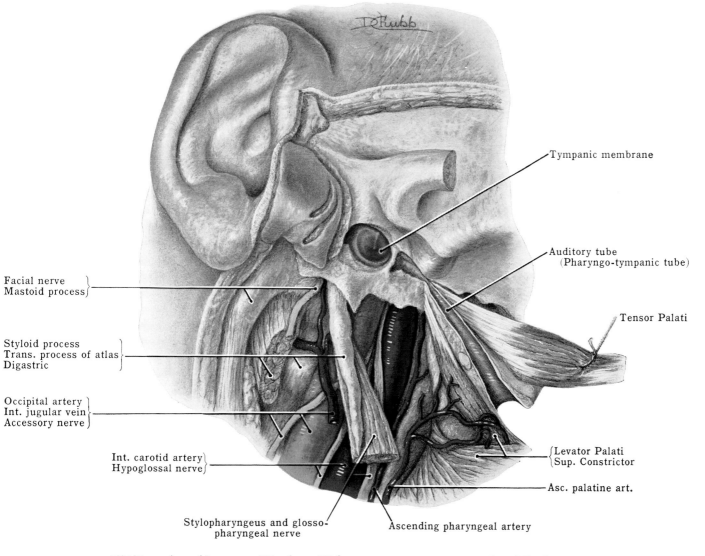

Facial nerve
Mastoid process

Styloid process
Trans. process of atlas
Digastric

Occipital artery
Int. jugular vein
Accessory nerve

Int. carotid artery
Hypoglossal nerve

Stylopharyngeus and glossopharyngeal nerve

Tympanic membrane

Auditory tube
(Pharyngo-tympanic tube)

Tensor Palati

Levator Palati
Sup. Constrictor

Asc. palatine art.

Ascending pharyngeal artery

577   Auditory Tube (Pharyngo-tympanic Tube)

Note:

1. The anterior wall of the cartilaginous part of the external acoustic meatus has two fissures—
two unchondrified areas—which are closed with fibrous tissue.

2. The anterior wall of the bony part of the meatus has been ground away.

3. The tympanic membrane lies at the bottom of the meatus. It faces laterally, downwards,
and forwards as though to catch sounds reflected from the ground, as one advances. The
central part of the membrane is in-drawn (towards the tympanic cavity), the umbo or
bottom of the concavity being at the end of the handle of the malleus. The peripheral part
of the membrane is thickened at its attachment to the tympanic bone.

4. The auditory tube has been opened from pharyngeal end to tympanic end by excising its
lateral membranous wall, but Tensor Palati, which arises in part from the tube, was first
reflected. The tympanic segment of the tube is short and bony; the pharyngeal segment is
long and cartilaginous. The two segments meet at an angle, and there the tube is narrowest.
The lateral wall of the pharyngeal or cartilaginous segment of the tube is, in reality, fibrous;
this wall has been excised.

5. The ascending palatine branch of the facial artery ascends on the outer surface of Superior
Constrictor to its free upper border and then descends on its medial surface with Levator
Palati.

6. The last 4 cranial nerves are close together between the internal jugular vein and the internal carotid artery. The vagus, however, is concealed by the hypoglossal nerve.

7. In this specimen, the stylo-mastoid artery (not labelled), which accompanies the facial
nerve, springs from the occipital artery—not the posterior auricular artery as in figure 550.

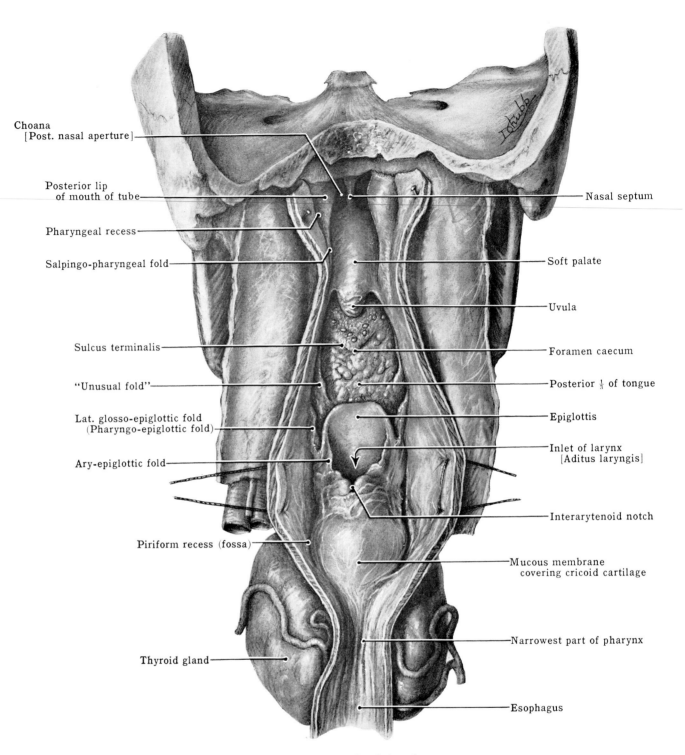

Choana
[Post. nasal aperture]

Posterior lip
of mouth of tube

Pharyngeal recess

Salpingo-pharyngeal fold

Sulcus terminalis

"Unusual fold"

Lat. glosso-epiglottic fold
(Pharyngo-epiglottic fold)

Ary-epiglottic fold

Piriform recess (fossa)

Thyroid gland

Nasal septum

Soft palate

Uvula

Foramen caecum

Posterior $\frac{1}{3}$ of tongue

Epiglottis

Inlet of larynx
[Aditus laryngis]

Interarytenoid notch

Mucous membrane
covering cricoid cartilage

Narrowest part of pharynx

Esophagus

578 Interior of the Pharynx, from behind

Observe:

1. The pharynx extending from the base of the skull to the lower border of the cricoid cartilage where it narrows to become the esophagus.

2. The soft palate ending postero-inferiorly in the uvula, and the larynx ending above at the tip of the epiglottis.

3. The 3 parts of the pharynx—nasal, oral, laryngeal.

4. The nasal part (naso-pharynx) lying above the level of the soft palate and continuous in front, through the choanae, with the nasal cavities.

5. The oral part, lying between the levels of the soft palate and

larynx, communicating in front with the oral cavity, and having the posterior $\frac{1}{3}$ of the tongue as its anterior wall. This part of the tongue is studded with lymph follicles (collectively called the lingual tonsil), and is demarcated from the anterior $\frac{2}{3}$ by the foramen caecum and the V-shaped sulcus terminalis.

6. The laryngeal part lying behind the larynx, and communicating with the cavity of the larynx through the oblique inlet or aditus. On each side of the inlet and separated from it by the ary-epiglottic fold is a piriform recess—the leader pointing to the recess is here too low.

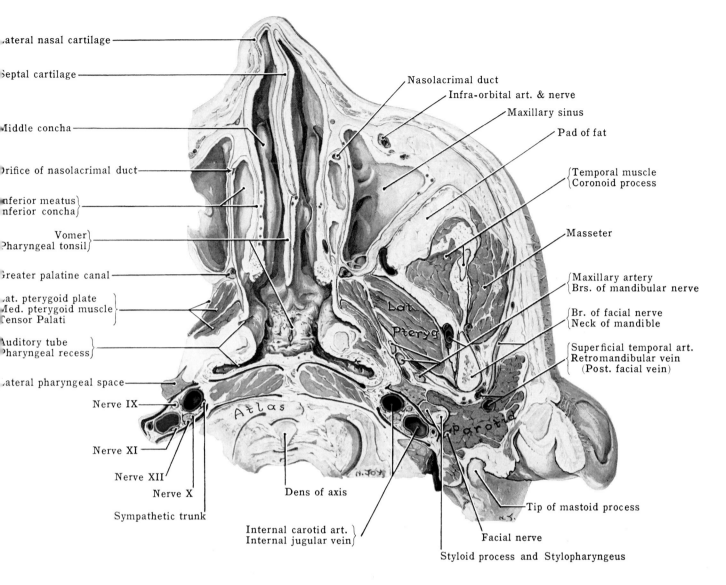

Lateral nasal cartilage

Septal cartilage

Middle concha

Orifice of nasolacrimal duct

Inferior meatus
Inferior concha

Vomer
Pharyngeal tonsil

Greater palatine canal

Lat. pterygoid plate
Med. pterygoid muscle
Tensor Palati

Auditory tube
Pharyngeal recess

Lateral pharyngeal space

Nerve IX

Nerve XI

Nerve XII

Nerve X

Sympathetic trunk

Nasolacrimal duct

Infra-orbital art. & nerve

Maxillary sinus

Pad of fat

Temporal muscle
Coronoid process

Masseter

Maxillary artery
Brs. of mandibular nerve

Br. of facial nerve
Neck of mandible

Superficial temporal art.
Retromandibular vein
(Post. facial vein)

Lat. Pteryg

Atlas

Parotid

Dens of axis

Tip of mastoid process

Internal carotid art.
Internal jugular vein

Facial nerve

Styloid process and Stylopharyngeus

579   Cross Section of Face and Neck, through the Nasal Cavities, viewed from below

Observe:

1. The septal cartilage continuous with the lateral nasal cartilages.
2. An unusual spur from the nasal septum pushing into the middle concha.
3. The pharyngeal tonsil somewhat overgrown (adenoids).
4. The nasolacrimal duct within the mucous membrane of the inferior meatus on one side, and its orifice on the other side.
5. The posterior ends of the inferior conchae, overgrown.
6. The pharyngeal recess spreading widely behind the mouth of the tube.
7. The mucous membrane of one maxillary sinus much thickened. The infra-orbital nerve and artery in front; the greater palatine nerve and artery behind.
8. The carotid sheath at the base of the skull, postero-lateral

to the pharynx, containing the internal carotid, the internal jugular, and 5 nerves (fig. 573).

9. Around the temporal muscle, fatty tissue which is continuous with the buccal pad of fat.
10. Lateral Pterygoid passing obliquely from the medial wall (lat. pterygoid plate) of the infratemporal fossa to the lateral wall (neck of jaw).
11. The parotid gland, its deep relations, the facial nerve largely deep to it.
12. The lateral pharyngeal fatty-areolar "space" (pale green) having the pharynx medially, the carotid sheath posteriorly, the styloid process and its 3 muscles (one at this high level) laterally, branches of the mandibular nerve in a fascial septum anteriorly, and separated from the pharyngeal process of the parotid gland by the stylomandibular lig. (not labelled).

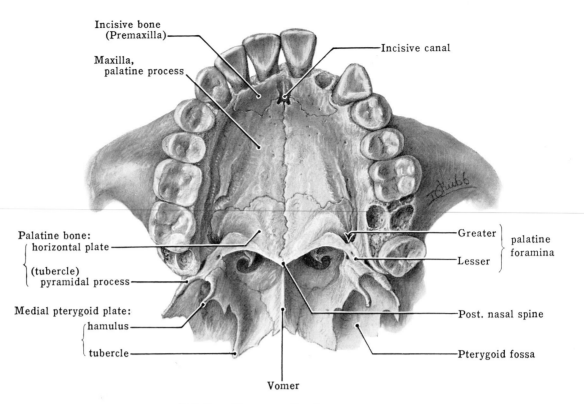

Incisive bone (Premaxilla)

Incisive canal

Maxilla, palatine process

Palatine bone:
  horizontal plate

  (tubercle)
  pyramidal process

Medial pterygoid plate:
  hamulus

  tubercle

Vomer

Greater ⎫ palatine
Lesser ⎭ foramina

Post. nasal spine

Pterygoid fossa

580 Bony Palate—I

(See also figure 570)

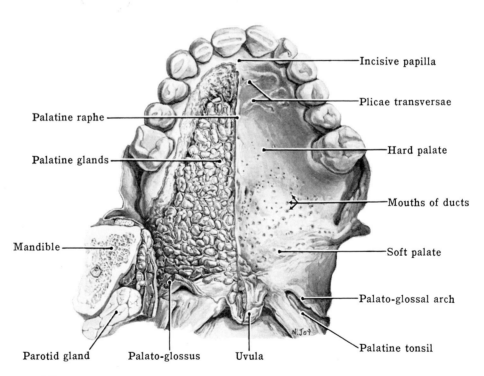

Palatine raphe

Palatine glands

Mandible

Parotid gland

Palato-glossus

Uvula

Incisive papilla

Plicae transversae

Hard palate

Mouths of ducts

Soft palate

Palato-glossal arch

Palatine tonsil

581 Palate—II

Observe:

1. On the right side of the page—the transverse palatine folds, which are so conspicuous in the dog; and the orifices of the ducts of the palatine glands which give the mucous membrane an orange-skin appearance.

2. On the left side—the palatine glands, forming a very thick layer in the soft palate; a thin one in the hard palate; and absent in the region of the incisive bone and anterior part of the median raphe.

3. Posteriorly, the palate ending medially in the uvula, and on each side in the palato-pharyngeal arch. The Palato-glossus and the palato-glossal arch extending to the under surface of the soft palate.

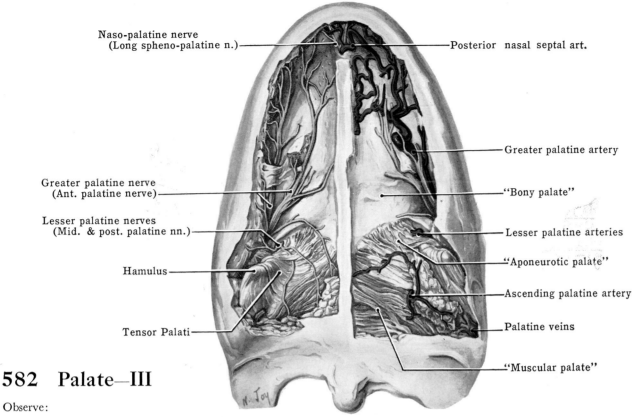

Naso-palatine nerve
(Long spheno-palatine n.)

Posterior nasal septal art.

Greater palatine artery

Greater palatine nerve
(Ant. palatine nerve)

"Bony palate"

Lesser palatine nerves
(Mid. & post. palatine nn.)

Lesser palatine arteries

"Aponeurotic palate"

Hamulus

Ascending palatine artery

Palatine veins

Tensor Palati

"Muscular palate"

582   Palate—III

Observe:

1. The palate in this edentulous specimen having bony, aponeurotic, and muscular parts.
2. Tensor Palati hooking round the hamulus to join the palatine aponeurosis.
3. Septa descending from the aponeurosis to enclose the palatine glands.
4. A crest on the bony palate, having a branch of the greater palatine nerve on each side and the artery on the lateral side. (Commonly the artery follows closely the pattern of the nerve.)

5. The lateral branch of the nerve expended mainly on the gums; the medial branch on the hard palate; the naso-palatine nerve in the incisive region; and the lesser palatine nerves in the soft palate.
6. Four palatine arteries, 2 being on the hard palate and 2 on the soft: (a) the greater palatine artery which anastomoses through the incisive canal with (b) the posterior septal artery (fig. 607), (c) lesser palatine arteries, and (d) the ascending palatine artery (fig. 577) which enters the soft palate with Levator Palati.

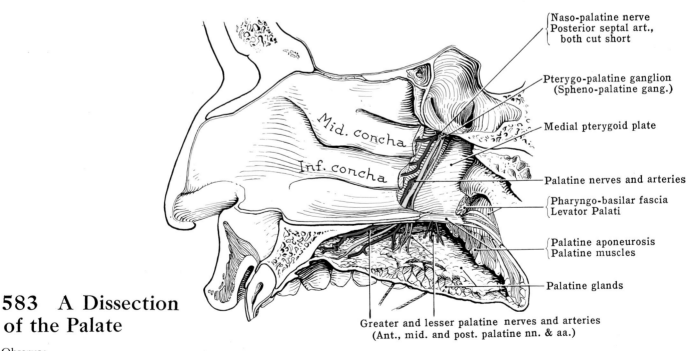

Naso-palatine nerve
Posterior septal art.,
both cut short

Pterygo-palatine ganglion
(Spheno-palatine gang.)

Mid. concha

Medial pterygoid plate

Inf. concha

Palatine nerves and arteries

Pharyngo-basilar fascia
Levator Palati

Palatine aponeurosis
Palatine muscles

Palatine glands

Greater and lesser palatine nerves and arteries
(Ant., mid. and post. palatine nn. & aa.)

583   A Dissection of the Palate

Observe:

1. From before backwards the basis of the palate is—bony, aponeurotic, muscular.
2. From this basis the mucous membrane, containing a layer of mucous glands has been separated by blunt dissection. The layer of glands is thin on the bony palate where it is part of a muco-periosteum; it is very thick on the aponeu-

rotic part; but it is less thick on the muscular part (fig. 587).

3. The posterior ends ($\frac{1}{3}$") of the middle and inferior conchae are cut through; these and the muco-periosteum are peeled off the side wall of the nose as far as the posterior border of the medial pterygoid plate. The papery perpendicular plate of the palatine bone is broken through and the palatine nerves and arteries are thereby exposed.

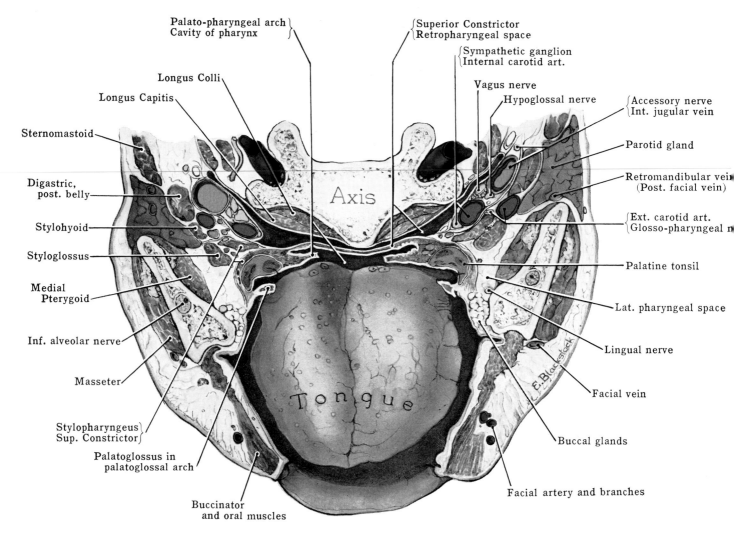

Palato-pharyngeal arch ⎱
Cavity of pharynx ⎰

⎰ Superior Constrictor
⎱ Retropharyngeal space

⎰ Sympathetic ganglion
⎱ Internal carotid art.

Vagus nerve

Hypoglossal nerve

⎰ Accessory nerve
⎱ Int. jugular vein

Longus Colli

Longus Capitis

Sternomastoid

Parotid gland

Retromandibular vein
(Post. facial vein)

Digastric,
post. belly

⎰ Ext. carotid art.
⎱ Glosso-pharyngeal n

Stylohyoid

Styloglossus

Palatine tonsil

Medial
Pterygoid

Lat. pharyngeal space

Inf. alveolar nerve

Lingual nerve

Masseter

Facial vein

Stylopharyngeus ⎱
Sup. Constrictor ⎰

Buccal glands

Palatoglossus in
palatoglossal arch

Facial artery and branches

Buccinator
and oral muscles

Axis

Tongue

E. Blackstock

584 Transverse Section of the Head, passing through the mouth, from the specimen used in figure 494

Observe:

1. The parotid gland filling its wedge-shaped bed or mould; the Digastric and Stylohyoid intervening between the parotid gland and the great vessels and nerves of the neck.

2. The Masseter inserted into one surface of the ramus of the jaw and the Medial Pterygoid inserted into the other.

3. The lingual nerve in contact with the ramus of the jaw.

4. Anterior to the ribbon-like Palatoglossus and its arch is the mouth; behind it is the pharynx.

5. The pharynx flattened antero-posteriorly, and the tonsil in its wall.

6. The tonsil bed formed by Superior Constrictor and Palatopharyngeus, an areolar space intervening, and limited in front and behind by the palatine arches. The carotid arteries well behind the bed.

7. The retropharyngeal space, here opened up, which allows the pharynx to contract and relax during swallowing. It is closed laterally at the carotid sheath and is limited posteriorly by the prevertebral fascia.

8. The three styloid muscles, viz., Stylohyoid, Styloglossus, and Stylopharyngeus; Stylopharyngeus being deepest and about to blend with Palatopharyngeus (Fig. 589).

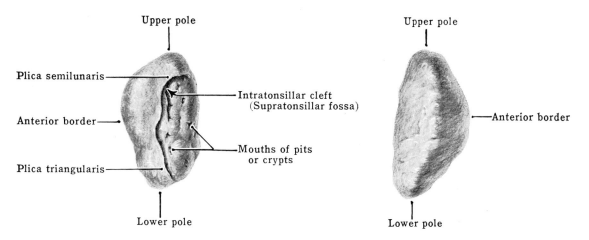

Upper pole

Plica semilunaris

Intratonsillar cleft
(Supratonsillar fossa)

Anterior border

Mouths of pits
or crypts

Plica triangularis

Lower pole

Upper pole

Anterior border

Lower pole

585 Palatine Tonsil ("The Tonsil"), medial and lateral views

Observe:

1. The long axis running vertically.
2. The fibrous capsule forming the lateral or attached surface of the tonsil. In removing the tonsil, the loose areolar tissue lying between the capsule and the thin pharyngobasilar fascia, which forms the immediate bed of the tonsil, was easily torn through.
3. The capsule extending round the anterior border and

slightly over the medial surface as a thin, free fold which was covered with mucous membrane on both surfaces. The upper part of this fold is called the plica semilunaris; the lower, the plica triangularis.

4. On the medial or free surface, the dozen stellate orifices of the testtube-like crypts that extend right through the organ to the capsule. The intratonsillar cleft that extends towards the upper pole.

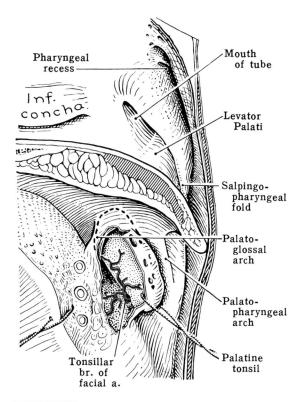

Pharyngeal recess

Inf. concha

Mouth of tube

Levator Palati

Salpingo-pharyngeal fold

Palato-glossal arch

Palato-pharyngeal arch

Palatine tonsil

Tonsillar br. of facial a.

FIRST STAGE

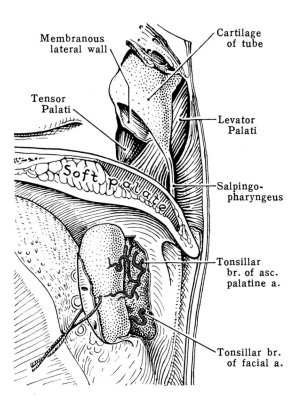

Membranous lateral wall

Cartilage of tube

Tensor Palati

Levator Palati

Salpingo-pharyngeus

Tonsillar br. of asc. palatine a.

Tonsillar br. of facial a.

SECOND STAGE

586 Removal of the Tonsil. The Arterial Supply

(*Dissections by Dr. P. G. Ashmore.*)

The mucous membrane has been incised along the palatoglossal arch, and the areolar space lateral to the fibrous capsule of the tonsil has been entered.

With the point and the rounded handle of the knife, the anterior border of the tonsil has been freed and the upper part, which extends far into the palate, has been shelled out. The mucous membrane along the palatopharyngeal arch is now cut through.

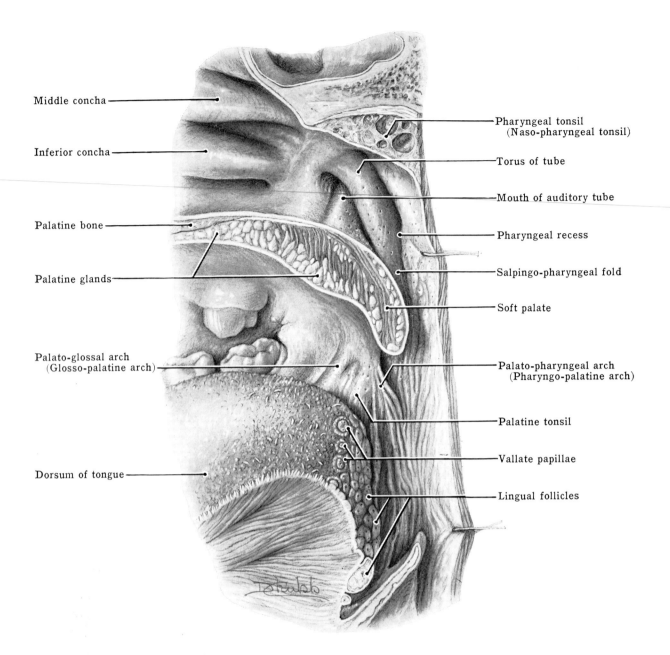

Middle concha

Inferior concha

Palatine bone

Palatine glands

Palato-glossal arch
(Glosso-palatine arch)

Dorsum of tongue

Pharyngeal tonsil
(Naso-pharyngeal tonsil)

Torus of tube

Mouth of auditory tube

Pharyngeal recess

Salpingo-pharyngeal fold

Soft palate

Palato-pharyngeal arch
(Pharyngo-palatine arch)

Palatine tonsil

Vallate papillae

Lingual follicles

587 Interior of the Pharynx, side view—I

Observe:

1. The numerous pinpoint orifices of the ducts of mucous glands.
2. The prominent torus (superior and posterior lips) of the auditory tube and the salpingo-pharyngeal fold that descends from the torus.
3. The location of the orifice of the tube—about $\frac{1}{2}''$ behind the inferior concha.
4. The ridge or torus produced by Levator Palati which has the appearance of being poured out of the tube.
5. The deep pharyngeal recess behind the torus of the tube.

6. The pharyngeal tonsil, better seen in figure 579 where deep clefts extend into the lymphoid tissue.
7. The considerable proportion of glandular tissue in the soft palate and its disposition.
8. The palato-glossal and the palato-pharyngeal arches which, in this specimen are not the sharp folds commonly seen, and the somewhat inconspicuous palatine tonsil between them.
9. The lingual follicles, each with the duct of a mucous gland opening on to its surface. Collectively, the follicles are known as the lingual tonsil.

Mouth of auditory tube

Tensor Palati

Ascending palatine art.

Palato-glossus
(Glosso-palatinus)

Paratonsillar vein
Tonsillar branch
of facial artery

Tongue retracted

Cartilage of tube

Pharyngo-basilar fascia

Levator Palati

Salpingo-pharyngeus

Musculus Uvulae

Palato-pharyngeus
(Pharyngo-palatinus)

Superior Constrictor

Middle Constrictor

Axis

C.3

588   Interior of the Pharynx dissected, side view—II

The palatine and pharyngeal tonsils and the mucous membrane are removed. The submucous pharyngo-basilar fascia, which attaches the pharynx to the basilar part of the occipital bone, is thick above and thin below. It too has been removed, except at the upper arched border of Superior Constrictor.

Observe:

1. The curved cartilage of the auditory tube; its free, upper and posterior lips at the pharyngeal orifice of the tube; and Salpingo-pharyngeus descending from the posterior lip to join Palato-pharyngeus.

2. The ascending palatine branch of the facial artery descending with Levator Palati to the soft palate (fig. 577).

3. The 5 muscles of the palate (paired)—Tensor Palati (see fig. 590), Levator Palati providing most of the muscle fibres seen in the cross section of the soft palate; Musculus Uvulae arising largely from the palatine aponeurosis: Palatoglossus,

here a substantial band, but commonly a wisp of muscle with free anterior and posterior borders; and Palato-pharyngeus, described with figure 589.

4. The tonsil bed from which a thin sheet of pharyngo-basilar fascia has been removed thereby exposing Palato-pharyngeus and Superior Constrictor.

Note: The bed of the palatine tonsil extends far into the soft palate; the tonsillar branch of the facial artery is here long and large; the paratonsillar vein, descending from the soft palate to join the pharyngeal plexus of veins, is a close lateral relation of the tonsil.

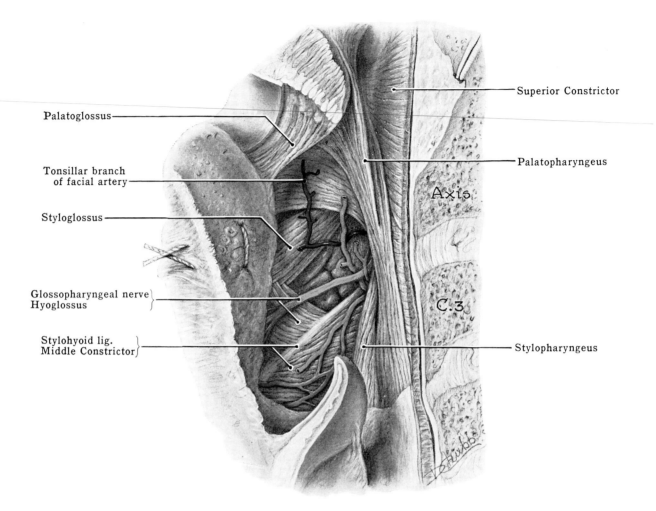

Palatoglossus

Tonsillar branch
of facial artery

Styloglossus

Glossopharyngeal nerve
Hyoglossus

Stylohyoid lig.
Middle Constrictor

Superior Constrictor

Palatopharyngeus

Axis

C.3

Stylopharyngeus

589 Deep Dissection of the Tonsil Bed—III

The tongue is pulled forward and the lower or lingual origin of Superior Constrictor is cut away.

Observe:

1. Styloglossus passing to the anterior ⅔ of the tongue, where its bundles interdigitate with those of Hyoglossus, and therefore anterior to the glossopharyngeal nerve which is passing to the posterior ⅓ of the tongue. This nerve, in turn lying anterior to Stylopharyngeus which descends along the anterior border of Palatopharyngeus.

2. The tonsillar branch of the facial artery, here sending a large branch (cut short) to accompany the glossopharyngeal nerve to the tongue. Lateral to the artery and the para-

tonsillar vein the submandibular salivary gland is seen.

Note: (a) In the region of the tonsil bed, Palatopharyngeus is commonly not well differentiated from Superior Constrictor, which makes it difficult or even arbitrary to decide where the lower border of Palatopharyngeus is. Elsewhere its borders are easily defined.

(b) Palatopharyngeus and Stylopharyngeus forming the longitudinal coat of the pharynx; the Constrictors form the circular coat.

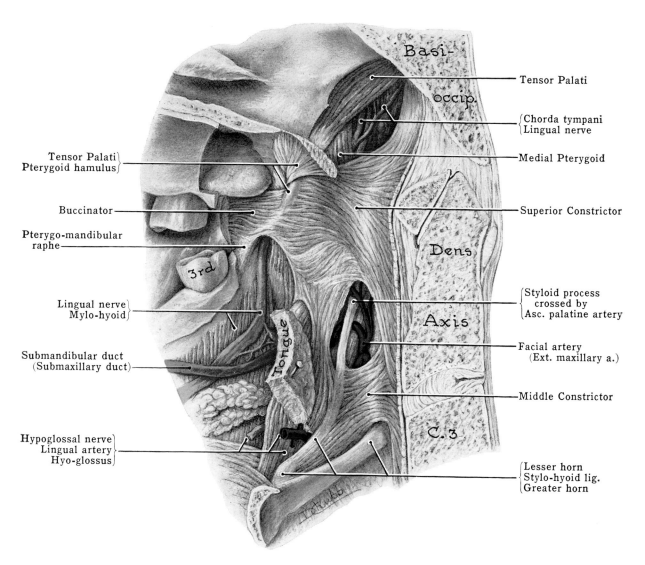

Tensor Palati

Chorda tympani
Lingual nerve

Medial Pterygoid

Superior Constrictor

Styloid process
  crossed by
Asc. palatine artery

Facial artery
  (Ext. maxillary a.)

Middle Constrictor

Lesser horn
Stylo-hyoid lig.
Greater horn

Tensor Palati
Pterygoid hamulus

Buccinator

Pterygo-mandibular
raphe

Lingual nerve
Mylo-hyoid

Submandibular duct
(Submaxillary duct)

Hypoglossal nerve
Lingual artery
Hyo-glossus

Basi-occip.

Dens

Axis

C. 3

Tongue

3rd

590 Superior and Middle Constrictors of the Pharynx, from within—IV

Observe:

1. Superior Constrictor arising from the pterygo-mandibular raphe which unites it to Buccinator, and from the bone at each end of the raphe (viz., the hamulus of the medial pterygoid plate superiorly and the mandible inferiorly) and also from the root of the tongue.

2. The arched upper and lower borders of Superior Constrictor extending to the median plane where the muscle meets its fellow of the opposite side.

3. Middle Constrictor arising from the angle formed by the greater and lesser horns or cornua of the hyoid bone and from the stylohyoid lig. In this specimen, the styloid process is long (fig. 568) and is therefore a lateral relation of the tonsil.

4. The facial artery arching over the posterior belly of Digastric, and the loop of the lingual artery just below it.

5. The tendon of Tensor Palati hooking around the hamulus and then ascending to blend with the palatine aponeurosis, i.e., it takes a recurrent course.

6. The lingual nerve joined by the chorda tympani, disappearing at the posterior border of Medial Pterygoid, reappearing at the anterior border, and applied to the mandible.

Superior sagittal sinus

Skin
Subcutaneous tissue
Galea aponeurotica
[Epicranial aponeurosis]

Subaponeurotic space

Pericranium

Diploe

Dura mater

Auricularis Anterior

Greater wing
of sphenoid

Temporal fascia

Temporalis

Zygoma

Masseter

(Ant.) Facial vein

Vestibule of mouth

Buccinator

Inferior alveolar
nerve and artery

591 Coronal Section of the Head

(For legend see figure 592.)

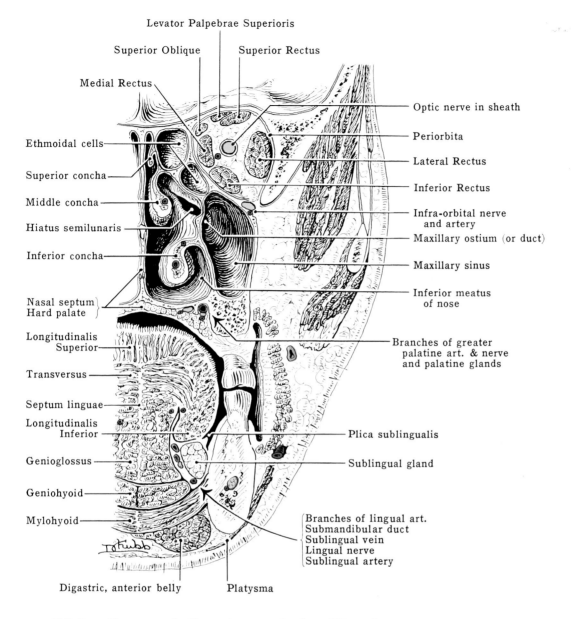

Levator Palpebrae Superioris

Superior Oblique

Superior Rectus

Medial Rectus

Ethmoidal cells

Superior concha

Middle concha

Hiatus semilunaris

Inferior concha

Nasal septum
Hard palate

Longitudinalis Superior

Transversus

Septum linguae

Longitudinalis Inferior

Genioglossus

Geniohyoid

Mylohyoid

Optic nerve in sheath

Periorbita

Lateral Rectus

Inferior Rectus

Infra-orbital nerve and artery

Maxillary ostium (or duct)

Maxillary sinus

Inferior meatus of nose

Branches of greater palatine art. & nerve and palatine glands

Plica sublingualis

Sublingual gland

Branches of lingual art.
Submandibular duct
Sublingual vein
Lingual nerve
Sublingual artery

Digastric, anterior belly   Platysma

592   Coronal Section of the Head

Observe:

1. By reference to figure 521, that the section passes through the optic nerve and therefore through the posterior half of the orbital cavity.
2. The subarachnoid space between the optic nerve and its sheath; the orbital fat, the surrounding muscles, and the easily detachable periorbita.
3. The nasal cavity wide at the floor, but very narrow at the roof.
4. The middle concha sheltering the hiatus semilunaris into which the maxillary ostium opens.
5. The layer of glands in the mucoperiosteum of the palate; the vessels and nerves deep to the glands.
6. The median or sucking groove on the tongue which becomes deeper on forceful sucking, as may be tested with one's finger.
7. How in chewing, the tongue pushes food between the molar or millstone teeth into the vestibule and the Buccinator pushes it back again.
8. The hairs of the beard extending through the skin into the fat of the cheek and chin.

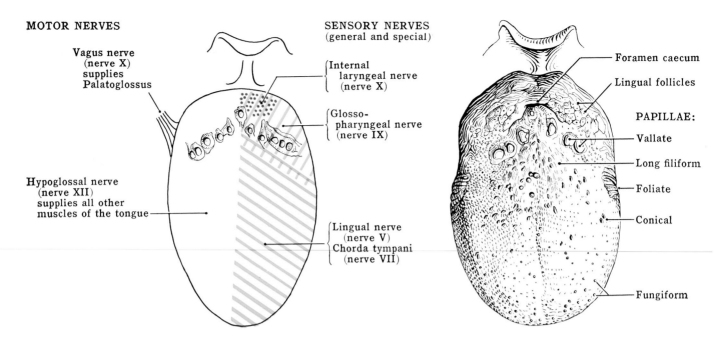

MOTOR NERVES

Vagus nerve
(nerve X)
supplies
Palatoglossus

Hypoglossal nerve
(nerve XII)
supplies all other
muscles of the tongue

SENSORY NERVES
(general and special)

Internal
laryngeal nerve
(nerve X)

Glosso-
pharyngeal nerve
(nerve IX)

Lingual nerve
(nerve V)
Chorda tympani
(nerve VII)

Foramen caecum

Lingual follicles

PAPILLAE:

Vallate

Long filiform

Foliate

Conical

Fungiform

593 Diagram of the Nerve Supply of the Tongue

594 Dorsum of the Tongue

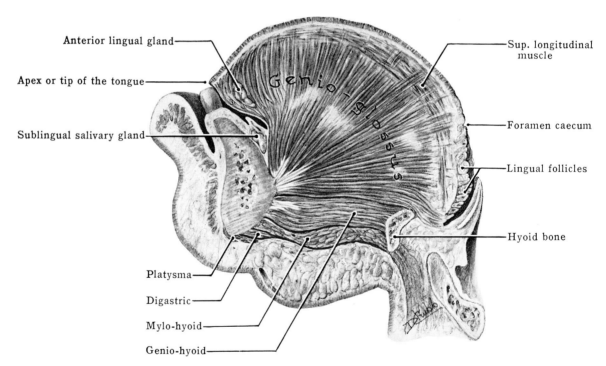

Anterior lingual gland

Apex or tip of the tongue

Sublingual salivary gland

Sup. longitudinal
muscle

Foramen caecum

Lingual follicles

Hyoid bone

Platysma

Digastric

Mylo-hyoid

Genio-hyoid

595 Tongue and Floor of the Mouth, on median section

Observe:

1. The 11 vallate papillae in figure 593 and the 7 in figure 594.

2. In figure 594, the foramen caecum, which is the patent upper end of the primitive thyro-glossal duct, and the limbs of the V-shaped sulcus terminalis, which diverge from the foramen, lie slightly behind the vallate papillae, and demarcate the developmentally different, posterior $\frac{1}{3}$ of the tongue from the anterior $\frac{2}{3}$.

3. The claw-like, conical papillae and the long filiform papillae which are directed postero-medially.

4. In figure 595 parts of the median septum of the tongue which appear as whitish areas. The anterior lingual gland, covered with a layer of muscle. The several ducts of this mixed muco-serous gland open below the tongue, but are not in view.

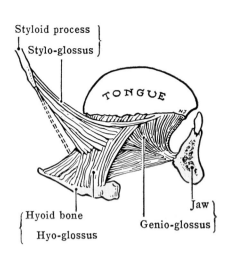

596   Hyoid Bone, showing attachments of muscles

596.1   Diagram of the 3 extrinsic lingual muscles to show their attachments, shapes, and directions.

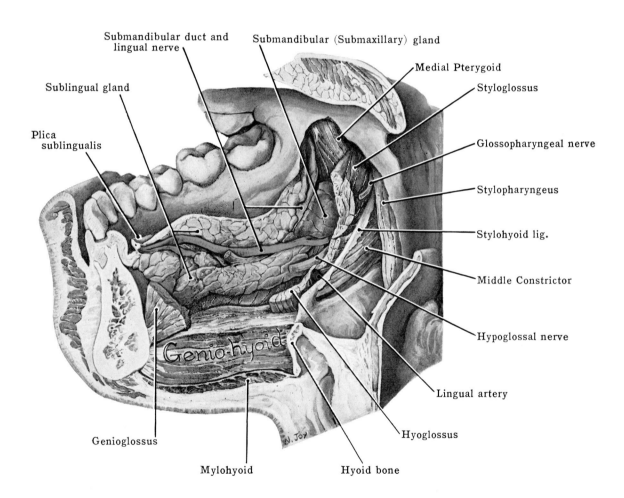

597   Floor and Side of Mouth, from which tongue is excised

Observe:

1. Undisturbed: Geniohyoid inferiorly, Middle Constrictor posteriorly, and the cut edge of the mucous membrane superiorly.

2. Three divided muscles: Genioglossus anteriorly, Hyoglossus inferiorly, and Styloglossus posteriorly.

3. Other 3 divided structures: lingual nerve, hypoglossal nerve, and lingual artery. The lingual nerve appearing between Medial Pterygoid and the ramus of the jaw and making three quarters of a spiral around the submandibular duct, being first superolateral, then in turn lateral, inferior, medial, and supero-medial. The hypoglossal nerve separated from the lingual artery by Hyoglossus.

4. The deep or oral part of the submandibular gland lying in the angle between the lingual nerve and the submandibular duct, which separate it from the sublingual gland. The orifice of the duct is seen at the anterior end of the plica sublingualis.

5. The submandibular duct adhering to the medial side of the sublingual gland, and here receiving, as it sometimes does, a large accessory duct from the lower part of the sublingual gland. For the lesser ducts see figure 547.

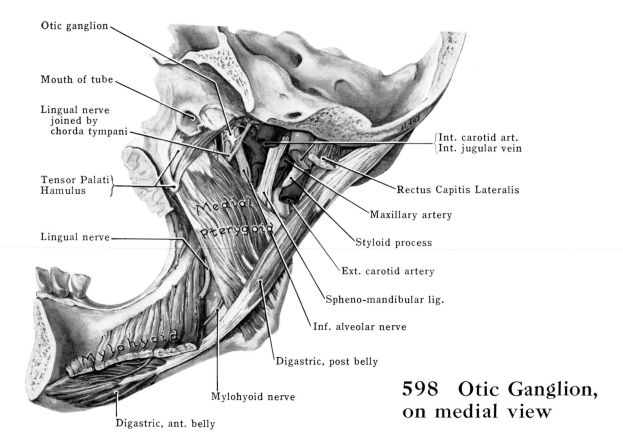

Otic ganglion

Mouth of tube

Lingual nerve
joined by
chorda tympani

Tensor Palati
Hamulus

Lingual nerve

Medial Pterygoid

Mylohyoid

Digastric, ant. belly

Mylohyoid nerve

Digastric, post belly

Mylohyoid nerve

Inf. alveolar nerve

Spheno-mandibular lig.

Ext. carotid artery

Styloid process

Maxillary artery

Rectus Capitis Lateralis

Int. carotid art.
Int. jugular vein

598 Otic Ganglion, on medial view

Observe:

1. Mylohyoid with thick, free, posterior border thinning anteriorly where, below the genial muscles, it must be almost functionless and may be deficient, as here, with resulting thin, free, anterior border.

2. Medial Pterygoid taking much the same direction on the medial side of the ramus as Masseter takes on the lateral.

3. Tensor Palati, here sending some fibres to the hamulus.

4. The lingual nerve, joined above Medial Pterygoid by the chorda tympani and appearing in the mouth at the anterior border of that muscle.

5. The otic ganglion lying medial to the mandibular nerve, and between foramen ovale above and Medial Pterygoid below. Tensor Palati usually covers the ganglion (fig. 659).

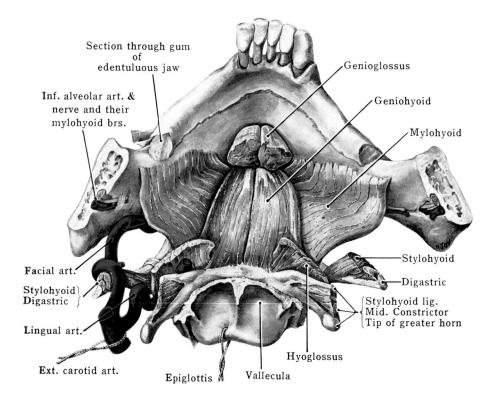

Section through gum
of
edentuluous jaw

Inf. alveolar art. &
nerve and their
mylohyoid brs.

Facial art.

Stylohyoid
Digastric

Lingual art.

Ext. carotid art.

Epiglottis

Vallecula

Hyoglossus

Stylohyoid lig.
Mid. Constrictor
Tip of greater horn

Digastric

Stylohyoid

Mylohyoid

Geniohyoid

Genioglossus

599 Muscles of the Floor of the Mouth

Observe:

1. Geniohyoid, paired, triangular, and occup[ing] a horizontal plane, with apex at the me[n]tal spine, base at the body of the hy[oid] bone, medial border in contact with its f[el]low, and lateral border in contact with M[y]lohyoid.

2. Mylohyoid arising from the mylohyoid li[ne] of the jaw; having a thick, free, poster[ior] border; thinning as it is traced forwards; a[nd] ending in a delicate, free, anterior border [as] it nears the origin of the genial muscles.

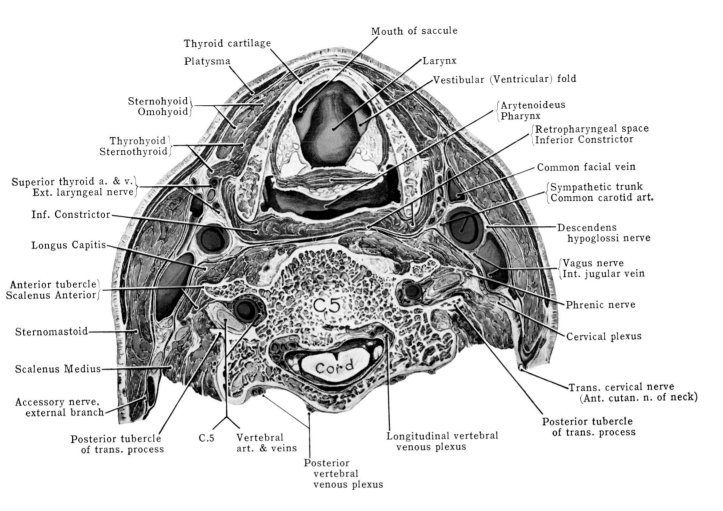

Mouth of saccule

Thyroid cartilage

Platysma

Larynx

Vestibular (Ventricular) fold

Sternohyoid
Omohyoid

{Arytenoideus
Pharynx

{Retropharyngeal space
Inferior Constrictor

Thyrohyoid
Sternothyroid

Common facial vein

Superior thyroid a. & v.
Ext. laryngeal nerve

{Sympathetic trunk
Common carotid art.

Inf. Constrictor

Descendens
hypoglossi nerve

Longus Capitis

{Vagus nerve
Int. jugular vein

Anterior tubercle
Scalenus Anterior

Phrenic nerve

C.5

Sternomastoid

Cervical plexus

Scalenus Medius

Cord

Accessory nerve,
external branch

Trans. cervical nerve
(Ant. cutan. n. of neck)

Posterior tubercle
of trans. process

Posterior tubercle
of trans. process

C.5   Vertebral
art. & veins

Longitudinal vertebral
venous plexus

Posterior
vertebral
venous plexus

600   Cross section of the Neck, through the middle of the Larynx, viewed from below

Observe:

1. The thyroid cartilage shielding the larynx and the pharynx.

2. The vestibular folds, seen from below, and lateral to them the mouths of the saccules of the larynx.

3. Arytenoideus (cut obliquely, hence appearing wide) attached to the posterior surface of the arytenoid cartilage and in continuity with Thyro-arytenoideus (not labelled).

4. Inferior Constrictor, curving round the posterior borders of the laminae of the thyroid cartilage to be attached to the oblique line. Sternothyroid and Thyrohyoid sharing the oblique line.

5. The superior thyroid vessels and the external laryngeal nerve applied to Inferior Constrictor.

6. The 3 contents of the carotid sheath—the common carotid

artery, the internal jugular vein and, in the posterior angle between them, the vagus nerve.

7. The sympathetic trunk, behind the carotid artery and medial to the vagus. The descendens hypoglossi in front of the carotid artery.

8. The retropharyngeal space, between the pharyngeal fascia, which covers Inf. Constrictor, and the prevertebral fascia, which covers Longi Colli et Capitis. This areolar space extending laterally to the carotid sheath and readily opened up beyond it. The phrenic nerve deep to the prevertebral fascia.

9. The vertebral artery, surrounded with a plexus of veins (which inferiorly becomes the vertebral vein) and the ventral ramus of a cervical nerve (C.5) crossing behind it.

10. Internal and external parts of the vertebral venous plexus.

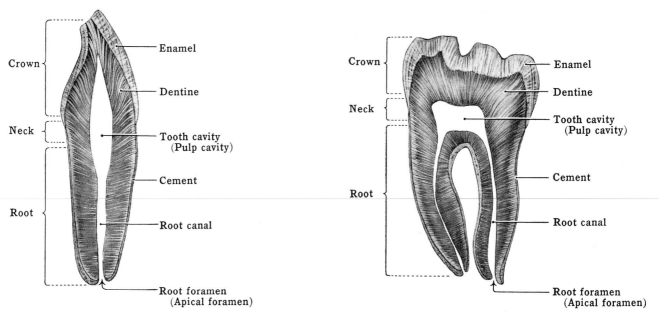

**601 An Incisor Tooth,
longitudinal section**

**601.1 A Molar Tooth,
longitudinal section**

601.2 Permanent Teeth and Their Sockets

Observe:

1. There are 32 permanent teeth, of which 8 are on each side of each dental arch—2 incisors, 1 canine, 2 premolars, and 3 molars. Hence the formula reads:

$$\frac{3.2.1.2.}{3.2.1.2.} \quad \frac{2.1.2.3.}{2.1.2.3.}$$

2. Upper or maxillary incisor teeth are larger than lower or mandibular incisor teeth. The upper central incisors are the largest of the incisors and the lower central are the smallest. In each dental arch the 1st molar tooth is usually the largest molar and the 3rd molar is the smallest, though the 3rd lower molar may be very large, as here.

3. Crowns: An incisor tooth has a cutting edge; a canine tooth (cuspid) has one cusp on its crown; a premolar tooth (bicuspid) has 2 (or 3) cusps; and a molar tooth has from 3 to 5 cusps. The crowns of the upper molars are either square or rhomboidal. The 1st usually has 4 cusps; the 2nd either 4 or 3; and the 3rd 3.
The crowns of the lower molars are oblong. The 1st has 5 cusps; the 2nd 4; and the 3rd from 3 to 5. The crowns are, here, well worn.

01.3 Roots of the Permanent Teeth, labial (buccal) view

Their empty sockets are shown in figure 601.2

Their empty sockets are shown in figure 601.2

Observe:

1. Lower or mandibular teeth: The incisor, canine, and premolar (bicuspid) teeth have each one root, whereas the molars have each 2 roots, a mesial (anterior) and a distal (posterior). The mesial roots generally have 2 root canals. The roots are flattened mesiodistally (i.e., from central incisor backwards to the 3rd molar).
    The sockets for the lower incisor teeth are near the labial surface of the mandible, whereas those for the lower molars are near the lingual surface.

2. Upper or maxillary teeth: The incisor and canine teeth have each one root. The premolars have each either one or 2 roots, the first premolar usually having 2, a lingual and a labial, and the second usually having one—though sometimes, as here, both premolars have 2 roots. Each of the 3 molars has 3 roots, one being lingual and 2 being labial (buccal). The roots are flattened mesio-distally, except the root of the central incisor and the lingual root of each of the 3 molars which are circular on cross section.

01.4 Permanent Teeth, in situ, with roots exposed by removal of the lateral alveolar wall

Observe:

1. The upper canine ("eye tooth") has the longest root; indeed, this is the longest tooth.
2. The roots of the upper premolars, in this specimen, are at some distance from the maxillary sinus or antrum, but the roots of the 3 molars almost penetrate into the sinus (see figs. 616 and 616.3).
3. The root of the 2nd lower premolar, very long in this specimen, does not usually extend below the level of the mental foramen.
4. The roots of the 2nd lower molar have been removed, thereby revealing the cribriform nature of the wall of a socket.
5. The upper and lower 3rd molars are not yet fully developed. The lower is more advanced than the upper—the root foramina of the lower are still large; whereas the roots of the upper have not yet formed.

601.5 Permanent Teeth, in occlusion

Observe:

1. The upper and lower teeth begin flush, or nearly so, on one side and end flush on the other.
2. The lower central incisor is the smallest of the incisors, and the 3rd upper molar is the smallest of the molars. Except for these 2 teeth—the first in the lower row and the last in the upper—all teeth, when in occlusion, bite on two opposing teeth.
3. The upper dental arch overlaps the lower dental arch.
4. The lower incisors bite against the lingual surface of the upper incisors (fig. 458) and not edge-to-edge as in prehistoric man. As a variant there may be a considerable overbite (fig. 601.4).

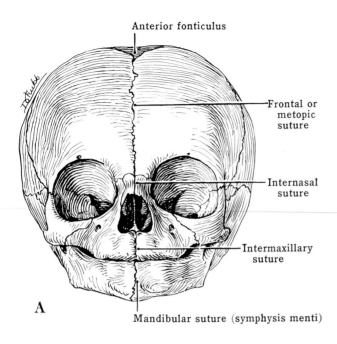

Anterior fonticulus

Frontal or metopic suture

Internasal suture

Intermaxillary suture

Mandibular suture (symphysis menti)

A

D Mandible at Birth, from above

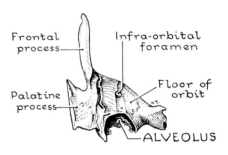

Frontal process

Infra-orbital foramen

Palatine process

Floor of orbit

ALVEOLUS

E Maxilla at Birth, posterior view

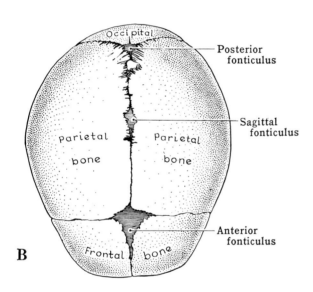

Occipital

Posterior fonticulus

Parietal bone

Parietal bone

Sagittal fonticulus

Anterior fonticulus

Frontal bone

B

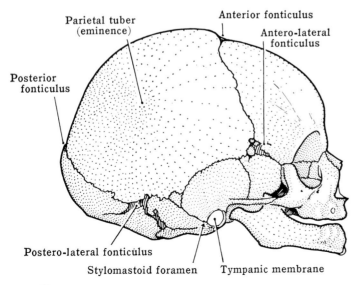

Parietal tuber (eminence)

Anterior fonticulus

Antero-lateral fonticulus

Posterior fonticulus

Postero-lateral fonticulus

Stylomastoid foramen

Tympanic membrane

C

602 Skull, Mandible, and Maxilla at Birth

Note:

1. The teeth have not erupted; hence, the air sinuses are rudimentary, the maxilla and mandible are small, the angle of the mandible is obtuse and so the ramus and body of the mandible are nearly in line. The orbital cavities are large and round but the nasal cavities are not deep. The face is indeed small.

2. The mandibular suture and the frontal suture, which close during the 2nd year, are still open.

3. The tuber of the parietal bone—like that of the frontal bone—is conical. Ossification, which starts at the tubers and spreads in centrifugal waves, has not yet reached the four angles of the parietal bone. Accordingly, these are still membranous and the membrane is blended with the pericranium externally and dura mater internally to form the fonticuli. Of the fonticuli, the anterior and largest closes during the 2nd year. It is shaped like a flat kite, the long angle and tail tapering between the two halves of the frontal bone.

4. There being no mastoid process until the 2nd year, the stylomastoid foramen, which transmits the facial nerve, opens beneath the surface of the skin. The external acoustic meatus having no length, the tympanic membrane is close to the surface of the skull.

5. The maxillary antrum or sinus being very small, the floor of the orbital cavity is also the "ceiling" of the alveolus in which the rudimentary primary molar teeth lie.

6. Each half of the mandible has 5 sockets or alveoli for 5 primary teeth. The course of the inferior alveolar nerve is indicated, but the branch to the canine and incisor teeth is not shown.

2nd molar   1st molar   canine   lateral incisor   central incisor

602.1 Primary Teeth

There are 20 primary, deciduous, temporary, or milk teeth, 5 being in each half of the mandible and 5 in each maxilla. They are named: central incisor, lateral incisor, canine, 1st molar, and 2nd molar. The formula reads

$$\frac{2.1.2.}{2.1.2.} \quad \frac{2.1.2.}{2.1.2.}$$

Of these 20 primary teeth the first to erupt through the gums are the lower central incisors, about the 7th month, and the last to erupt are the 2nd upper molars, about the end of the 2nd year. The 3 roots of the upper or maxillary molars and the 2 roots of the lower or mandibular molars are spread to grasp the developing Permanent Premolars (fig. 604).

M 1

m 2

Socket for m 1

canine

central and lateral incisors

canine

m 1

m 2

M 1

M 2

602.2 Primary Dentition, aged under 2 years

The anterior fonticulus has disappeared. Only traces of the frontal and mandibular sutures remain.

(The Permanent Teeth are colored yellow.)

Observe:

1. The canines have not fully erupted, the 2nd molars have just started to erupt—the sequence of eruption being incisors, 1st molars, canines, 2nd molars.
2. The 2nd molars have much larger crowns than the 1st molars.
3. The socket for the 3-pronged root of the 1st upper molar is seen.
4. The foramina, seen on the lingual side of the primary incisors, lead to the alveoli for the Permanent Incisors.
5. The crowns of the unerupted 1st and 2nd Permanent Molars are partly visible.

Aged 6 to 7 years **Aged 8 years** **Aged 12 years**

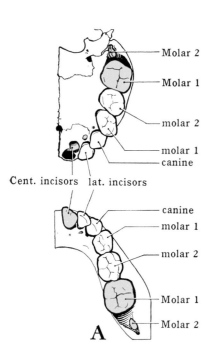

A

- Molar 2
- Molar 1
- molar 2
- molar 1
- canine

Cent. incisors lat. incisors

- canine
- molar 1
- molar 2
- Molar 1
- Molar 2

B

- M 3
- M 2
- M 1
- m 2
- m 1
- canine

Incisors

- canine
- m 1
- m 2
- M 1
- M 2
- M 3

C

- M 3
- M 2
- M 1
- Pm 2
- Pm 1
- C

I 1 I 2

- C
- Pm 1
- Pm 2
- M 1
- M 2
- M 3

603 Progress in the Eruption of Permanent Teeth

Between the 6th and 12th years the primary teeth are shed and are succeeded by Permanent Teeth.

A. The 1st Molars (6th-year Molars) have fully erupted. The primary central incisors have been shed. The Lower Central Incisors have nearly fully erupted and the Upper Central Incisors are moving downwards into the empty sockets.

B. All the Permanent Incisors have erupted, the Upper and Lower Central and the Upper Lateral fully and the Lower Lateral partially. Note that the alveolus has not yet closed around the Upper Lateral Incisors.

(Here, the root of the left lower lateral primary incisor has not been resorbed, so the tooth has not been shed. It needs the aid of a dentist.)

C. The 20 primary teeth have been replaced by 20 Permanent Teeth, and the 1st Molars and the 2nd Molars (12th-year Molars) have erupted. But, the Canines, 2nd Premolars, and 2nd Molars—especially those in the upper jaw—have not erupted fully nor have their bony sockets closed around them.

A

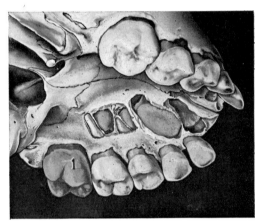

B

604 Mixed Dentition, labial and lingual views

(From the same specimen as fig. 603 A, after the removal of bone.)

The crowns of the Permanent Teeth are fully formed at the time of eruption (i.e., they grow no larger). The Permanent Incisors and Canines develop and erupt on the lingual side of the primary incisors and canines, the Lateral Incisors being the most posterior. Indeed, the Upper Lateral Incisors extend into the bony palate. The Premolar Teeth develop between the spread roots of the primary molars. The Permanent Molars have no predecessors.

C

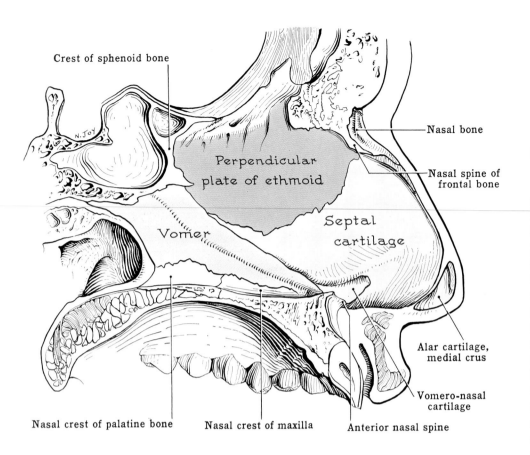

Crest of sphenoid bone

Perpendicular plate of ethmoid

Nasal bone

Nasal spine of frontal bone

Vomer

Septal cartilage

Alar cartilage, medial crus

Vomero-nasal cartilage

Nasal crest of palatine bone

Nasal crest of maxilla

Anterior nasal spine

605 Septum of Nose

Like the palate, the septum of the nose has a hard part and a soft or mobile part. The skeleton or basis of the hard septum consists of 3 parts—perpendicular plate of ethmoid, septal cartilage, vomer—and, around the circumference of these, the adjacent bones (frontal, nasal, maxillary, palatine, and sphenoid) make minor contributions. The mobile septum comprises (a) the medial limbs (crura) of the U-shaped alar cartilages (figs. 468 and 611), and (b) the skin and soft tissues between the tip of the nose and the anterior nasal spine. Behind the vomer, an extension of the muco-periosteum of the septum forms a second, though unimportant, mobile septum.

606 Diagram of the Nerve Supply of the Lateral Wall of the Nose

(See also figures 655 and 656.)

Olfactory bulb

Postero-lateral nasal branches

Anterior ethmoidal nerve

Internal nasal branches

External nasal branch

Nasal branch of ant. superior alveolar nerve

Internal nasal branch of infra-orbital nerve

Naso-palatine nerve

Ridge over maxillary nerve

Ridge over nerve of pterygoid canal

Pharyngeal nerve

Pterygo-palatine ganglion (Spheno-palatine gang.)

Lesser (Mid., Post.)

Greater (Anterior)

palatine nerves

507 Arteries of the Walls of the Nasal Cavity

Observe:

1. Anterior ethmoidal and posterior ethmoidal branches of the ophthalmic a. entering through the cribriform plate. Only these are derived from the internal carotid, all others being from the external carotid.

2. The sphenopalatine a. as the main supply. Entering through the sphenopalatine foramen (fig. 608.1), it sends (a) lateral nasal branches forwards on both surfaces of the conchae, partly in bony canals, and the posterior septal a. which crosses the roof of the nose below the anterior part of the floor of the sphenoidal sinus and anastomoses through the incisive foramen.

3. The facial a. via 3 branches: (a) the septal branch of the superior labial a.; (b) twigs from the lateral nasal a. that pierce the ala to supply the vestibular region; and (c) anastomoses from the ascending palatine a.

Arteries of the Septum.

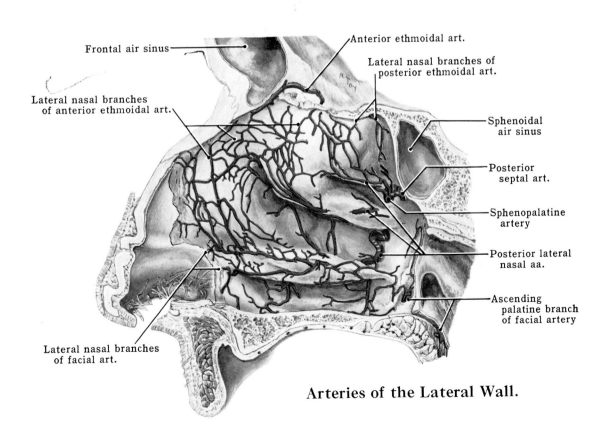

Arteries of the Lateral Wall.

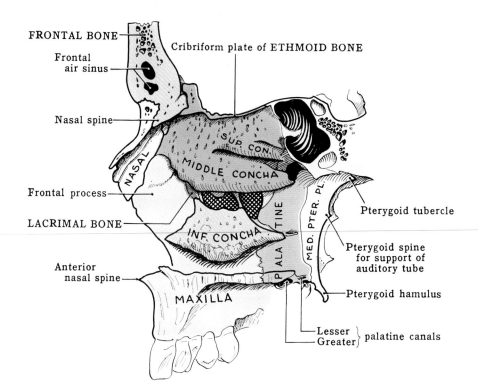

FRONTAL BONE

Frontal air sinus

Nasal spine

Frontal process

LACRIMAL BONE

Anterior nasal spine

Cribriform plate of ETHMOID BONE

SUP CON.

MIDDLE CONCHA

NASAL

INF. CONCHA

PALATINE

MED. PTER. PL.

MAXILLA

Pterygoid tubercle

Pterygoid spine for support of auditory tube

Pterygoid hamulus

Lesser } palatine canals
Greater }

608 Bones of the Lateral Wall of the Nose—I

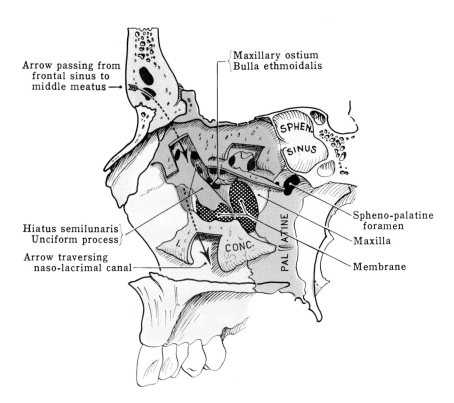

Arrow passing from frontal sinus to middle meatus

Maxillary ostium
Bulla ethmoidalis

SPHEN. SINUS

Hiatus semilunaris }
Unciform process }

Arrow traversing naso-lacrimal canal

I. CONC.

PALATINE

Spheno-palatine foramen

Maxilla

Membrane

608.1 Dissection of the Bones of the Lateral Wall of the Nose—II

Note:

1. The superior and middle conchae are parts of the ethmoid bone, whereas the inferior concha is a bone of itself.

2. The pterygoid process is part of the sphenoid bone. Its medial plate forms the posterior part of the lateral wall of the bony nasal cavity.

3. The fragile, perpendicular plate of the palatine bone has a notch at its upper border, which, when in articulation with the body of the sphenoid bone, forms the spheno-palatine foramen.

4. The groove on the nasal bone is for the external nasal branch of the anterior ethmoidal nerve (fig. 606).

5. The hiatus semilunaris is bounded below by the unciform process of the ethmoid bone. The maxillary ostium opens on to the hiatus. Accessory maxillary ostia may occur in the membrane that closes the maxillary hiatus.

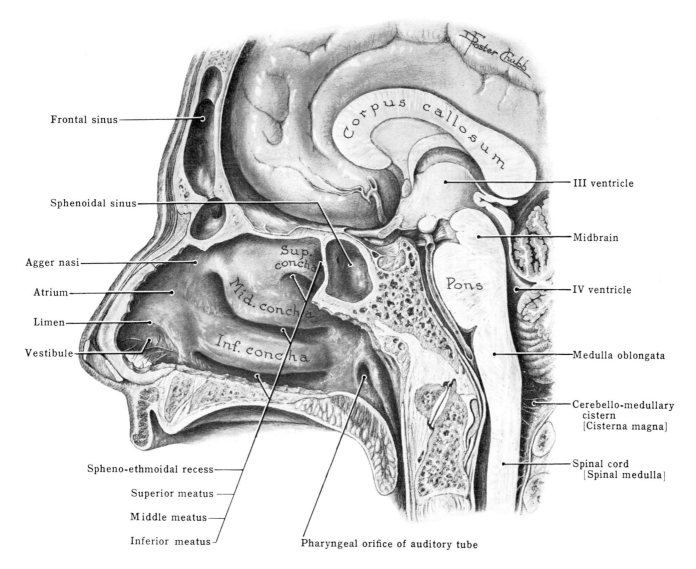

Frontal sinus

Sphenoidal sinus

Agger nasi

Atrium

Limen

Vestibule

Corpus callosum

Sup. concha

Mid. concha

Inf. concha

Pons

III ventricle

Midbrain

IV ventricle

Medulla oblongata

Cerebello-medullary cistern [Cisterna magna]

Spinal cord [Spinal medulla]

Spheno-ethmoidal recess

Superior meatus

Middle meatus

Inferior meatus

Pharyngeal orifice of auditory tube

609   Lateral Wall of the Nose—I

Observe:

1. The vestibule, above the nostril or naris and in front of the inferior meatus. The hairs growing from its skin-lined surface, spreading in all directions.

2. The atrium, above the vestibule and in front of the middle meatus.

3. The inferior and middle conchae, curving downwards and medially from the lateral wall, dividing it into 3 nearly equal parts, and covering the inferior and middle meatuses respectively.

4. The superior concha, small and in front of the sphenoidal sinus. The middle concha, with an angled lower border, ending below the sphenoidal sinus. The inferior concha, with

a slightly curved lower border, ending below the middle concha, $\frac{1}{3}''$ to $\frac{1}{2}''$ in front of the orifice of the tube—i.e., about the width of the medial pterygoid plate (fig. 608).

5. The floor of the nose, inclined slightly downwards and backwards, at the level of the atlas.

6. The roof comprising (a) an anterior sloping part, corresponding to the bridge of the nose; (b) an intermediate horizontal part, formed by the delicate cribriform plate; (c) a perpendicular part in front of the sphenoidal sinus and, (d) a curved part, below the sinus, which is confluent with the roof of the naso-pharynx.

7. The pons and the fourth ventricle at the level of the sphenoidal sinus.

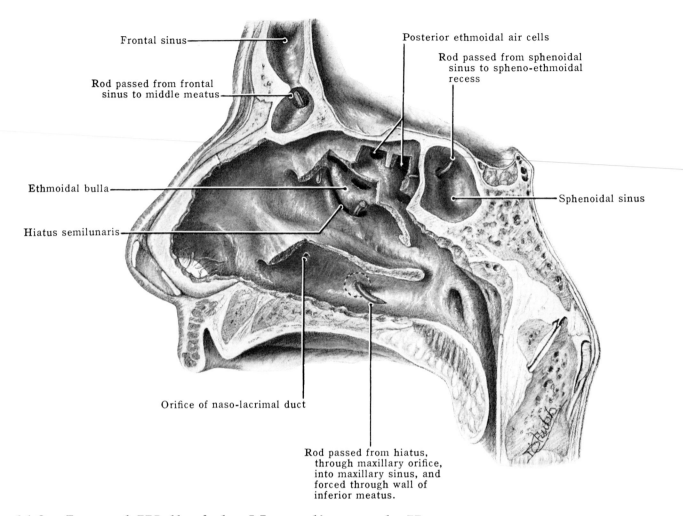

Frontal sinus

Rod passed from frontal
sinus to middle meatus

Ethmoidal bulla

Hiatus semilunaris

Orifice of naso-lacrimal duct

Posterior ethmoidal air cells

Rod passed from sphenoidal
sinus to spheno-ethmoidal
recess

Sphenoidal sinus

Rod passed from hiatus,
through maxillary orifice,
into maxillary sinus, and
forced through wall of
inferior meatus.

610   Lateral Wall of the Nose, dissected—II

Parts of the superior, middle, and inferior conchae are cut away.

Observe:

1. The sphenoidal sinus, in the body of the sphenoid bone; its orifice, above the middle of its anterior wall, opening into the spheno-ethmoidal recess.

2. The orifices of posterior ethmoidal cells opening into the superior meatus.

3. A cell, in this specimen, opening on to the upper surface of the ethmoidal bulla.

4. The attachment of the inferior concha, steep in its anterior $\frac{1}{3}$, but gently sloping in its posterior $\frac{2}{3}$. The orifice of the naso-lacrimal duct, a short (variable) distance below the angle of union of the anterior $\frac{1}{3}$ and posterior $\frac{2}{3}$.

5. The sharp probe forced through the thinnest portion of the medial wall of the maxillary sinus, well above the level of the floor of the nose.

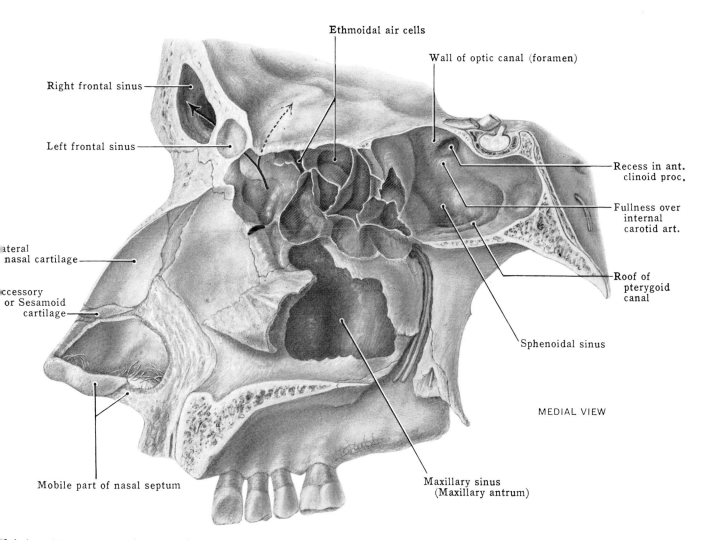

Right frontal sinus

Left frontal sinus

Lateral
nasal cartilage

Accessory
or Sesamoid
cartilage

Mobile part of nasal septum

Ethmoidal air cells

Wall of optic canal (foramen)

Recess in ant.
clinoid proc.

Fullness over
internal
carotid art.

Roof of
pterygoid
canal

Sphenoidal sinus

Maxillary sinus
(Maxillary antrum)

MEDIAL VIEW

511 Paranasal Air Sinuses, opened

Observe:

The ethmoidal cells (pink), collectively called a sinus, like a honey-comb, and having the thin orbital plate of the frontal bone for a roof (figs. 520 & 617).

An anterior ethmoidal cell (blue) invading the diploe of the squama of the frontal bone to become a frontal sinus. It is ethmoidal in origin, but frontal in location. An offshoot (broken arrow) invades the orbital plate of the frontal bone.

The sphenoidal sinus (blue) here, very extensive—compare with figure 610—extending (a) backwards below the hypophysis cerebri to the dorsum sellae, (b) laterally, below the optic nerve, into the anterior clinoid process, and (c) downwards to the pterygoid process, but leaving the pterygoid canal rising as a ridge on the floor of the sinus.

The maxillary sinus (yellow) pyramidal in shape; its base (largely nibbled away), contributing to the lateral wall of the nose; its apex being in the zygomatic process; and its orifice being at its highest point.

R. & L. frontal sinus

L.
maxillary
sinus

FRONT VIEW

611.1

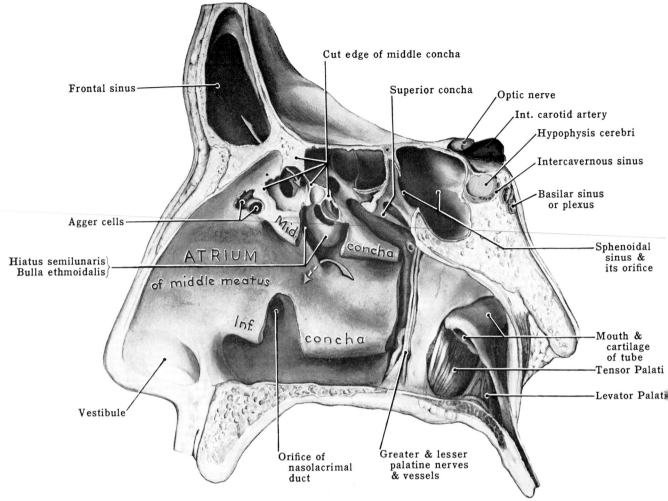

Frontal sinus

Cut edge of middle concha

Superior concha

Optic nerve

Int. carotid artery

Hypophysis cerebri

Intercavernous sinus

Basilar sinus or plexus

Sphenoidal sinus & its orifice

Agger cells

Hiatus semilunaris
Bulla ethmoidalis

ATRIUM

of middle meatus

Mid.

concha

Inf.

concha

Mouth & cartilage of tube

Tensor Palati

Levator Palati

Vestibule

Orifice of nasolacrimal duct

Greater & lesser palatine nerves & vessels

612 Paranasal Air Sinuses

Note:

1. The frontal sinus with its outlet at its lowest point, leading into the middle meatus medial to the hiatus semilunaris. The hiatus ends blindly in front as an anterior ethmoidal cell, and posteriorly as the maxillary orifice, indicated by an arrow.

2. Lateral to the agger nasi, there are 2 agger cells: one is a diverticulum from the frontal sinus; the other from the hiatus.

3. The sphenoidal sinus of average size, and with a very large orifice.

4. A bullar cell with its orifice above.

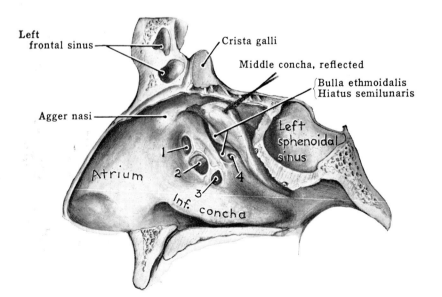

Left frontal sinus

Crista galli

Middle concha, reflected

Bulla ethmoidalis
Hiatus semilunaris

Agger nasi

Atrium

Left sphenoidal sinus

1
2
3
4

Inf. concha

613 Accessory Maxillary Orifices

Note:

1. In addition to the primary or normal ostium (not in view), there are here present 4 secondary or acquired ostia resulting from the breaking down of the membrane shown in cross hatching in figure 608.1.

2. The septum between the right and the left sphenoidal sinus, here occupies the median plane—it is usually deflected to one side or other.

Crista galli — Cribriform plate

LABYRINTH

Nasal cavity — Perpendicular plate

614　Scheme of the Ethmoidal Air Cells, collectively called a sinus

The ethmoidal air cells may be likened to a number of rubber balloons projecting into an oblong box and variously inflated to the full capacity of the box. Indeed, one (occasionally more) of the anterior balloons bursts through the lid of the box (i.e., the roof of the ethmoidal labyrinth) and invades the neighbouring territory (i.e., the frontal bone) to a variable extent and acquires the name "frontal air sinus".

Sphenoidal

Ethmoidal:
Posterior

Anterior

Frontal

Sphenoidal

Ethmoidal:
Posterior

Anterior

Frontal

614.1　Air Sinuses Surrounding the Cribriform Plate, from above

Right frontal sinus

Left frontal sinus

Anterior ethmoidal cell

Posterior ethmoidal cell

Anterior ethmoidal cell

Posterior ethmoidal cell

614.2　Frontal Air Sinuses, from the front

The orifices of the sinuses are at the lowest points of the sinuses.

614.3　Frontal Air Sinuses, from below

The right frontal air sinus is here, as usual, an extension of an anterior ethmoidal cell. The corresponding left cell (blue) is small, but the next cell behind it has invaded the diploe of the frontal bone and so become a frontal sinus.

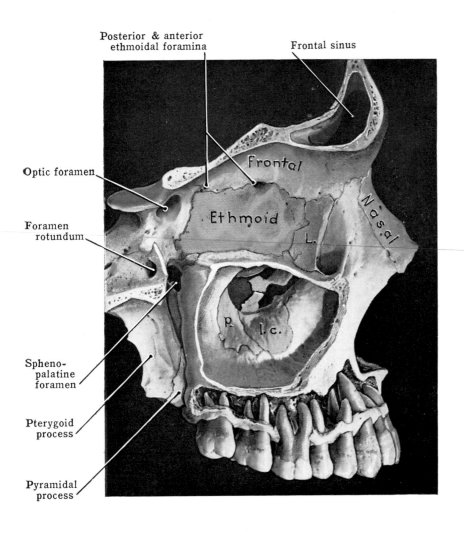

Posterior & anterior
ethmoidal foramina

Frontal sinus

Optic foramen

Foramen
rotundum

Spheno-
palatine
foramen

Pterygoid
process

Pyramidal
process

Frontal

Ethmoid

Nasal

L.

P. I.c.

615 Medial Wall of Orbital Cavity and of Maxillary Sinus

Ic.—inferior concha (green)
L.—lacrimal bone (blue)
P.—palatine bone (yellow)

Note:

1. The site of the hiatus semilunaris between bulla of the ethmoid bone above and the un (= hook-like) process below.

2. The pterygo-palatine fossa between pter process, maxilla, palatine bone, and sph bone. The foramen rotundum opens into the from the middle cranial fossa and the sp palatine foramen opens into the nasal cavity

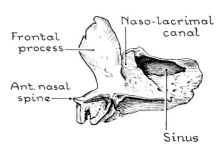

Frontal
process

Naso-lacrimal
canal

Ant. nasal
spine

Sinus

615.1 Maxilla at birth, medial view

Lacrimal sulcus

for ethmoid bone
(red)

for palatine bone
(yellow)

Crest for
middle concha

Frontal process

Crest for
inferior concha

Anterior
nasal spine

Incisive &
nasal crests

Sinus

C   *1*   *2*

Palatine process

Alveolar
process

for palatine
vessels &
nerves

615.2 Medial Aspect of Maxilla

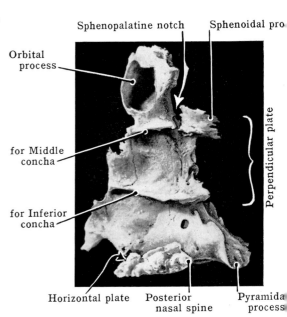

Orbital
process

Sphenopalatine notch

Sphenoidal pro

for Middle
concha

for Inferior
concha

Perpendicular plate

Horizontal plate

Posterior
nasal spine

Pyramida
process

615.3 Medial Aspect of Palatine Bone

Note:

1. The pyramidal process has 2 grooves for the pteryg process.

2. The cell in the orbital process is an extension of eit the maxillary sinus, an ethmoidal cell, or the sphenoi sinus.

616 Maxillary Sinus, left side, lateral view

Note:

The roots of the teeth are, here, at some distance from the sinus.

Contrast this figure with figures 601.4 and 615 where the roots of the teeth come closer to the floor of the bony sinus, and with figure 616.3 where they penetrate it.

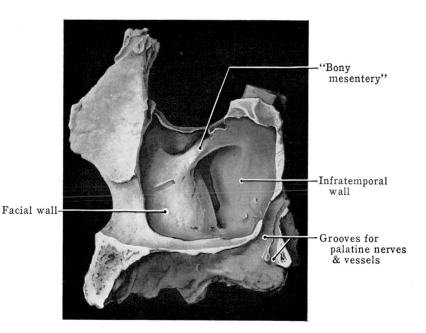

616.1 Maxillary Sinus, medial view

Note:

1. The "bony mesentery" for the infra-orbital nerve and vessels, here, projecting, not from the roof, but from the lateral wall.
2. The anterior or facial wall pushing far into the sinus.
3. The grooves for the greater and lesser palatine nerves.

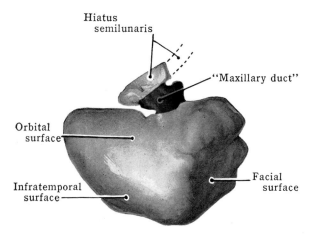

616.2 Cast of the right Maxillary Sinus, lateral view

Note:

The so-called orifice or ostium, which opens into the hiatus semilunaris, is usually a duct, in shape flattened oval or slit-like, and of the following average dimensions: Length of the duct along its anterior wall, 6.0 mm, and along its posterior wall, 3.5 mm; similarly, the long diameter of the oval, 6.0 mm, and the short diameter, 3.5 mm. J.C.B.G.

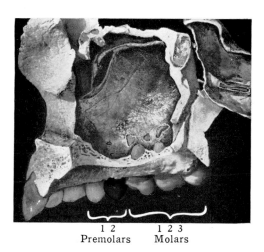

616.3 Maxillary Sinus, medial view

Note:

The roots of 3 teeth, here, penetrate the bony floor.

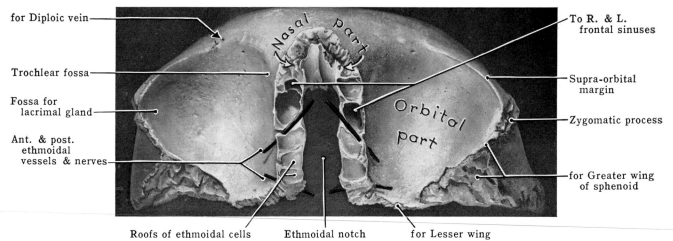

for Diploic vein

Trochlear fossa

Fossa for lacrimal gland

Ant. & post. ethmoidal vessels & nerves

Nasal part

Orbital part

To R. & L. frontal sinuses

Supra-orbital margin

Zygomatic process

for Greater wing of sphenoid

Roofs of ethmoidal cells   Ethmoidal notch   for Lesser wing

617   Frontal Bone, inferior aspect

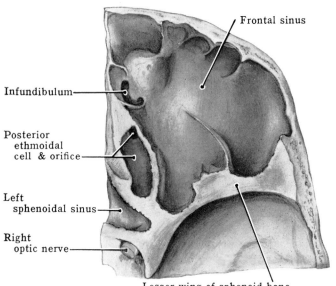

Frontal sinus

Infundibulum

Posterior ethmoidal cell & orifice

Left sphenoidal sinus

Right optic nerve

Lesser wing of sphenoid bone

from above

617.1   Extensive Frontal Sinus

This sinus occupies the entire orbital part of the frontal bone.

An anterior ethmoidal cell bulges dome-like into the floor, of the frontal sinus.

The left sphenoidal sinus crosses the median plane and helps to form the roof of the right optic canal.

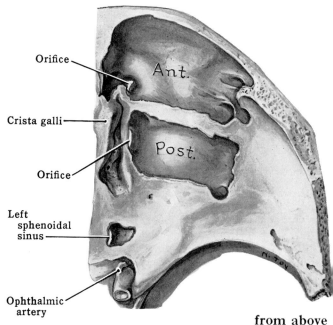

Orifice

Ant.

Crista galli

Post.

Orifice

Left sphenoidal sinus

Ophthalmic artery

from above

617.2   Extensive Ethmoidal Cell

This cell occupies the hinder half of the orbital part of the frontal bone, behind an average sized frontal sinus

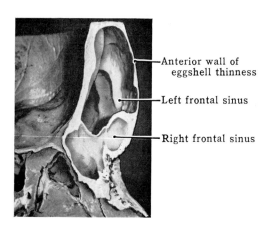

Anterior wall of eggshell thinness

Left frontal sinus

Right frontal sinus

617.3   A Frontal Sinus, with thin anterior wall

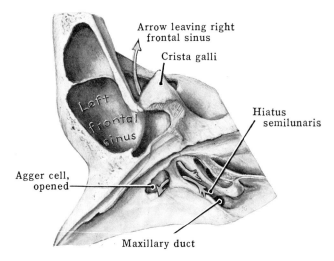

Arrow leaving right frontal sinus

Crista galli

Left frontal sinus

Hiatus semilunaris

Agger cell, opened

Maxillary duct

617.4   A Frontal Sinus in the Crista Galli

The left sinus here extends far across the median plane.
The right sinus opens at the summit of the hiatus.
The agger cell is here a diverticulum from the hiatus.

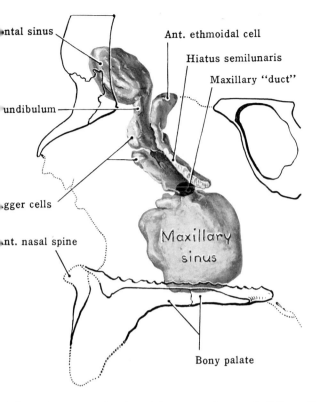

ntal sinus

Ant. ethmoidal cell

Hiatus semilunaris

Maxillary "duct"

undibulum

gger cells

nt. nasal spine

Maxillary sinus

Bony palate

18   Cast of the Frontal and Maxillary inuses, medial view

te :

The frontal sinus lies above the orbital cavity and has its opening at its lowest point, whereas the maxillary sinus lies below the orbital cavity and has its opening on a level with its highest point.

Had this frontal sinus failed to develop, the anterior ethmoidal cell (shown) would have taken its place in default.

Frontal sinus

Ethmoid

Uncinate process   Frontal process of maxilla

618.1   Frontonasal Duct

From figure 615 after removal of the lacrimal bone.

The golden arrow suggests that, if there were fluid in the frontal sinus, it would drain through the infundibulum ethmoidale, (situated at the lowest point of the sinus) into the hiatus semilunaris and thence into the maxillary sinus via its orifice or duct (618), situated on a level with its highest point.

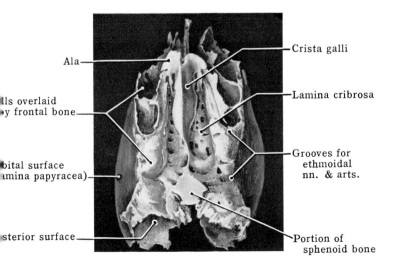

Ala

lls overlaid y frontal bone

bital surface amina papyracea)

sterior surface

Crista galli

Lamina cribrosa

Grooves for ethmoidal nn. & arts.

Portion of sphenoid bone

18.2   Ethmoid Bone, superior aspect

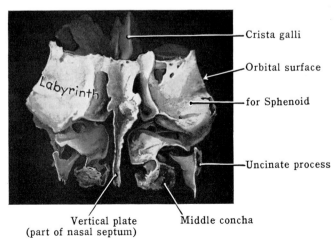

Labyrinth

Crista galli

Orbital surface

for Sphenoid

Uncinate process

Vertical plate (part of nasal septum)   Middle concha

618.3   Ethmoid Bone, posterior aspect

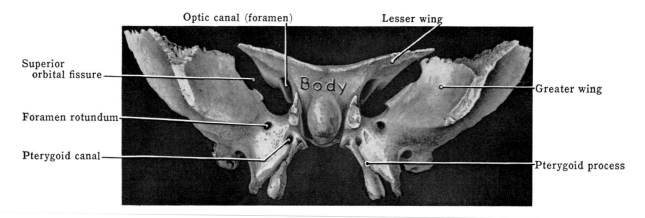

Optic canal (foramen) Lesser wing
Superior orbital fissure Body
Foramen rotundum Greater wing
Pterygoid canal Pterygoid process

619   Sphenoid Bone of a Child

Nerves { III IV VI V¹ Symp } superior orbital fissure

Nerve II–optic canal   Olfactory tract (Nerve I)   Lesser wing

Nerve V²—for. rotundum

Nerve of pterygoid canal —pterygoid canal

Spine of sphenoid

Middle meningeal a —for. spinosum

Nerve V³—for. ovale

Right & left orifices

Temporal
Orbital
Infratemporal
Pterygopalatine
} surfa

Pterygoid process
Lateral plate
Notch for pyramidal process
Hamulus

619.1   Sphenoid Bone of an Adult

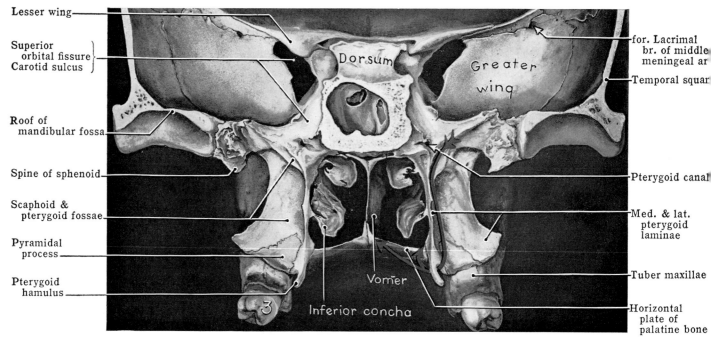

Lesser wing

Superior orbital fissure Carotid sulcus }

Roof of mandibular fossa

Spine of sphenoid

Scaphoid & pterygoid fossae

Pyramidal process

Pterygoid hamulus

Dorsum   Greater wing

for. Lacrimal br. of middle meningeal ar

Temporal squar

Pterygoid canal

Med. & lat. pterygoid laminae

Tuber maxillae

Horizontal plate of palatine bone

Vomer
Inferior concha

619.2   A Coronal Section of the Skull

619 Sphenoid Bone of a Young Child, front view

The right and left sphenoidal sinuses do not invade the body until about the 4th year.

619.1 Sphenoid Bone of an Adult, front view

Note:

On each side 6, or 50%, of the 12 cranial nerves are closely related to the sphenoid, nerve V piercing it in 3 divisions. The nerve of the pterygoid canal and the middle meningeal artery pierce the bone.

The parts coloured pink are the sphenoidal conchae.

619.2 A Coronal Section of the Skull, showing the sphenoid bone and surroundings, posterior view

Note:

1. The 2 posterior nasal apertures [choanae] separated from each other by the vomer, and each bounded below by the horizontal plate of the palatine bone, laterally by the medial pterygoid lamina, and above by the ala of the vomer and the vaginal process of the medial pterygoid lamina (not labelled). The inferior and middle conchae are visible within.
2. The pterygoid fossa, bounded medially by the medial pterygoid lamina, which extends upwards to the pterygoid canal and which ends below the level of the palate, as the hamulus (i.e. the pulley of the Tensor Palati). The Tensor (scarlet arrow) arises from the canoe-shaped scaphoid fossa.
3. The very thin (even translucent) roof of the mandibular fossa.
4. The occasional foramen through which the middle meningeal and lacrimal arteries anastomose.

620.1 Extensive Sphenoidal Sinus, left side $\longrightarrow$

Note:

1. This very extensive sinus extends laterally between the maxillary nerve and the nerve of the pterygoid canal, inflating the greater wing of the sphenoid bone and the pterygoid process. It extends forwards into the lateral wall of the orbital cavity, backwards to the mandibular nerve which passes through the foramen ovale, laterally to the temporal fossa, and downwards to the roof and medial walls of the infratemporal fossa.
2. The greater (superficial) petrosal nerve is seen leaving the hiatus facialis, running above the carotid canal, descending through the foramen lacerum and, when joined by sympathetic fibres (not shown), it becomes the nerve of the pterygoid canal (fig. 657).

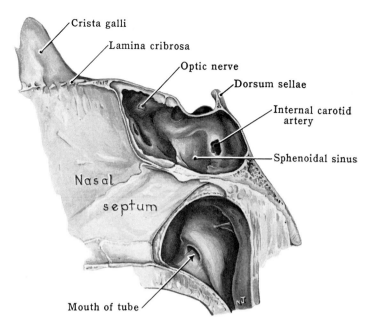

Crista galli — Lamina cribrosa — Optic nerve — Dorsum sellae — Internal carotid artery — Sphenoidal sinus — Nasal septum — Mouth of tube

620 Right Sphenoidal Sinus, very large and thin walled

Note:

1. The sinus extends from an average-sized orifice placed half way down the anterior wall, to the dorsum sellae and basi-occipital. It passes below the chiasmatic sulcus and the hypophyseal fossa (fig. 612).
2. The internal carotid artery and the optic nerve have a papery covering of bone and project in relief from the lateral wall.
3. Between nerve and artery a diverticulum leads into the anterior clinoid process.

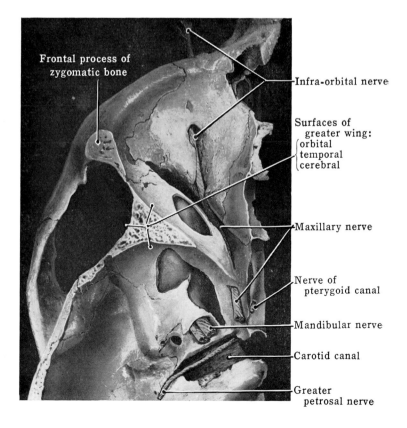

Frontal process of zygomatic bone — Infra-orbital nerve — Surfaces of greater wing: orbital, temporal, cerebral — Maxillary nerve — Nerve of pterygoid canal — Mandibular nerve — Carotid canal — Greater petrosal nerve

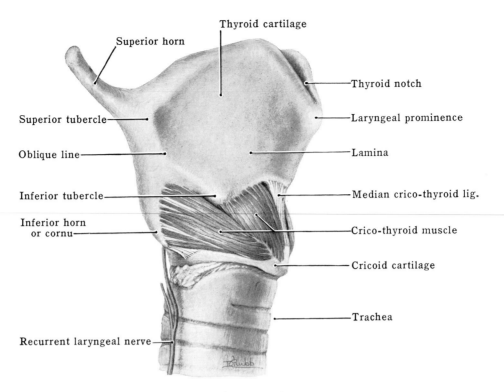

621 Thyroid Cartilage: Crico-thyroideus

Observe:

The Cricothyroid arising from the outer surface of the arch

of the cricoid cartilage and having 2 parts—

(a) a straight, which is inserted into the lower border of the lamina of the thyroid cartilage, and

(b) an oblique, which is inserted into the anterior border of the inferior horn.

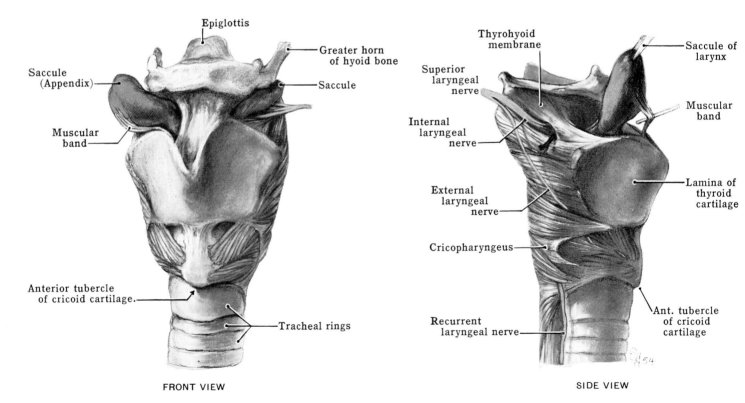

FRONT VIEW

SIDE VIEW

622 Large Laryngeal Saccules (Appendices)

The saccule shown in fig. 628 may be very large, as here. In certain apes it is enormous.

Although the sac is applied to the internal laryngeal nerve, these 2 structures, namely the sac and the nerve, perforate the thyrohyoid membrane through separate apertures.

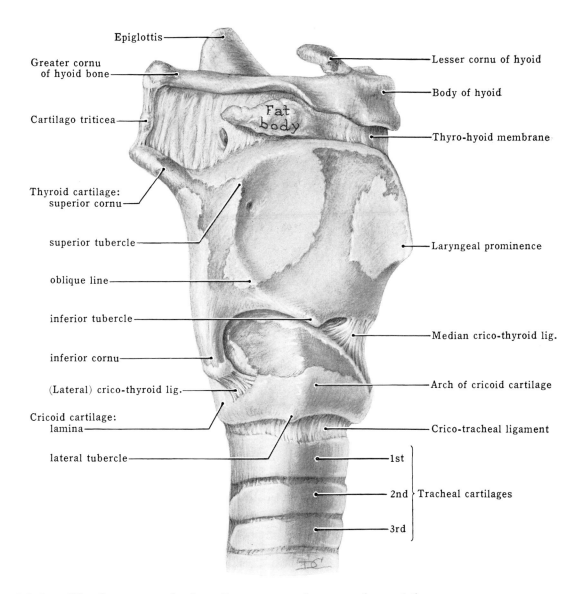

Epiglottis

Greater cornu
of hyoid bone

Cartilago triticea

Thyroid cartilage:
superior cornu

superior tubercle

oblique line

inferior tubercle

inferior cornu

(Lateral) crico-thyroid lig.

Cricoid cartilage:
lamina

lateral tubercle

Fat
body

Lesser cornu of hyoid

Body of hyoid

Thyro-hyoid membrane

Laryngeal prominence

Median crico-thyroid lig.

Arch of cricoid cartilage

Crico-tracheal ligament

1st
2nd Tracheal cartilages
3rd

623   Skeleton of the Larynx, from the side

The larynx extends vertically from the tip of the epiglottis to the lower border of the cricoid cartilage. The hyoid bone or tongue bone is not regarded as part of the larynx.

Observe:

1. The lesser cornu of the hyoid bone, still partly cartilaginous, and not yet fused with the body. The thyroid and cricoid cartilages, on the other hand, partly ossified.

2. The right lamina of the thyroid cartilage, projecting anteriorly above the point of union with its fellow to form the laryngeal prominence. Its posterior border, prolonged into a superior and an inferior cornu; of these, the inferior articulates with the cricoid cartilage. The oblique line (for the attachment of 3 muscles—Inferior Constrictor, Sterno-thyroid, Thyro-hyoid) curving from the superior tubercle to the inferior tubercle.

3. The cricoid cartilage, having 2 parts—an arch anteriorly, and a lamina posteriorly.

4. The thyro-hyoid membrane (a) attaching the whole length of the upper border of the thyroid lamina to the upper border (not lower, see fig. 629) of the body and greater cornu of the hyoid bone; (b) thickened posteriorly to form the thyro-hyoid ligament which contains a nodule of cartilage; (c) pierced by the internal laryngeal nerve and companion vessels; and (d) evaginated by a fat body.

5. The median cricothyroid ligament, uniting the median parts of the adjacent borders of the cricoid and thyroid cartilages. The remainder of the lower border of the thyroid cartilage gives attachment to the Cricothyroid (fig. 621); whereas, the remainder of the upper border of the arch of the cricoid cartilage gives attachment to the Lateral Crico-arytenoid (fig. 628) and the cricothyroid ligament (fig. 629).

6. The upper border of the arch of the cricoid, inclined; the lower border, resembling that of the thyroid cartilage and projecting anteriorly beyond the trachea.

Epiglottic cartilage

Tip of greater horn of hyoid bone

Cartilago triticea

Superior cornu (horn) of thyroid cartilage

Cuneiform cartilage

Corniculate cartilage

Arytenoid cartilage: posterior surface

muscular process

Inferior cornu (horn) of thyroid cartilage

Occasional muscle

Lamina of cricoid

Posterior free ends of tracheal rings

Thyro-hyoid membrane

Quadrangular membrane

Posterior ligament of crico-arytenoid joint

Ligaments of crico-thyroid joint: postero-superior

antero-inferior

Crico-tracheal ligament

624 Skeleton of the Larynx, from behind (Cartilages, membranes, and ligaments)

Observe:

1. The thyroid cartilage, shielding the smaller cartilages of the larynx (epiglottic, arytenoid, corniculate, and cuneiform); and the hyoid bone—though not a part of the larynx—doing the same for the upper part of the epiglottic cartilage at a higher level. The rounded posterior border of the thyroid cartilage, prolonged into an upper and a lower cornu; the lower cornu articulating with the cricoid cartilage by means of a synovial joint (figs. 628 & 629), the capsule of which is reinforced by 2 distinct mooring bands (postero-superior and antero-inferior) and not uncommonly by a muscle, as shown.

2. The quadrangular membrane, connecting the border of the epiglottic cartilage to the arytenoid and corniculate cartilages, having a free upper border, and ending below as the vestibular ligament (fig. 632).

3. The posterior, concave surface of the 3-sided, pyramidal arytenoid cartilage.

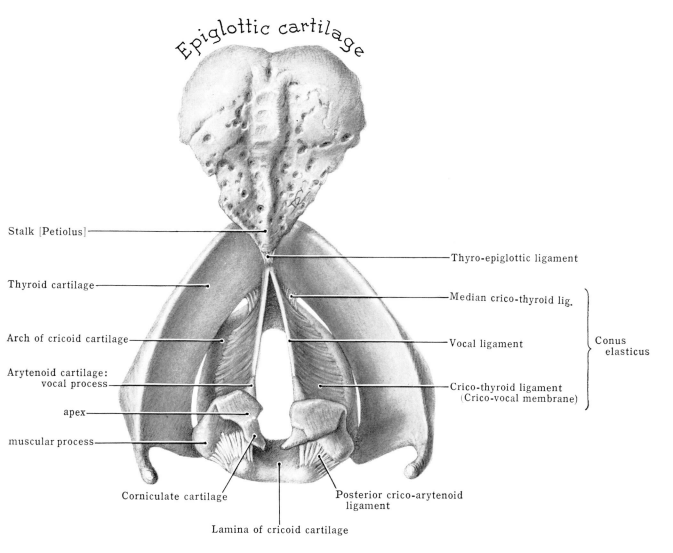

Epiglottic cartilage

Stalk [Petiolus]

Thyroid cartilage

Arch of cricoid cartilage

Arytenoid cartilage:
vocal process

apex

muscular process

Thyro-epiglottic ligament

Median crico-thyroid lig.

Vocal ligament

Crico-thyroid ligament
(Crico-vocal membrane)

Conus
elasticus

Corniculate cartilage

Posterior crico-arytenoid
ligament

Lamina of cricoid cartilage

625 Skeleton of the Larynx, from above

Observe:

1. The right and the left lamina of the thyroid cartilage, united anteriorly at an "angle" of about 60° in the male and 90° in the female (cf. the subpubic angle, figs. 218 & 220).

2. The epiglottic cartilage, shaped like a bicycle saddle, pitted for discrete mucous and serous glands, and attached at its apex by ligamentous fibres to the angle of the thyroid cartilage above the vocal ligaments.

3. The arytenoid cartilage (paired), having a blunt apex prolonged as the corniculate cartilage; a rounded, lateral, basal angle called the muscular process; and a sharp, anterior basal angle, called the vocal process, for the attachment of the vocal ligament.

4. The strong posterior crico-arytenoid ligament, which prevents the arytenoid cartilage from falling into the larynx.

5. The vocal ligament, which forms the skeleton of the vocal fold, extending from the vocal process to the "angle" of the thyroid cartilage, and there joining its fellow below the thyro-epiglottic ligament.

6. The crico-thyroid ligament blending in front with the median crico-thyroid ligament (fig. 623), and sweeping upwards from the upper border of the arch of the cricoid cartilage to the vocal ligament. Hence, when the vocal ligaments are in apposition, the membranes of opposite sides form a roof for the infraglottic section of the larynx below them. The 3 ligaments—median cricothyroid lig., cricothyroid lig., and vocal lig.—are sometimes referred to as the *conus elasticus*, but the term is indefinite.

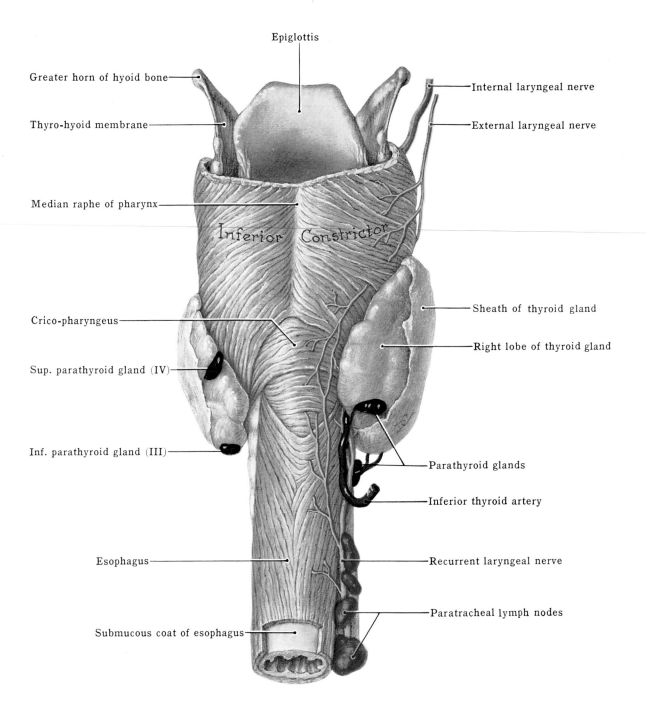

Epiglottis

Greater horn of hyoid bone

Thyro-hyoid membrane

Internal laryngeal nerve

External laryngeal nerve

Median raphe of pharynx

Inferior Constrictor

Crico-pharyngeus

Sheath of thyroid gland

Right lobe of thyroid gland

Sup. parathyroid gland (IV)

Inf. parathyroid gland (III)

Parathyroid glands

Inferior thyroid artery

Esophagus

Recurrent laryngeal nerve

Paratracheal lymph nodes

Submucous coat of esophagus

626 Thyroid Gland, the Parathyroid Glands, and the Three Laryngeal Nerves, from behind

Observe:

1. The right and left lobes of the thyroid gland, unequal in size, applied to the Inferior Constrictor of the pharynx, the trachea, and the esophagus.

2. The superior parathyroid gland, here, as usual, fusiform in shape and lying in a crevice on the posterior border of the lateral lobe of the thyroid gland. The inferior gland, more circular and applied to the lower pole of the thyroid gland. On the right side, both parathyroid glands are rather low, the inferior gland (verified histologically) being altogether below the thyroid gland. Both glands are supplied by the inferior thyroid artery.

3. The internal laryngeal nerve, which is sensory (see fig. 627). The external laryngeal nerve, supplying Inferior Constrictor and Crico-thyroid (see figs. 530 & 532). The recurrent laryngeal nerve, which is mixed, supplying esophagus, trachea (fig. 534), and Inferior Constrictor, dividing into 2 branches which ascend variously related to the branches of the inferior thyroid artery.

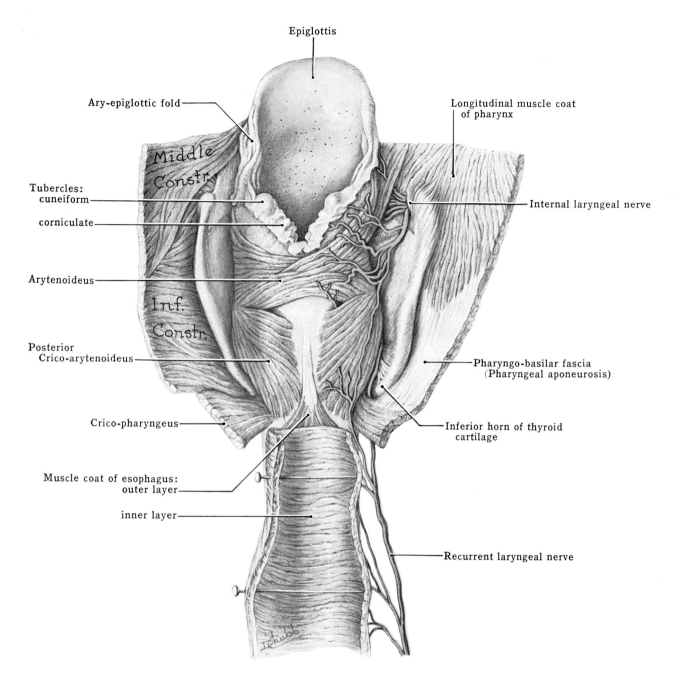

Epiglottis

Ary-epiglottic fold

Longitudinal muscle coat
of pharynx

Middle
Constr.

Tubercles:
cuneiform

Internal laryngeal nerve

corniculate

Arytenoideus

Inf.
Constr.

Posterior
Crico-arytenoideus

Pharyngo-basilar fascia
(Pharyngeal aponeurosis)

Crico-pharyngeus

Inferior horn of thyroid
cartilage

Muscle coat of esophagus:
outer layer

inner layer

Recurrent laryngeal nerve

627 Muscles of the Pharynx, Larynx, and Esophagus, posterior view

The mucous membrane of the pharynx and esophagus is
removed; on the left side, Palato-pharyngeus also is removed and the Middle and Inferior Constrictors are
thereby uncovered.

Observe:

1. On the epiglottis, the pinpoint orifices of the glands that
occupy the pits on the epiglottic cartilage (fig. 625).

2. Palato-pharyngeus and Stylo-pharyngeus together constituting the inner or longitudinal muscle coat of the pharynx
and inserted into the pharyngo-basilar fascia and into the
thyroid cartilage.

3. The esophagus, having inner or circularly arranged muscle
fibres and outer or longitudinally arranged fibres; the latter
suspending the esophagus from the cricoid cartilage.

4. Inferior Constrictor, attached not to the posterior border of
the thyroid cartilage (but to the oblique line and the tubercles, fig. 623). Its lowest fibres, called Crico-pharyngeus,
which act as a sphincter, attached to the cricoid cartilage.

5. The fan-shape of Crico-arytenoideus Posterior. Its upper
fibres rotate the arytenoid cartilage laterally; its lower fibres
pull the cartilage downwards.

6. Arytenoideus (Interarytenoideus), having transverse fibres;
and also oblique fibres which are continued into the ary-
epiglottic fold as Ary-epiglotticus.

7. The recurrent laryngeal nerve (mixed—motor and sensory),
entering the larynx as two branches of which the anterior
runs immediately behind the crico-thyroid joint.

8. The internal laryngeal nerve (sensory) piercing the thyro-
hyoid membrane as several diverging branches.

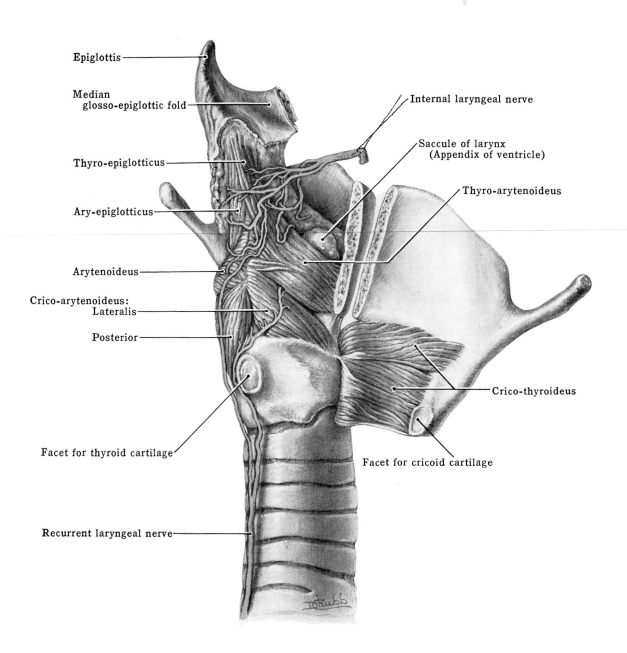

Epiglottis

Median glosso-epiglottic fold

Thyro-epiglotticus

Ary-epiglotticus

Arytenoideus

Crico-arytenoideus:
Lateralis

Posterior

Facet for thyroid cartilage

Recurrent laryngeal nerve

Internal laryngeal nerve

Saccule of larynx
(Appendix of ventricle)

Thyro-arytenoideus

Crico-thyroideus

Facet for cricoid cartilage

628 and 628.1 Muscles, Nerves and Arteries of the Larynx and the Cricothyroid Joint, side view

The thyroid cartilage is cut through to the right of the median plane; the crico-thyroid joint is laid open; the right lamina of the thyroid cartilage is turned forwards, stripping Crico-thyroideus off the arch of the cricoid cartilage.

Observe:

1. Crico-arytenoideus Lateralis, arising from the upper border of the arch of the cricoid cartilage, and inserted with Crico-arytenoideus Posterior into the muscular process of the arytenoid cartilage.
2. Thyro-arytenoideus, inserted with Arytenoideus into the lateral border of the arytenoid cartilage; and its uppermost fibres continued to (or towards) the epiglottis as Thyro-epiglotticus.
3. The blind upper end of the laryngeal saccule, see also figure 622.
4. The internal and recurrent laryngeal nerves, described with figure 627.
5. The anastomoses between (a) the superior laryngeal artery, which is a branch of the sup. thyroid art., and (b) the inferior laryngeal artery, which is a branch of the inf. thyroid art. Arterial twigs piercing the epiglottic cartilage at the sites of the pits for glands.

Epiglottic cartilage

Aryepiglottic fold

Cuneiform tubercle

Corniculate cartilage

Arytenoid cartilage: triangular pit

vocal process

muscular process

Lamina of cricoid cartilage

Facet for thyroid cartilage

Hyo-epiglottic ligament

Hyoid bone

Thyrohyoid membrane

Vestibular fold (Ventricular fold)

Ventricle of larynx

{Vocalis muscle Vocal fold

Cricothyroid ligament (Cricovocal memb.)

Median cricothyroid lig.

Arch of cricoid

Fatty pad

Epiglottis

ɔi-glottic cartil.

ryepi-glottic fold

stibular fold

cal fold

Pharyngo-epiglottic fold

Internal laryngeal nerve

Superior laryngeal art.

Fractured superior horn

Lamina of thyroid cartilage

Post. Crico-arytenoid

Inferior laryngeal art.

28.1

629 Larynx, side view

Above the vocal folds (vocal cords), the larynx is sectioned near the median plane and the interior of its left side is seen. Below this level, the right side of the larynx is dissected.

Observe:

1. The hyo-epiglottic ligament and the thyrohyoid membrane, both attached to the upper part of the body of the hyoid bone. The space behind the body of the hyoid for the subhyoid bursa.
2. The fatty pad and the collection of glands (not labelled) filling the triangular space between ligament, membrane, and epiglottic cartilage.
3. The antero-lateral surface of the arytenoid cartilage and most of the features of this cartilage, including the pit for the attachment of the vestibular ligament and of the cuneiform cartilage. Figure 624 shows the concave posterior surface (covered with Arytenoideus). Figure 632 shows the flat medial surface (covered with mucous membrane).
4. The lateral aspect of the cricoid cartilage—the flat circular facet for the inferior cornu of the thyroid cartilage, placed between the lamina and the arch; above this, the end of the sloping facet for the arytenoid cartilage; the nearly horizontal lower border; and the oblique upper border of the arch.
5. The triangular membrane, called the cricothyroid ligament, having the vocal lig. (fig. 632) for its upper border, blending with the median cricothyroid lig. antero-inferiorly, attached in front to the angle of the thyroid cartilage between these two structures, and below to the cricoid cartilage.

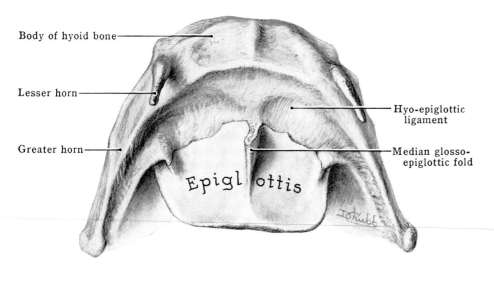

Body of hyoid bone

Lesser horn

Greater horn

Hyo-epiglottic ligament

Median glosso-epiglottic fold

Epiglottis

630 Hyo-epiglottic Ligament, from above

Observe:

1. The hyo-epiglottic ligament, uniting the glottic cartilage to the hyoid bone.
2. The three parts of the hyoid bone, and the asy metry of the greater and lesser horns or cor of opposite sides. (Hyoid bone, see fig. 596.)

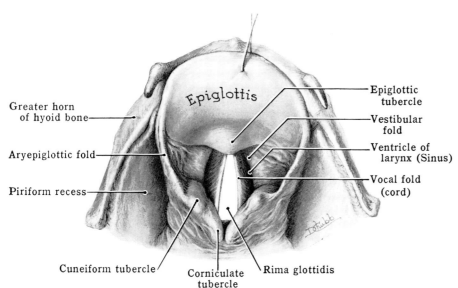

Epiglottis

Greater horn of hyoid bone

Aryepiglottic fold

Piriform recess

Epiglottic tubercle

Vestibular fold

Ventricle of larynx (Sinus)

Vocal fold (cord)

Cuneiform tubercle

Corniculate tubercle

Rima glottidis

631 Larynx, from abov

Observe:

1. The inlet or aditus to the larynx, bounde front by the free, curved edge of the epigl behind, by the arytenoid cartilages, the corr late cartilages, which cap them, and the i arytenoid fold which unites them; and, on side, by the aryepiglottic fold, which con the upper end of the cuneiform cartilage.
2. The vocal folds, closer together than the ve ular folds (false cords) and, therefore, vi below them. The sharpness of the vocal f the fullness of the vestibular folds.
3. The mucous membrane, smooth and adhe in the epiglottic region and over the v folds, but loose and even wrinkled posteri where movement is free.

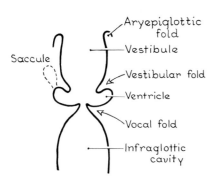

Aryepiglottic fold

Vestibule

Saccule

Vestibular fold

Ventricle

Vocal fold

Infraglottic cavity

631.1 Diagram of the 3 compartments of the larynx, on coronal section

These are—a vestibule, a middle compart-ment having a right and a left ventricle, and an infraglottic cavity.

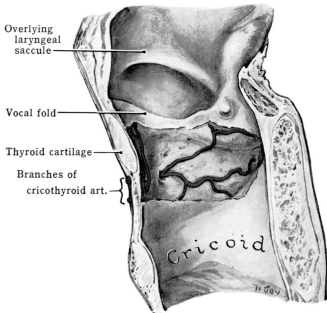

Overlying laryngeal saccule

Vocal fold

Thyroid cartilage

Branches of cricothyroid art.

Cricoid

631.2 Distribution of Cricothyroid Arter

This branch of the superior thyroid art. anastomoses with its fellow i front of the median cricothyroid lig., as shown in figure 528. Lymp vessels accompany it.

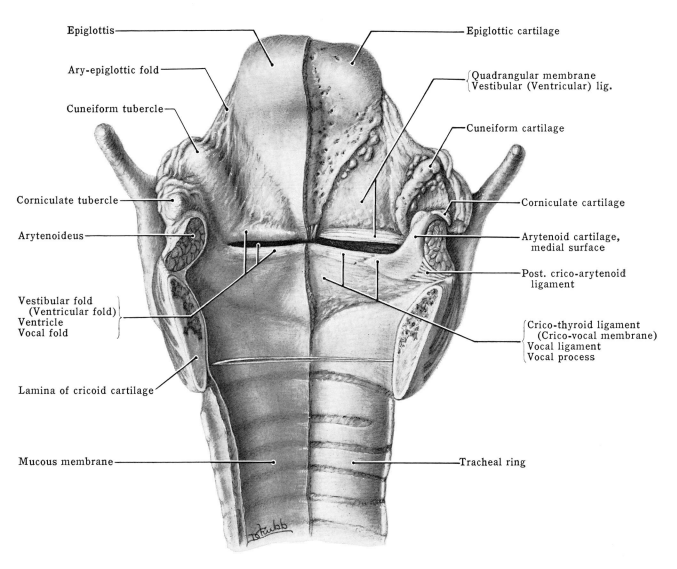

Epiglottis

Ary-epiglottic fold

Cuneiform tubercle

Corniculate tubercle

Arytenoideus

Vestibular fold
(Ventricular fold)
Ventricle
Vocal fold

Lamina of cricoid cartilage

Mucous membrane

Epiglottic cartilage

Quadrangular membrane
Vestibular (Ventricular) lig.

Cuneiform cartilage

Corniculate cartilage

Arytenoid cartilage,
medial surface

Post. crico-arytenoid
ligament

Crico-thyroid ligament
(Crico-vocal membrane)
Vocal ligament
Vocal process

Tracheal ring

632   Interior of the Larynx, posterior view

The posterior wall of the larynx is split medianly, and the two sides are held apart. On the left side, the mucous membrane, which is the innermost coat of the larynx, is intact; on the right side, the mucous and submucous coats are peeled off and the next coat, consisting of cartilages, ligaments and a fibro-elastic membrane, is thereby laid bare.

Observe:

1. Arytenoideus and the lamina of the cricoid cartilage, divided posteriorly.
2. The entrance to the larynx to be oblique; the lower limit, at the lower border of the cricoid cartilage where the trachea begins, to be horizontal.
3. The 3 compartments of the larynx—(a) the uppermost compartment or vestibule, above the level of the vestibular folds; (b) the middle, between the levels of the vestibular and vocal folds, and having a right and a left canoe-shaped depression, the ventricles; and (c) the lowest or infraglottic cavity, below the level of the vocal folds.

4. The mucous membrane, particularly smooth and adherent over the epiglottic cartilage and vocal ligaments; and particularly loose and wrinkled about the arytenoid cartilages, where movement is free.

5. The two parts of the fibro-elastic membrane—(a) an upper quadrangular, and (b) a lower triangular. The upper part, the quadrangular membrane, which is thickened below to form the vestibular ligament. The lower part, the crico-thyroid ligament (conus elasticus), which begins below as the strong median cricothyroid ligament and ends above as the vocal ligament. Between the vocal and the vestibular ligament, the membrane, lined with mucous membrane, is evaginated to form the wall of the ventricle.

6. The cuneiform cartilage; (a) more club-shaped than wedge-shaped, (b) composed of elastic cartilage and pitted for, and surrounded with, glands, like the epiglottic cartilage of which it is a detached part, and (c) attached to the arytenoid cartilage beside the posterior end of the vestibular ligament.

7. The posterior ligament of the crico-arytenoid joint, anchoring the arytenoid cartilage. The flat, medial, submucous surface of the arytenoid cartilage.

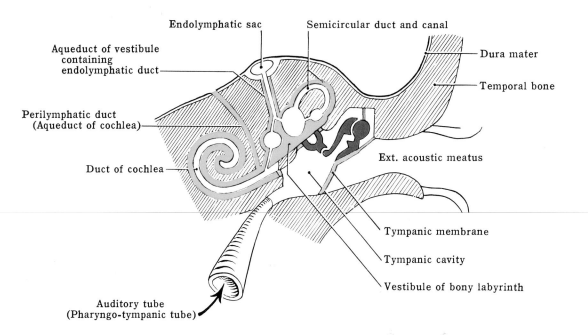

Endolymphatic sac

Semicircular duct and canal

Aqueduct of vestibule
containing
endolymphatic duct

Dura mater

Temporal bone

Perilymphatic duct
(Aqueduct of cochlea)

Ext. acoustic meatus

Duct of cochlea

Tympanic membrane

Tympanic cavity

Vestibule of bony labyrinth

Auditory tube
(Pharyngo-tympanic tube)

633   General Scheme of the Ear

The ear is divisible into 3 parts—external, middle, internal.

The external ear comprises (a) the auricle and (b) the external acoustic meatus, the medial end of which is closed by the tympanic membrane.

The tympanic membrane is set obliquely and is slightly conical, its most in-drawn point or umbo being at the lower end of the handle of the malleus which is attached to the membrane.

The middle ear or tympanum lies between the tympanic membrane and the internal ear.

Three ossicles (red)—malleus, incus, stapes—stretch from the lateral to the medial wall of the tympanum. Of these, the malleus is attached to the tympanic membrane; the stapes is attached by an annular ligament to the oval opening, called the fenestra vestibuli; and the incus connects these two ossicles.

The part of the tympanic cavity that lies above the level of the external acoustic meatus is the epitympanic recess (not labelled). It contains the upper ends of the malleus and incus.

The auditory tube opens into the anterior wall of the tympanic cavity; the aditus ad antrum opens from the epitympanic recess backwards to the mastoid antrum (fig. 639).

The internal ear comprises a closed system of membranous tubes and bulbs, called the membranous labyrinth, which are filled with fluid, called endolymph, and are bathed in surrounding fluid called perilymph (blue). The perilymph is contained within the bony labyrinth, but this system is not a closed one, for, as represented in fig. 633, perilymph and cerebrospinal fluid are confluent in the posterior cranial fossa. There is, however, good evidence that this system also is closed, the perilymphatic duct ending as a perilymphatic sac. (Wharton Young.)

When the tympanic membrane vibrates, the malleus vibrates with it and transmits the vibrations via the incus to the stapes. The stapes, being attached to the margins of the fenestra vestibuli (oval window) by an annular ligament, transmits the vibrations to the perilymph within the vestibule.

A secondary tympanic membrane which closes the fenestra cochleae (round window), receiving the vibrations transmitted to the incompressible perilymph, is itself made to vibrate in turn.

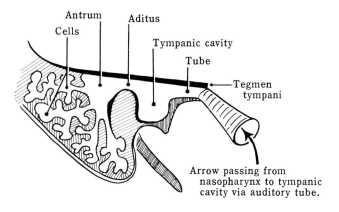

Antrum

Cells

Aditus

Tympanic cavity

Tube

Tegmen
tympani

Arrow passing from
nasopharynx to tympanic
cavity via auditory tube.

633.1   Diagram of Tegmen Tympani

The mastoid air cells are in communication with the outside air via the mastoid antrum, aditus ad antrum, tympanic cavity, and bony and cartilaginous parts of the auditory tube.

A thin plate of bone, called the tegmen tympani, forms a roof for these.

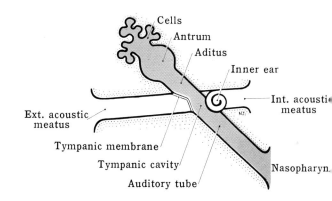

Cells

Antrum

Aditus

Inner ear

Int. acoustic
meatus

Ext. acoustic
meatus

Tympanic membrane

Tympanic cavity

Auditory tube

Nasopharynx

633.2   Scheme of Meatuses and Airway

showing the line of the meatuses and the line of the airway (from nasopharynx to mastoid cells) intersecting at the tympanic cavity.

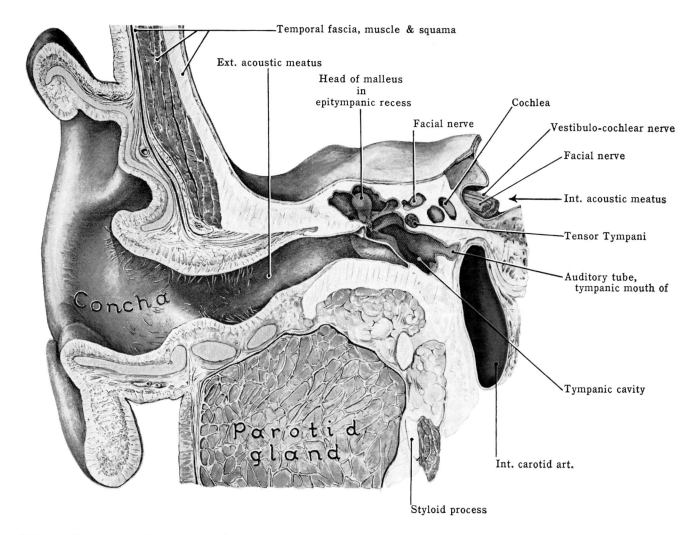

Temporal fascia, muscle & squama

Ext. acoustic meatus

Head of malleus
in
epitympanic recess

Cochlea

Facial nerve

Vestibulo-cochlear nerve

Facial nerve

Int. acoustic meatus

Tensor Tympani

Auditory tube,
tympanic mouth of

Tympanic cavity

Concha

Parotid gland

Int. carotid art.

Styloid process

634 Ear on Coronal Section, anterior view

(Inner ear tinted blue; mucous membrane of the middle ear pink.)

Observe:

1. The external acoustic (auditory) meatus which from tragus to ear drum is 1¼″ long, half the length being cartilaginous and half bony. Narrowest near the drum due to the rise on the floor, hence the "well" where fluid might collect at the medial end of the meatus.

2. The cartilaginous or mobile part of the external meatus, lined with thick skin and having hairs and the mouths of many glands; the bony part lined with a thin epithelium which adheres to the periosteum and also forms the outermost layer of the tympanic membrane.

3. The obliquity of the tympanic membrane which meets the roof of the meatus at an obtuse angle and the floor at an acute one.

4. The middle ear or tympanic cavity, extending above the level of the drum as the epitympanic recess, and the recess extending laterally above the bony meatus.

5. The tympanic cavity widest above, narrow below, and narrowest at the level of the umbo where the membrane is indrawn and faces the promontory of the cochlea.

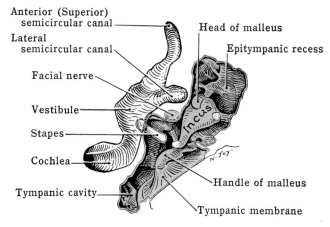

Anterior (Superior)
semicircular canal

Lateral
semicircular canal

Facial nerve

Vestibule

Stapes

Cochlea

Tympanic cavity

Head of malleus

Epitympanic recess

INCUS

Handle of malleus

Tympanic membrane

(Inset from another specimen, posterior view.)

6. The thin shell of bone covering the facial nerve. The grooved anterior crus of the stapes and the anterior half of its base closing the fenestra vestibuli. The long axis of the stapes inclined upwards and medially—not lying horizontally.

7. The lateral canal, above facial nerve (fig. 637).

635 Tympanic Membrane, on lateral view

(Exposed by grinding away the bony exterior meatus.)

Observe:

1. The tympanic membrane, oval rather than round, and shaped like a funnel with rolled rim and a depressed part, called the umbo, at the tip of the handle of the malleus which is situated antero-inferior to the centre of the membrane.

2. The stria mallearis, which overlies the handle of the malleus, extending upwards to the prominentia, which overlies the lateral process of the malleus.

3. Above the prominentia the membrane is thin and is called the pars flaccida. The pars flaccida lacks the radial and circular fibres present in the remainder of the membrane (pars tensa). The junction between the two parts, flaccid and tense, is marked by an anterior and a posterior line which run from the prominentia to the free ends of the horseshoe-shaped tympanic ring (fig. 646).

4. The pars flaccida forms the lateral wall of the superior recess (fig. 641) of the tympanic cavity.

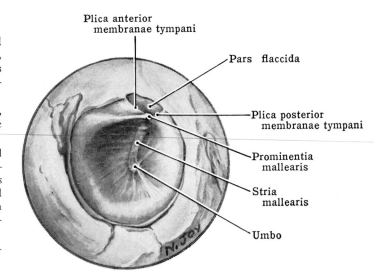

Plica anterior membranae tympani

Pars flaccida

Plica posterior membranae tympani

Prominentia mallearis

Stria mallearis

Umbo

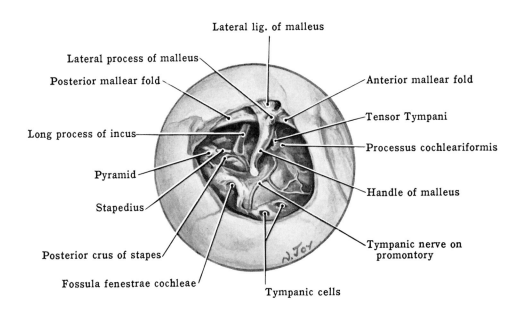

Lateral lig. of malleus

Lateral process of malleus

Posterior mallear fold

Long process of incus

Pyramid

Stapedius

Posterior crus of stapes

Fossula fenestrae cochleae

Anterior mallear fold

Tensor Tympani

Processus cochleariformis

Handle of malleus

Tympanic nerve on promontory

Tympanic cells

636 Tympanic Cavity, infero-lateral view, after removal of the tympanic membrane

Observe:

1. The direction of the handle of the malleus and of the long process of the incus which lies behind it; also the posterior and anterior mallear folds of mucous membrane in which the chorda tympani passes between the two bones (fig. 641).

2. The fulness of the promontory with grooves for the tympanic nerve (a branch of the glossopharyngeal nerve) and its connections.

3. The end of a fossula at the deep end of which is the fenestra cochleae or round window, closed by the secondary tympanic membrane (not in view).

4. The tendon of Stapedius passing forwards to the neck of the stapes; the tendon of Tensor Tympani passing laterally to the neck of the malleus.

5. The lateral ligament of the malleus and the neck of the malleus forming the medial wall of the superior recess of the tympanic membrane (fig. 641).

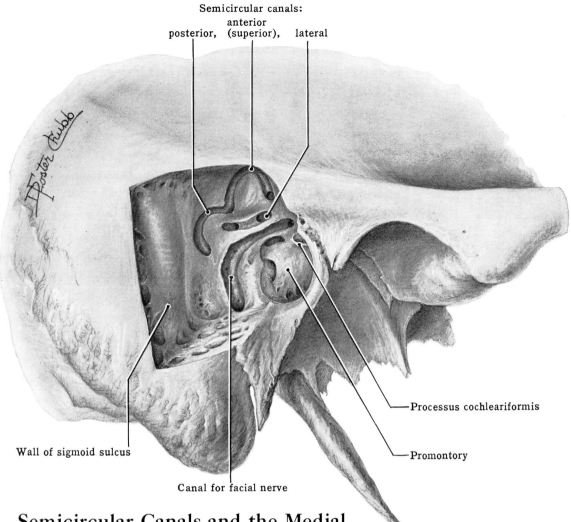

Semicircular canals:
anterior
posterior, (superior), lateral

Processus cochleariformis

Promontory

Wall of sigmoid sulcus

Canal for facial nerve

637 Semicircular Canals and the Medial Wall of the Tympanic Cavity, lateral view

The mastoid cells, seen in coronal section in figure 643, are largely removed and the inner table of the skull, here forming the semi-tubular wall of the sigmoid sulcus, is exposed. The posterior wall of the external acoustic meatus and the mastoid antrum are removed.

Observe:

1. The 3 semicircular canals, lying in the 3 planes of space, are opened.
2. The anterior and posterior canals, placed vertically and at right angles to each other. The lateral canal, placed horizontally and at right angles to the anterior and posterior canals.
3. The medial end of the anterior canal and the upper end of the posterior canal, uniting to form the crus commune. The lateral canal lying in the medial wall of the aditus ad antrum.
4. The features of the medial or labyrinthine wall of the tympanic cavity:
    (a) The promontory, lying 2 mm deep to the umbo, and overlying the basal turn of the cochlea.
    (b) The processus cochleariformis, at the end of the canal for Tensor Tympani. It acts as a pulley for the Tensor.
    (c) The fenestra vestibuli, close behind the pulley and medial to it. It is closed by the foot-plate of the stapes, which is bound to its margin by an annular ligament.
    (d) The fossula leading to the fenestra cochleae, below the vestibular window and separated from it by a rounded bar which projects backwards from the promontory.
    (e) The facial canal (opened) running horizontally backwards, between the vestibular window and the lateral semicircular canal, to the junction of the medial and posterior walls, then descending in the posterior wall to its orifice, the stylomastoid foramen.

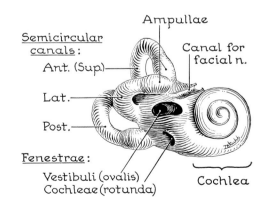

Semicircular canals:
Ant. (Sup.)
Lat.
Post.

Ampullae

Canal for facial n.

Cochlea

Fenestrae:
Vestibuli (ovalis)
Cochleae (rotunda)

637.1 Bony Inner Ear, lateral view

To aid in orientation of fig. 637.

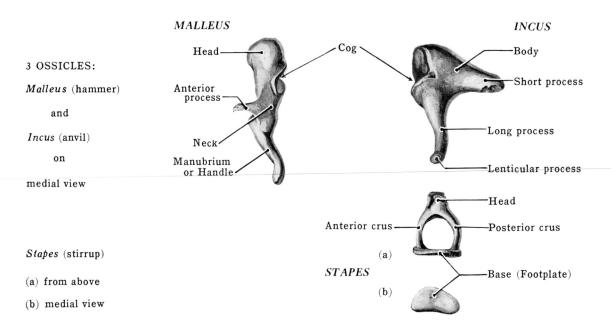

MALLEUS

INCUS

Head

Cog

Body

Short process

3 OSSICLES:

Malleus (hammer)

and

Incus (anvil)

on

medial view

Anterior process

Neck

Manubrium or Handle

Long process

Lenticular process

Head

Anterior crus

Posterior crus

Stapes (stirrup)

(a) from above

(b) medial view

(a)

STAPES

(b)

Base (Footplate)

3 Ossicles of the middle ear in their relative positions.

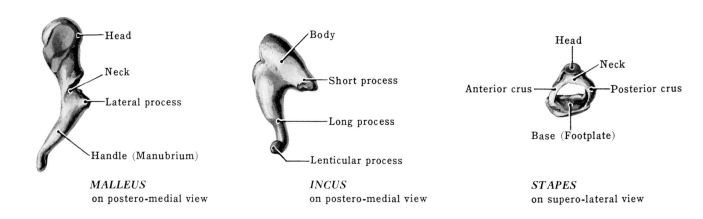

Head

Neck

Lateral process

Handle (Manubrium)

MALLEUS
on postero-medial view

Body

Short process

Long process

Lenticular process

INCUS
on postero-medial view

Head

Neck

Anterior crus

Posterior crus

Base (Footplate)

STAPES
on supero-lateral view

638 Ossicles of the Middle Ear

(Malleus, Incus, and Stapes)

The head of the malleus and the body and short process of the incus lie in the epitympanic recess.

The saddle-shaped articular surface of the head of the malleus and the reciprocally saddle-shaped articular surface of the body of the incus form the incudo-mallear synovial joint.

The anterior process of the malleus and the short process of the incus (it might better have been called the posterior process) are in line and are moored fore and aft by ligaments.

The handle of the malleus, from lateral process to tip, is imbedded in the tympanic membrane.

The end of the long (vertical) process of the incus has a convex articular facet for articulation with the head of the stapes, at the incudo-stapedial synovial joint.

The hole in the stapes in the embryo transmits an artery, the stapedial artery. It is now closed by an obturator. The upper border of the footplate is convex; and it is deeper anteriorly than posteriorly. The two crura are grooved. The anterior crus is the more slender and straighter and it is fixed to a small area on the plate; the posterior crus is attached to the whole depth of the plate.

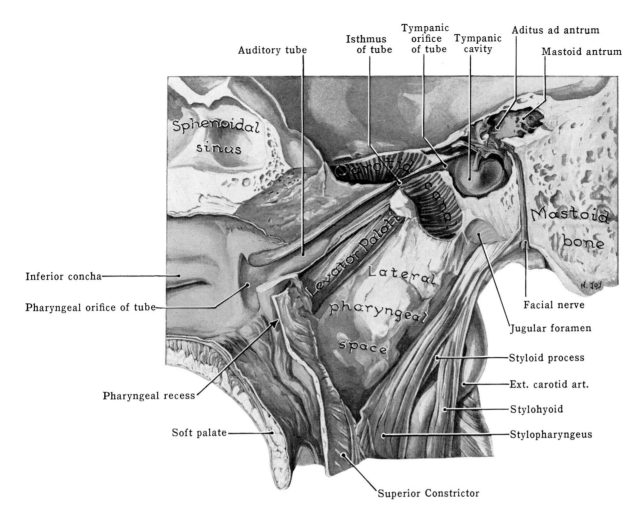

Auditory tube — Isthmus of tube — Tympanic orifice of tube — Tympanic cavity — Aditus ad antrum — Mastoid antrum

Inferior concha

Pharyngeal orifice of tube

Pharyngeal recess

Soft palate

Facial nerve

Jugular foramen

Styloid process

Ext. carotid art.

Stylohyoid

Stylopharyngeus

Superior Constrictor

639 Auditory Tube (Pharyngo-tympanic Tube), exposed from the medial or pharyngeal aspect

Observe:

1. The general direction of the tube—upwards, backwards, and laterally from nasopharynx to tympanic cavity.

2. The funnel-shaped pharyngeal orifice of the tube, situated $\frac{1}{2}''$ behind the inferior concha of the nose.

3. The cartilaginous part of the tube, 1″ long, resting throughout its length on Levator Palati, but affording it almost no origin.

4. The bony part of the tube passing lateral to the carotid canal, $\frac{1}{2}''$ long, narrow at the isthmus where it joins the cartilaginous part, wider at its tympanic orifice, and less steep than the cartilaginous part.

5. Tensor Tympani, lying above a bony ledge, called the processus cochleariformis, and inserted into the neck of the malleus.

6. The chorda tympani lying in a "mesentery", the anterior and posterior mallear folds, and the anterior and posterior recesses of the tympanic membrane lateral to the respective folds.

7. The anterior mallear fold acting as a mesentery for Tensor Tympani also, and continuous with a fold that passes forwards from the head of the malleus.

8. The upper half of the lateral pharyngeal space, seen on cross section in figures 579 & 584.

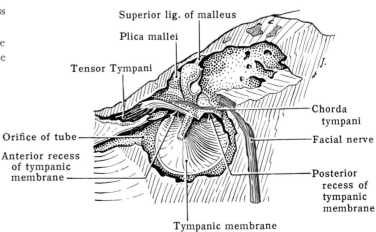

Superior lig. of malleus

Plica mallei

Tensor Tympani

Orifice of tube

Anterior recess of tympanic membrane

Chorda tympani

Facial nerve

Posterior recess of tympanic membrane

Tympanic membrane

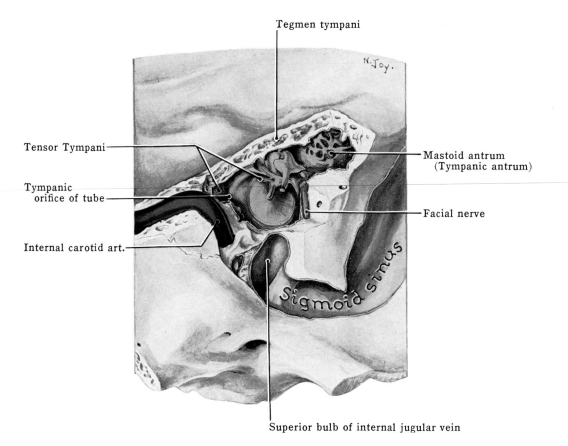

Tegmen tympani

N. Joy.

Tensor Tympani

Tympanic orifice of tube

Internal carotid art.

Mastoid antrum (Tympanic antrum)

Facial nerve

Sigmoid sinus

Superior bulb of internal jugular vein

640 Walls of the Tympanic Cavity or Middle Ear

(Exposed with a drill, from the medial aspect.)

Observe:

1. The tegmen tympani forming the roof of the tube, tympanic cavity, and antrum, here fairly thick but commonly papery in thinness.

2. The int. carotid artery as the main feature of the anterior wall; the int. jugular vein the main feature of the floor; and the facial nerve the main feature of the posterior wall.

3. The supero-lateral part of the anterior wall leading to the auditory tube and Tensor Tympani; the supero-lateral part of the posterior wall leading to the mastoid antrum.

4. The tympanic membrane forming much of the lateral wall. Above it is the epitympanic recess in which are housed the greater parts of the malleus and incus.

5. A ligament suspending the malleus from the tegmen tympani; the short process of the incus moored by ligaments to the fossa incudis in the floor of the aditus to the antrum.

6. The chorda tympani passing between incus and malleus.

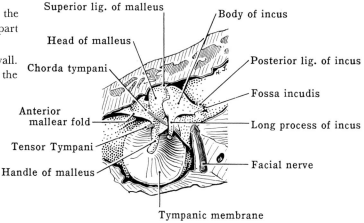

Superior lig. of malleus

Head of malleus

Chorda tympani

Anterior mallear fold

Tensor Tympani

Handle of malleus

Body of incus

Posterior lig. of incus

Fossa incudis

Long process of incus

Facial nerve

Tympanic membrane

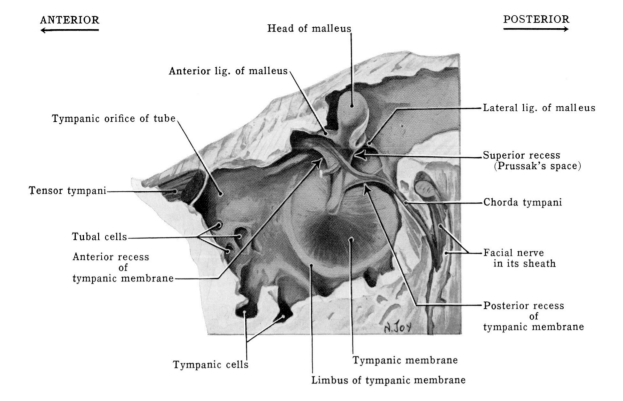

Head of malleus

Anterior lig. of malleus

Tympanic orifice of tube

Tensor tympani

Tubal cells

Anterior recess
of
tympanic membrane

Lateral lig. of malleus

Superior recess
(Prussak's space)

Chorda tympani

Facial nerve
in its sheath

Posterior recess
of
tympanic membrane

Tympanic cells

Tympanic membrane

Limbus of tympanic membrane

641   Lateral Wall of the Tympanic Cavity, medial view

Observe:

1. The oval tympanic membrane, with a greater vertical than horizontal diameter (9 mm. x 8 mm.).

2. The handle of the malleus incorporated in the membrane, its end being at the umbo.

3. The anterior process of the malleus anchored forwards by the anterior lig. This lig. is almost continuous through the petro-tympanic fissure with the spheno-mandibular lig.

4. The facial nerve within its tough periosteal tube. The chorda tympani leaving the facial nerve, and as it goes to the front wall (a) lying within 2 crescentic folds of mucous membrane, the anterior and posterior mallear folds, which, so to speak, suspend it from the tympanic membrane at the junction of its flaccid and tense parts, (b) crossing the neck of the malleus above the tendon of Tensor, and (c) following the anterior process and anterior lig.

5. The 3 recesses of the membrane—the anterior and the posterior recess, which extend upwards between the mallear folds and the pars tensa of the membrane, and thirdly the superior recess. The superior recess extends forwards (see arrow) between the neck of the malleus and the pars flaccida, and it is limited below by the short process of the malleus and above by the lateral lig. (fig. 636). This space may open posteriorly, lateral to the incus, as here, or it may open downwards into the posterior recess.

6. The fibro-cartilaginous margin or limbus of the membrane which fastens it to the sulcus in the tympanic bone.

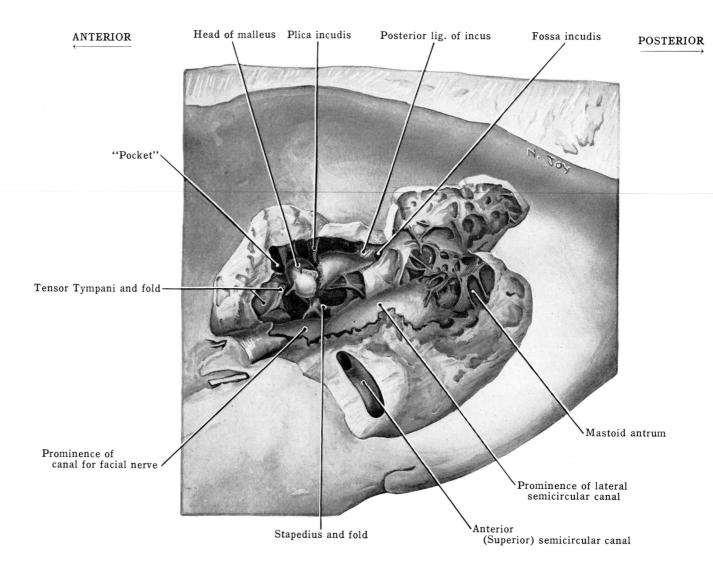

ANTERIOR   Head of malleus   Plica incudis   Posterior lig. of incus   Fossa incudis   POSTERIOR

"Pocket"

Tensor Tympani and fold

Prominence of canal for facial nerve

Stapedius and fold

Mastoid antrum

Prominence of lateral semicircular canal

Anterior (Superior) semicircular canal

642   Tympanic Cavity and Mastoid Antrum, from above

The bony roof, or tegmen tympani, has been removed with the aid of an electric drill.

Observe:

1. Extensive folds, strands, "mesenteries", and pockets of mucous membrane.
2. The mesentery for Tensor Tympani (commonly perforated) and the mesentery for Stapedius and stapes.
3. The head of the malleus and the body and short crus of the incus in the epitympanic recess. The short process of the incus moored by two ligamentous bands to the sides of the fossa incudis on the floor of the aditus ad antrum.
4. The strand from the body of the incus to the lateral wall is commonly an extensive fold as in fig. 648 and the result is a pocket. The superior ligament of the malleus (not labelled) is cut short.

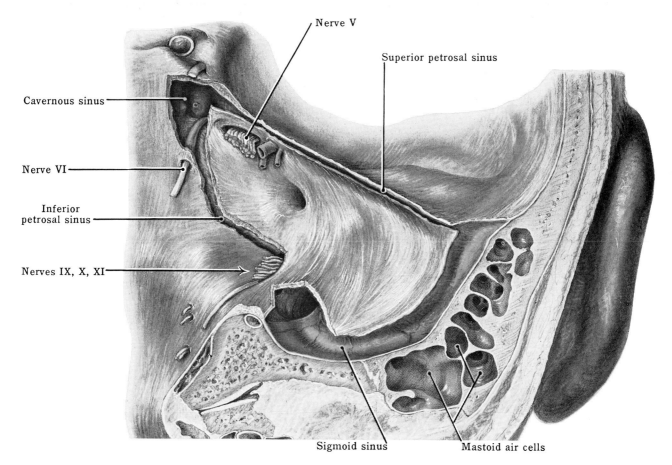

Nerve V

Superior petrosal sinus

Cavernous sinus

Nerve VI

Inferior petrosal sinus

Nerves IX, X, XI

Sigmoid sinus

Mastoid air cells

643 Mastoid Air Cells—Dural Sinuses

Observe:

1. Mastoid cells (pink), lined with mucous membrane, and occupying the diploe (fig. 633.1). The branching ducts through which these cells communicate with the antrum. The two lowest cells almost bursting through the outer table of the skull.

2. The posterior surface of the petrous bone encircled with 3 sinuses—sigmoid, superior petrosal, and inferior petrosal.

The two petrosal sinuses draining the cavernous sinus.

3. The sup. petrosal sinus, at the attached margin of the tentorium, bridging nerve V. The sigmoid sinus, nerves IX, X, and XI, and the inf. petrosal sinus disappearing into the jugular foramen.

4. Nerve VI, passing through the inf. petrosal sinus and bending forwards to enter the cavernous sinus. (Fig. 514.)

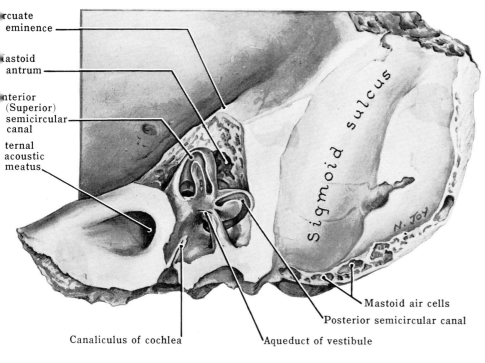

Arcuate eminence

Mastoid antrum

Anterior (Superior) semicircular canal

Internal acoustic meatus

Sigmoid sulcus

N. Joy

Mastoid air cells

Posterior semicircular canal

Canaliculus of cochlea

Aqueduct of vestibule

644 Semicircular Canals and the Aqueducts, postero-superior view

Observe:

1. The anterior semicircular canal, set vertically, below the arcuate eminence, and making a right angle with the posterior surface of the petrous bone.

2. The posterior semicircular canal, nearly parallel to the posterior surface of the bone, close to that surface, and only 5 mm. from the sigmoid sulcus.

3. The aqueduct of the vestibule, which contains the ductus endolymphaticus and opens medial to the posterior canal.

4. The canaliculus of the cochlea, which contains the perilymphatic duct (aqueduct of cochlea) and opens at the apex of the depression for the ganglion of nerve IX.

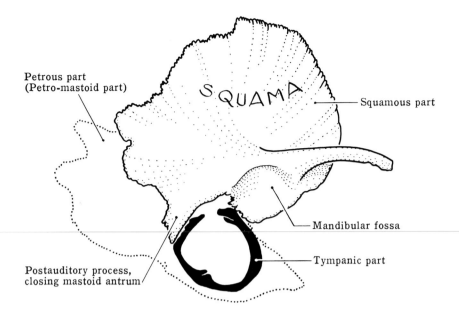

Petrous part
(Petro-mastoid part)

Squamous part

Mandibular fossa

Tympanic part

Postauditory process,
closing mastoid antrum

645   Temporal Bone at Birth, lateral view

Note:

1. The 3 parts of the temporal bone—squamous, petrous, tympanic—separable at birth.
2. The mandibular fossa is shallow. The postauditory process, descending from the squamous part, closes the mastoid antrum laterally.
3. No mastoid process has yet appeared on the petrous part, there being as yet no mastoid cells.
4. The tympanic part is a ring that is incomplete above; no tympanic plate has yet grown to give length to the external acoustic meatus; hence the tympanic membrane is close to the surface of the skull.

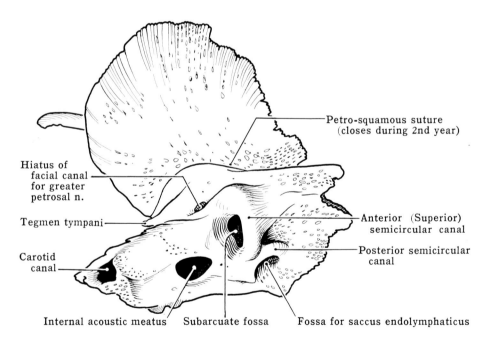

Petro-squamous suture
(closes during 2nd year)

Hiatus of
facial canal
for greater
petrosal n.

Tegmen tympani

Anterior (Superior)
semicircular canal

Posterior semicircular
canal

Carotid
canal

Internal acoustic meatus   Subarcuate fossa   Fossa for saccus endolymphaticus

645.1   Temporal Bone at Birth, posterior view

Note:

1. The hollows round about the anterior and posterior semicircular canals are not yet filled in with bone; hence, these canals project as bony rims.
2. The subarcuate fossa, within the arc of the anterior semicircular canal, is large and looks medially. The fossa within the arc of the posterior canal is likewise large; it looks downwards and laterally and lodges the endolymphatic sac, shown in figure 650.

546 Temporal Bone during the first year of life, lateral view

(The mastoid antrum has been opened.)

Note:

1. There is a mastoid antrum, but no mastoid process, and accordingly no mastoid cells.

2. The tympanic bone is a ring, incomplete above. It has no length, but sprouting from its lateral border are two spines.

3. The stylo-mastoid foramen, from which the facial nerve emerges, is near the skin surface.

4. The tympanic cavity is large.

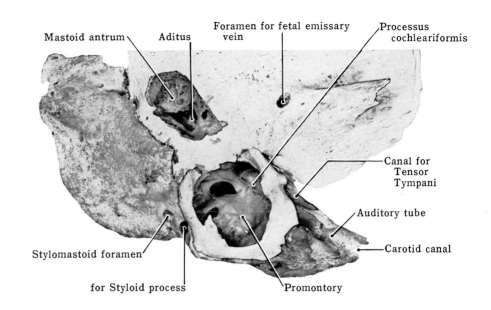

Mastoid antrum   Aditus   Foramen for fetal emissary vein   Processus cochleariformis

Canal for Tensor Tympani

Auditory tube

Carotid canal

Stylomastoid foramen for Styloid process   Promontory

547 Temporal Bone during the third or fourth year, lateral view

(The mastoid antrum and the epitympanic recess have been opened.)

Note:

1. The mastoid process is appearing. The walls of the antrum are like a honeycomb.

2. The enlarging spines on the tympanic ring are nearer to meeting and so to enclosing a temporary foramen (closed by membrane) in what is becoming the tympanic plate. This plate will form the anterior and the inferior, and part of the posterior, wall of the external acoustic meatus (fig. 558).

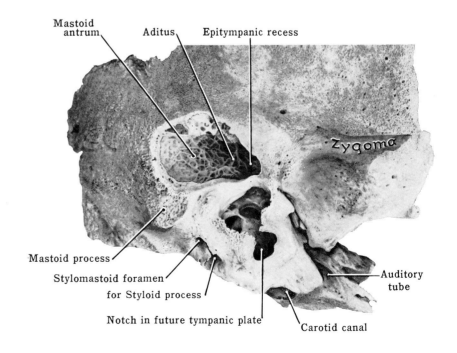

Mastoid antrum   Aditus   Epitympanic recess

Zygoma

Mastoid process

Stylomastoid foramen for Styloid process

Notch in future tympanic plate

Auditory tube

Carotid canal

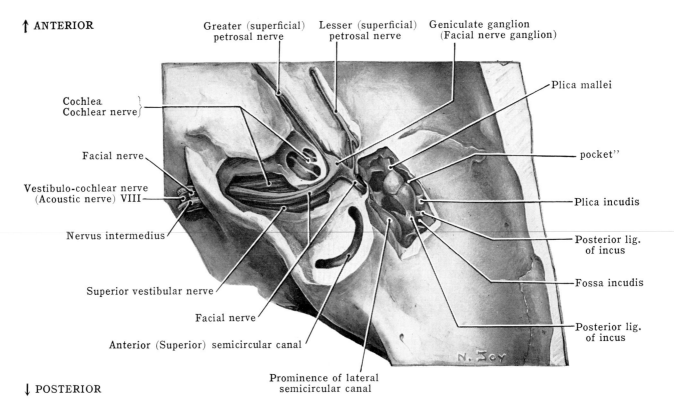

Greater (superficial) petrosal nerve

Lesser (superficial) petrosal nerve

Geniculate ganglion (Facial nerve ganglion)

Cochlea
Cochlear nerve

Facial nerve

Vestibulo-cochlear nerve (Acoustic nerve) VIII

Nervus intermedius

Superior vestibular nerve

Facial nerve

Anterior (Superior) semicircular canal

Plica mallei

pocket"

Plica incudis

Posterior lig. of incus

Fossa incudis

Posterior lig. of incus

Prominence of lateral semicircular canal

↓ POSTERIOR

648 Geniculate Ganglion, from above

(The Ganglion of the Facial Nerve.)

Observe:

1. The facial nerve, the nervus intermedius, and the vestibulo-cochlear nerve, entering and traversing the internal acoustic meatus. The facial nerve, joined by the nervus intermedius, running close behind the cochlea and, therefore, across the roof of the vestibule (fig. 649) to the geniculate ganglion and at the ganglion making a right angle bend, called the genu, and then curving downwards and backwards within its bony canal, called the facial canal, whose papery lateral wall separates it from the tympanic cavity.

2. The petrosal branch of the middle meningeal artery, which enters the canal at the hiatus (fig. 513), running with the nerve.

3. The geniculate ganglion, which is the cell station of fibers of general sensation and of taste (fig. 657), situated at the genu and in line with the internal acoustic meatus. Through the ganglion run forward fibers of the greater (superficial) petrosal nerve on their way to the pterygopalatine ganglion; from the facial nerve, beyond the ganglion, goes a communicating branch to the lesser (superficial) petrosal nerve on its way to the otic ganglion. Further on, but not in view, the chorda tympani leaves the facial nerve and joins the lingual which conducts it to the submandibular ganglion.

MEDIAL

LATERAL

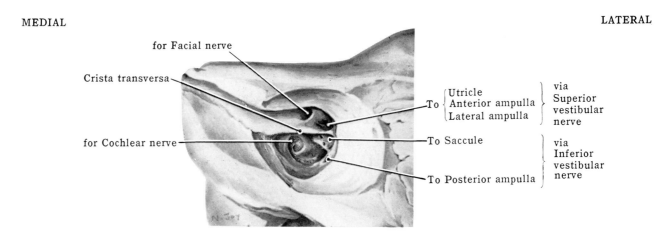

for Facial nerve

Crista transversa

for Cochlear nerve

To { Utricle / Anterior ampulla / Lateral ampulla } via Superior vestibular nerve

To Saccule

To Posterior ampulla

} via Inferior vestibular nerve

648.1 Fundus of the Internal Acoustic Meatus

(The walls of the meatus have been ground away.)

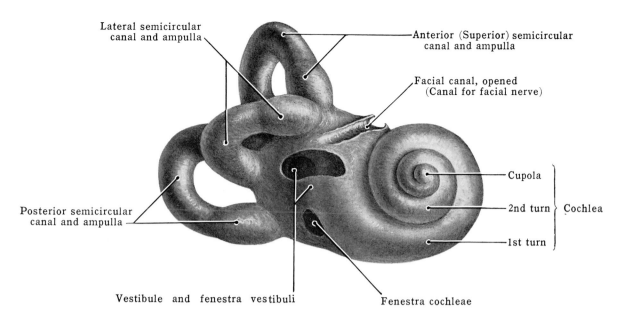

649 **Bony Labyrinth, lateral view, right side**

Observe:

1. The 3 parts of the bony internal ear or bony labyrinth—cochlea, in front; vestibule in the middle; semicircular canals, behind.

2. The 2½ turns or coils of the cochlea; the first or basal coil, which lies deep to the medial wall of the tympanic cavity, communicating with the tympanic cavity through the fenestra cochleae (round window). In life this fenestra is closed by the secondary tympanic membrane.

3. The vestibule, crossed above by the facial canal and communicating with the tympanic cavity through the fenestra vestibuli (oval window). In life this window is closed by the base or foot-piece of the stapes.

4. The 3 semicircular canals—anterior, posterior, lateral. The anterior and posterior canals set vertically and at right angles to each other; the lateral canal set horizontally and at a right angle to the two others. Each canal, forming about ⅔ of a circle, and each having an ampulla at one end. The lateral canal is the shortest; the posterior canal is the longest. The non-ampullated ends of the anterior and posterior canals joining to form a crus commune, seen through the arc of the lateral canal; hence, the 3 canals open into the vestibule by 5 openings.

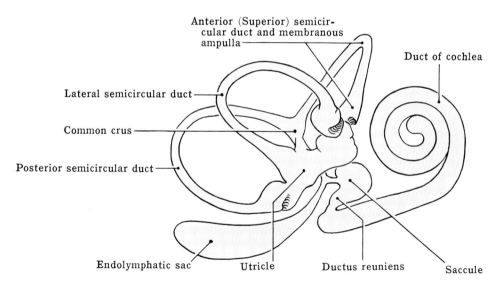

650 **Membranous Labyrinth, lateral view, right side**

From a reconstruction made by Dr. Milne Dickie and Dr. J. S. Fraser.

Note:

The membranous labyrinth or membranous internal ear is contained within the bony labyrinth or bony internal ear.

It is a closed system of ducts and chambers, filled with endolymph and surrounded with, or bathed in, perilymph.

It has 3 parts—the duct of the cochlea, within the cochlea; the saccule and the utricle, within the vestibule; the 3 semicircular ducts, within the 3 semicircular canals.

One end of the duct of the cochlea is closed; the other end communicates with the saccule through the ductus reuniens.

The saccule in turn communicates with the utricle through the utriculo-saccular duct (not labelled). From this duct springs the endolymphatic duct, which occupies the aqueduct of the vestibule and ends in the endolymphatic sac (fig. 633). Into the utricle the 3 semicircular ducts open by 5 openings.

The Cranial Nerves
and the Dermatomes

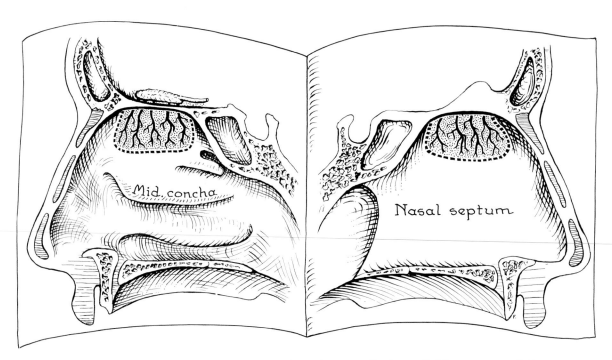

651　Scheme of the Distribution of the Olfactory Nerve

(Cranial Nerve I)

The olfactory area is usually much smaller than that shown here, and it is irregular in outline due to streamer-like invasion by non-olfactory, ciliated, columnar epithelium. The decrease in size is believed to result mainly from the destruction of the sensory olfactory neurons in the course of recurring infections of the nasal mucosa.

A study of the olfactory nerves in 143 adults (over 21 years of age) revealed that only 12% had a full complement of olfactory nerve fibres, that 8% had lost all fibres on one side, and that 5% had lost all fibres on both sides.

There is considerable variation in the number of olfactory nerve fibres in individuals of a given age, but on the average there is a loss of 1% of fibres per year during postnatal life, i.e., at the age of 50 years the average person has lost 50% of fibres and at the age of 75 years, 75% of fibres. (*C. G. Smith.*)

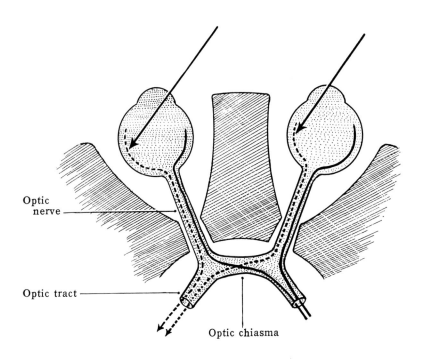

652　Scheme of the Distribution of the Optic Nerve

(Cranial Nerve II)

Rays of light from the right half of the visual field impinge on the left half of each retina, and impulses set up there travel along nerve fibres that pass to the left optic tract. Similarly, rays of light from the left half of the visual field set up impulses that reach the right optic tract. Thus, the nerve fibres from the nasal half of each retina are the ones that cross in the optic chiasma; those from the temporal half of each retina remain uncrossed.

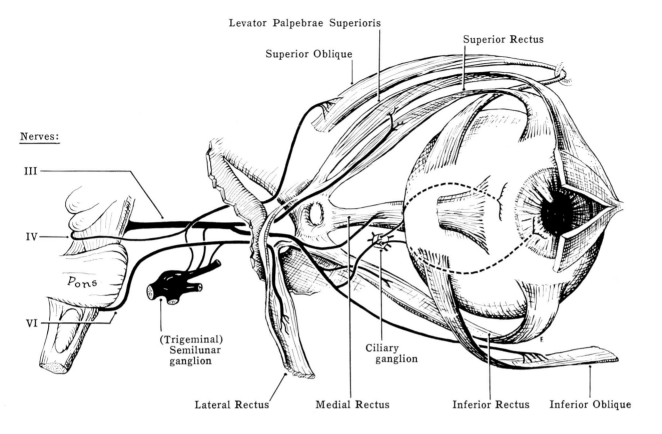

Levator Palpebrae Superioris

Superior Oblique

Superior Rectus

Nerves:

III

IV

Pons

VI

(Trigeminal)
Semilunar
ganglion

Ciliary
ganglion

Lateral Rectus

Medial Rectus

Inferior Rectus

Inferior Oblique

653 Scheme of the Distribution of the Oculomotor, Trochlear, and Abducent Nerves

(Cranial Nerves III, IV, and VI)

These 3 motor nerves, after receiving proprioceptive fibers from the trigeminal nerve, supply the orbital muscles. Nerves IV and VI each supply one muscle and nerve III supplies the remaining five muscles.

The trochlear nerve supplies Superior Oblique—the muscle that passes through a trochlea or pulley; the abducent nerve supplies Lateral Rectus—the muscle that abducts; and the oculomotor nerve supplies Levator Palpebrae Superioris, Superior Rectus, Medial Rectus, Inferior Rectus, and Inferior Oblique and, via the ciliary ganglion, it supplies the ciliary muscle and the Sphincter Pupillae.

Sympathetic fibres (not shown) from segments T.1 and 2, via the superior cervical sympathetic ganglion, supply the Dilator Pupillae and also involuntary muscle fibres (a) in the upper lid, (b) in the lower lid, and (c) bridging the inferior orbital fissure.

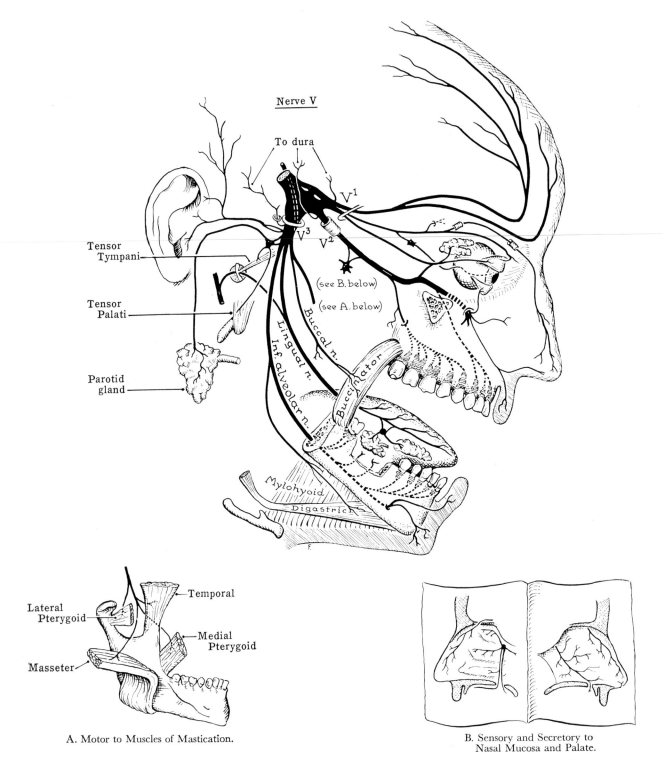

Nerve V

To dura

Tensor Tympani

Tensor Palati

Parotid gland

V¹

V³ V²

(see B. below)

(see A. below)

Buccal n.

Lingual n.

Inf. alveolar n.

Buccinator

Mylohyoid

Digastric

Lateral Pterygoid

Masseter

Temporal

Medial Pterygoid

A. Motor to Muscles of Mastication.

B. Sensory and Secretory to Nasal Mucosa and Palate.

654, 655, 656 Scheme of the Distribution of the Trigeminal Nerve

(Cranial Nerve V)

The cutaneous distribution of the 3 divisions of nerve V is shown in figure 470.1. Each division supplies not the skin surface only but also the whole thickness of tissue from skin surface to mucous surface.

Each of the 3 divisions sends a twig to the dura mater—V¹ to the tentorium cerebelli; V² & V³ to the floor and side wall of the middle cranial fossa.

Each of the 3 divisions is connected with a parasympathetic ganglion—V¹ with the ciliary, V² with the pterygopalatine, and V³ with the submandibular and otic. These ganglia are excitor cell stations whose preganglionic fibres travel with nerves III, VII, and IX. The postganglionic fibres are distributed with the branches of nerve V to smooth muscles of the eyeball and to glands.

The ophthalmic nerve (V¹) is sensory: (a) to the eyeball and cornea via the ciliary nerves (fig. 520); hence, if paralysed, the ocular conjunctiva is insensitive to touch; (b) to the frontal, ethmoidal, and sphenoidal

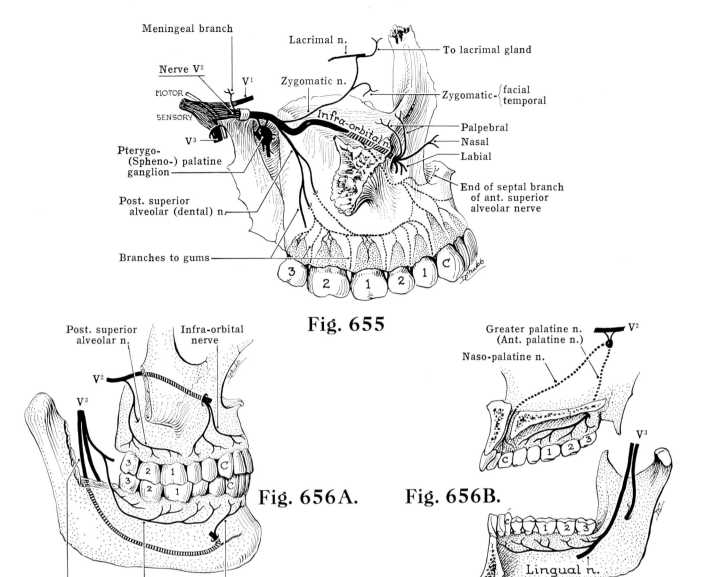

Meningeal branch

Nerve V²

MOTOR
SENSORY

V¹

V³

Pterygo-
(Spheno-) palatine
ganglion

Post. superior
alveolar (dental) n.

Branches to gums

Lacrimal n.

Zygomatic n.

Infra-orbital n.

To lacrimal gland

Zygomatic- {facial
          {temporal

Palpebral
Nasal
Labial

End of septal branch
of ant. superior
alveolar nerve

3 2 1 2 1 C

Fig. 655

Post. superior
alveolar n.

Infra-orbital
nerve

V²

V³

3 2 1 C
3 2 1 C
     2 1

Fig. 656A.

Inf. alveolar n.   Buccal n.   Mental n.

Greater palatine n.
(Ant. palatine n.)

Naso-palatine n.

V²

V³

C 1 2 3

c 1 2 3

Lingual n.

Fig. 656B.

air sinuses via the supra-orbital and ethmoidal nerves; and (c) to the skin and conjunctival surfaces of the upper eyelid and to the skin and mucous surfaces of the external nose (fig. 606).

The maxillary nerve (V²) is sensory: (a) to the upper teeth and gums (see below); (b) to the face, both surfaces of the lower lid, the skin of the side and vestibule of the nose, and both surfaces of the upper lip (fig. 470); (c) via the pterygopalatine ganglion (fig. 606) to the mucoperiosteum of the nasal cavity, palate, and roof of the pharynx; and (d) to the maxillary, ethmoidal, and sphenoidal air sinuses; (e) secretory fibres from this ganglion pass with the zygomatic and then with the lacrimal nerve to the lacrimal gland (fig. 655).

The mandibular nerve (V³) is motor: (a) to the 4 muscles of mastication—but not to Buccinator; (b) to the 2 Tensores (Tympani and Palati) via the otic ganglion; and (c) to Mylohyoid and anterior belly of Digastric. It is sensory: (a) to the lower teeth and gums (see below); (b) to both surfaces of the lower lip by the mental nerve; (c) to the auricle and temporal region by the auriculotemporal nerve which also sends twigs

to the external meatus and outer surface of the ear drum, and conveys secretory fibres from the otic ganglion to the parotid gland; (d) to the mucous membrane of the cheek by the buccal nerve (fig. 559); and (e) to the anterior two-thirds of the tongue, floor of the mouth, and gums by the lingual nerve which also distributes the chorda tympani.

The gums and teeth—Nerve V² subserves sensation to the upper gums by 4 branches (fig. 656) and to the upper teeth by 2 branches, viz., the posterior and anterior superior alveolar (dental) nerves (fig. 655). Nerve V³ subserves the lower gums by 3 branches and the lower teeth by one branch, viz., inferior alveolar. The gums are also supplied by twigs that perforate the alveoli (fig. 655). The territory of any of these gingival and dental nerves may either be extended or contracted, e.g., twigs of the mental and lingual nerves may cross the median plane to supply the gums of the opposite side, and the inferior alveolar nerves may decussate in the mandibular canal to supply the incisors of the opposite side.

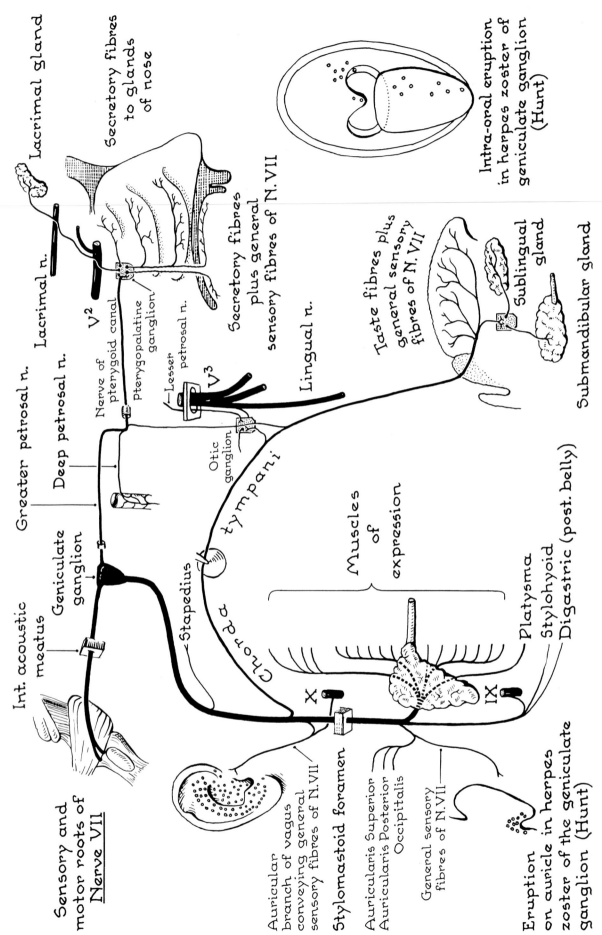

Lacrimal gland

Secretory fibres to glands of nose

Intra-oral eruption in herpes zoster of geniculate ganglion (Hunt)

Secretory fibres plus general sensory fibres of N. VII

Lacrimal n.

Greater petrosal n.

V²

Nerve of pterygoid canal

Pterygopalatine ganglion

Deep petrosal n.

Lesser petrosal n.

V³

Lingual n.

Taste fibres plus general sensory fibres of N. VII

Sublingual gland

Submandibular gland

Int. acoustic meatus

Geniculate ganglion

Otic ganglion

Chorda tympani

Muscles of expression

Platysma

Stylohyoid

Digastric (post. belly)

Sensory and motor roots of Nerve VII

Stapedius

X

Auricular branch of vagus conveying general sensory fibres of N. VII

Stylomastoid foramen

IX

Auricularis Superior
Auricularis Posterior
Occipitalis

General sensory fibres of N. VII

Eruption on auricle in herpes zoster of the geniculate ganglion (Hunt)

657 Scheme of the Distribution of the Facial Nerve

(Cranial Nerve VII)

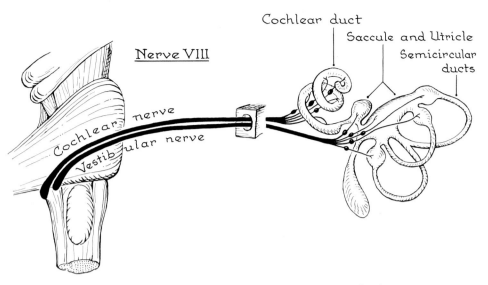

Cochlear duct

Saccule and Utricle

Semicircular ducts

Nerve VIII

Cochlear nerve

Vestibular nerve

658   Scheme of the Distribution of the Vestibulo-cochlear Nerve

(Auditory or acoustic nerve. Cranial Nerve VIII)

This nerve has two parts: (a) the cochlear nerve, or nerve of hearing, whose fibres transmit impulses from the spiral organ of Corti in the cochlear duct; and (b) the vestibular nerve, or nerve of balancing, whose fibres transmit impulses from the maculae of the saccule and utricle and in the ampullae of the three semicircular ducts.

657   Scheme of the Distribution of the Facial Nerve

Motor to the muscles of expression—i.e., muscles around the eye, nose, mouth, and ear; of the scalp above and the platysma below. It also supplies Stapedius, Stylohyoid, and Digastric (post. belly). Levator Palpebrae is not of this group, but Buccinator is. Hence, if the facial nerve is paralysed (a) the "eye" remains open and cannot close, and (b) food collects in the vestibule of the mouth, pushed there by the tongue, and the Buccinator cannot return it (fig. 591).

Secretory (1) via the greater superficial petrosal nerve and nerve of the pterygoid canal to the pterygopalatine ganglion, thence by relay to the glands of the nose and palate and to the lacrimal gland; (2) via the chorda tympani (a) to the submandibular (submaxillary) ganglion whence fibres are relayed to the submandibular and sublingual salivary glands; and, (b) via its connection with the otic ganglion, it activates the parotid gland.

Sensory fibres, with cell stations in the geniculate ganglion, carry impulses (a) from the deep tissues of the face, (b) from the external meatus, the auricle, and, (c) via the chorda tympani and greater petrosal nerve, from the tongue and palate.

Taste fibres, with cell stations in the geniculate ganglion, pass (a) from the palate non-stop through the pterygopalatine ganglion, nerve of the pterygoid canal, and greater petrosal nerve to the geniculate ganglion; and (b) from the anterior two-thirds of the tongue two routes are followed: (1) via the chorda tympani to the facial nerve and so to the geniculate ganglion, and (2) by a branch of the chorda that traverses the otic ganglion to join the greater petrosal nerve and so to the geniculate ganglion. As evidence of this double route is the fact that the chorda tympani may be cut without any loss of taste, whereas cutting the greater petrosal nerve may result in loss of taste. (*Schwartz, H. G., and Weddell, G., 1938.*)

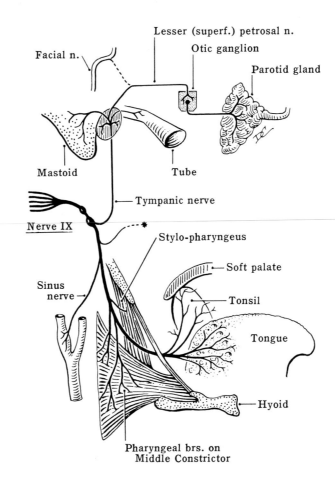

Facial n.

Lesser (superf.) petrosal n.

Otic ganglion

Parotid gland

Mastoid

Tube

Tympanic nerve

Nerve IX

Stylo-pharyngeus

Sinus nerve

Soft palate

Tonsil

Tongue

Hyoid

Pharyngeal brs. on
Middle Constrictor

659   Scheme of the Distribution of the Glossopharyngeal Nerve

(Cranial Nerve IX)

Motor fibres supply one muscle—Stylopharyngeus.

Secretory fibres travel via the tympanic and lesser (superficial) petrosal nerves to the otic ganglion, there to be relayed in the auriculotemporal nerve to the parotid gland. It has been observed that cutting the chorda tympani reduces permanently the secretion not only of the submandibular gland but also of the parotid. Cutting the glossopharyngeal nerve above the connecting branch it sends to the nerve to Digastric (post. belly) also reduces secretion in the three large salivary glands. Hence, it is surmised that secretory fibres travel down nerve IX, through the connecting branch to the nerve to Digastric (indicated by a star in fig. 659 and shown in fig. 657), thence up the stem of nerve VII and along the chorda (a) to the submandibular ganglion where the impulses are relayed to the submandibular and sublingual glands, and (b) to the otic ganglion where the impulses are relayed to the parotid gland. (Reichert, F. L., and Poth, E. J.)

General sensory fibres supply almost the entire one half of the pharyngeal wall, including the oro-pharyngeal isthmus (i.e., under surface of the soft palate, tonsil, pharyngeal arches, and posterior third of the tongue). They also supply the dorsum of the soft palate, the auditory tube, tympanum, medial surface of the ear drum, mastoid antrum, and mastoid air cells. The pharyngeal branch of the maxillary nerve (fig. 606) attends to the roof of the pharynx; the lesser palatine nerves (fig. 582) to the anterior parts of the soft palate; and the internal laryngeal nerve to the lowest part of the pharynx (fig. 627) and somewhat to the surroundings of the laryngeal orifice (fig. 593).

Taste fibres supply the posterior third of the tongue including the vallate papillae (fig. 593).

The sinus nerve is afferent from the carotid sinus and carotid body.

Note: (1) The glossopharyngeal nerve, like the facial nerve, activates each of the three large salivary glands. (2) Clinical evidence is undecided as to the share taken by nerves VII, IX, and X in conveying sensation from the auricle and external meatus and in supplying the muscles of the palate.

660 Scheme of the Distribution of the Vagus Nerve

(Cranial Nerve X)

Motor: (a) The fibres received from the cranial root of the accessory nerve (fig. 661) supply the muscles of the pharynx (Stylopharyngeus excepted), of the palate (Tensor Palati excepted, but including Palatoglossus), and of the larynx (without exception). The foregoing are skeletal muscles.

    (b) Inhibitory to the cardiac muscle.

Motor to all smooth muscle, secretory to all glands, and afferent from all mucous surfaces in the following parts—pharynx (lowest part), larynx, trachea, bronchi and lungs; esophagus (entire), stomach, and gut down to the left colic flexure; liver, gall gladder and bile passages; pancreas and pancreatic ducts; and perhaps spleen and kidney.

Taste: from the few taste buds about the epiglottis.

    Branches arise from the vagus thus:

In the jugular fossa—(a) a meningeal branch to the dura of the posterior cranial fossa; and (b) an auricular branch to the outer surface of the ear drum, the external acoustic meatus, and the back of the auricle (figs. 551 & 552).

In the neck—(a) the pharyngeal branch is motor to Superior and Middle Constrictors and muscles of the soft palate; (b) the superior laryngeal nerve, via the internal laryngeal nerve, is sensory to the larynx above the vocal cords and to the lowest part of the pharynx (fig. 627) and, via the external laryngeal nerve, motor to Inferior Constrictor and Cricothyroid (figs. 532 & 626), (c) a twig (sinus nerve) to the carotid sinus, and (d) two cardiac branches.

In the thorax—(a) the recurrent nerve sends a motor branch to Inferior Constrictor, is motor to all the laryngeal muscles (excepting Cricothyroid), and is both afferent and efferent to the larynx below the level of the cords, as well as to the upper part of the esophagus; (b, c, and d) cardiac and pulmonary branches and the esophageal plexus.

In the abdomen—see figure 133.

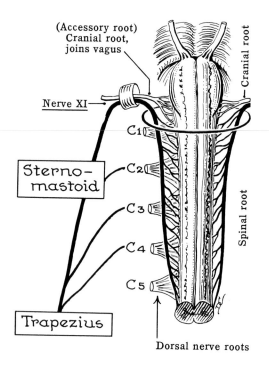

661   Scheme of the Distribution of the Spinal Part of the Accessory Nerve

(Cervical Nerve XI)

The spinal root of the accessory nerve, joined by fibres from the ventral ramus of C.2, supplies Sternomastoid and, joined by fibres from the ventral rami of C.3 & 4, supplies Trapezius. Experiments on lower animals (cat, rabbit and monkey) give evidence that the ventral rami fibres of cervical nerves 2, 3, & 4 are proprioceptive, that is, sensory only. (*K. B. Corbin and F. Harrison.*) In man, however, there is clinical evidence (both surgical and medical) that these contributions from C.2, 3, & 4 convey motor as well as sensory fibres. (*H. W. Wookey; K, G. McKenzie; W. Haymaker and B. Woodhall.*) The spinal root of the accessory nerve usually passes through the dorsal root ganglion of C.1 and may receive sensory fibres from it (*A. A. Pearson*).

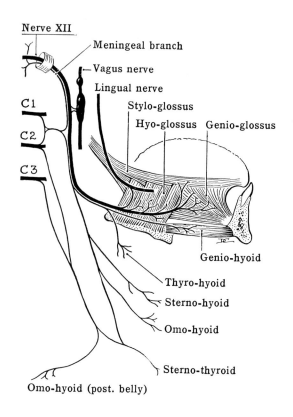

662   Scheme of the Distribution of the Hypoglossal Nerve

(Cranial Nerve XII)

This efferent nerve supplies all the intrinsic (longitudinal, transverse, and vertical) and extrinsic (Styloglossus, Hyoglossus, and Genioglossus) muscles of the tongue, Palatoglossus excepted.

It receives a mixed (motor and sensory) branch from the loop between the ventral rami of C.1 and 2. The sensory or afferent fibres in part take a recurrent course and end in the dura mater of the posterior cranial fossa. The motor or efferent branch supplies Geniohyoid and Thyrohyoid, and it provides a descending branch which unites with a descending branch of C.2 and 3 to form a loop, the ansa cervicalis. This and the ansa supply the remaining depressor muscles of the hyoid bone.

663 Dermatomes of the Upper and and Lower Limbs

(Modified, after Keegan, J. J., and Garrett, F. D.)

According to the clinical, surgical, and experimental findings of Keegan and Garrett, the dermatomes of the limbs from the 5th cervical to the 1st thoracic, and from the 3rd lumbar to the 2nd sacral extend as a series of bands from the mid-dorsal line of the trunk into the limbs, as illustrated. When the function of even a single dorsal nerve root is interrupted, faint but definite diminution of sensitivity can be demonstrated in the dermatome. The best method to detect and plot the area of diminished sensitivity is by the use of light pin scratch for pain sensation, although it can be found for temperature and for tactile sensation also.

Note: Pearson, A. A. and Bass, J. J. find that in the human embryo it is unusual for the dorsal rami of C. 6, 7 and 8 to possess cutaneous branches, for only about 10% do; and that C.5 and T.1 possess them in only 67% and 82% respectively. In contrast, they do find that in rabbit embryos each of these dorsal rami (C.5—T.1) possesses a cutaneous branch.

664 Dermatomes of the Upper Parts of the Body

(Modified, from Fender, after Foerster)

A dermatome is an area of skin supplied by the dorsal (sensory) root of a spinal nerve.

The dermatomes were determined by plotting (a) the areas of vasodilation that resulted on stimulation of individual dorsal nerve roots, and (b) the areas of "remaining sensibility" after cutting three roots above and three roots below a given nerve root. The areas plotted represent the average finding for each dorsal root based on pain sensation. Areas determined for temperature sensation have similar limits, but those for touch are more extensive.

Note that there is considerable overlapping of contiguous dermatomes; that is to say, each segmental nerve overlaps the territories of its neighbours. As a result, no anesthesia results unless two or more consecutive dorsal roots have lost their functions.

The 7th cervical dermatome (not depicted) begins lower on the upper arm than the 6th and includes most, or all, of the hand.

665 Dermatomes of the Lower Limb
(Modified, from Fender, after Foerster)

References

Figure

27   Barlow, R. N. The sternalis muscle in American whites and Negroes. Anat. Rec., *61:* 413, 1935.

27   Seib, G. A. The musculus pectoralis minor in American whites and American Negroes. Am. J. Phys. Anthropol., *23:* 389, 1938.

28   J. C. B. G. Data collected by the author.

42   C. G. S. Data collected by Carleton G. Smith.

47   Terry, R. J. A study of the supracondyloid process in the living. Am. J. Phys. Anthropol., *4:* 129, 1921.

47   Terry, R. J. On the racial distribution of the supracondyloid variation. Am. J. Phys. Anthropol., *14:* 459, 1930.

48   Trotter, M. Septal apertures in the humerus of American whites and Negroes. Am. J. Phys. Anthropol., *19:* 213, 1934.

48.1   Hazlett, J. W. The superficial ulnar artery with references to accidental intra-arterial injection. Canad. M. A. J., *61:* 289, 1949.

85   Appleton, A. B. A case of abnormal distribution of the musculocutaneous nerve. J. Anat. & Physiol., *46:* 89, 1911.

85   Hutton, W. K. Remarks on the innervation of the dorsus manus with special reference to certain rare abnormalities. J. Anat. & Physiol., *40:* 326, 1906.

85   Learmonth, J. R. A variation in the distribution of the "radial nerve." J. Anat., *53:* 371, 1919.

85   Stopford, J. S. B. The variation in distribution of the cutaneous nerves of the hands and digits. J. Anat., *53:* 14, 1918.

89   Landsmeer, J. M. F. The anatomy of the dorsal aponeurosis of the human finger and its functional significance. Anat. Rec., *104:* 31, 1949.

97-D   R. K. G. Data collected by R. K. George.

98   McKern, T. W., and Stewart, T. D. Skeletal age changes in young American males. Quartermaster Research & Development Center, Natick, Mass., U. S. A., 1957.

Figure

98   Francis, C. C., and Werle, P. P. The appearance of centers of ossification from birth to 5 years. Anat. Rec., *24:* 273, 1939.

98   Francis, C. C. The appearance of centers of ossification from 6 to 15 years. Anat. Rec., *27:* 127, 1940.

98   Pryor, J. W. Differences in the time of development of centers of ossification in the male and female skeleton. Anat. Rec., *8:* 252, 1922.

104   Pryor, J. W. Time of ossification of the bones of the hand of the male and female. Am. J. Phys. Anthropol., *8:* 401, 1925.

104   Greulich, W. W., and Pyle, S. I. Radiographic Atlas of Skeletal Development of the Hand and Wrist, 2nd ed. Stanford University Press, 1959.

132   Michels, N. A. Blood Supply and Anatomy of the Upper Abdominal Organs. J. B. Lippincott Company, Philadelphia, 1955.

133   McCrea, E. A. The abdominal distribution of the vagus. J. Anat., *59:* 18, 1924.

133   Mitchell, G. A. G. Innervation of the stomach. *In* Anatomy of the Autonomic Nervous System, p. 281. E. & S. Livingstone, Ltd., Edinburgh, 1953.

135   Falconer, C. W. A., and Griffiths, E. The anatomy of the blood vessels in the region of the pancreas. Brit. J. Surg., *37:* 334, 1950.

137–140   Hjortsjo, C. H. The topography of the intrahepatic duct systems (and of the portal vein). Acta anat., *11:* 599, 1951.

137–140   Hjortsjo, C. H. The intrahepatic ramifications of the portal vein. Lunds Universitets Arsskrift, *52:* 20, 1956.

137–140   Healey, J. E., Schroy, P. C., and Sorensen, R. J. The intrahepatic artery in man. J. Internat. Coll. Surgeons, *20:* 133, 1953.

137–140   Healey, J. E., and Schroy, P. C. Anatomy of the biliary ducts within the human liver. A. M. A. Arch. Surg., *66:* 599, 1953.

Figure

137–140 SCHMIDT, H., AND GUTTMAN, E. Systematische Anatomie der Gallengange des Menschen. Acta anat. 28: 1, 1956.

137–140 ELIAS, H., AND PETTY, D. Gross anatomy of the blood vessels and ducts within the human liver. Am. J. Anat., 90: 59, 1952.

137–140 ELIAS, H. Nomenklatur der intrahepatischen Gefasse. Anat. Anzeiger, 102: 1/4, 73, 1955.

143 DASELER, E. H., ANSON, B. J., HAMBLEY, W. C., AND REIMANN, A. F. The cystic artery and constituents of the hepatic pedicle. Surg. Gynec. & Obst., 85: 47, 1947.

144 J. C. B. G. From data collected by the author.

145 MICHELS, N. A. Blood Supply and Anatomy of the Upper Abdominal Organs. J. B. Lippincott Company, Philadelphia, 1955.

152 CURTIS, G. M., AND MOVITZ, D. The surgical significance of the accessory spleen. Ann. Surg., 123: 276, 1946.

152 HALPERT, B., AND GYORKEY, F. Accessory spleen in the tail of the pancreas. A. M. A. Arch. Path., 64: 266, 1957.

152 HALPERT, B., AND GYORKEY, F. Lesions observed in accessory spleens of 311 patients. Am. J. Clin. Path., 32: 165, 1959.

157 MILLBOURN, E. On the excretory ducts of the pancreas in man, with special reference to their relations to each other, to the common bile duct and to the duodenum: radiological and anatomical study. Acta anat., 9: 1, 1950.

157 HORSEY, W. J., AND PAUL, W. Personal observations.

158 WOODBURNE, R. T., AND OLSEN, L. L. The arteries of the pancreas. Anat. Rec., 111: 255, 1951.

158 PIERSON, J. M. The arterial blood supply of the pancreas. Surg. Gynec. & Obst., 77: 426, 1943.

161 BOYDEN, E. A. The "Phrygian cap" in cholecystography; congenital anomaly of the gall-bladder. Am. J. Roentgenol., 33: 589, 1935.

161 BOYDEN, E. A. The accessory gall-bladder. Am. J. Anat., 38: 177, 1926.

162 BASMAJIAN, J. V. The marginal anastomoses of the arteries to the large intestine. Surg. Gynec. & Obst., 99: 614, 1954.

162 BASMAJIAN, J. V. The main arteries of the large intestine. Surg. Gynec. & Obst., 101: 585, 1955.

170.1 JAY, G. D., III, MARGULIS, R. R., McGRAW, A. B., AND NORTHRIP, R. R. Meckel's diverticulum: survey of 103 cases. Arch. Surg., 61: 158, 1950.

172 WAKELEY, C. P. G. The position of the vermiform appendix as ascertained by the analysis of 10,000 cases. J. Anat., 67: 277, 1933.

180 CLARK, K. The blood vessels of the adrenal gland. J. Roy. Coll. Surgeons, Edin., 4: 257, 1959.

183.1 GRAVES, F. T. The anatomy of the intrarenal arteries and its application to segmental resection of the kidney. Brit. J. Surg., 42: 132, 1954.

Figure

183.1 GRAVES, F. T. The anatomy of the intrarenal arteries in health and disease. Brit. J. Surg., 43: 605, 1956.

183.1 RICHES, E. W. The present status of renal angiography. Brit. J. Surg., 42: 462, 1955.

186 LOWSLEY, O. S. Postcaval ureter—operation for its correction. Surg. Gynec. & Obst., 82: 549, 1946.

186 PICK, J. W., AND ANSON, B. J. Retrocaval ureter. J. Urol., 43: 672, 1940.

187 BELL, E. T. Anomalies. In Renal Diseases, p. 55. Lea & Febiger, Philadelphia, 1946.

187 LLOYD, L. W. The renal artery in whites and American Negroes. Am. J. Phys. Anthropol., 20: 153, 1935.

187 MERKLIN, R. J., AND MICHELS, N. A. The variant renal and suprarenal blood supply with data on the inferior phrenic, ureteral and gonadal arteries. J. Internat. Coll. Surgeons, 29: 41, 1958.

187 ADACHI, B. Multiple renal arteries. In Das Arteriensystem der Japaner. Kyoto, 1928.

187 CAMPBELL, M. Ureteral reduplication (double ureter). In Urology, vol. 1, p. 309. W. B. Saunders Company, Philadelphia, 1954.

187 ANDERSON, G. A., RICE, G. G., AND HARRIS, B. A. Pregnancy and labor complicated by pelvic ectopic kidney anomalies; a review. Obst. & Gynec. Surv., 4: 737, 1949.

188.3 SEIB, G. A. The azygos system of veins in American whites and American Negroes, including observations on inferior caval venous system. Am. J. Phys. Anthropol., 19: 39, 1934.

196 WILDE, F. R. The anal intermuscular septum. Brit. J. Surg., 36: 279, 1949.

214 LEARMONTH, J. E. A contribution to the neurophysiology of the urinary bladder in man. Brain, 54: 147, 1931.

214 LANGWORTHY, O. R., KOLB, L. C., AND LEWIS, L. G. In Physiology of Micturition. The Williams & Wilkins Company, Baltimore, 1940.

255 BASMAJIAN, J. V. The distribution of valves in the femoral, external iliac and common iliac veins and their relationship to varicose veins. Surg. Gynec. & Obst., 95: 537, 1952.

257 FLEMING, J. F. R., AND LEVY, L. F. Personal observations.

279 WOLCOTT, W. E. The evolution of the circulation in the developing femoral head and neck. Surg. Gynec. & Obst., 77: 61, 1943.

279 TRUETA, J., AND HARRISON, M. H. M. Normal vascular anatomy of the femoral head in adult man. J. Bone & Joint Surg., 35B: 442, 1953.

309 R. K. G. Data collected by R. K. George.

Figure

323   J. C. B. G. Data collected by the author.

324   SENIOR, H. D. An interpretation of the recorded arterial anomalies of the human leg and foot. J. Anat., *53:* 130, 1919.

324   QUAIN, R. The Anatomy of the Arteries of the Human Body. Taylor and Walton, London, 1844.

350   FRANCIS, C. C., AND WERLE, P. P. See reference for Figure 98.

350   McKERN, T. W., AND STEWART, T. D. See reference for Figure 98.

356   C. E. S. Data collected by Charles E. Storton.

356   HARRIS, R. I., AND BEATH, T. Army Foot Survey, vol. 1, p. 52. National Research Council of Canada, Ottawa, 1947.

373.1 McKERN, T. W., AND STEWART, T. D. See reference for Figure 98.

378   HO, G. T. Personal observations.

382   ROWE, G. G., AND ROCHE, M. B. The etiology of separate neural arch. J. Bone & Joint Surg., *35A:* 102, 1953.

382   STEWART, T. D. The age incidence of neural-arch defects in Alaskan natives considered from the standpoint of etiology. J. Bone & Joint Surg., *35A:* 937, 1953.

390   BATSON, O. V. The function of the vertebral veins and their role in the spread of metastases. Ann. Surg., *112:* 138, 1940.

390   BATSON, O. V. The vertebral vein system. Am. J. Roentgenol., *78:* 195, 1957.

394   TROTTER, M. Synostosis between manubrium and body of the sternum in whites and Negroes. Am. J. Phys. Anthropol., *18:* 439, 1934.

394   McKERN, T. W., AND STEWART, T. D. See reference for Figure 98.

400   ADSON, A. W. Cervical ribs: symptoms, differential diagnosis and indications for section of insertion of scalenus anticus muscle. J. Internat. Coll. Surgeons, *16:* 546, 1951.

403   KROPP, B. N. The lateral costal branch of the internal mammary artery. J. Thoracic Surg., *21:* 421, 1951.

424   JACKSON, C. L., AND HUBER, J. F. Correlated applied anatomy of the bronchial tree and lungs with a system of nomenclature. Dis. Chest, *9:* 319, 1943.

425   BOYDEN, E. A. Segmental Anatomy of the Lungs. McGraw-Hill Book Company, New York, 1954.

425   BOYDEN, E. A. The nomenclature of the bronchopulmonary segments and their blood supply. Dis. Chest, *39:* 1, 1961.

415.1 WALLS, E. W. Dissection of the atrioventricular node and bundle in the human heart. J. Anat., *79:* 45, 1945.

446.4 ADACHI, B. Das Arteriensystem der Japaner. Kyoto, 1928.

446.4 QUAIN, R. The Anatomy of the Arteries of the Human Body. Taylor and Walton, London, 1844.

446.4 THOMSON, A. Third Annual Report of the Committee of Collective Investigation of the Anatomical Society of Great Britain and Ireland for the Year 1891–1892. J. Anat. & Physiol., *27:* 191, 1893.

464.4 LOTH, E. Anatomie des Partes Molles. Masson et Cie, Paris, 1931.

447.1 McDONALD, J. J., AND ANSON, B. J. Variations in origin of arteries derived from the aortic arch in American whites and Negroes. Am. J. Phys. Anthropol., *27:* 91, 1940.

447.1 ANSON, B. J. *In* Callander's Surgical Anatomy, 4th ed., p. 318. W. B. Saunders Company, Philadelphia, 1957.

455   SEIB, G. A. See reference for Figure 188.3.

471   WHITNALL, S. E. *In* Anatomy of the Human Orbit. Oxford Medical Publications, London, 1921.

471.5 HUELKE, D. F. A study of the transverse cervical and dorsal scapular arteries. Anat. Rec., *132:* 233, 1958.

471.5 ADACHI, B. A. transversa scapulae and a. transversa colli. *In* Das Arteriensystem der Japaner, vol. 1, pp. 147 and 182. Kyoto, 1928.

471.5 READ, W. T., AND TROTTER, M. The origins of transverse cervical and of transverse scapular arteries in American whites and Negroes. Am. J. Phys. Anthropol., *28:* 239, 1941.

471.5 MacINTOSH, D., AND SMITH, G. G. Personal observations.

484   SUH, T. H., AND ALEXANDER, L. Vascular system of the human spinal cord (radicular vessels). Arch. Neurol. & Psychiat., *41:* 659, 1939.

484   MacDONALD, I. B., McKENZIE, K. G., AND BOTTERELL, E. H. Anterior rhizotomy. J. Neurosurg., *3:* 421, 1946.

484   SMITH, C. G. Changes in length and position of the segments of the spinal cord with changes in posture in the monkey. Radiology, *66:* 259, 1956.

484.1 JIT, I., AND CHARNAKIA, V. M. The vertebral level of the termination of the spinal cord. J. Anat. Soc. India, *8:* 93, 1959.

484.1 REIMANN, A. F., AND ANSON, B. J. Vertebral level of termination of the spinal cord with a report of a case of a sacral cord. Anat. Rec. 88: 127, 1944. *Also in* Callander's Surgical Anatomy, 4th ed., p. 771. W. B. Saunders Company, Philadelphia, 1958.

499   STILES, H. J. *In* Cunningham's Textbook of Anatomy, 4th ed., p. 1359. Oxford Medical Press, London, 1913.

511   McKERN, T. W., AND STEWART, T. D. See reference for Figure 98.

566.1 LEWIS, G. F. Personal observations.

Figure

566.2 MacIntosh, D., and Smith, C. G. Personal observations.

567 Adachi, B. Arteria vertebralis. *In* Das Arteriensystem der Japaner, vol. 1, p. 138. Kyoto, 1928.

567 Bell, R. H., Swigart, L. L., and Anson, B. J. The relation of the vertebral artery to the cervical vertebrae. Quart. Bull. Northwestern Univ. M. School, *24*: no. 3, 184, 1950.

567 Cobb, W. M. The ossa suprasternalia in whites and American Negroes and the form of the superior border of the manubrium. J. Anat., Pt 2, *71*: 245, 1937.

624 Hetherington, J. The kerato-cricoid muscle in the American white and Negro. Am. J. Phys. Anthropol., *19*: 209, 1934.

633 Young, M. W. The termination of the perilymphatic duct. Anat. Rec., *112*: 404, 1952.

651 Smith, C. G. Incidence of atrophy of the olfactory nerves in man. Arch. Otolaryng., *34*: 533, 1941.

657 Schwartz, H. G., and Wedell, G. Observations on the pathways transmitting the sensation of taste. Brain, *61*: 99, 1938.

657 Hunt, J. R. Geniculate neuralgia. Arch. Neurol. & Psychiat., *37*: 253, 1937.

659 Reichert, F. L., and Poth, E. J. Recent knowledge

Figure

regarding the physiology of the glossopharyngeal nerve in man with analysis of its sensory, motor, gustatory and secretory functions. Bull. Johns Hopkins Hosp., *53*: 131, 1933.

661 Corbin, K. B., and Harrison, F. The sensory innervation of the spinal accessory and tongue musculature in the rhesus monkey. Brain, *62*: 191, 1939.

661 Haymaker, W., and Woodhall, B. Peripheral Nerve Injuries, 2nd ed. W. B. Saunders Company, Philadelphia, 1953.

661 Pearson, A. A. The spinal accessory nerve in human embryos. J. Comp. Neurol., *68*: 243, 1938.

663 Fender, F. A. Foerster's scheme of the dermatomes. Arch. Neurol. & Psychiat., *41*: 688, 1939.

665 Keegan, J. J., and Garrett, F. D. The segmental distribution of the cutaneous nerves in the limbs of man. Anat. Rec., *102*: 409, 1948.

665 Pearson, A. A., and Bass, J. J. Cutaneous branches of the posterior primary rami of the cervical nerves. Anat. Rec., *139*: 263, 1961.

665 Pearson, A. A., and Bass, J. J. Further observations on the cutaneous branches of the posterior primary rami of the cervical nerves in embryos. Anat. Rec., *142*: 266, 1962.

Index